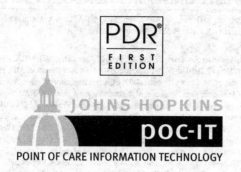

PDR®
FIRST
EDITION

JOHNS HOPKINS

poc-it

POINT OF CARE INFORMATION TECHNOLOGY

THE ABX GUIDE
DIAGNOSIS & TREATMENT OF INFECTIOUS DISEASES

Edited By: John G. Bartlett, M.D.
Paul G. Auwaerter, M.D., M.B.A.
Paul A. Pham, Pharm.D.

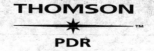

THOMSON

PDR

Johns Hopkins University School of Medicine

POC-IT Center

PDR

Thomson PDR

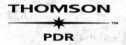

ISBN: 1-56363-519-4

TABLE OF CONTENTS

APPENDIX II: GENERAL THERAPEUTIC TABLES

ANTIBIOTIC SENSITIVITY CHART   Inside Back Cover

The "ABX Guide," largely the product of the Division of Infectious Diseases at Johns Hopkins University School of Medicine, launched in 2000 as a website and was then adapted for use with handheld devices in April 2001. Presenting comprehensive material for patient management in a format concise enough to fit the small screen of a handheld device forced extraordinary discipline in economy of language, restricting the authors to include only the most practical and important issues of clinical practice. The adaptation of this material for this new print publication—*The PDR/Johns Hopkins ABX Guide: Diagnosis & Treatment of Infectious Diseases*—now captures these important features.

The goal of this guide is to provide timely and accurate recommendations for the management of the most common infectious diseases. It comes at a time when the field is sizzling from our recent experiences with SARS, MRSA, *Acinetobacter*, West Nile virus, prion diseases, and anthrax, just to name a few hot topics. A great concern is the evolution of resistance—the inevitable consequence of antibiotic use and abuse. This concern is now compounded by the relative paucity of new antimicrobial agents, which is sometimes referred to as the "dry pipeline." We are in a period during which physicians are challenged to be particularly careful in antibiotic use. In some instances, physicians will need to resort to antibiotics that have been used infrequently for years or decades, such as colistin and minocycline.

Several features of this book are worth special emphasis. First, and possibly most important, is credibility. Each topic is written by an experienced clinician, someone who actually practices medicine and has been asked to write a monograph based on his or her experience, augmenting the piece with recommendations from authoritative sources when these exist. Thus, most of the recommendations are based on guidelines from the Centers for Disease Control, scholarly societies, reviews by the Cochrane Library, BMJ reviews, HCRQ reviews, and more. Once completed, these documents are reviewed by at least three other professionals in order to ensure consistency and accuracy. At one point we offered $1,000 to anyone who could find a mistake that would result in patient mismanagement. There was only one response, but because it was simply a typographical error no payment was made.

Another important attribute of the guide is timeliness. All of medicine seems to change rather rapidly, but no field moves with the same velocity as infectious diseases in terms of diagnostic testing, recognition of new pathogens, surprising new pathogens and epidemics, and changes in management guidelines. Most of the monographs included here were originally written between 2000 and 2002, but all have been updated through mid 2005.

The presentation of information is the one we have found most useful for guidance in the field of infectious diseases for primary care practitioners, the professional group that writes 80% of scripts for antibiotics. Each of the four sections—anti-infectives, diagnoses, vaccines, and pathogens—has a standardized format designed to provide the most important information relevant to patient care in terms of management decisions, thus answering many common practitioner queries.

In sum, this book is designed as an authoritative resource dealing with virtually all important antimicrobial agents, the vast majority of infectious diseases, and commonly encountered pathogens. The recommendations are based on reliable sources, the information is timely, and the format permits easy, rapid access to clinically relevant information.

John G. Bartlett, M.D.
Chief, Division of Infectious Diseases
Johns Hopkins University
School of Medicine

How to Use This Book

Clinicians need accurate, concise, and easy-to-use information at point-of-care. The *PDR/Johns Hopkins ABX Guide: Diagnosis & Treatment of Infectious Diseases* is all that and more. In this one convenient book, you've got an authoritative decision support tool for infectious diseases that allows you to make fast, appropriate choices for your patients' care.

This guide is organized in four sections that cover drug therapy, vaccines, diagnoses, and pathogens. The first section—Anti-infectives—is organized alphabetically. Each drug monograph covers indications, dosing and dosing adjustments, drug interactions, information regarding use during pregnancy and breastfeeding, and a chart that shows the available forms of the drug as well as the brand names, route of administration, and estimated costs. In addition, each monograph includes important notes about the drug and, in somes cases, a list of related references for further reading.

Please note that prices listed in the charts under the "cost" column represent cost per unit specified and are representative of "Average Wholesale Price" (AWP). AWP prices were obtained and gathered using manufacturers' information and Thomson Healthcare's *Red Book®* database. Please refer to the AWP Policy at the end of this section as you review the pricing information contained in *The ABX Guide*.

The second section on vaccines consists of an alphabetically arranged collection of monographs covering common vaccines. Each one lists diagnostic criteria, treatment regimens, and important clinical points about the vaccine.

The third section—Diagnoses—is also organized alphabetically. Each monograph includes diagnostic criteria, common pathogens, and a thorough treatment regimen section that includes adjunctive therapy. Additional information includes expert commentary regarding the condition and treatment options, as well as important points and further reading references.

The fourth section is comprised of pathogen monographs, organized alphabetically with class, that cover clinical relevance of the organism, sites of infection, and treatment regimens according to infection site. This section also includes important points and references for further reading.

An appendix of relevant tables, charts, and algorithms includes both material referenced under specific monographs, as well as material of general interest.

Finally, conveniently situated right inside the back cover is a fold-out antibiotic sensitivity chart. You can see at a glance how the most commonly used antibiotics act against a wide range of pathogens.

RED BOOK® AWP POLICY

The Average Wholesale Price (AWP) as published by Thomson Healthcare is in most cases the manufacturer's[1] suggested AWP and does not necessarily reflect the *actual* AWP charged by a wholesaler. Thomson Healthcare bases the AWP data it publishes on the following:

- AWP is reported by the manufacturer, **or**
- AWP is calculated based on a markup specified by the manufacturer. This markup is typically based on the Wholesale Acquisition Cost (WAC) or Direct Price (DP), as provided by the manufacturer, but may be based on other pricing data provided by the manufacturer.

When the manufacturer does not provide an AWP or markup formula from which AWP can be calculated, the AWP will be calculated by applying a standard 20% markup over the manufacturer-supplied WAC. If a WAC is not provided, the standard markup will be applied to the DP.

Please note that Thomson Healthcare does not perform any independent analysis to determine or calculate the *actual* AWP paid by providers[2] to wholesalers. Thomson Healthcare also does not independently investigate the *actual* WAC paid by wholesalers to manufacturers or DP paid by providers to manufacturers. Thomson Healthcare relies on the manufacturers to report the values for these categories as described above.

Thomson Healthcare provides a list of the manufacturers that do not provide the AWP or a markup formula. The list of these manufacturers and products is available at the following website: *http://www.micromedex.com/products/redbook/awp/.* Additionally, an ASCII text file with this same information is available to download. For more information on this file and instructions on downloading, please contact Thomson Healthcare Technical Support at *http://www.micromedex.com/support/request/.*

[1] The term "manufacturer" includes manufacturers, repackagers, and private labelers.
[2] The term "provider" includes retailers, hospitals, physicians, and others buying either from the wholesaler or directly from the manufacturer for distribution to a patient.

KEY TO DRUG NAME ABBREVIATIONS

Abbreviation	Drug
3TC	Lamivudine
5-FC	Flucytosine
ABC	Abacavir
ABV	Vincristine/vinblastine
ADR	Adverse drug reaction
AMB	Amphotericin B
APV	Amprenavir
ASA	Aspirin
ATV	Atazanavir
Azithro	Azithromycin
AZT	Zidovudine
d4T	Stavudine
ddC	Zalcitabine
ddI	Didanosine
DLV	Delavirdine
EFV	Efavirenz
EMB	Ethambutol
ENF (T-20)	Enfuvirtide
EPO	Erythropoietin
FPV	Fosamprenavir
FQ	Fluoroquinolone
FTC	Emtricitabine
FTV	*Fortovase*
G-CSF	Filgrastim
GM-CSF	*Prokine*
GAZT	AZT-glucuronide
HU	Hydroxyurea
IDV	Indinavir
INH	Isoniazid
INV	*Invirase*
LPV	Lopinavir
LPV/r	Lopinavir/Ritonavir
NNRTI	Non-nucleoside reverse transcriptase inhibitor
NRTI	Nucleoside reverse transcriptase inhibitor
NSAID	Nonsteroidal anti-inflammatory drug
NFV	Nelfinavir
NVP	Nevirapine
PCN	Penicillin
PI	Protease inhibitor
PZA	Pyrazinamide
RB	Rifabutin
RTV	Ritonavir
SM	Streptomycin
SMX	Sulfamethoxazole
SQV	Saquinavir
TDF	Tenofovir
TMP	Trimethoprim
TMP-SMX	Trimethoprim-Sulfamethoxazole
TZV	Trizivir

KEY TO DRUG ADMINISTRATION AND GENERAL ABBREVIATIONS

Abbreviation	Term/Phrase	Abbreviation	Term/Phrase
μL	microliter	mmol	millimole
μmol	micromole	mo, mos	month, months
Abnl	abnormal	mU	milliunits
Abx	antibiotic(s)	N	normal (solution) or total sample size
Ac	before meal		
admin	administered	ng	nanogram
All	allergy, allergic	nm	nanometer
ART	antiretroviral therapy	OI	opportunistic infection
bid	twice per day	OTC	over-the-counter
Bx, Bxp	biopsy	oz	ounce
c	copies	PE	physical exam
ca	cancer	Plt	platelet
caps	capsules	PO	by mouth
cg	centigram	PRN or prn	as needed
cm	centimeter	PSI	pounds per square inch
cm²	square centimeters		
cx	culture	Pt	patient
d/c	discontinue, discharge	pt-yrs	patient-years
Ddx	differential diagnosis	qd	every day
dL	deciliter	qid	four times a day
DS	double strength	qmo	every month
dx	diagnosis	qod	every other day
Dz	disease	qwk	every week
g	gram	RBC	red blood cell
H₂O	water	r/o	rule out
HAART	highly active anti-retroviral therapy	Rx	treatment, prescription
		rxn	reaction
Hg	mercury	s	second
hr, hrs	hour, hours	sol'n	solution
hs	hours of sleep	SQ	subcutaneously
hx	history	SS	single strength
IM	intramuscular	sx	symptoms
Infxn	infection	tid	three times per day
IU	international unit	tiw	three times per week
IV	intravenous	tx	treatment
kg	kilogram	Txf	transfusion
L	liter	Txp	transplant
m	meter	U	unit
m²	square meters	vol	volume
Mc	megacycle	w/	with
mcg or μg	microgram	w/i	within
mEq	milliequivalent	w/o	without
mg	milligram	WBC	white blood cell
min, mins	minute, minutes	wk, wks	week, weeks
mL	milliliter	wnl	within normal limits
mm	millimeter	x	times
mm3	cubed millimeters	yr., yrs.	year, years

ANTI-INFECTIVES

Note: All monographs written by John G. Bartlett, M.D., and Paul A. Pham, Pharm.D.

For all protease inhibitors and NNRTIs, healthcare professionals should refer to the New York state guidelines, the Johns Hopkins online HIV guide (www.hopkins-hivguide.org), or the U.S. Department of Health and Human Services guidelines for a more comprehensive list of drug interactions and management recommendations.

ABACAVIR (ABC)

FDA INDICATIONS

- HIV infection treatment in combination with other antiretrovirals

USUAL ADULT DOSING: ABC 300mg PO bid; ABC 600mg PO qd (based on pharmacokinetic data); Epzicom (ABC 600mg/3TC 300mg) 1 tab qd; Trizivir (ABC 300mg/3TC 150mg/AZT 300mg bid)

Dosing Adjustments

GFR 50-80 mL/min: Usual dose

GFR 10-50 mL/min: No data-Usual dose likely

GFR<10 mL/min: No data-Usual dose likely: HD-No data-Usual dose likely

Hemodialysis: No data-Usual dose likely

Peritoneal Dialysis: No data-Usual dose likely

ADVERSE DRUG REACTIONS: Hypersensitivity rxn: fever, rash, fatigue, malaise, GI symptoms, and arthralgia (noted in 2-3% of patients). Mandatory d/c with hypersensitivity rxn. DO NOT RECHALLENGE. Rare cases of LACTIC ACIDOSIS +/- hepatomegaly w/ steatosis. **Rare:** Tubular injury

DRUG INTERACTIONS

Alcohol: Increases ABC levels by 41%, no effect on alcohol levels (clinical significance unknown).

PREGNANCY RISK: C--Rodent studies demonstrated placental passage. Teratogenic in rodent studies resulting in anasarca, skeletal malformation at 1000mg/kg dose (35 times human therapeutic levels) during organogenesis. However rabbit studies using 8.5 times human therapeutic levels did not result in fetal malformation. No adequate human data; placental passage was 32-66%.

BREAST FEEDING: No human data. Breast feeding is not recommended in the U.S. in order to avoid post-natal transmission of HIV to the child, who may not yet be infected.

COMMENTS: The most potent nucleoside analogue. Generally a well-tolerated antiretroviral but rare (2-3%) cases of hypersensitivity reaction that can be fatal with re-challenge requires close monitoring (Re-challenge is contraindicated). Triple NRTI combination of TDF/ABC/3TC and ABC/ddI/d4T are not recommended due to early virologic failure.

FORMS

Brand name	Preparation	Mfr.	Route	Form	Strength	Cost (AWP)
Ziagen	Abacavir (ABC)	GlaxoSmithKline	PO	solution	20mg/mL	$2.45 per 5mL
			PO	tablet	300mg	$7.46
Trizivir	Abacavir/Zidovudine/Lamivudine	GlaxoSmithKline	PO	tablet	300mg ABC/ 300mg AZT/ 150mg 3TC	$19.51
Epzicom	ABC/3TC	GlaxoSmithKline	PO	tablet	ABC 600mg and 3TC 300mg	$26.03

SELECTED READINGS

Mallal S, Nolan D, Witt C et al. Association between presence of HLA-B*5701, HLA-DR7, and HLA-DQ3 and hypersensitivity to HIV-1 reverse-transcriptase inhibitor abacavir. Lancet 2002 Mar 2;359 (9308):727-32

ACYCLOVIR

FDA INDICATIONS

- Herpes infections (initial and recurrent episodes, immunocompromised patients)
- Herpes simplex encephalitis
- Herpes zoster (immunocompromised patients)
- Varicella (immunocompetent patients if started w/i 48h of rash onset; American Academy of Pediatrics does not recommend use for uncomplicated chickenpox in healthy children)
- Initial episodes of herpes genitalis (immunocompetent patients)
- Herpes labialis (cream, but questionable efficacy)

USUAL ADULT DOSING: Mild HSV: 200mg 5x/day or 400mg PO tid. Suppressive, recurrent genital HSV (>6x/yr): 400mg PO bid. Severe HSV: 5mg/kg IV q8h. Extensive cutaneous, visceral HSV/VZV or encephalitis: 10mg/kg IV q8h. Zoster: 800mg PO 5x/d (valacyclovir preferred).

Dosing Adjustments

GFR 50-80 mL/min: 5-10 mg/kg IV q8h; 200-800mg PO 5x per day
GFR 10-50 mL/min: 5-10 mg/kg IV q12-24h; 200-800mg PO q8h
GFR<10 mL/min: 2.5-5mg/kg IV q24h; 200-800mg PO q12h
Hemodialysis: 2.5-5mg/kg IV q24h, dose after HD
Peritoneal Dialysis: 2.5-5mg/kg IV q24h

ADVERSE DRUG REACTIONS: Generally well tolerated with minor irritation at infusion site. **Occasional:** Rash, nausea & vomiting; diarrhea; renal toxicity (esp w/ rapid IV infusion, dehydration, prior renal disease & nephrotoxic drugs), dizziness, elevated LFTs; pruritis, headache.

DRUG INTERACTIONS

Probenecid: No dose adjustment needed. Increase in acyclovir levels due to competitive tubular secretion by probenecid.
Meperidine: may increase nor-meperidine levels.
Theophylline: May increase theophylline plasma concentration.

PREGNANCY RISK: C-not a teratogen but potential to cause chromosomal damage at high dose. CDC recommends use of acyclovir for life-threatening disease but does not advocate use for treatment or prophylaxis of genital herpes.

BREAST FEEDING: Acyclovir is concentrated at high levels in breast milk. Acyclovir has been used in newborns to treat HSV infection without adverse events. The American Academy of Pediatrics considers acyclovir to be compatible with breast feeding.

COMMENTS: Oral and parenteral antiviral agent with activity against HSV and VZV. Main use is for treatment and prevention of H. simplex infections and in varicella zoster. The drug is well tolerated. Topical use is not effective. Monitor for crystalluria when large IV doses given to patients with dehydration and/or renal insufficiency.

FORMS

Brand name	Preparation	Mfr.	Route	Form	Strength	Cost (AWP)
Zovirax	Acyclovir	GlaxoSmithKline	IV	vial	500mg	$78.56 per vial
			PO	cap	200mg	$2.02
			PO	susp	200mg/5mL	$1.56 per 5mL
			PO	tab	400mg; 800mg	$3.45; $6.70
Zovirax	Acyclovir	Biovail	topical	cre	5% (2g); 5% (5g)	$38.89; $90.44

SELECTED READINGS

Spruance SL et al. Acyclovir Cream for Treatment of Herpes Simplex Labialis: Results of Two Randomized, Double-Blind, Vehicle-Controlled, Multicenter Clinical Trials. AAC 2002;46:2238

Shafran SD, Tyring SK, Ashton R. Once, twice, or three times daily famciclovir compared with aciclovir for the oral treatment of herpes zoster in immunocompetent adults: a randomized, multicenter, double-blind clinical trial . J Clin Virol. 2004;29:248-53

ADEFOVIR

FDA INDICATIONS

- Chronic hepatitis B (pts w/ clinical evidence of lamivudine-resistant HBV with either compensated or decompensated liver function)

USUAL ADULT DOSING: 10mg qd (with or without food) x 48-92 weeks

Dosing Adjustments

GFR 50-80 mL/min: 10mg qd

GFR 10-50 mL/min: 20-49mL/min:10mg q48h; 10-19mL/min: 10mg q72 hours

Hemodialysis: 10mg q7 days following HD

↓ *Hepatic Function:* 10mg qd

ADVERSE DRUG REACTIONS: Generally well tolerated. **Occasional:** Increased creatinine (w/ underlying renal insufficiency); asthenia, abd pain; h/a; fever; n/v/d; exacerbation of hepatitis (with discontinuation of therapy); pruritus; rash; cough. **Rare:** NEPHROTOXICITY, LACTIC ACIDOSIS

DRUG INTERACTIONS

Ibuprofen: Increases adefovir AUC by 23%.

Probenecid: Drugs that inhibit tubular secretion may increase adefovir serum level.

PREGNANCY RISK: C- IV adefovir, when given at 20mg/kg (systemic exposure 38 times human), resulted in embryotoxicity and fetal malformations. No human data.

BREAST FEEDING: No data. Not recommended

COMMENTS: Adefovir is an effective tx of chronic HBV infection. In HIV-co-infected pts, a concern w/ the use of low dose adefovir is the potential for the development of cross-resistance w/ nucleoside analogues &/or future activity of tenofovir. Preliminary data didn't show selection of adefovir mutations. Entecavir may be a better choice due to potency & lack of potential of cross-resistance in HIV-coinfected pts.

FORMS

Brand name	Preparation	Mfr.	Route	Form	Strength	Cost (AWP)
Hepsera	Adefovir dip-ivoxil	Gilead	PO	tab	10mg	$19.85

SELECTED READINGS

Peters MG, Hann Hw H, Martin P et al. Adefovir dipivoxil alone or in combination with lamivudine in patients with lamivudine-resistant chronic hepatitis B. Gastroenterology. 2004;126:91-101.

ALBENDAZOLE

FDA INDICATIONS

- Neurocysticercosis caused by Taenia solium
- Hydatid disease caused by Echinococcus granulosus

USUAL ADULT DOSING: Microsporidiosis: 400mg PO bid with meals. Hookworm: 400mg x 1. Hydatid disease: 400mg bid with meals x 28 d followed by a 14-d drug-free interval x 3 cycles. Neurocysticercosis: 400mg bid w/ with meals for 8 to 30 days with steroid during 1st wk.

Dosing Adjustments

GFR 50-80 mL/min: Usual dose

GFR 10-50 mL/min: Usual dose

GFR<10 mL/min: Usual dose

Hemodialysis: Not removed in hemodialysis; use usual dose

ADVERSE DRUG REACTIONS: Occasional: Diarrhea, abdominal pain. **Rare:** Leukopenia; alopecia; increased LFTs; hypersensitivity; dizziness.

DRUG INTERACTIONS

Dexamethasone: Increased in albendazole concentration. Monitor for albendazole toxicity, dose may need to be decreased. In some case reports through concentration of albendazole it was increased up to 56%.

Praziquantel: Increased albendazole concentration. Monitor for adverse events of albendazole. Dose of albendazole may need to be decreased. In some case reports mean plasma concentration of albendazole was increased up to 50%.

PREGNANCY RISK: C-Teratogenicity demonstrated in laboratory animals.

BREAST FEEDING: Unknown

COMMENTS: Well-tolerated oral agent, broad-spectrum anti-helminthic. Agent of choice over praziquantel for neurocysticercosis due to higher eradication rate in parenchymal brain cysts.

FORMS

Brand name	Preparation	Mfr.	Route	Form	Strength	Cost (AWP)
Albenza	Albendazole	GlaxoSmithKline	PO	tab	200mg	$1.58

SELECTED READINGS

Legesse M, Erko B, Medhin G et al. Efficacy of albendazole and mebendazole in the treatment of Ascaris and Trichuris infections. Ethiop Med J. 2002 Oct;40(4):335-43.

AMANTADINE

FDA INDICATIONS

- Influenza A (prophylaxis and treatment)
- Parkinsonism

USUAL ADULT DOSING: Influenza treatment: 100mg PO q12h (within 48 hours of symptoms) x 5 days. Influenza prophylaxis: 100mg PO q12h continued for at least 10 days after exposure or 2-4 weeks after vaccination.

Dosing Adjustments

GFR 50-80 mL/min: 100mg q24-48h

GFR 10-50 mL/min: 100mg q48-72h

GFR<10 mL/min: 100mg q7d

Hemodialysis: 100mg q7d, no supplement needed post-dialysis

Peritoneal Dialysis: 100mg q7d, no supplement needed post-dialysis

ADVERSE DRUG REACTIONS: Frequent: Insomnia, lethargy, dizziness, inability to concentrate. **Occasional:** GI intolerance, esp nausea; rash, depression; confusion; livedo reticularis

DRUG INTERACTIONS

Anticholinergic agents: May increase the incidence of CNS side effects. Avoid concurrent administration, or decrease dose of anticholinergic if atropine-like adverse reaction occurs.

Trimethoprim: Decreased renal clearance of amantadine; may enhance CNS side effects (confusion, tremors, seizures). Monitor for CNS side effects; may need to reduce amantadine dose.

PREGNANCY RISK: C-Embryotoxic and teratogenic in animal studies. Of 51 exposures during the first trimester in a Michigan Medicaid surveillance study, the incidence of defects was 9.8%; though high, the numbers of exposures were too small to draw any conclusions.

BREAST FEEDING: Excreted in low concentration in breast milk, potential for urinary retention, vomiting and skin rash.

COMMENTS: Oral agent for prophylaxis and treatment of influenza A (but not active against influenza B). CNS side effects may be bothersome, esp in elderly patients and in patients with renal impairment. Due to CNS toxicity, may prefer rimantidine or neuraminidase inhibitors which are more expensive.

FORMS (◆ DENOTES AVAILABLE GENERICALLY)

Brand name	Preparation	Mfr.	Route	Form	Strength	Cost (AWP)
Symmetrel	Amantadine HCl	◆ Endo	PO	tab	100mg	$1.46
Amantadine HCl	Amantadine HCl	◆ Hi-Tech Phar-macal	PO	syrup	50mg/5mL	$0.70 per 5mL

SELECTED READINGS

T. O. Jefferson, et al. Cochrane Review. The Cochrane Library, Oxford, February 1999 as reviewed in the ACP Journal Club, 1999;131:68

AMIKACIN

FDA INDICATIONS

- Amikacin sulfate indicated in the short-term treatment of serious infections due to susceptible organisms
- Bacterial septicemia (including neonatal sepsis)
- Respiratory tract infections
- Bones and joint infections
- Central nervous system infections
- Skin and soft tissue infections
- Intra-abdominal infections
- Burns
- Post-operative infections
- Complicated and recurrent urinary tract infections

USUAL ADULT DOSING: 15mg/kg/day IV qd or divided q12h or q8h. Target peak: 15-30mcg/mL (30mcg/mL for pulmonary & serious infections). Don't use qd dosing in pts w/ unstable renal function, CrCl <60mL/min, endocarditis, meningitis, or increased Vd (pregnancy, ascites, edema, burns, and shock).

Dosing Adjustments

GFR 50-80 mL/min: 60-90% of usual dose q12h or 100% of usual dose q12-24 hrs. (monitor levels, redose when trough <8mg/L)

GFR 10-50 mL/min: 30-70% of usual dose q 12-18h or 100% of usual dose q24-48 hrs (monitor levels, redose when trough <8mg/L)

GFR<10 mL/min: Dose based on serum level, redose when trough <8mg/L
Hemodialysis: 2.5-3.75 mg/kg post dialysis
Peritoneal Dialysis: 9-20mg per Liter of dialysate exchange per day. Aminoglycosides given for prolonged periods to patients receiving continuous peritoneal dialysis have been associated with high rates of ototoxicity. Monitor level after loading dose and follow for symptoms

ADVERSE DRUG REACTIONS: Frequent: Renal failure (usually reversible) **Occasional:** Vestibular and auditory damage [usually irreversible, genetic predisposition possible-- check family for aminoglycoside ototoxicity hx]

DRUG INTERACTIONS

Loop diuretics: (bumetanide, furosemide, ethacrynic acid, torsemide) Ototoxicity (auditory) may be increased. The co-administration of aminoglycoside with loop diuretics may have an additive or synergistic ototoxicity effect. Ototoxicity appears to be dose dependent and may be increased with renal dysfunction. Irreversible ototoxicity has been reported. Avoid concomitant administration, if used together careful dose adjustments needed in patients with renal failure and close monitoring for ototoxicity required.
Nephrotoxic agents: (amphotericin B, foscarnet, cidofovir) Additive nephrotoxicity. Avoid co-administration, if used together monitor renal function closely and discontinue if warranted.
Nondepolarizing muscle relaxants: (atracurium, pancuronium, tubocurarine, gallamine triethiodide) Possible enhanced action of nondepolarizing muscle relaxant resulting in possible respiratory depression. Avoid co-administration, if concurrent administration is needed titrate the nondepolarizing muscle relaxant slowly and monitor neuromuscular function closely.
Penicillins: In vitro inactivation (possible). Do not mix together before administration (i. e., running in the same line or concurrent intraperitoneal administration). In vivo patients with poor renal function where renal excretion of the drugs is delayed (where the ratio of penicillin to aminoglycoside is greater than 50 to 1 there is a potential for drug inactivation). Amikacin may be less affected by this interaction compared to gentamicin and tobramycin.
Vancomycin: controversial, but may increase nephrotoxicity.

PREGNANCY RISK: D-No reports linking the use of amikacin to congenital defects have been located. Ototoxicity has not been reported as an effect of in utero exposure to amikacin, however, eighth cranial nerve toxicity in the fetus is well known following exposure to other aminoglycosides (kanamycin and streptomycin) and could potentially occur with amikacin.

BREAST FEEDING: Only a trace amount of amikacin was found in some nursing infants. Due to the poor absorption of aminoglycoside the systemic toxicity should not occur, but alteration in normal bowel flora may occur in nursing infants.

COMMENTS: Amikacin is an aminoglycoside that is active against many gram-negative bacteria resistant to gentamicin and tobramycin. Amikacin should be restricted to infections with organisms resistant to other aminoglycosides. Desired peak 15-30mcg/mL (high peak for serious, pulmonary, and pseudomonal infections).

FORMS (◆ DENOTES AVAILABLE GENERICALLY)

Brand name	Preparation	Mfr.	Route	Form	Strength	Cost (AWP)
Amikacin	Amikacin sulfate	◆ Bedford	IV	vial	1000mg/4mL; 500mg/2mL	$15.60; $7.80
Amikacin	Amikacin sulfate pediatric	◆ Bedford	IV	vial	100mg/2mL	$7.80

SELECTED READINGS

Baron EJ; Young LS. Amikacin, ethambutol, and rifampin for treatment of disseminated Mycobacterium avium-intracellulare infections in patients with acquired immune deficiency syndrome. Diagn Microbiol Infect Dis 1986 Sep;5(3):215-20

Love LJ; Schimpff SC; Hahn DM et al. Randomized trial of empiric antibiotic therapy with ticarcillin in combination with gentamicin, amikacin or netilmicin in febrile patients with granulocytopenia and cancer. Am J Med 1979 Apr;66(4):603-10

Holm SE; Hill B; Lowestad A et al. A prospective, randomized study of amikacin and gentamicin in serious infections with focus on efficacy, toxicity and duration of serum levels above the MIC. J Antimicrob Chemother 1983 Oct;12(4):393-402

ATS and IDSA. Guidelines for the Management of Adults with Hospital-acquired, Ventilator-associated, and Healthcare-associated Pneumonia . Am J Respir Crit Care Med 2005;171:388

AMOXICILLIN

FDA INDICATIONS

- Bronchopulmonary infections
- Urinary tract infections (cystitis, pyelonephritis)
- Duodenal ulcer caused by H. pylori (in combination with clarithromycin and a PPI)
- Sinusitis
- Uncomplicated gonorrhea (currently not the drug of choice)
- Otitis media (Haemophilus influenzae, nonbetalactamase producer)
- Proteus mirabilis infections
- Lower respiratory infection (PCN-sensitive CAP)
- Skin and skin structure infections

USUAL ADULT DOSING: CAP: 500mg PO tid. UTI: 250-500mg PO tid (consider 875mg q12h). SSTI: 250mg-500mg PO tid (consider 875mg q12h). Up to 3-4g/day for some intermediately resistant pneumococcal infections.

Dosing Adjustments
GFR 50-80 mL/min: 0.25g-0.5g q12h
GFR 10-50 mL/min: 0.25g-0.5g q12-24h
GFR<10 mL/min: 0.25g-0.5g q12-24h
Hemodialysis: 0.25g post dialysis.
Peritoneal Dialysis: 250mg q12h

ADVERSE DRUG REACTIONS: Frequent: Rash (esp. w/ mononucleosis). **Occasional:** Diarrhea; C. difficile; hypersensitivity rxns; Jarisch-Herxheimer reaction with spirochetal infection. **Rare:** Coombs' test positive, hemolytic anemia; interstitial nephritis; pancytopenia; drug fever.

DRUG INTERACTIONS

Tetracyclines: In vitro antagonism when co-administered. Bactericidal effect of penicillins may be diminished in vivo. Avoid concurrent administration. In two studies involving a total of 79 patients with pneumococcal meningitis treated with either penicillin plus tetracyclines or penicillin monotherapy there was a higher mortality rate (79-85%) in the combination therapy compared to penicillin monotherapy (30-33%). (Arch Intern Med 1951:88:489, Ann Intern Med 1961; 55:545). However there was not a difference in mortality between penicillin monotherapy and penicillin plus tetracycline in the treatment of pneumococcal pneumonia. (Arch Intern Med 1953; 91:197).

PREGNANCY RISK: B-Several collaborative perinatal project reports involving over 12,000 exposures to penicillin derivatives during the first trimester indicated no association between penicillin derivative drugs and birth defects.

BREAST FEEDING: Excreted in breast milk at low concentrations. The American Academy of Pediatrics considers amoxicillin compatible with breast feeding.

COMMENTS: Oral aminopenicillin derivative w/ comparable gram-positive & gram-negative coverage to ampicillin, but better absorption & GI tolerance with oral administration. This is the preferred oral penicillin for all infections w/ possible exception of strep pharyngitis & shigellosis. Rash seen w/ amox use in setting of infectious mono does not preclude future use of drug (i.e., not actual pen allergy).

FORMS (◆ DENOTES AVAILABLE GENERICALLY)

Brand name	Preparation	Mfr.	Route	Form	Strength	Cost (AWP)
Amoxil	Amoxicillin trihydrate	◆ GlaxoSmithK-line	PO	chew tab	200mg; 400mg	0.51; 0.62
			PO	susp	200mg/5mL; 400mg/5mL	0.51 per 5mL; 0.55 per 5mL
			PO	tab	500mg; 875mg	0.55; 0.97
Amoxicillin	Amoxicillin trihydrate	◆ Teva	PO	susp	125mg/5mL; 250mg/5mL	0.20 per 5mL; 0.30 per 5mL

SELECTED READINGS

J. W. Williams Jr, et al. Antimicrobial Therapy for Acute Maxillary Sinusitis. Cochrane Review, May 26, 1999

S. Bent, et al. Antibiotics in Acute Bronchitis: A Meta-Analysis. Am J Med 1999;107:62

AMOXICILLIN + CLAVULANATE

FDA INDICATIONS

- Lymphadenitis
- Mastitis
- Otitis media
- Pharyngitis
- Community-acquired pneumonia (XR)
- Acute bacterial sinusitis (XR and IR)
- Skin and skin-structure infections (carbuncles, cellulitis, subcutaneous abscess)
- Tonsillitis
- Urinary-tract infection

USUAL ADULT DOSING: 250-500mg PO tid. 875/125mg PO bid. XR: 2 tablets (2000mg:125mg) PO bid.

Dosing Adjustments

GFR 50-80 mL/min: Usual dose

GFR 10-50 mL/min: 0.25g-0.5g q12h

GFR<10 mL/min: 0.25g-0.5g q24-36h

Hemodialysis: 0.5g (amoxicillin)+ 0.125g (CA) halfway through and another dose at the end.

Peritoneal Dialysis: Usual regimen

ADVERSE DRUG REACTIONS: Frequent: GI intolerance and diarrhea including C. difficile. **Occasional:** Hypersensitivity reaction, rash (esp with EBV inf.) **Rare:** Coombs' test positive, hemolytic anemia, Jarisch-Herxheimer reaction, hepatitis, pancytopenia, interstitial nephritis.

DRUG INTERACTIONS

Tetracyclines: In vitro antagonism when co-administered. Bactericidal effect of penicillins may be diminished in vivo. Avoid concurrent administration. In two studies involving a total of 79 patients with pneumococcal meningitis treated with either penicillin plus tetracyclines or penicillin monotherapy there was a higher mortality rate (79-85%) in the combination therapy compared to penicillin monotherapy (30-33%). (Arch Intern Med 1951:88:489, Ann Intern Med 1961; 55:545). However there was not a difference in mortality between penicillin monotherapy and penicillin plus tetracycline in the treatment of pneumococcal pneumonia. (Arch Intern Med 1953; 91:197).

PREGNANCY RISK: B-In surveillance study of Michigan Medicaid recipients, 556 newborns were exposed to clavulanate/penicillin during the first trimester; there were no associations between birth defects and clavulanate/penicillin.

BREAST FEEDING: No studies with clavulanate.

COMMENTS: Oral betalactam w/ activity against common bacteria that produce beta-lactamases: e.g., H. influenzae, MSSA, Moraxella and all PCN-resistant anaerobes. Diarrhea is common due to both clavulanate & amoxicillin. The IDSA recommends amox/clav if anaerobes or H. influenzae are suspected [CID 2000; 31:347]. No advantage using Augmentin XR over amox 1g PO tid for intermediately-resistant S. pneumoniae.

FORMS (♦ DENOTES AVAILABLE GENERICALLY)

Brand name	Preparation	Mfr.	Route	Form	Strength	Cost (AWP)
Augmentin	Amoxicillin + Clavulanate	♦ GlaxoSmithKline	PO	chew tab	125:31 ; 250:62	$1.51; $2.88
			PO	susp	125mg/ 31.25mg per 5mL; 250mg/ 62.5mg per 5mL	$1.51 per 5mL; $2.88 per 5mL
			PO	tab	250:125; 500:125; 875:125	$3.20; $4.71; $6.28
Augmentin ES	Amoxicillin + Clavulanate	GlaxoSmithKline	PO	tab	600mg/42.9mg per 5mL	$2.68 per 5mL
Augmentin XR	amoxicillin + clavulanate	GlaxoSmithKline	PO	tab, ER	1000mg/ 62.5mg	$3.01

SELECTED READINGS

R Dagan, et al. Bacteriologic and Clinical Efficacy of Amoxicillin/Clavulanate vs Azithromycin in Acute Otitis Media. Ped Infect Dis J 2000;19:95

A. Freifeld et al. A Double-Blind Comparison of Empiric Oral and Intravenous Antibiotic Therapy for Loss Risk Febrile Patients with Neutropenia During Cancer Chemotherapy. NEJM 1999;341:305

AMPHOTERICIN B CHOLESTERYL SULFATE COMPLEX (ABCD)

FDA INDICATIONS

• Invasive aspergillosis in patients who are refractory to or intolerant of amphotericin B deoxycholate therapy

USUAL ADULT DOSING: 3-4mg/kg/day

Dosing Adjustments

GFR 50-80 mL/min: Usual

GFR 10-50 mL/min: Usual

GFR<10 mL/min: Usual

Hemodialysis: Not removed in dialysis, no supplement needed post HD. Usual dose.

Peritoneal Dialysis: Usual

ADVERSE DRUG REACTIONS: Frequent: Fever, chills & rigor (worse than conventional AmB & other lipid ampho formulations); anemia; phlebitis & pain at infusion site. **Occasional:** Serum creatinine increase; hypokalemia; hypomagnesemia; hypocalcemia; hypotension; n/v; metallic taste; h/a.

DRUG INTERACTIONS

Digoxin: Potential increase in digitalis toxicity secondary to ampho-induced potassium depletion. Monitor potassium, supplementation may be needed.
Diuretics and **steroids:** May increase risk of hypokalemia.

PREGNANCY RISK: B- There is limited data on the use of amphotericin B cholesteryl sulfate complex in pregnancy, therefore the use should be limited to patients where the benefit outweighs the risk.

BREAST FEEDING: No data available.

COMMENTS: Parenteral lipid amphotericin that is the least expensive of all lipid formulations, but with increased incidence of infusion-related side effects compared to standard amphotericin B and other lipid amphotericin formulations.

FORMS

Brand name	Preparation	Mfr.	Route	Form	Strength	Cost (AWP)
Amphotec	Amphotericin B cholesteryl sulfate complex (ABCD)	Intermune	IV	vial	50mg; 100mg	$93.33; $160 per vial

SELECTED READINGS

JD Sobel, et al. Practice Guidelines for the Treatment of Fungal Infections. CID 2000; 30:652

White MH, et al. Randomized, double-blind clinical trial of amphotericin B colloidal dispersion vs. amphotericin B in the empirical treatment of fever and neutropenia . Clin Infect Dis 1998 Aug;27 (2):296-302

Bowden R et al. A Double-Blind, Randomized, Controlled Trial of Amphotericin B Colloidal Dispersion versus Amphotericin B for Treatment of Invasive Aspergillosis in Immunocompromised Patients. CID 2002;35:359

AMPHOTERICIN B DEOXYCHOLATE

FDA INDICATIONS

- Aspergillosis
- Blastomycosis
- Disseminated candidiasis
- Leishmaniasis
- Cryptococcosis
- Histoplasmosis
- Cryptococcal meningitis (treatment and suppression)
- Meningitis caused by organisms such as Coccidioides immitis, candida species, Sporothrix schenckii, and aspergillus species.
- Coccidioidomycosis
- Disseminated sporotrichosis

USUAL ADULT DOSING: Systemic fungal infections: 0.5-1.5 mg/kg/d over 2-4 hrs w/ pre and post hydration. Candida esophagitis: 0.3-0.5 mg/kg/day IV. Cryptococcal meningitis: 0.7mg/kg IV qd (+/- 5FC) x 10-14 d followed by fluconazole.

Dosing Adjustments

GFR 50-80 mL/min: Usual

GFR 10-50 mL/min: Usual
GFR<10 mL/min: Usual
Hemodialysis: Usual dose, no supplement needed post HD.
Peritoneal Dialysis: Usual

ADVERSE DRUG REACTIONS: Frequent: Nephrotoxicity; renal tubular acidosis; fever & chills; hypokalemia; anemia; phlebitis (improved with addition of 1000 units heparin to infusion). **Occasional:** Hypomagnesemia; hypocalcemia; hypotension; n/v (reduce w/ compazine), metallic taste; H/A.

DRUG INTERACTIONS

Digoxin: Potential increase in digitalis toxicity secondary to ampho-induced potassium depletion.

Diuretics and **steroids:** May increase risk of hypokalemia.

Nephrotoxic agents (Foscarnet, aminoglycosides, IV contrast, etc.): additive nephrotoxicity.

PREGNANCY RISK: B-A Collaborative Perinatal Project identified 9 first-trimester exposures to amphotericin and found no adverse fetal effects. Animal studies demonstrated amphotericin to be harmless in pregnancy.

BREAST FEEDING: No data available.

COMMENTS: Parenteral use is complicated by high rate of infusion related reactions, anemia, electrolyte imbalance and renal failure. A switch to the lipid formulation is often not recommended until the creatinine is elevated to an arbitrary threshold (Scr >2.5 used at Hopkins). Infusion related side effects is worst with Amphotec [CID 2002; 35: 359]

FORMS (◆ DENOTES AVAILABLE GENERICALLY)

Brand name	Preparation	Mfr.	Route	Form	Strength	Cost (AWP)
Amphotericin B	Amphotericin B	◆ Abbott	IV	vial	50mg	$11.64 per vial

SELECTED READINGS

van der Horst CM, Saag MS, Cloud GA, et al. Treatment of cryptococcal meningitis associated with the acquired immunodeficiency syndrome. N Engl J Med 1997 Jul 3;337(1):15-21

Patterson TF, et al. Invasive Aspergillosis: Disease Spectrum, Treatment Practices, and Outcomes. Medicine 2000; 79: 250

JD Sobel, et al. Practice Guidelines for the Treatment of Fungal Infections. CID 2000; 30:652

AMPHOTERICIN B LIPID COMPLEX (ABLC)

FDA INDICATIONS

- Aspergillosis infections in patients who are refractory to or intolerant of conventional amphotericin B therapy

USUAL ADULT DOSING: 5mg/kg/day

Dosing Adjustments

GFR 50-80 mL/min: Usual
GFR 10-50 mL/min: Usual
GFR<10 mL/min: Usual
Hemodialysis: Not removed in dialysis, no supplement needed post HD. Usual dose.
Peritoneal Dialysis: Usual

ADVERSE DRUG REACTIONS: Frequent: Fever & chills; anemia; phlebitis & pain at infusion site. **Occasional:** Creatinine increase; hypokalemia; hypomagnesemia; hypocalcemia;

hypotension; nausea, vomiting, metallic taste; headache; increased LFTs; increased bilirubin (1.5x).

DRUG INTERACTIONS

Digoxin: Potential increase in digitalis toxicity secondary to ampho-induced potassium depletion. Monitor potassium, supplementation may be needed.
Diuretics and **steroids:** May increase risk of hypokalemia.

PREGNANCY RISK: B- There is limited data on the use of Amphotericin B lipid complex in pregnancy therefore the use should be limited to patients where the benefit outweighs the risk.

BREAST FEEDING: No data available.

COMMENTS: Abelcet has comparable cost to Amphotec but generally better tolerated with less infusion related reactions. Compared to Ambisome, Abelcet resulted in a higher incidence of nephrotoxicity and infusion related side effects.

FORMS

Brand name	Preparation	Mfr.	Route	Form	Strength	Cost (AWP)
Abelcet	Amphotericin B lipid complex (ABLC)	Enzon	IV	vial	5mg/mL	$240 per vial

SELECTED READINGS

Sharkey PK, et al. Amphotericin B lipid complex compared with amphotericin B in the treatment of cryptococcal meningitis in patients with AIDS . Clin Infect Dis 1996 Feb;22(2):315-21

JD Sobel. Practice Guidelines for the Treatment of Fungal Infections. CID 2000; 30:652

John R. Wingard et al. A Randomized, Double-Blind Comparative Trial Evaluating the Safety of Liposomal Amphotericin B vs. Amphotericin B Lipid Complex in the Empirical Treatment of Febrile Neutropenia. CID 2000; 31:1155-63

Fleming RV et al. Comparison of ABLC vs. Ambisome in the Treatment of Suspected or Documented Fungal Infection in Patients with Leukemia. Leukemia and Lymphoma 2001; 405: 511

AMPHOTERICIN B LIPOSOMAL

FDA INDICATIONS

- Aspergillosis (in patients refractory to or intolerant of amphotericin B deoxycholate)
- Candidiasis (in patients refractory to or intolerant of amphotericin B deoxycholate)
- Cryptococcosis (in patients refractory to or intolerant of amphotericin B deoxycholate)
- Empiric therapy for presumed fungal infection in patients with febrile neutropenia
- Visceral leishmaniasis

USUAL ADULT DOSING: Empiric treatment of fever in neutropenic pts not responding to abx: 3mg/kg/day. Cryptococcal meningitis (alternative): 4mg/kg IV qd. Aspergillosis: 5mg/kg IV qd.

Dosing Adjustments
GFR 50-80 mL/min: Usual
GFR 10-50 mL/min: Usual
GFR<10 mL/min: Usual

ADVERSE DRUG REACTIONS: Frequent: Fever, chills (premedicate w/hydrocortisone, NSAID, ASA, APAP, meperidine), anemia; phlebitis, pain at infusion site. **Occasional:** Creatinine rise; hypokalemia; hypomagnesemia; hypocalcemia;hypotension; nausea, vomiting; metallic taste; h/a.

DRUG INTERACTIONS

Digoxin: Potential increase in digitalis toxicity secondary to ampho-induced potassium depletion. Monitor potassium, supplementation may be needed.
Diuretics and **steroids:** May increase risk of hypokalemia.

PREGNANCY RISK: B- There is limited data on the use of Amphotericin B liposomal complex in pregnancy therefore the use should be limited to patients where the benefit outweighs the risk.

BREAST FEEDING: No data available

COMMENTS: The only truly liposomal amphotericin that is also the most expensive of the lipid formulations (but cost will vary between institutions). Compared to Abelcet, Ambisome resulted in less nephrotoxicity and fewer infusion related side effects. No difference in efficacy compared to conventional amphoB, w/ the possible exception of disseminated histo in AIDS pts (Ann Intern Med 2002; 137:105-9).

FORMS

Brand name	Preparation	Mfr.	Route	Form	Strength	Cost (AWP)
AmBisome	Amphotericin B liposomal	Astellas	IV	vial	50mg	$188.40 per vial

SELECTED READINGS

Sobel JD, et al. Practice Guidelines for the Treatment of Fungal Infections. Clin Infect Dis. 2000 Apr;30 (4):652

Leenders AC, et al. Liposomal amphotericin B compared with amphotericin B deoxycholate in the treatment of documented and suspected neutropenia-associated invasive fungal infections. Br J Haematol 1998 Oct;103(1):205-12

Leenders AC, et al. Liposomal amphotericin B (AmBisome) compared with amphotericin B both followed by oral fluconazole in the treatment of AIDS-associated cryptococcal meningitis . AIDS 1997 Oct;11(12):1463-71

Tollemar J, et al. Liposomal amphotericin B prevents invasive fungal infections in liver transplant recipients. A randomized, placebo-controlled study . Transplantation 1995 Jan 15;59(1):45-50

Philip CJ, Wheat LJ, Cloud GA et al. Safety and Efficacy of Liposomal Amphotericin B Compared with Conventional Amphotericin B for Histoplasmosis. Annals of Internal Med. 2002; 137:105

AMPICILLIN

FDA INDICATIONS

- Diverticulitis (in combination with metronidazole)
- Gonorrhea (in combination with probenecid, however currently not recommended due to high failure rate)
- Streptococcal infections (Group A streptococcal pharyngitis, Group B streptococci)
- Otitis media (Haemophilus influenzae due to beta-lactamase negative strains)
- Enteric infections (Proteus mirabilis infections, salmonellosis, shigellosis)
- Urinary tract infections
- Bacterial vaginosis

USUAL ADULT DOSING: 250-500mg PO qid; 1-2g IV q4-6h

Dosing Adjustments

GFR 50-80 mL/min: Usual dose
GFR 10-50 mL/min: 1g-2g IV q8h; no dose adjustment needed for oral administration
GFR<10 mL/min: 1g-2g IV q12h; no dose adjustment needed for oral administration.
Hemodialysis: 1g-2g IV q12h. On HD days, give post HD.

Peritoneal Dialysis: 250mg q12h

ADVERSE DRUG REACTIONS: Frequent: GI intolerance & diarrhea (more common than amox) incl. C. difficile; hypersensitivity rxns; maculopapular rash esp w/ primary EBV (not urticarial). **Rare:** Drug fever; Coombs' test +, hemolytic anemia; Jarisch-Herxheimer rxn w/ spirochetal dz.

DRUG INTERACTIONS

Allopurinol: Incidence of skin rash increased to 14-22% when the two are co-administered compared to 6-8% with ampicillin when administered alone or 2% when allopurinol is administered alone. Use alternative therapy if possible, if not beware of the increased incidence of rash when ampicillin and allopurinolare co-administered.

Tetracyclines: In vitro antagonism when co-administered. Bactericidal effect of penicillins may be diminished in vivo. Avoid concurrent administration. In two studies involving a total of 79 patients with pneumococcal meningitis treated with either penicillin plus tetracyclines or penicillin monotherapy there was a higher mortality rate (79-85%) in the combination therapy compared to penicillin monotherapy (30-33%). (Arch Intern Med 1951;88:489, Ann Intern Med 1961; 55:545). However there was not a difference in mortality between penicillin monotherapy and penicillin plus tetracycline in the treatment of pneumococcal pneumonia. (Arch Intern Med 1953; 91:197).

PREGNANCY RISK: B-Several collaborative perinatal project reports involving over 12,000 exposures to penicillin derivatives during the first trimester indicated no association between penicillin derivative drugs and birth defects.

BREAST FEEDING: Excreted in breast milk at low concentrations.

COMMENTS: Oral and parenteral betalactam. Due to inferior absorption of ampicillin, amoxicillin has replaced oral ampicillin for all infections except shigellosis. IV ampicillin is the drug of choice for infections involving ampicillin sensitive enterococci.

FORMS (♦ DENOTES AVAILABLE GENERICALLY)

Brand name	Preparation	Mfr.	Route	Form	Strength	Cost (AWP)
Ampicillin	ampicillin	♦ Sandoz	IV	vial	2g	$20.10
			PO	cap	250mg; 500mg	$0.23; $0.40
Ampicillin	ampicillin	♦ Stada	PO	susp	125mg/5mL; 250mg/5mL	$0.25 per 5mL; $0.35 per 5mL

SELECTED READINGS

Bennish ML; Salam MA; Haider R; Barza M . Therapy for shigellosis. II. Randomized, double-blind comparison of ciprofloxacin and ampicillin. J Infect Dis 1990 Sep;162(3):711-6

AMPICILLIN + SULBACTAM

FDA INDICATIONS

- Gynecologic infections
- Intra-abdominal infections
- Skin and soft tissue infections

USUAL ADULT DOSING: Mild to moderate infections: 1.5g (1g ampicillin/0.5g sulbactam)IV q6h. Moderate to severe infections: 3g (2g ampicillin/1g sulbactam) IV q6h

Dosing Adjustments

GFR 50-80 mL/min: 1g-2g q8h

GFR 10-50 mL/min: 1g-2g q8h

GFR<10 mL/min: 1g-2g q12h

Hemodialysis: 1g q12h with 2g ampicillin post dialysis.

Peritoneal Dialysis: Usual regimen

ADVERSE DRUG REACTIONS: Occasional: Hypersensitivity reaction, maculopapular rash (not urticarial); GI intolerance; phlebitis at infusion sites and sterile abscesses at IM sites. **Rare:** Drug fever; Coomb's test positive; Jarisch-Herxheimer reaction.

DRUG INTERACTIONS

Allopurinol: Incidence of skin rash increased to 14-22% when the two are co-administered compared to 6-8% with ampicillin when administered alone or 2% when allopurinol is administered alone. Use alternative therapy if possible, if not beware of the increased incidence of rash when ampicillin and allopurinolare co-administered.

Tetracyclines: In vitro antagonism when co-administered. Bactericidal effect of penicillins may be diminished in vivo. Avoid concurrent administration. In two studies involving a total of 79 patients with pneumococcal meningitis treated with either penicillin plus tetracyclines or penicillin monotherapy there was a higher mortality rate (79-85%) in the combination therapy compared to penicillin monotherapy (30-33%). (Arch Intern Med 1951;88:489, Ann Intern Med 1961; 55:545). However there was not a difference in mortality between penicillin monotherapy and penicillin plus tetracycline in the treatment of pneumococcal pneumonia. (Arch Intern Med 1953; 91:197).

PREGNANCY RISK: B-Several collaborative perinatal project reports involving over 12,000 exposures to penicillin derivatives during the first trimester indicated no association between penicillin derivative drugs and birth defects. The safety of sulbactam has not been evaluated in humans. There was no adverse effect reported in animal data.

BREAST FEEDING: Excreted in breast milk at low concentrations.

COMMENTS: Parenteral betalactam/betalactamase inhibitor. Sulbactam increases the activity of ampicillin, but inducible chromosomal B-lactamases produced by Citrobacter, Enterobacter, Proteus, Pseudomonas, & Serratia are not generally inhibited by sulbactam. Active vs. H. influenzae, MSSA, most anaerobes and many GNB. Sulbactam is active against most strains of Acinetobacter. Contains Na+ 5 Meq/1.5 g

FORMS (♦ DENOTES AVAILABLE GENERICALLY)

Brand name	Preparation	Mfr.	Route	Form	Strength	Cost (AWP)
Unasyn	Ampicillin + Sulbactam	♦ Pfizer	IV	vial	1g:0.5g ; 2g:1g	$9.50; $16.86

SELECTED READINGS

Talan DA, et al. Ampicillin/Sulbactam and Cefoxitin in the Treatment of Cutaneous and Other Soft-Tissue Abscesses in patients With or Without Histories of Injection Drug Abuse . CID 2000;31:464

AMPRENAVIR (APV)

FDA INDICATIONS

• HIV infection (in combination with other antiretrovirals)

USUAL ADULT DOSING: Amprenavir liquid (only form available in US) APV 1200mg PO bid; liquid APV 1400mg PO BID. Combination dosing: APV 1200mg qd w/ RTV 200mg qd. APV 600mg bid + RTV 100mg bid + EFV 600mg qhs. LPV-r 533/100mg bid + APV 750mg bid.

Dosing Adjustments

GFR 50-80 mL/min: Usual dose

GFR 10-50 mL/min: Usual dose likely

GFR<10 mL/min: Usual dose likely. Avoid liquid formulation.

Hemodialysis: No data, usual dose likely

Peritoneal Dialysis: No data, usual dose likely

↓ *Hepatic Function:* Some recommend 450mg bid with liver disease and 300mg bid with severe cirrhosis based on PK data but this has not been evaluated in clinical trials

ANTI-INFECTIVES

ADVERSE DRUG REACTIONS: GI intolerance most common (N/V/D); oral paresthesias; headache; rash (11%); lipodystrophy syndrome; hyperglycemia; increased triglycerides and/or cholesterol; transaminase elevation. TOXICITY FROM PROPYLENE GLYCOL IN THE ORAL SOLUTION.

DRUG INTERACTIONS

Substrate, inhibitor, and likely inducer of CYP3A4. CYP3A4 inhibitors may increase APV serum levels. CYP3A4 inducers may decrease APV serum levels. APV may increase or decrease serum levels of CYP3A4 substrates.

Contraindicated with: terfenadine, astemizole, cisapride, ergot alkaloid, rifampin, bepridil, pimozide, flecainide, propafanone, St. Johns Wort, midazolam and triazolam.

PREGNANCY RISK: C-Placental passage unknown. Rat studies using half the human dose, resulted in thymic elongation and incomplete ossification of bones. Rabbit studies using one-twentieth of human therapeutic doses were associated with abortions and skeletal abnormalities.

BREAST FEEDING: No human data, breast milk excretion in animal studies. Breast feeding is not recommended in the U.S. in order to avoid post-natal transmission of HIV to the child, who may not yet be infected.

COMMENTS: Avoid long term use of APV oral solution due to propylene glycol content. Fosamprenavir is the preferred formulation due to lower pill burden and better bioavailability.

FORMS

Brand name	Preparation	Mfr.	Route	Form	Strength	Cost (AWP)
Agenerase	Amprenavir	GlaxoSmithKline	PO	cap	50mg	$0.54
			PO	sol	15mg/mL	$0.80 per 5mL

ATAZANAVIR (ATV)

FDA INDICATIONS

• Indicated for the treatment of HIV-1 infection in combination with other antiretroviral agents.

USUAL ADULT DOSING: ATV 400mg qd w/ food (FDA-approved dose--use in PI-naive pts only) ATV300mg/RTV100mg qd w/ food (author's preferred dose, especially for PI-experienced patients). When co-administered with EFV 600mg qhs dose ATV300mg/RTV100mg qd.

Dosing Adjustments

GFR 50-80 mL/min: No data. Usual dose likely.

GFR 10-50 mL/min: No data. Usual dose likely.

GFR<10 mL/min: No data. Usual dose likely.

Hemodialysis: No data. Usual dose likely.

↓ *Hepatic Function:* ATV AUC increased by 45% w/ mild to mod hepatic insuf. Consider decrease. ATV to 300mg/day in those subjects (but no clinical data). No human data.

ADVERSE DRUG REACTIONS: Common: Reversible benign hyperbilirubinemia (grade 3-4 occurring in 35-47% of patients), jaundice, and scleral icterus. **Occasional:** Nausea, vomiting, abdominal pain, lipodystrophy, rash, h/a, and mild transaminase elevation (unrelated to UGT 1A1 inhibition).

DRUG INTERACTIONS

Substrate and inhibitor of CYP3A4. Weak inhibitor of CYP1A2 and CYP2C9 *in vitro* but clinical significance unknown. Inhibitor of phase II conjugation (UGT1A1). CYP3A4 inhibitors may increase ATV levels. CYP3A4 inducers may decrease ATV levels. ATV may increase levels of CYP3A4 substrates.

Contraindicated with: rifampin, irinotecan, ergot Alkaloid, cisapride, St. Johns wort, midazolam, triazolam, bepridil, pimozide, simvastatin, lovastatin, indinavir, and all proton pump-inhibitors.

PREGNANCY RISK: B No human data. In animal studies, ATV did not result in embryonic or fetal toxicity when given maternally toxic doses.

BREAST FEEDING: No data

COMMENTS: The benefit in terms of lipid profile is consistently shown. This may offer a distinct advantage to patients with established CV disease risks, high lipid levels at baseline or high levels post-therapy with other PIs. Benign increase in indirect bilirubin may be bothersome to some pts.

FORMS

Brand name	Preparation	Mfr.	Route	Form	Strength	Cost (AWP)
Reyataz	Atazanavir	Bristol-Myers Squibb	PO	cap	200mg; 100mg; 150mg	$14.29; $14.29; $14.29

SELECTED READINGS

Murphy R, Pokrovsky V, Rozenbaum W, et al. Long-term efficacy and safety of atazanavir with stavudine and lamivudine in patients previously treated with nelfinavir or ATV: 180 weeks results of BMS study 008/044. 10th CROI, Boston, 2/03, Abstract 555

Squires K, Thiry A, Giordano M. Atazanavir (ATV) qd and efavirenz (EFV) qd with fixed dose ZDV-3TC. 42nd ICAAC, San Diego, 2002, Abstract H1076

ATOVAQUONE

FDA INDICATIONS

- Prevention of Pneumocystis jiroveci pneumonia (patients intolerant to TMP-SMX)
- Treatment of mild-to-moderate Pneumocystis jiroveci pneumonia.
- Prevention and treatment of malaria due to Plasmodium falciparum (including chloroquine-resistant strains) in adults and pediatric patients weighing 5-11 kg (in combination with proguanil [Malarone]) .

USUAL ADULT DOSING: PCP prophylaxis 750mg PO bid or 1500mg PO qd with food. P. falciparum treatment: Malarone 4 tabs/d (1000mg/400mg) x 3 d with food. Malaria prophylaxis: Malarone 1 tab (250mg/100 mg) qd with food (1-2d before and ending 1wk after travel).

Dosing Adjustments
GFR 50-80 mL/min: Usual dose
GFR 10-50 mL/min: Usual dose
GFR<10 mL/min: Usual dose
Hemodialysis: Usual dose
Peritoneal Dialysis: Usual dose

ADVERSE DRUG REACTIONS: Common: Rash; GI intolerance (diarrhea). **Rare:** Stevens-Johnson syndrome was reported with malarone (CID 2003;37:E5-7)

DRUG INTERACTIONS

Metoclopromide: may decrease atovaquone levels.
Rifampin and **rifabutin:** May decrease atovaquone serum level. Avoid co-administration.
Tetracyline: decreases atovaquone by 40%. Avoid co-administration.

PREGNANCY RISK: C-Not teratogenic in animal studies; no studies in humans.

BREAST FEEDING: No human data, breast milk excretion in animal studies.

ANTI-INFECTIVES

COMMENTS: High cost and GI distress make dapsone a better second line agent for PCP prophylaxis. Weekly mefloquine is more convenient, less expensive yet equivalent to daily atovaquone/proguanil for malaria prophylaxis. FDA approved for treatment of mild-to-moderately severe PCP, but generally not recommended since it is inferior to TMP/SMX. Must be taken with food for absorption.

FORMS

Brand name	Preparation	Mfr.	Route	Form	Strength	Cost (AWP)
Mepron	Atovaquone	GlaxoSmithKline	PO	susp	750mg/5mL	$18.54 per 5mL
Malarone	Atovaquone/ Chloro- quanide	GlaxoSmithKline	PO	tab	62.5mg/125mg; 250mg/100mg	$2; $5

SELECTED READINGS

Krause PJ, et al. Atovaquone and Azithromycin for the Treatment of Babesiosis. NEJM 2000;343:1454

Hughes W, Leoung G, Kramer F. Comparison of atovaquone (566C80) with trimethoprim-sulfamethoxazole to treat Pneumocystis carinii pneumonia in patients with AIDS. NEJM 1993; 329(16): 1207

Chirgwin K et al. Randomized Phase II Trial of Atovaquone with Pyrimethamine or Sulfadiazine for Treatment of Toxoplasmic Encephalitis in Patients with Acquired Immunodeficiency Syndrome: ACTG 237/ANRS 039 Study. Clin Infect Dis 2002;34:1243

ATOVAQUONE + PROGUANIL

FDA INDICATIONS

• P. falciparum malaria prophylaxis and treatment

USUAL ADULT DOSING: Treatment of acute malaria: atovaquone 1000mg/proguanil 400mg (4 tabs, single dose) qd x 3 d. Prevention of malaria: atovaquone 250mg/proguanil 100mg (1 tab) qd beginning 1-2d before travel and continuing for 1 wk after leaving endemic area.

Dosing Adjustments

GFR 50-80 mL/min: Usual dose

GFR<10 mL/min: No data: may need to be decreased.

Hemodialysis: No data: unlikely to be removed.

Peritoneal Dialysis: No data: unlikely to be removed.

↓ *Hepatic Function:* No data: may need to be decreased with severe hepatic dysfunction.

ADVERSE DRUG REACTIONS: Malarone side effect profile comparable to the placebo in studies. Abdominal pain, n/v/d, headache, asthenia, anorexia & dizziness can occur with treatment doses. Reversible elevation LFTs. Stevens-Johnson syndrome reported [CID 2003;37:E5].

DRUG INTERACTIONS

Atovaquone: Tetracycline (decreased atovaquone by 40%).

Metoclopramide: Decreased atovaquone level.

Proguanil component: No significant interactions noted.

Rifampin: Decreased atovaquone by 50%; rifabutin decreases atovaquopne by 34%.

PREGNANCY RISK: C- atovaquone not teratogenic in rat studies. Maternal and fetal toxicities (decreased fetal weight, early fetal resorption and post-implantation fetal loss) reported in rabbits. No human data. Proguanil: not teratogenic in rat studies. In a study of 200 pregnant Nigerian women in the first two trimesters, proguanil 100mg/day resulted in reduction of parasitemia from 35% to 2%, reduction of anemia from 18% to 3% and increases in mean birth weights by 132g. [Lancet 1990; 335(8680):45].

BREAST FEEDING: No data

COMMENTS: Malarone offers a well-tolerated alternative to mefloquine for the treatment and prevention of chloroquine-resistant P. falciparum. Disadvantages of Malarone include a higher price and the need for daily administration.

FORMS

Brand name	Preparation	Mfr.	Route	Form	Strength	Cost (AWP)
Malarone	atovaquone/ proguanil	Glaxo Wellcome	PO	tab	62.5mg/25mg; 250mg/100mg	$1.83; $4.94

SELECTED READINGS

Camus D, Djossou F, Schilthuis HJ et al. Atovaquone-proguanil versus chloroquine-proguanil for malaria prophylaxis in nonimmune pediatric travelers: results of an international, randomized, open-label study. Clin Infect Dis. 2004;38:1716-23

Borrmann S, Faucher JF, Bagaphou T et al. Atovaquone and proguanil versus amodiaquine for the treatment of Plasmodium falciparum malaria in African infants and young children. Clin Infect Dis. 2003;37:1441-7

Schlagenhauf P, Tschopp A, Johnson R, et al. Tolerability of malaria chemoprophylaxis in non-immune travellers to sub-Saharan Africa: multicentre, randomised, double blind, four arm study. BMJ. 2003;327 (7423):1078.

Petersen E. The safety of atovaquone/proguanil in long-term malaria prophylaxis of nonimmune adults. J Travel Med. 2003;10 Suppl 1:S13-5; discussion S21

van Vugt M, Leonardi E, Phaipun L et al. Treatment of uncomplicated multidrug-resistant falciparum malaria with artesunate-atovaquone-proguanil . Clin Infect Dis. 2002;35:1498-1504

AZITHROMYCIN

FDA INDICATIONS

- Acute bacterial exacerbations of chronic obstructive pulmonary disease (ZPAK and TRI-PAK).
- Pharyngitis/tonsillitis
- Uncomplicated Skin and skin structure infections
- Urethritis and cervicitis (GC and non-GC)
- Genital ulcer disease caused by H. ducreyi
- Community-acquired pneumonia
- Treatment and prophylaxis of disseminated M. avium infection (treatment requires co-administration with ethambutol)
- Acute otitis media
- PID (due to C. trachomatis)

USUAL ADULT DOSING: CAP: 500mg/d, then 250mg qd PO x 4d (ZPAK); 500mg IV qd. AECB: 500mg PO x 3d (TRI-PAK, only indication FDA approved). MAC prophylaxis: 1200mg PO q week. MAC Rx: 600mg PO qd + ethambutol 15mg/kg/d. Non-GC urethritis/cervicitis: 1g PO x 1.

Dosing Adjustments

GFR 50-80 mL/min: Usual dose

GFR 10-50 mL/min: No data, but usual dose likely due to high biliary excretion.

GFR<10 mL/min: No data, but usual dose likely due to high biliary excretion.

Hemodialysis: No data, usual dose likely.

Peritoneal Dialysis: Usual regimen

↓ *Hepatic Function:* No dose adjustment [Mazzei. JAC 1993; 31(Suppl E): 57]

ADVERSE DRUG REACTIONS: Occasional: GI intolerance (in 4% of patients, but better tolerated than erythromycin); diarrhea, nausea, abdominal pain; vaginitis; reversible hearing loss in 5% of pts with mean exposure of 59g.

DRUG INTERACTIONS

Cyclosporin: Azithromycin may (in one case report) interfere with the metabolism of cyclosporin therefore increasing the level of cyclosporin. Increase in cyclosporin level may increase risk nephrotoxicity and neurotoxicity. With concurrent administration, close monitoring of cyclosporin level is indicated with dose adjustment when needed. Azithromycin did not affect cyclosporin levels in a report involving 6 patients. (Nephron 1996:73:724).

Pimozide: Possible increased in pimozide concentration, which may result in QT prolongation and cardiac arrhythmia. Contraindicated by manufacturer. Do not co-administer.

PREGNANCY RISK: B - animal studies show no harm to the fetus. No human data available

BREAST FEEDING: Accumulates in breast milk. The American Academy of Pediatrics considers erythromycin compatible with breast feeding.

COMMENTS: An oral and parenteral macrolide with convenient once daily dosing (half-life of 68 hrs). Expanded spectrum includes improved activity against H. influenzae compared to erythromycin. In contrast to other macrolides, azithromycin is not likely to interact with drugs metabolized by CYP3A4.

FORMS

Brand name	Preparation	Mfr.	Route	Form	Strength	Cost (AWP)
Zithromax	Azithromycin	Pfizer	IV	vial	500mg	$29.46
			PO	pwdr packet	1g	$25.79
			PO	susp	100mg/5mL; 200mg/5mL	$11.72 per 5mL; $11.72 per 5mL
			PO	tab	250mg; 500mg; 600mg	$8.30; $16.61; $19.93
			PO	TRI-PAK	500mg x 3 tabs	$49.83 per pack
			PO	ZPAK	250mg x 6 tabs	$49.80 per pack

SELECTED READINGS

Stamm WE, Hicks CB, Martin DH, et al. Azithromycin for empirical treatment of the nongonococcal urethritis syndrome in men. A randomized double-blind study . JAMA 1995 Aug 16;274(7):545-9

Martin DH, Sargent SJ, Wendel GD Jr, et al. Comparison of azithromycin and ceftriaxone for the treatment of chancroid. Clin Infect Dis. 1995 Aug;21(2):409-14

Luft BJ; Dattwyler RJ; Johnson RC, et al. Azithromycin compared with amoxicillin in the treatment of erythema migrans. A double-blind, randomized, controlled trial. Ann Intern Med. 1996 May 1;124 (9):785-91

Kinasewitz G, Wood RG, et al. Azithromycin versus cefaclor in the treatment of acute bacterial pneumonia . Eur J Clin Microbiol Infect Dis 1991 Oct;10(10):872-7

Hoepelman IM; Mollers MJ; van Schie MH, et al. A short (3-day) course of azithromycin tablets versus a 10-day course of amoxycillin-clavulanic acid (co-amoxiclav) in the treatment of adults with lower respiratory tract infections. Int J Antimicrob Agents 1997 Jan;9(3):141-6

AZTREONAM

FDA INDICATIONS

- Gram-negative bacterial pneumonia
- Skin and soft tissue infections

- Complicated and uncomplicated urinary tract infections
- Intra-abdominal infections (in combination with clindamycin)
- Septicemia
- Gynecologic infections

USUAL ADULT DOSING: Gram-negative infections: 1-2g IV q8h. UTI: 0.5-1g IV q12h-q8h. Serious infections and meningitis: 2.0g IV q8-6h.

Dosing Adjustments
GFR 50-80 mL/min: 1g-2g q8-12h
GFR 10-50 mL/min: 1g-2g q12-18h
GFR<10 mL/min: 1g-2g q24h.
Hemodialysis: 250mg post-dialysis
Peritoneal Dialysis: 1-2g loading dose, then 250-500mg q8h. May be given intraperitoneal: loading dose of 1g, then 250mg per liter exchange.
↓ *Hepatic Function:* Some recommend dose reduction of 20-25%

ADVERSE DRUG REACTIONS: Frequent: LFTs elevation; transient eosinophilia (can be used in PCN allergic patients). **Occasional:** Phlebitis at infusion site; rash; diarrhea; nausea

DRUG INTERACTIONS
No significant interactions noted.

PREGNANCY RISK: B-animal studies show no harm to the fetus. No human data available.

BREAST FEEDING: Excreted in breast milk at low concentration. The American Academy of Pediatrics considers aztreonam to be compatible with breast feeding.

COMMENTS: A parenteral monobactam for infections caused by gram-negative bacteria that can be used in penicillin-allergic patients. Isolated cross-reactivity described in ceftazidime-allergic patients. Spectrum of activity includes Pseudomonas but no reliable activity against gram-positive bacteria or anaerobes.

FORMS

Brand name	Preparation	Mfr.	Route	Form	Strength	Cost (AWP)
Azactam	Aztreonam	Elan	IV	vial	500mg; 1000mg; 2000mg	$12.55; $25.18; $50.44

SELECTED READINGS

Murase T. Aztreonam or gentamicin combined with piperacillin as empiric antibiotic therapy during neutropenia of patients with hematologic diseases . Kansenshogaku Zasshi 1992 Feb;66(2):121-6

Conrad DA; Williams RR; Couchman TL; et al. Efficacy of aztreonam in the treatment of skeletal infections due to Pseudomonas aeruginosa. Rev Infect Dis 1991 May-Jun;13 Suppl 7:S634-9

Bosso JA; Black PG. Controlled trial of aztreonam vs. tobramycin and azlocillin for acute pulmonary exacerbations of cystic fibrosis. Pediatr Infect Dis J 1988 Mar;7(3):171-6

BACITRACIN

FDA INDICATIONS
- Prevention of infection in minor cuts, scrapes, and burns.

USUAL ADULT DOSING: 10,000-25,000 units IM q6h (painful injection); 25,000 units PO q6h (C. difficile colitis), topical administration to affected area 1-5 times/day.

Dosing Adjustments
GFR 50-80 mL/min: avoid systemic use
GFR 10-50 mL/min: avoid systemic use

GFR<10 mL/min: avoid systemic use.

ADVERSE DRUG REACTIONS: Frequent: Nephrotoxicity with IM use (proteinuria; oliguria; azotemia); pain with IM use

DRUG INTERACTIONS

Nondepolarizing muscle relaxants (atracurium, vecuronium, pancuronium, tubocurarine): Neuromuscular blockade may be enhanced with IM use. Avoid co-administration, if concurrent administration is needed titrate the nondepolarizing muscle relaxant slowly and monitor neuromuscular function closely.

PREGNANCY RISK: C-One report listed 18 patients exposed to bacitracin (route was not specified) during the first trimester; there was no association with malformation found.

BREAST FEEDING: No data available

COMMENTS: Bacitracin 25,000 units q6h is a cost-effective alternative to oral vancomycin or metronidazole in the treatment of C. difficile, but has not been as well studied as either drug. Often used for topical therapy of wounds, but most authorities are unconvinced that topical antibiotics have established merit in promoting wound healing, preventing infection or treating infection.

FORMS (◆ DENOTES AVAILABLE GENERICALLY)

Brand name	Preparation	Mfr.	Route	Form	Strength	Cost (AWP)
Bacitracin	Bacitracin	◆ Pharmacia	IM	vial	50,000U	$11.40
Bacitracin	Bacitracin	◆ Fougera	oph-thalmic	oint	500U/g	$4.75 per 3.5g
			topical	oint	500U/g	$2.90 per 15g; $4.24 per 30g

SELECTED READINGS

Leyden JJ; Bartelt NM. Oral bacitracin vs vancomycin therapy for Clostridium difficile-induced diarrhea. A randomized double-blind trial. Arch Intern Med 1986 Jun;146(6):1101-4

Dudley MN; McLaughlin JC; Carrington G et al. Oral bacitracin vs vancomycin therapy for Clostridium difficile-induced diarrhea. A randomized double-blind trial. Arch Intern Med 1986 Jun;146(6):1101-4

Leyden JJ; Bartelt NM. Comparison of topical antibiotic ointments, a wound protectant, and antiseptics for the treatment of human blister wounds contaminated with Staphylococcus aureus. J Fam Pract 1987 Jun;24(6):601-4

CARBENICILLIN INDANYL SODIUM

FDA INDICATIONS
- Upper and lower UTI caused by Enterobacter, Escherichia coli, Proteus (indole positive infections), P. aeruginosa
- Prostatitis

USUAL ADULT DOSING: Uncomplicated UTI: 382-764mg PO q6h

Dosing Adjustments
GFR 50-80 mL/min: Usual dose
GFR 10-50 mL/min: 0.5g-1g q8h
GFR<10 mL/min: Avoid use
Hemodialysis: 0.75-2g post-dialysis
Peritoneal Dialysis: 2g q 6-12h
↓ *Hepatic Function:* Maximum dose is 2g/day for patients with severe h

ADVERSE DRUG REACTIONS: **Frequent:** Hypersensitivity reactions; rash. **Occasional:** GI intolerance; drug fever; Coombs' test positive, hemolytic anemia; phlebitis at infusion sites and sterile abscesses at IM sites; Jarisch-Herxheimer reaction

DRUG INTERACTIONS

Tetracyclines: In vitro antagonism when co-administered. Bactericidal effect of penicillins may be diminished in vivo. Avoid concurrent administration. In two studies involving a total of 79 patients with pneumococcal meningitis treated with either penicillin plus tetracyclines or penicillin monotherapy there was a higher mortality rate (79-85%) in the combination therapy compared to penicillin monotherapy (30-33%). (Arch Intern Med 1951:88:489, Ann Intern Med 1961; 55:545). However there was not a difference in mortality between penicillin monotherapy and penicillin plus tetracycline in the treatment of pneumococcal pneumonia. (Arch Intern Med 1953; 91:197).

Warfarin: Carbenicillin-induced inhibition of ADP-mediated platelet aggregation in addition to warfarin-induced hypoprothrombinemia may prolong bleeding time. Monitor INR closely and adjust warfarin dose accordingly.

PREGNANCY RISK: B-Several collaborative perinatal project reports involving over 12,000 exposures to penicillin derivatives during the first trimester indicated no association between penicillin derivative drugs and birth defects.

BREAST FEEDING: Excreted in breast milk at low concentrations.

COMMENTS: Oral betalactam that should be restricted to uncomplicated urinary tract infections including those caused by Pseudomonas and proteus. Use is largely supplanted by fluoroquinolones. Sodium content is 5-6 meq per gram.

FORMS

Brand name	Preparation	Mfr.	Route	Form	Strength	Cost (AWP)
Geocillin	Carbenicillin indanyl sodium	Pfizer	PO	tab	382mg	$2.53

CASPOFUNGIN ACETATE

FDA INDICATIONS

- Invasive aspergillosis in patients who are refractory or intolerant to other anti-fungal therapy.
- Candidemia and the following Candida infections: intra-abdominal abscesses, peritonitis and pleural space infections.
- Esophageal candidiasis (author's opinion: would reserve caspofungin for azole-resistant cases)
- Empiric treatment of presumed fungal infections in febrile neutropenic patients

USUAL ADULT DOSING: 70mg IV load on day 1, then 50mg IV qd (infuse over 1 hour). Dosing for Child-Pugh score of 7-9, after initial 70mg load on day 1, decrease daily dose to 35mg qd.

Dosing Adjustments

GFR 50-80 mL/min: Usual dose

GFR 10-50 mL/min: Usual dose

GFR<10 mL/min: Usual dose

Hemodialysis: Not dialyzable, thus no supplemental doses needed post dialysis. Usual dose.

Peritoneal Dialysis: No data, usual dose likely

↓ *Hepatic Function:* For Child-Pugh score of 7-9, after initial 70mg load on day 1, decrease daily dose to 35mg qd.

Adverse Drug Reactions: Generally well tolerated. **Occasional:** Histamine-mediated sx including rash, facial swelling, pruritus & sensation of warmth (consider antihistamine). **Rare:** Fever, phlebitis, nausea, vomiting, headache, eosinophilia, proteinuria, increased alk phos & hypokalemia.

Drug Interactions

Cyclosporin: Increased caspofugin AUC by 35%. Co-administration not recommended, close monitoring of liver enzyme recommended with co-administration.
Tacrolimus: AUC decreased by 20% with caspofugin co-administration. Monitor tacrolimus levels closely.

Pregnancy Risk: C No human data. Animal data with exposure similar to a 70mg-dose in human resulted in incomplete ossification of skull, torso, cervical ribs and talus/calcaneous.

Breast Feeding: No data

Comments: Caspofungin offers clinicians an alternative to voriconazole and liposomal amphotericin for the treatment of invasive aspergillosis that is refractory or intolerant to first line therapy. It has established efficacy as an alternative to amphotericin for Candida esophagitis and invasive candidiasis, but must be given IV--is clearly second line to (oral) azoles for most candida infections.

Forms

Brand name	Preparation	Mfr.	Route	Form	Strength	Cost (AWP)
Cancidas	Caspofungin Acetate	Merck	IV	vial	50mg; 70mg	$395.36 ; $509.33

Selected Readings

Walsh TJ, Teppler H, Donowitz GR et al. Caspofungin versus liposomal amphotericin B for empirical antifungal therapy in patients with persistent fever and neutropenia . N Engl J Med. 2004;351(14):1391-402

Mora-Duarte J et al. Comparison of caspofungin and amphotericin B for invasive candidiasis . N Engl J Med 2002;347:2020

CEFACLOR

FDA Indications

- Skin and skin-structure infections (impetigo, cellulitis, pyoderma, skin ulcers)
- Streptococcal tonsillitis
- Upper respiratory tract infections (otitis media, pharyngitis)
- Lower respiratory tract infections
- Urinary tract infections (cystitis, pyelonephritis)

Usual Adult Dosing: 250-500mg PO q6-8h (regular release); 375mg or 500mg PO q12h with food (sustained release).

Dosing Adjustments
GFR 50-80 mL/min: Usual dose
GFR 10-50 mL/min: Usual dose
GFR<10 mL/min: Usual dose
Hemodialysis: 500mg post-dialysis
Peritoneal Dialysis: Usual regimen

Adverse Drug Reactions: Occasional: Allergic reactions; diarrhea and C. difficile colitis; eosinophilia; positive Coombs' test. **Rare:** Anaphylaxis rare; hemolytic anemia; serum sickness (0.1-0.5%)

DRUG INTERACTIONS

Probenecid: Increase in cephalosporin serum concentration due to inhibition of tubular secretion by probenecid. Monitor for potential cephalosporin toxicity, interaction may be beneficial if high serum concentration is desired.

PREGNANCY RISK: B-Cephalosporins are usually considered safe to use during pregnancy.

BREAST FEEDING: Excreted in breast milk at low concentrations. The American Academy of Pediatrics classifies cephalosporin antibiotics as compatible with breast feeding.

COMMENTS: Oral 2nd generation cephalosporin that has poor activity against S. pneumoniae, and therefore is not an ideal agent in the treatment of respiratory tract infections. This drug is a favorite for pediatricians because it wins the taste test. Higher rate of serum sickness reported compared to the other cephalosporins. Cefaclor CD should be taken with food.

FORMS (◆ DENOTES AVAILABLE GENERICALLY)

Brand name	Preparation	Mfr.	Route	Form	Strength	Cost (AWP)
Ceclor	Cefaclor	◆ Eli Lilly	PO	pulvules	250mg; 500mg	$2.33; $4.65
			PO	susp	125mg/5mL; 187mg/5mL; 250mg/5mL; 375mg/5mL	$1.04 per 5mL; $1.56 per 5mL; $1.88 per 5mL; $2.82 per 5mL
Raniclor	cefaclor	Ranbaxy	PO	tab, chew-able	125mg; 187mg; 250mg; 375mg	$1; $1.60; $1.90; $2.90

CEFADROXIL

FDA INDICATIONS

- Streptococcal pharyngitis and tonsillitis.
- Skin and soft tissue infections
- Urinary tract infections

USUAL ADULT DOSING: Soft tissue infection: 0.5g PO bid or 1g PO qd. Pharyngitis: 0.5g PO bid or 1g PO qd x 10 days. UTI: 1g PO qd or 1g PO bid.

Dosing Adjustments
GFR 50-80 mL/min: Usual dose
GFR 10-50 mL/min: 0.5g q12-24h
GFR<10 mL/min: 0.5g q36h
Hemodialysis: 0.5-1.0g post-dialysis
Peritoneal Dialysis: 0.5g/day

ADVERSE DRUG REACTIONS: Occasional: Allergic reactions (anaphylaxis rare); diarrhea and C. difficile colitis; eosinophilia; positive Coombs' test

DRUG INTERACTIONS

Probenecid: Increase in cephalosporin serum concentration due to inhibition of tubular secretion by probenecid. Monitor for potential cephalosporin toxicity, interaction may be beneficial if high serum concentration is desired.

PREGNANCY RISK: B-Cephalosporins are usually considered safe to use during pregnancy.

BREAST FEEDING: Excreted in breast milk at low concentrations. The American Academy of Pediatrics classifies cephalosporin antibiotics as compatible with breast feeding.

COMMENTS: Oral 1st generation cephalosporin with good oral bioavailability and long half-life allowing for once or twice a day dosing, but more expensive than comparable agents (i.e., cephalexin)

FORMS (◆ DENOTES AVAILABLE GENERICALLY)

Brand name	Preparation	Mfr.	Route	Form	Strength	Cost (AWP)
Duricef	Cefadroxil	◆ Warner Chilcott Labs	PO	cap	500mg	$9.48
			PO	susp	250mg; 500mg/5mL	$3.38 per 5mL; $4.68 per 5mL
			PO	tab	1000mg	$17.84

SELECTED READINGS

Bucko AD, Hunt BJ, Kidd SL et al. Randomized, double-blind, multicenter comparison of oral cefditoren 200 or 400mg BID with either cefuroxime 250mg BID or cefadroxil 500mg BID for the treatment of uncomplicated Skin and skin-structure infections. Clin Ther. 2002;24(7):1134-47.

CEFAMANDOLE

FDA INDICATIONS

- Bone and joint infections
- Lower respiratory infections
- Peritonitis
- Pneumonia
- Surgical prophylaxis
- Urinary tract infections

USUAL ADULT DOSING: 0.5-3.0g IM or IV q4-6h (up to 12g per day)

Dosing Adjustments
GFR 50-80 mL/min: 0.5g-2.0g q6h
GFR 10-50 mL/min: 1g-2g q8h
GFR<10 mL/min: 0.5g-0.75g q12h
Hemodialysis: 1-2g post-dialysis
Peritoneal Dialysis: 0.5-1.0g q12h

ADVERSE DRUG REACTIONS: Frequent: Phlebitis at infusion sites. **Occasional:** Allergic reactions (anaphylaxis rare); hypoprothrombinemia; diarrhea and C. difficile colitis; eosinophilia; positive Coombs' test

DRUG INTERACTIONS

Ethanol: Methyltetrazolethiol moiety inhibits aldehyde dehydrogenase resulting in acetaldehyde accumulation and disulfiram-like reactions. Avoid ethanol consumption while on cephalosporins with the methyltetrazolethiol moiety.

Probenecid: Increase in cephalosporin serum concentration due to inhibition of tubular secretion by probenecid. Monitor for potential cephalosporin toxicity, interaction may be beneficial if high serum concentration is desired.

Warfarin: Warfarin anticoagulation effect may be enhanced. Monitor INR closely and adjust warfarin dose accordingly.

PREGNANCY RISK: B-Cephalosporins are usually considered safe to use during pregnancy.

BREAST FEEDING: Excreted in breast milk at low concentrations. The American Academy of Pediatrics classifies cephalosporin antibiotics as compatible with breast feeding.

COMMENTS: Parenteral second-generation cephalosporin with broad activity against most common respiratory pathogens. Contains the N-methylthiotetrazole (NMTT) side chain, may result in prolongation of prothrombin time and disulfiram-like reaction. Alternative second-generation cephalosporins with a more favorable safety profile are often preferred.

FORMS

Brand name	Preparation	Mfr.	Route	Form	Strength	Cost (AWP)
Mandol	Cefamandole	Eli Lilly	IV	vial	1g ; 2g	$9.06; $18.13

CEFAZOLIN

FDA INDICATIONS

- Bacterial infections
- Staphylococcal endocarditis
- Pneumococcal pneumonia
- Surgical prophylaxis (i.e., thoracic, appendectomy)
- Respiratory infections
- Skin infections (staphylococcal and streptococcal)
- Traumatic wound
- Urinary tract infections

USUAL ADULT DOSING: 0.5-2.0g IV q6-8h

Dosing Adjustments

GFR 50-80 mL/min: 0.5g-1.5g q8h

GFR 10-50 mL/min: 0.5g-1.0g q8-12h

GFR<10 mL/min: 0.25g-0.75g q18-24h

Hemodialysis: HD: 1.0g post dialysis [Fogel MA et al. Am J Kidney Dis. 1998;32:401]

Peritoneal Dialysis: 0.5g q12h

↓ *Hepatic Function:* No data. Usual dose likely.

ADVERSE DRUG REACTIONS: **Frequent:** Minimal phlebitis at infusion sites. **Occasional:** Allergic reactions (anaphylaxis rare); diarrhea and C. difficile colitis; eosinophilia; positive Coombs' test

DRUG INTERACTIONS

Probenecid: Increase in cephalosporin serum concentration due to inhibition of tubular secretion by probenecid. Monitor for potential cephalosporin toxicity, interaction may be beneficial if high serum concentration is desired.

Warfarin: Warfarin anticoagulation effect may be enhanced. Monitor INR closely and adjust warfarin dose accordingly.

PREGNANCY RISK: B-cephalosporins are usually considered safe to use during pregnancy.

BREAST FEEDING: Excreted in breast milk at low concentrations. The American Academy of Pediatrics classifies cephalosporin antibiotics as compatible with breast feeding.

COMMENTS: Parenteral first-generation cephalosporin with relatively long half-life that can be given IV or IM. This is the preferred cephalosporin for meth-sensitive S. aureus and for many forms of surgical prophylaxis with the exception of colorectal procedures.

FORMS (◆ DENOTES AVAILABLE GENERICALLY)

Brand name	Preparation	Mfr.	Route	Form	Strength	Cost (AWP)
Ancef	Cefazolin	◆ Abbott	IV or IM	vial	1g; 10g	$5.59; $43.83 per vial

SELECTED READINGS

Bratzler DW et al. Antimicrobial prophylaxis for surgery: an advisory statement from the National Surgical Infection Prevention Project. Clin Infect Dis. 2004 Jun 15;38:1706-15

CEFDINIR

FDA INDICATIONS
- Upper respiratory tract infections (otitis media, acute sinusitis, chronic sinusitis, chronic bronchitis, pharyngitis, tonsillitis)
- Community-acquired pneumonia (CAP)
- Skin and skin structure infections

USUAL ADULT DOSING: CAP and soft tissue infections: 300mg PO bid. Upper respiratory tract infections: 300mg PO bid or 600mg PO qd

Dosing Adjustments
Hemodialysis: Remove in dialysis; dose after dialysis.

ADVERSE DRUG REACTIONS: Occasional: Allergic reactions (anaphylaxis rare); diarrhea; C. difficile colitis; eosinophilia; positive Coombs' test

DRUG INTERACTIONS

Probenecid: Increase in cephalosporin serum concentration due to inhibition of tubular secretion by probenecid. Monitor for potential cephalosporin toxicity, interaction may be beneficial if high serum concentration is desired.

PREGNANCY RISK: B-Cephalosporins are usually considered safe to use during pregnancy.

BREAST FEEDING: Excreted in breast milk at low concentrations. The American Academy of Pediatrics classifies cephalosporin antibiotics as compatible with breast feeding.

COMMENTS: Oral 3rd generation cephalosporin that has activity against many gram-negative organisms, but not active against Enterobacter and Pseudomonas. Activity against gram-positive bacteria is good and is similar to cefpodoxime, which includes relatively good activity against S. pneumoniae.

FORMS

Brand name	Preparation	Mfr.	Route	Form	Strength	Cost (AWP)
Omnicef	Cefdinir	Abbott	PO	susp	125mg/5mL ; 250mg/5mL	$3.75 per 5mL; $7.32 per 5mL
			PO	tab	300mg	$4.75

SELECTED READINGS

Drehobl M, Bianchi P, Keyserling CH et al. Comparison of cefdinir and cefaclor in treatment of community-acquired pneumonia. Antimicrob Agents Chemother. 1997;41:1579-83.

Tack KJ, Littlejohn TW, Mailloux G et al. Cefdinir versus cephalexin for the treatment of Skin and skin-structure infections. The Cefdinir Adult Skin Infection Study Group. Clin Ther. 1998;20(2):244-56.

CEFDITOREN

FDA INDICATIONS
- Acute bacterial exacerbations of chronic bronchitis
- Pharyngitis/tonsillitis
- Uncomplicated skin and skin-structure infections
- Community-acquired pneumonia

USUAL ADULT DOSING: Uncomplicated soft tissue infection: 200mg PO bid. Community-acquired pneumonia, pharyngitis, and tonsillitis: 400mg PO bid x10-14d.

Dosing Adjustments
GFR 50-80 mL/min: Usual dose

GFR 10-50 mL/min: 200mg bid (max)

GFR<10 mL/min: <30mL/min=200mg qd

Hemodialysis: 200mg PO qd, dose post-HD on days of HD (30% removed in HD)

↓ *Hepatic Function:* Usual dose

ADVERSE DRUG REACTIONS: Common: Nausea, abdominal pain, and diarrhea. LFT and alkaline phosphatase elevation. **Occasional:** Rash and mild eosinophilia; C. difficile colitis. **Rare:** Anaphylaxis; carnitine deficiency with prolonged therapy (monitor for muscle weakness)

DRUG INTERACTIONS

Antacid and **H2 receptor blocker:** Do not co-administer. Serum concentration of cefditoren decreased.

Probenecid: Serum concentration of cefditoren increased.

PREGNANCY RISK: B Not teratogenic in animal studies. No human data.

BREAST FEEDING: Excreted in breast milk. Use with caution.

COMMENTS: Oral third-generation cephalosporin with spectrum of activity similar to cefpodoxime and cefdinir that includes good activity against S. pneumoniae, H. influenzae and M. catarrhalis. A short half-life makes a twice-a-day dosing a concern for severe infections.

FORMS

Brand name	Preparation	Mfr.	Route	Form	Strength	Cost (AWP)
Spectracef	Cefditoren pivoxil	Purdue Pharma	PO	cap	200mg	$2.08

SELECTED READINGS

Roux JL, Fata L, Palo W et al. Cefditoren is Effective Treatment for Community-Acquired Pneumonia in Adults. ICCAC 2001, poster 852

Bucko AD, Hunt BJ, Kidd SL et al. Randomized, double-blind, multicenter comparison of oral cefditoren 200 or 400mg BID with either cefuroxime 250mg BID or cefadroxil 500mg BID for the treatment of uncomplicated skin and skin-structure infections. Clin Ther. 2002;24(7):1134-47.

CEFEPIME

FDA INDICATIONS

- Pneumonia (nosocomial)
- Cellulitis
- Febrile neutropenia, empiric therapy
- Intra-abdominal infections
- Bronchitis
- Skin and skin structure infections
- Uncomplicated and complicated urinary tract infections (pyelonephritis)

USUAL ADULT DOSING: 1-2g IV q12h. Pseudomonas and/or CNS infections: 1-2g q8h. Mild to moderate UTI: 0.5-1g IV or IM q12h.

Dosing Adjustments

GFR 50-80 mL/min: 0.5g-2g q24h

GFR 10-50 mL/min: 0.5g-1.0g q24h

GFR<10 mL/min: 0.25g-0.5g q24h

Hemodialysis: 1-2g post-dialysis

Peritoneal Dialysis: 1-2g q48h

ANTI-INFECTIVES

ADVERSE DRUG REACTIONS: **Frequent:** Phlebitis at infusion sites. **Occasional:** Antibiotic-associated diarrhea. **Rare:** Encephalopathy, myoclonus, and seizure; allergic reaction; fever.

DRUG INTERACTIONS

Probenecid: Increase in cephalosporin serum concentration due to inhibition of tubular secretion by probenecid. Monitor for potential cephalosporin toxicity, interaction may be beneficial if high serum concentration is desired.

PREGNANCY RISK: B-Cephalosporins are usually considered safe to use during pregnancy.

BREAST FEEDING: Excreted in breast milk at low concentrations. The American Academy of Pediatrics classifies cephalosporin antibiotics as compatible with breast feeding.

COMMENTS: Parenteral 4th generation cephalosporin with activity against P. aeruginosa comparable to ceftazidime and activity against GPC comparable to cefotaxime. Resistant to hydrolysis by many expanded spectrum beta-lactamases (ESBLs).

FORMS

Brand name	Preparation	Mfr.	Route	Form	Strength	Cost (AWP)
Maxipime	Cefepime	Elan	IV	vial	1000mg; 2000mg; 500mg	$20.88; $40.06; $9.78

SELECTED READINGS

Wang FD; Liu CY; Hsu HC; et al. A comparative study of cefepime versus ceftazidime as empiric therapy of febrile episodes in neutropenic patients. Chemotherapy. 1999 Sep-Oct;45(5):370-9.

Saez-Llorens X; Castano E; Garcia R; et al. Prospective randomized comparison of cefepime and cefotaxime for treatment of bacterial meningitis in infants and children. Antimicrob Agents Chemother 1995 Apr;39(4):937-40

Hoepelman AI; Kieft H; Aoun M; et al. International comparative study of cefepime and ceftazidime in the treatment of serious bacterial infections. J Antimicrob Chemother 1993 Nov;32 Suppl B:175-86

ATS and IDSA. Guidelines for the Management of Adults with Hospital-acquired, Ventilator-associated, and Healthcare-associated Pneumonia . Am J Respir Crit Care Med 2005;171:388

CEFIXIME

FDA INDICATIONS

- Uncomplicated Gonococcal infection
- Otitis media
- Respiratory tract infections (sinusitis and AECB)
- Urinary tract infections (cystitis)

USUAL ADULT DOSING: 400mg PO qd. Uncomplicated GC: 400mg PO x 1.

Dosing Adjustments
GFR 50-80 mL/min: Usual dose
GFR 10-50 mL/min: 300mg/day
GFR<10 mL/min: 200mg/day
Hemodialysis: 300 mg/day
Peritoneal Dialysis: 200 mg/day

ADVERSE DRUG REACTIONS: **Frequent:** Diarrhea and nausea. **Occasional:** Allergic reactions; C.difficile colitis; eosinophilia; positive Coombs' test. **Rare:** Anaphylaxis.

DRUG INTERACTIONS

Probenecid: Increase in cephalosporin serum concentration due to inhibition of tubular secretion by probenecid. Monitor for potential cephalosporin toxicity, interaction may be beneficial if high serum concentration is desired.

PREGNANCY RISK: B-Cephalosporins are usually considered safe to use during pregnancy.

BREAST FEEDING: Excreted in breast milk at low concentrations. The American Academy of Pediatrics classifies cephalosporin antibiotics as compatible with breast feeding.

COMMENTS: Oral thrid-generation cephalosporin. Poor activity vs S. aureus and S. pneumoniae, therefore a poor agent for empiric use in respiratory tract infection. First line oral agent for uncomplicated GC.

FORMS

Brand name	Preparation	Mfr.	Route	Form	Strength	Cost (AWP)
Suprax	Cefixime	Lupin	PO	susp	100mg/5mL	$4.54 per 5mL

SELECTED READINGS

Kiani R; Johnson D; Nelson B. Comparative, multicenter studies of cefixime and amoxicillin in the treatment of respiratory tract infections. Am J Med 1988 Sep 16;85(3A):6-13

Raz R; Rottensterich E; Leshem Y et al. Double-blind study comparing 3-day regimens of cefixime and ofloxacin in treatment of uncomplicated urinary tract infections in women. Antimicrob Agents Chemother 1994 May;38(5):1176-7

Portilla I; Lutz B; Montalvo M et al. Oral cefixime versus intramuscular ceftriaxone in patients with uncomplicated gonococcal infections. Sex Transm Dis 1992 Mar-Apr; 19(2):94-8

CEFOTAXIME

FDA INDICATIONS

- Bacteremia
- Bone and joint infections
- Central nervous system infections (ventriculitis, meningitis)
- Genitourinary infections
- Gynecologic infection (endometritis, pelvic cellulitis, pelvic inflammatory disease)
- Intra-abdominal infections
- Lower respiratory tract infections (pneumonia)
- Peritonitis
- Septicemia
- Skin and skin structure infections

USUAL ADULT DOSING: Moderate to severe infections: 1-2g IV q8h. Meningitis: 2g IV q4-6h. GC (urethritis and cervicitis): 500mg x 1. GC (rectal) 1g x1.

Dosing Adjustments

GFR 50-80 mL/min: Usual dose
GFR 10-50 mL/min: 1g-2g q6-12h
GFR<10 mL/min: 1g-2g q12h
Hemodialysis: 1-2g qd plus 1g post dialysis
Peritoneal Dialysis: 0.5-2g qd

ADVERSE DRUG REACTIONS: Frequent: Phlebitis at infusion sites. **Occasional:** Allergic reactions; diarrhea and C.difficile colitis; eosinophilia; positive Coombs' test. **Rare:** Anaphylaxis; hemolytic anemia.

DRUG INTERACTIONS

Probenecid: Increase in cephalosporin serum concentration due to inhibition of tubular secretion by probenecid. Monitor for potential cephalosporin toxicity, interaction may be beneficial if high serum concentration is desired.

PREGNANCY RISK: B-Cephalosporins are usually considered safe to use during pregnancy.

BREAST FEEDING: Excreted in breast milk at low concentrations. The American Academy of Pediatrics classifies cephalosporin antibiotics as compatible with breast feeding.

COMMENTS: A parenteral 3rd generation cephalosporin with reliable CNS penetration when dosed at 2g IV q4h. Cefotaxime and ceftriaxone are the preferred parenteral cephalosporins for serious pneumococcal infections, but 3-5% of strains are resistant. Although less convenient dosing schedule, cefotaxime is therapeutically equivalent to ceftriaxone usually with a lower cost.

FORMS

Brand name	Preparation	Mfr.	Route	Form	Strength	Cost (AWP)
Claforan	Cefotaxime	Abbott	IV	vial	500mg; 1000mg; 2000mg; 10g	$8.62; $13.26; $24.18; $188.66
Claforan	Cefotaxime	Abbott	IV	vial	1g/50mL; 2g/50mL	$12.76; $21.42 per vial

SELECTED READINGS

Garber GE; Auger P; Chan RM; Conly JM; Shafran SD; Gerson M. A multicenter, open comparative study of parenteral cefotaxime and ceftriaxone in the treatment of nosocomial lower respiratory tract infections. Diagn Microbiol Infect Dis 1992 Jan;15(1):85-8

Peltola H; Anttila M; Renkonen OV. Randomised comparison of chloramphenicol, ampicillin, cefotaxime, and ceftriaxone for childhood bacterial meningitis. Lancet 1989 Jun 10;1(8650):1281-1287

Pfister HW; Preac-Mursic V; Wilske B; Schielke E; Sorgel F; Einhaupl. Randomized comparison of ceftriaxone and cefotaxime in Lyme neuroborreliosis. J Infect Dis 1991 Feb;163(2):311-8

CEFOTETAN

FDA INDICATIONS

- Bone/joint infections
- Surgical prophylaxis: C-section, abd & vaginal hysterectomy, transurethral, biliary tract and GI surgery.
- Endometritis
- Gynecologic infections
- Intra-abdominal infections
- Intrapelvic cellulitis
- Parametritis
- Skin and skin structure infections
- Lower respiratory tract infections
- UTIs

USUAL ADULT DOSING: UTI: 0.5g to 1g IV or IM q12h. Mild to moderate infections: 1g IV q12h. Severe infections: 2-3g IV q12h (max 6g/24hrs).

Dosing Adjustments

GFR 50-80 mL/min: Usual dose

GFR 10-50 mL/min: 1g-2g q24h

GFR<10 mL/min: 1g-2g q48h

Hemodialysis: .5-1g qd plus 1g post dialysis

Peritoneal Dialysis: 1g qd

ADVERSE DRUG REACTIONS: Frequent: Phlebitis at infusion sites. **Occasional:** Allergic reactions; hypoprothrombinemia; diarrhea and C. difficile colitis; eosinophilia; positive Coombs' test. **Rare:** Anaphylaxis; hemolytic anemia.

DRUG INTERACTIONS

Ethanol: Methyltetrazolethiol moiety inhibits aldehyde dehydrogenase resulting in acetaldehyde accumulation and disulfiram-like reactions. Avoid ethanol consumption while on cephalosporins with the methyltetrazolethiol moiety.

Probenecid: Increase in cephalosporin serum concentration due to inhibition of tubular secretion by probenecid. Monitor for potential cephalosporin toxicity, interaction may be beneficial if high serum concentration is desired.

Warfarin: Warfarin anticoagulation effect may be enhanced. Monitor INR closely and adjust warfarin dose accordingly.

PREGNANCY RISK: B-Cephalosporins are usually considered safe to use during pregnancy.

BREAST FEEDING: Excreted in breast milk at low concentrations. The American Academy of Pediatrics classifies cephalosporin antibiotics as compatible with breast feeding.

COMMENTS: Parenteral cephamycin second-generation cephalosporin w/ anaerobic activity, but up to 44% of B. fragilis may be resistant (while 5.8% resistance w/ cefoxitin). Longer half-life allows q12h dosing compared to cefoxitin. Contains the N-methylthiotetrazole (NMTT) side chain that may result in prolonged hypoprothrombinemia & disulfiram-like reactions. In short supply due to manufacturing problems (March 2005).

FORMS

Brand name	Preparation	Mfr.	Route	Form	Strength	Cost (AWP)
Cefotan	Cefotetan	Astra-Zeneca	IV	vial	1000mg; 2000mg; 1g/ 50mL; 2g/50mL	$15; $29; $16.72; $33.42

SELECTED READINGS

Snydman DR et al. National Survey on the Susceptibility of Bacteroides fragilis Group: Report and Analysis of Trends for 1997-2000 . CID 2002;35:Suppl 1:S126

Bratzler DW, Houck PM. Antimicrobial Prophylaxis for Surgery: An Advisory Statement from the National Surgical Infection Prevention Project. Clin Infect Dis. 2004;38:1706-1715

CEFOXITIN

FDA INDICATIONS

- Bone and joint infections
- Gonococcal (cervicitis)
- Gynecologic infections (endometritis, pelvic cellulitis, pelvic inflammatory disease)
- Intra-abdominal infections
- Skin and skin structure infections
- Surgical prophylaxis (GI, abdominal hysterectomy, vaginal hysterectomy, Cesarean section)
- Urinary tract infections

USUAL ADULT DOSING: UTI or mild uncomplicated infections: 1.0g IV or IM q6-8h. Moderate infections: 2g IV q6h. Severe infections: 2g IV q4h or 3g q6h(up to 12g/day).

Dosing Adjustments

GFR 50-80 mL/min: 1g-2g q8-12h

GFR 10-50 mL/min: 1g-2g q12-24h

> *GFR<10 mL/min:* 0.5g-1g q12-48h
> *Hemodialysis:* 1-2g post-dialysis
> *Peritoneal Dialysis:* 1 g/day

Adverse Drug Reactions: Frequent: Phlebitis at infusion sites. **Occasional:** Allergic reactions; diarrhea and C. difficile colitis; eosinophilia; positive Coombs' test. **Rare:** Anaphylaxis rare; hemolytic anemia.

Drug Interactions

Probenecid: Increase in cephalosporin serum concentration due to inhibition of tubular secretion by probenecid. Monitor for potential cephalosporin toxicity, interaction may be beneficial if high serum concentration is desired.

Warfarin: Warfarin anticoagulation effect may be enhanced. Monitor INR closely and adjust warfarin dose accordingly.

Pregnancy Risk: B-Cephalosporins are usually considered safe to use during pregnancy.

Breast Feeding: Excreted in breast milk at low concentrations. The American Academy of Pediatrics classifies cephalosporin antibiotics as compatible with breast feeding.

Comments: Parenteral cephamycin second-generation cephalosporin with good anaerobic activity including B. fragilis (but 5.8% may be resistant). Preferred over cefotetan for B. fragilis coverage but requires more frequent administration.

Forms (◆ denotes available generically)

Brand name	Preparation	Mfr.	Route	Form	Strength	Cost (AWP)
Mefoxin	Cefoxitin	◆ Merck	IV	vial	1g/50mL; 2g/50mL	$15.30; $27.19 per vial

Selected Readings

Talan DA, et al. Ampicillin/Sulbactam and Cefoxitin in the Treatment of Cutaneous and Other Soft-Tissue Abscesses in patients With or Without Histories of Injection Drug Abuse . CID 2000;31:464

Snydman DR et al. National Survey on the Susceptibility of Bacteroides fragilis Group: Report and Analysis of Trends for 1997-2000 . CID 2002;35:Suppl 1:S126

CEFPODOXIME PROXETIL

FDA Indications

- Upper respiratory infections (acute maxillary sinusitis, bronchitis, otitis media, pharyngitis, tonsillitis)
- Lower respiratory infections (pneumonia)
- Skin and skin structure infections
- Uncomplicated urinary tract infections
- Uncomplicated GC (men and women) and rectal gonococcal infections (women)

Usual Adult Dosing: Uncomplicated GC: 400mg x 1. CAP and sinusitis: 200mg PO bid. Soft tissue infection: 400mg PO bid.

Dosing Adjustments

GFR 50-80 mL/min: 200mg-400mg q12h
GFR 10-50 mL/min: 200mg-400mg q16-24h
GFR<10 mL/min: 200mg-400mg q24-48h
Hemodialysis: 200-400mg 3x/week
Peritoneal Dialysis: 200-400mg q24h

Adverse Drug Reactions: Occasional: Allergic reactions; diarrhea and C. difficile colitis; eosinophilia; positive Coombs' test. **Rare:** Anaphylaxis

DRUG INTERACTIONS

Probenecid: Increase in cephalosporin serum concentration due to inhibition of tubular secretion by probenecid. Monitor for potential cephalosporin toxicity, interaction may be beneficial if high serum concentration is desired.

PREGNANCY RISK: B-Cephalosporins are usually considered safe to use during pregnancy.

BREAST FEEDING: Excreted in breast milk at low concentrations. The American Academy of Pediatrics classifies cephalosporin antibiotics as compatible with breast feeding.

COMMENTS: Oral third-generation cephalosporin with greatest in vitro activity among oral cephalosporins against S. pneumoniae and moderate Staphylococcal activity. Effective for the management of uncomplicated GC but more extensive clinical data with cefixime.

FORMS (◆ DENOTES AVAILABLE GENERICALLY)

Brand name	Preparation	Mfr.	Route	Form	Strength	Cost (AWP)
Vantin	Cefpodoxime proxetil	◆ Pharmacia	PO	susp	50mg/5mL; 100mg/5mL	$2.65 per 5mL; $5.05 per 5mL
			PO	tab	100mg; 200mg	$4.71; $6.22

SELECTED READINGS

Safran C. Cefpodoxime proxetil: dosage, efficacy and tolerance in adults suffering from respiratory tract infections. J Antimicrob Chemother 1990 Dec;26 Suppl E:93-101

Novak E; Paxton LM; Tubbs HJ et al. Orally administered cefpodoxime proxetil for treatment of uncomplicated gonococcal urethritis in males: a dose-response study. Antimicrob Agents Chemother 1992 Aug;36(8):1764-5

CEFPROZIL

FDA INDICATIONS

- Upper respiratory tract infections (acute bronchitis, chronic bronchitis, otitis media, pharyngitis, sinusitis, tonsillitis)
- Uncomplicated skin and skin structure infections

USUAL ADULT DOSING: URTI and Uncomplicated soft tissue infection: 250mg-500mg PO q12h.

Dosing Adjustments
GFR 50-80 mL/min: Usual dose
GFR 10-50 mL/min: 0.25g-0.5g q24h
GFR<10 mL/min: 0.25g q12-24h
Hemodialysis: 250-500mg post-dialysis
Peritoneal Dialysis: 0.25g q12-24h

ADVERSE DRUG REACTIONS: Occasional: Allergic reactions (anaphylaxis rare); diarrhea and C. difficile colitis; eosinophilia; positive Coombs' test. **Rare:** Anaphylaxis. Avoid cefprozil oral solution in patients with phenylketonuria since it contains 28mg of phenylalanine per 5mL.

DRUG INTERACTIONS

Probenecid: Increase in cephalosporin serum concentration due to inhibition of tubular secretion by probenecid. Monitor for potential cephalosporin toxicity, interaction may be beneficial if high serum concentration is desired.

PREGNANCY RISK: B-Cephalosporins are usually considered safe to use during pregnancy.

BREAST FEEDING: Excreted in breast milk at low concentrations. The American Academy of Pediatrics classifies cephalosporin antibiotics as compatible with breast feeding.

COMMENTS: Oral second-generation cephalosporin with good activity against S. pneumoniae but not FDA indicated for pneumonia.

FORMS

Brand name	Preparation	Mfr.	Route	Form	Strength	Cost (AWP)
Cefzil	Cefprozil	Bristol-Myers Squibb	PO	susp	125mg/5mL; 250mg/5mL	$2.23 per 5mL; $4.04 per 5mL
			PO	tab	250mg; 500mg	$4.67; $9.51

SELECTED READINGS

Adelglass J, Bundy JM, Woods R. Efficacy and tolerability of cefprozil versus amoxicillin/clavulanate for the treatment of adults with severe sinusitis. Clin Ther. 1998;20(6):1115-29.

CEFTAZIDIME

FDA INDICATIONS

- Septicemia
- Bone and joint infections
- CNS infections
- Gram-negative infections (Escherichia coli, Klebsiella pneumoniae, Proteus indole positive infections, Serratia, Pseudomonas aeruginosa)
- Gynecologic infections (endometritis, pelvic cellulitis)
- Intra-abdominal infections
- Lower respiratory tract infections (pneumonia)
- Meningitis
- Peritonitis
- Skin and soft-tissue infections

USUAL ADULT DOSING: Mild to moderate infections: 1g q8-12h. UTI: 500mg q12h-q8h. Severe infections or meningitis: 2g IV q8 (up to 8g per day)

Dosing Adjustments
GFR 50-80 mL/min: Usual dose
GFR 10-50 mL/min: 1g q12-24h
GFR<10 mL/min: 0.5g q24-48h
Hemodialysis: 1g loading, 1g post-dialysis
Peritoneal Dialysis: 0.5-1.0g loading, 250mg per each 2 Liter of dialysate exchange per day

ADVERSE DRUG REACTIONS: Frequent: Phlebitis at infusion sites. **Occasional:** Allergic reactions; diarrhea and C.difficile colitis; eosinophilia; positive Coombs' test. **Rare:** Anaphylaxis rare; hemolytic anemia

DRUG INTERACTIONS

Probenecid: Increase in cephalosporin serum concentration due to inhibition of tubular secretion by probenecid. Monitor for potential cephalosporin toxicity, interaction may be beneficial if high serum concentration is desired.

PREGNANCY RISK: B-Cephalosporins are usually considered safe to use during pregnancy.

BREAST FEEDING: Excreted in breast milk at low concentrations. The American Academy of Pediatrics classifies cephalosporin antibiotics as compatible with breast feeding.

COMMENTS: Parenteral third-generation cephalosporin with good P. aeruginosa activity but poor activity vs gram-positive cocci. Cefepime is equivalent to ceftazidime against GNB including P. aeruginosa and usually shows a lower cost.

FORMS (◆ DENOTES AVAILABLE GENERICALLY)

Brand name	Preparation	Mfr.	Route	Form	Strength	Cost (AWP)
Fortaz	Ceftazidime	◆ GlaxoSmithK-line	IV or IM	vial	500mg; 1g; 2g; 6g; 1g/50mL; 2g/50mL	$7.12; $14.71; $28.93; $82.80 per vial; $16.93; $31.15 per vial

SELECTED READINGS

ATS and IDSA. Guidelines for the Management of Adults with Hospital-acquired, Ventilator-associated, and Healthcare-associated Pneumonia . Am J Respir Crit Care Med 2005;171:388

CEFTIBUTEN

FDA INDICATIONS

- Acute exacerbation of chronic bronchitis
- Otitis media
- Pharyngitis and tonsillitis

USUAL ADULT DOSING: AECB, pharyngitis, tonsillitis, and otitis: 400mg PO qd

Dosing Adjustments

GFR 50-80 mL/min: Usual dose

GFR 10-50 mL/min: 200mg q day

GFR<10 mL/min: 100mg q day

Hemodialysis: 400mg post-dialysis

Peritoneal Dialysis: not removed in peritoneal dialysis. 100-200mg qd

ADVERSE DRUG REACTIONS: Occasional: Allergic reactions (anaphylaxis rare); headache, diarrhea and C. difficile colitis; eosinophilia; positive Coombs' test; serum sickness; 2% in clinical trials discontinued drug due to ADR

DRUG INTERACTIONS

Probenecid: Increase in cephalosporin serum concentration due to inhibition of tubular secretion by probenecid. Monitor for potential cephalosporin toxicity, interaction may be beneficial if high serum concentration is desired.

PREGNANCY RISK: B-Cephalosporins are usually considered safe to use during pregnancy.

BREAST FEEDING: Excreted in breast milk at low concentrations. The American Academy of Pediatrics classifies cephalosporin antibiotics as compatible with breast feeding.

COMMENTS: Oral third-generation cephalosporin. Poor activity against S. aureus and S. pneumoniae. Not hydrolyzed by some extended-spectrum Beta-lactamases. Alternative oral 3rd generation cephalosporin should be considered for CAP.

FORMS

Brand name	Preparation	Mfr.	Route	Form	Strength	Cost (AWP)
Cedax	Ceftibuten	Shionogi USA	PO	susp	90mg/5mL	$4.13 per 5mL
			PO	tab	400mg	$9.81

SELECTED READINGS

McAdoo MA, Rice K, Gordon GR et al. Comparison of ceftibuten once daily and amoxicillin-clavulanate three times daily in the treatment of acute exacerbations of chronic bronchitis. Clin Ther. 1998 Jan-Feb;20(1):88-100.

CEFTIZOXIME

FDA INDICATIONS

- Bacteremia
- Septicemia
- Gonorrhea (urethritis)
- Intra-abdominal infections
- Lower respiratory tract infections
- Meningitis
- Pelvic inflammatory disease
- Skin and skin-structure infections
- Soft tissue infections
- Bone and joint infections

USUAL ADULT DOSING: 1-2g IM or IV q8-12h. Severe infections: 2g IV q4h. GC 500mg IM x1.

Dosing Adjustments

GFR 50-80 mL/min: 0.5g-1.5g q8h
GFR 10-50 mL/min: 0.25g-1g q12h
GFR<10 mL/min: 0.25g-0.5g q24h
Hemodialysis: 1g post dialysis
Peritoneal Dialysis: 1 g/day

ADVERSE DRUG REACTIONS: Frequent: Phlebitis at infusion sites. **Occasional:** Allergic reactions (anaphylaxis rare); diarrhea and C. difficile colitis; eosinophilia; positive Coombs' test.

DRUG INTERACTIONS

Probenecid: Increase in cephalosporin serum concentration due to inhibition of tubular secretion by probenecid. Monitor for potential cephalosporin toxicity, interaction may be beneficial if high serum concentration is desired.

PREGNANCY RISK: B-Cephalosporins are usually considered safe to use during pregnancy.

BREAST FEEDING: Excreted in breast milk at low concentrations. The American Academy of Pediatrics classifies cephalosporin antibiotics as compatible with breast feeding.

COMMENTS: Parenteral third-generation cephalosporin with in vitro activity comparable to cefotaxime but with less S. pneumoniae activity but better B. fragilis activity.

FORMS

Brand name	Preparation	Mfr.	Route	Form	Strength	Cost (AWP)
Cefizox	Ceftizoxime	Astellas	IV	vial	1g; 2g; 10g; 1g/50mL; 2g/50mL	$13.44; $24.64; $104.44 per vial; $13.98; $23.74 per vial

SELECTED READINGS

Yangco et al. Comparative efficacy of ceftizoxime, cefotaxime, and latamoxef in the treatment of bacterial pneumonia in high risk patients. JAC 1987; 19: 239

CEFTRIAXONE

FDA INDICATIONS

- Bacterial septicemia
- Bone and joint infections

- Skin and skin structure infections
- Gonorrhea (urethral, cervical, pharyngeal, disseminated)
- Intra-abdominal infections
- Upper respiratory tract infections (otitis media
- Lower respiratory tract infections (pneumonia)
- Meningitis
- Complicated and uncomplicated urinary tract infections
- Pelvic inflammatory disease
- Shunt infections

USUAL ADULT DOSING: 1-2g IM or IV qd (up to 4g per day); 2g IV q12h (meningitis)

Dosing Adjustments
GFR 50-80 mL/min: Usual dose
GFR 10-50 mL/min: Usual dose
GFR<10 mL/min: Usual dose
Hemodialysis: 1-2g IV qd (No extra doses needed post dialysis)
Peritoneal Dialysis: Usual regimen
↓ *Hepatic Function:* Maximum dose is 2g with severe renal and hepatic impairment

ADVERSE DRUG REACTIONS: Frequent: Phlebitis at infusion sites. **Occasional:** Allergic reactions (anaphylaxis rare); diarrhea and C. difficile colitis; eosinophilia; pseudocholelithiasis with sludge in gallbladder by ultrasound. **Rare:** Positive Coombs' test w/ hemolysis.

DRUG INTERACTIONS

Probenecid: Increase in cephalosporin serum concentration due to inhibition of tubular secretion by probenecid. Monitor for potential cephalosporin toxicity, interaction may be beneficial if high serum concentration is desired.
Warfarin: Warfarin anticoagulation effect may be enhanced.

PREGNANCY RISK: B-Cephalosporins are usually considered safe to use during pregnancy.

BREAST FEEDING: Excreted in breast milk at low concentrations. The American Academy of Pediatrics classifies cephalosporin antibiotics as compatible with breast feeding.

COMMENTS: Parenteral third-generation cephalosporin with convenient once a day dosing often used for outpatient therapy. Cefotaxime is clinically equivalent, often with lower cost but given q6h. Excreted via biliary and urinary tract. May cause biliary sludging and cholecystitis. Cefotaxime and ceftriaxone are the preferred cephalosporins for serious pneumococcal infections, but 3%-5+% of strains are resistant.

FORMS

Brand name	Preparation	Mfr.	Route	Form	Strength	Cost (AWP)
Rocephin	Ceftriaxone	Roche	IV	vial	250mg; 500mg; 1g; 2g; 10g	$15.82; $28.68; $50.65; $100.04; $478.32
	Ceftriaxone	Roche	IV	vial	1g/50mL; 2g/50mL	$39.20; $68.84

CEFUROXIME AND CEFUROXIME AXETIL

FDA INDICATIONS

- Skin soft tissue infection
- Upper respiratory infection (acute bronchitis, chronic bronchitis, acute sinusitis, chronic sinusitis, pharyngitis, tonsillitis, otitis media, epiglottis)
- Lower respiratory tract infection (pneumonia)

- Bone and joint infections (septic arthritis)
- Gonorrhea
- Osteomyelitis
- Respiratory tract infections - lower
- Septic arthritis
- Sinusitis
- Skin and soft tissue infections (cellulitis)

USUAL ADULT DOSING: Mild to moderate infections: 0.75g IM or IV q8h. Severe infections: 1.5g IV q8h. Oral regimen: 250-500mg PO bid. Uncomplicated GC: 1000mg x 1 (but cefixime preferred).

Dosing Adjustments

GFR 50-80 mL/min: Usual dose

GFR 10-50 mL/min: 0.75g-1.5g IV q8-12h; No dosage change for oral administration

GFR<10 mL/min: 0.75g IV q24h; 250mg PO q24h

Hemodialysis: 750mg post dialysis

Peritoneal Dialysis: 750mg qd

ADVERSE DRUG REACTIONS: Frequent: Phlebitis at infusion sites. **Occasional:** Allergic reactions; diarrhea and C. difficile colitis; eosinophilia; positive Coombs' test. **Rare:** Anaphylaxis; hemolytic anemia; neutropenia, and leukopenia

PREGNANCY RISK: B-cephalosporins are usually considered safe to use during pregnancy.

BREAST FEEDING: Excreted in breast milk at low concentrations. The American Academy of Pediatrics classifies cephalosporin antibiotics as compatible with breast feeding.

COMMENTS: Second-generation oral and parenteral cephalosporin with convenient twice-a-day dosing schedule. Activity in vitro vs. S. pneumoniae is inferior to that of cefotaxime, ceftriaxone and cefprozil.

FORMS (♦ DENOTES AVAILABLE GENERICALLY)

Brand name	Preparation	Mfr.	Route	Form	Strength	Cost (AWP)
Ceftin	Cefuroxime axetil	♦ GlaxoSmithK-line	PO	suspension	250mg/5mL	$4.63 per 5mL
			PO	tab	250mg; 500mg; 125mg/5mL	$6.45; $11.76; $2.72 per 5mL
Zinacef	Cefuroxime sodium	♦ GlaxoSmithK-line	IV	vial	750mg ; 1.5g; 7.5g; 750mg/50mL; 1.5g/50mL	$7.24; $13.94; $65.94; $9.46; $16.16

CEPHALEXIN

FDA INDICATIONS

- Osteomyelitis
- Otitis media
- Streptococcal pharyngitis
- Prostatitis
- Respiratory infections
- Skin and skin structure infections
- Urinary tract infections

USUAL ADULT DOSING: Mild to moderate infections: 250mg PO qid. Severe infections: 500mg PO qid. Streptococcal pharyngitis and uncomplicated cystitis: consider 500mg PO q12h.

Dosing Adjustments
GFR 50-80 mL/min: Usual dose
GFR 10-50 mL/min: 0.25g-1.0g q8-12h
GFR<10 mL/min: 0.25g-1g q24-48h
Hemodialysis: 0.25-1.0g post-dialysis
Peritoneal Dialysis: 250mg tid

ADVERSE DRUG REACTIONS: Occasional: Allergic reactions; diarrhea and C. difficile colitis; eosinophilia; positive Coombs' test. **Rare:** Anaphylaxis; hemolytic anemia.

DRUG INTERACTIONS
Probenecid: Increase in cephalosporin serum concentration due to inhibition of tubular secretion by probenecid. Monitor for potential cephalosporin toxicity, interaction may be beneficial if high serum concentration is desired.

PREGNANCY RISK: B-Cephalosporins are usually considered safe to use during pregnancy.

BREAST FEEDING: Excreted in breast milk at low concentrations. The American Academy of Pediatrics classifies cephalosporin antibiotics as compatible with breast feeding.

COMMENTS: Well absorbed first-generation cephalosporin with good gram-positive coverage and a low price but q6-8h dosing may decrease patient compliance.

FORMS (♦ DENOTES AVAILABLE GENERICALLY)

Brand name	Preparation	Mfr.	Route	Form	Strength	Cost (AWP)
Keflex	Cephalexin	♦ Advantus Pharm	PO	cap	250mg; 500mg	$0.70; $1.50
Cephalexin	Cephalexin	♦ Ranbaxy	PO	cap	250mg; 500mg	$0.69; $1.38
			PO	susp	125mg/5mL; 250mg/5mL	$0.40 per 5mL; $0.80 per 5mL
Panixine Dis-perdose	Cephalexin	Ranbaxy	PO	tab	125mg; 250mg	$0.41; $0.81

SELECTED READINGS
Blaser MJ, Klaus BD, Jacobson JA et al. Comparison of cefadroxil and cephalexin in the treatment of community-acquired pneumonia. Antimicrob Agents Chemother. 1983;24:163-7.

CEPHALOTHIN

FDA INDICATIONS
- No longer available in the U.S.
- Bone and joint infections
- Gastrointestinal infections
- Meningitis
- Respiratory tract infections
- Skin and skin structure infections
- Soft tissue infections
- Surgical prophylaxis (cardiac, gastrointestinal, gynecologic, orthopedic, thoracic, vascular)
- Urinary tract infections

USUAL ADULT DOSING: 0.5-3.0g IV q4-8h (up to 12g per day)

Dosing Adjustments
GFR 50-80 mL/min: Usual dose
GFR 10-50 mL/min: 1mL-1.5g q6h
GFR<10 mL/min: 0.5g q8h

Hemodialysis: 1-2g post-dialysis

Peritoneal Dialysis: 0.5g q8h No supplementation needed for peritoneal dialysis.

ADVERSE DRUG REACTIONS: Frequent: phlebitis at infusion sites. **Occasional:** allergic reactions (anaphylaxis rare); diarrhea and C. difficile colitis; eosinophilia; positive Coombs' test

PREGNANCY RISK: B-Cephalosporins are usually considered safe to use during pregnancy.

BREAST FEEDING: Excreted in breast milk at low concentrations. The American Academy of Pediatrics classifies cephalosporin antibiotics as compatible with breast feeding.

COMMENTS: No longer available in the US. Parenteral 1st generation cephalosporin.

FORMS

Brand name	Preparation	Mfr.	Route	Form	Strength	Cost (AWP)
Keflin; Seffin	Cephalothin	No longer available in the U.S.	IV	vial	1000mg ; 200mg	N/A; N/A

CEPHRADINE

FDA INDICATIONS

- Surgical prophylaxis (appendectomy, cesarean section, hip replacement, vaginal hysterectomy, vascular surgery)
- Bone infections
- Nasal furunculosis
- Upper respiratory tract infection (otitis media, peritonsillitis, tonsillitis)
- Lower respiratory tract infection (pneumoccal pneumonia)
- Respiratory tract infections
- Septicemia
- Skin and skin-structure infections
- Urinary tract infection
- Otitis media

USUAL ADULT DOSING: 0.5-1.0g PO q6-12h; 0.5-2.0g IV or IM q6h (up to 8g per day)(parenteral formulation no longer available in the U.S.)

Dosing Adjustments

GFR 50-80 mL/min: 0.5g-1g IV q6h; No dosage adjustment needed for oral administration

GFR 10-50 mL/min: 0.5g-1g IV q6-24h; 0.5g PO q6h

GFR<10 mL/min: 0.5g-1g IV q24-72h; 0.25g PO q12h

Hemodialysis: 250mg at the start, 250mg 12 hours later, and 36 to 48 hours after the start of hemodialysis

Peritoneal Dialysis: 0.5g-1g IV q6-24h; 0.5g PO q6h

ADVERSE DRUG REACTIONS: Frequent: Phlebitis at infusion sites. **Occasional:** Allergic reactions (anaphylaxis rare); diarrhea and C. difficile colitis; eosinophilia; positive Coombs' test

DRUG INTERACTIONS

Probenecid: Increase in cephalosporin serum concentration due to inhibition of tubular secretion by probenecid. Monitor for potential cephalosporin toxicity, interaction may be beneficial if high serum concentration is desired.

PREGNANCY RISK: B-Cephalosporins are usually considered safe to use during pregnancy.

BREAST FEEDING: Excreted in breast milk at low concentrations. The American Academy of Pediatrics classifies cephalosporin antibiotics as compatible with breast feeding.

COMMENTS: Oral first-generation cephalosporin. Well-absorbed cephalosporin giving similar serum concentration compared to IM administration.

FORMS (◆ DENOTES AVAILABLE GENERICALLY)

Brand name	Preparation	Mfr.	Route	Form	Strength	Cost (AWP)
Velosef	Cephradine	◆ Bristol-Myers Squibb	PO	cap	250mg; 500mg	$0.95; $1.86
			PO	susp	250mg/5mL	$0.97 per 5mL

CHLORAMPHENICOL

FDA INDICATIONS

- Brain abscess
- Paratyphoid fever
- Q fever
- Rocky mountain spotted fever and other Typhus infections caused by Rickettsia species
- Ehrlichiosis
- Meningitis
- Typhoid fever

USUAL ADULT DOSING: 250-500mg PO qid (usual dose is 500mg PO qid); 50mg/kg IV in 4 divided doses (up to 100mg/kg/day)

Dosing Adjustments

GFR 50-80 mL/min: Usual dose

GFR 10-50 mL/min: Usual dose

GFR<10 mL/min: Usual dose

Hemodialysis: 500mg Dose post-dialysis

Peritoneal Dialysis: Usual regimen

↓ *Hepatic Function:* Use with caution with renal and/or hepatic failure; monitor serum levels to achieve levels between 5-20 mcg/mL

ADVERSE DRUG REACTIONS: Occasional: GI intol. with oral admin; dose related reversible bone marrow suppression (more likely with >4g per day or with serum level >25 mcg/mL. **Rare:** Aplastic anemia (not dose related)and "Gray baby syndrome" with cyanosis and circulatory collapse

DRUG INTERACTIONS

Iron supplements: Chloramphenicol may inhibit heme synthesis, reduce iron clearance and increase serum iron level. Monitor iron stores and change the dose of iron accordingly.

Phenobarbital: Phenobarbital may result in decreased plasma concentration of chloramphenicol. Monitor for therapeutic efficacy and blood concentration of chloramphenicol.

Rifampin: Enzyme induction by rifampin resulting in increased metabolism and decreased serum concentration of chloramphenicol. Monitor for therapeutic efficacy and blood concentration of chloramphenicol.

Sulfonylureas (chlorpropamide, tolbutamide): Chloramphenicol may inhibit hepatic metabolism of some sulfonyl ureas resulting in prolongation of half-life and resultant hypoglycemia. Monitor blood sugar closely, dose of sulfonyl ureas may need to be decreased accordingly.

Vitamin B12: Hematologic effects of vitamin B12 in patients with pernicious anemia may be decreased. Avoid combination. Use alternative antibiotic.

Warfarin (anticoagulant): Increased anticoagulant effect possibly due to chloramphenicol inhibition of warfarin hepatic metabolism or interference with intestinal bacterial producing vitamin K. Monitor INR closely when chloramphenicol is co-administered with warfarin.

PREGNANCY RISK: C--A collaborative perinatal project monitored 98 exposures during the first trimester, 348 exposures anytime during pregnancy found no evidence of relationship with chloramphenicol and malformation. Although apparently nontoxic to the fetus, chloramphenicol should not be used near term due to the potential of "Gray Baby Syndrome."

BREAST FEEDING: Excreted in breast milk. The American Academy of Pediatrics classifies chloramphenicol as an agent whose effect on the nursing infant as unknown but may be of concern because of the potential of idiosyncratic bone marrow suppression.

COMMENTS: Oral and parenteral broad spectrum drug that is infrequently used in the U.S. due to rare idiosyncratic toxicity of aplastic anemia (1:40,000) and the availability of alternative agents. May be used as a second line agent (with Vancomycin) for the empiric treatment of bacterial meningitis in PCN-allergic patients. Oral formulation unavailable in U.S.

FORMS (◆ DENOTES AVAILABLE GENERICALLY)

Brand name	Preparation	Mfr.	Route	Form	Strength	Cost (AWP)
Chloromycetin	Chloram-phenicol	◆ Monarch	IV	vial	1000mg	$7.59

SELECTED READINGS

Peltola H; Anttila M; Renkonen OV. Randomised comparison of chloramphenicol, ampicillin, cefotaxime, and ceftriaxone for childhood bacterial meningitis. Lancet 1989 Jun 10;1(8650):1281-1287

Lennard ES; Minshew BH; Dellinger EP; Wertz MJ; Heimbach DM; Counts GW; Schoenknecht FD; Coyle MB . Stratified outcome comparison of clindamycin-gentamicin vs chloramphenicol-gentamicin for treatment of intra-abdominal sepsis. Arch Surg 1985 Aug;120(8):889-98

CHLOROQUINE

FDA INDICATIONS

- Malaria prophylaxis and treatment (caused by P. vivax, P. malariae, P. ovale, and chloroquine-susceptible strains of P. falciparum)
- Amebic liver abscess

USUAL ADULT DOSING: P. vivax, P. ovale, P. malariae, & chloroquine-sensitive P. falciparum: chloroquine phosphate 1g salt (600mg base) once, then 500mgmg salt (300mg base) 6hr later, then 500mg at 24 h and 48h. Chloroquine HCL 160-200mg (base) IM or IV q6h (IV n/a in US).

Dosing Adjustments

GFR 50-80 mL/min: Usual

GFR 10-50 mL/min: Usual

GFR<10 mL/min: 150-300mg PO qd

↓ *Hepatic Function:* 30-50% decrease in dose is recommended

ADVERSE DRUG REACTIONS: Occasional: visual disturbances; GI intolerance; pruritus; weight loss; alopecia. **Rare:** H/A, confusion, dizziness, extraocular muscle palsies; psychosis; peripheral neuropathy; cardiac toxicity; hemolysis (G6PD deficiency).

DRUG INTERACTIONS

Aluminum salts and **magnesium salts:** Decrease absorption of chloroquine. Separate the administration time by 2-4 hours. The clinical significance of this interaction is not known.

Cimetidine: Possible increase in chloroquine blood concentration due to cimetidine inhibition of hepatic enzyme metabolism of chloroquine. Monitor for chloroquine toxicity, dose of chloroquine may need to be lowered.

PREGNANCY RISK: C-Embryotoxic and teratogenic in animals studies. In a report of 169 infants exposed to in utero to 300mg of chloroquine weekly throughout pregnancy, there was no increase in teratogenicity. Chloroquine is the antimalarial prophylaxis considered probably safe in pregnancy; there is no other antimalaria prophylaxis with enough data in pregnancy, therefore pregnant women should be strongly discouraged to travel in a chloroquine-resistant malarial region.

BREAST FEEDING: 2.8% of dose is excreted in breast milk. The American Academy of Pediatrics considers chloroquine to be compatible with breast feeding.

COMMENTS: Oral antimalarial agent. Effective as malaria prophylaxis in Mexico and Central America above the Panama Canal. Some chloroquine resistance in the Middle East. Substantial resistance in continental South America. Mefloquine recommended for travel to areas with chloroquine-resistant P. falciparum.

FORMS (◆ DENOTES AVAILABLE GENERICALLY)

Brand name	Preparation	Mfr.	Route	Form	Strength	Cost (AWP)
Aralen phosphate	Chloroquine phosphate	◆ Sanofi Syntholabo	PO	tab	250mg; 500mg	$2.50; $6.03
Plaquenil	Hydroxychloroquine	◆ Sanofi Syntholabo	PO	tab	200mg	$1.20

CIDOFOVIR

FDA INDICATIONS

- Cytomegalovirus retinitis

USUAL ADULT DOSING: CMV retinitis: induction 5mg/kg qwk x 2 wks, then q2 wks. Must give w/ probenecid: 2g given 3hrs prior to cidofovir, and 1g given 2 and 8 hrs after infusion. Hydrate with >1L NS immediately before cidofovir infusion.

Dosing Adjustments

GFR 50-80 mL/min: 5mg/kg

GFR 10-50 mL/min: Contraindicated for serum creatinine >1.5mg/dL or creatinine clearance < or = 55 mL/min

GFR<10 mL/min: Contraindicated for serum creatinine >1.5mg/dL or creatinine clearance < 55 mL/min

Hemodialysis: 52% +/- 11% cleared during high-flux hemodialysis. (Clin Pharm Ther 1999 Jan; 65(1):21-8. Dose post-HD.

Peritoneal Dialysis: Not significantly cleared

ADVERSE DRUG REACTIONS: Frequent: NEPHROTOXICITY (proteinuria, azotemia, proximal tubular dysfunction)-dose dependent, increased w/other nephrotoxins, reduced w/ hydration & probenecid. **Occasional:** GI intolerance; neutropenia; metabolic acidosis. **Rare:** Uveitis; ocular hypotony.

DRUG INTERACTIONS

Contraindicated with other nephrotoxic drugs: aminoglycoside, amphoteracin B, foscarnet, NSAIDs, pentamidine: One week wash out period of nephrotoxic drug before cidofovir administration recommended.

PREGNANCY RISK: C-CARCINOGENIC, TERATOGENIC AND CAUSES HYPOSPERMIA in animal studies, no human data available.

BREAST FEEDING: No data, avoid due to potential for severe toxicity.

COMMENTS: Parenteral antiviral agent used as second line drug for CMV infections. Convenience of every-other-week dosing for maintenance of CMV infections, but nephrotoxicity limits its routine use. Probenecid (which often causes severe side effects including chills, fever, headache, rash and nausea in 30-50% of patients) must be given concurrently to decrease the incidence of nephrotoxicity.

FORMS

Brand name	Preparation	Mfr.	Route	Form	Strength	Cost (AWP)
Vistide	Cidofovir	Gilead	IV	vial	75mg/mL (5mL)	$888.00 per vial

SELECTED READINGS

Lalezari JP, Holland GN, Kramer F, et al. Randomized, controlled study of the safety and efficacy of intravenous cidofovir for the treatment of relapsing cytomegalovirus retinitis in patients with AIDS . J Acquir Immune Defic Syndr Hum Retrovirol 1998 Apr 1;17(4):339-44

Lalezari J, Schacker T, Feinberg J, et al . A randomized, double-blind, placebo-controlled trial of cidofovir gel for the treatment of acyclovir-unresponsive mucocutaneous herpes simplex virus infection in patients with AIDS . J Infect Dis 1997 Oct;176(4):892-8

De Clercq E. Potential of acyclic nucleoside phosphonates in the treatment of DNA virus and retrovirus infections. Expert Rev Anti Infect Ther. 2003 Jun;1(1):21-43

CIPROFLOXACIN

FDA INDICATIONS

- Uncomplicated UTI (Cipro XR and Cipro); complicated UTI (Cipro).
- Prostatitis
- Endocervical and urethral infections caused N. gonorrhoeae (Note: high resistance rates reported in Hawaii and California).
- Gastroenteritis
- Pneumonia (nosocomial)
- Acute sinusitis
- Bone and joint infections
- Skin and soft tissue infections
- Empiric therapy for neutropenic fever (in combination with piperacillin)
- Post-exposure prophylaxis for inhalation anthrax. [CDC recommends as first line agent + 1-2 additional agents with in vitro activity (for inhalation anthrax, see "Anthrax" in the Diagnoses section")]

USUAL ADULT DOSING: Usual dose: 500mg PO bid. UTI: 250 PO bid or XR 500mg qd x 3d. Serious infections: 750mg PO bid or 400mg IV q8-12h. Nosocomial pneumonia 400mg IV q8h.

Dosing Adjustments

GFR 50-80 mL/min: Usual dose

GFR 10-50 mL/min: 0.4g IV q18h ; 0.25mL-0.5g PO q12h

GFR<10 mL/min: 0.4g IV q24h; 0.25mL-0.5g PO q18h

Hemodialysis: 250-500mg q24h post-dialysis (200-400 IV q24h)

Peritoneal Dialysis: 250-500mg qd (200-400 IV qd)

ADVERSE DRUG REACTIONS: Generally well tolerated. **Occasional:** GI intolerance; CNS-headache, malaise, insomnia, restlessness, and dizziness. **Rare:** Allergic reactions; diarrhea; photosensitivity; increased LFTs; tendon rupture; peripheral neuropathy; seizure.

DRUG INTERACTIONS

Antacids (magnesium, aluminum, calcium, Al-Mg buffer found in didanosine): Antacid binding to quinolone antibiotics resulting in decreased absorption and loss therapeutic efficacy.

Mexiletine: Quinolone may inhibit CYP450 1A2 resulting in increased mexiletine concentration.

Milk or dairy products: Decreased the GI absorption of ciprofloxacin by 36-47%.

Probenecid: Probenecid interferes with renal tubular secretion of ciprofloxacin; this may result in 50% increase in serum level of ciprofloxacin.

Sucralfate: Decrease absorption of fluoroquinolone due to the complexation of the aluminum ions contained in the sucralfate.

Theophylline: Increase theophylline concentration by 17-257%.

Vitamins and minerals containing divalent and trivalent cation such as zinc and iron: Formation of quinolone-ion complex results in decreased absorption of quinolones.

Warfarin: Case reports of ciprofloxacin enhancing anti-coagulation effect of warfarin. Monitor INR closely.

PREGNANCY RISK: C-In a prospective follow-up study conducted by the European Network of Teratology Information Services (ENTIS), 549 cases of fluoroquinolone exposure (majority of exposures were during 1st trimester) showed a congenital malformation rate of 4.8% (Schaefer et al). From previous epidemiologic data, the 4.8% did not exceed the background rate. Animal data demonstrated arthropathy in immature animals with erosions in joint cartilage. Because of the animal data, and the availability of alternative antimicrobial agents, the use of fluoroquinolones during pregnancy is considered contraindicated.

BREAST FEEDING: Fluoroquinolones are not recommended during breast feeding due to the potential for arthropathy (based on animal data).

COMMENTS: Oral and parenteral fluoroquinolone with a history of the best clinical and in vitro data against P. aeruginosa. Experience is favorable and extensive for nosocomial pneumonia, osteomyelitis, neutropenic fever, travelers diarrhea, chronic prostatitis and UTIs. Other fluoroquinolones (i.e., levofloxacin, gatifloxacin, moxifloxacin) are preferred for infections due to S. pneumoniae.

FORMS (◆ DENOTES AVAILABLE GENERICALLY)

Brand name	Preparation	Mfr.	Route	Form	Strength	Cost (AWP)
Cipro	Ciprofloxacin	◆ Schering	PO	susp	250mg/5mL; 500mg/5mL	$5.61 per 5mL; $6.56 per 5mL
			PO	tab	100mg; 250mg; 500mg; 750mg	$3.70; $5.28; $6.16; $6.46
Cipro IV	Ciprofloxacin	Bayer	IV	vial	10mg/mL; 200mg/100mL; 400mg/200mL	$0.65 per mL; $15.60 per vial; $30.01 per vial
CiproXR	Ciprofloxacin	Schering	PO	tab, ER	500mg; 1000mg	$8.32; $9.47
Ciloxan	Ciprofloxacin	Alcon	topical	ophthalmic oint; gtt	0.3%-3.5g; 0.3%-2.5mL; 5mL;10mL	$61.56; $53.16 per 5mL

SELECTED READINGS

A. Freifeld, et al. A Double-Blind Comparison of Empiric Oral and Intravenous Antibiotic Therapy for Loss Risk Febrile Patients with Neutropenia During Cancer Chemotherapy. NEJM 1999;341:305

Heldman AW, Hartert TV, Ray SC, et al. Oral antibiotic treatment of right-sided staphylococcal endocarditis in injection drug users: prospective randomized comparison with parenteral therapy. Am J Med 1996 Jul;101(1):68-76

D. A. Talan. Comparison of Ciprofloxacin (7 days) and Trimethoprim-Sulfamethoxazole (14 days) for Acute Uncomplicated Pyelonephritis in Women: A Randomized Trial. JAMA 2000;283:1583

Anon. Fluoroquinolone-Resistance in Neisseria gonorrhoeae, Hawaii, 1999, and Decreased Susceptibility to Azithromycin in N. gonorrhoeae, Missouri, 1999: . MMWR 2000;49:833

Adachi JA, et al. Empirical Antimicrobial Therapy for Traveler's Diarrhea. CID 2000;31:1079

CLARITHROMYCIN

FDA INDICATIONS

- Pharyngitis/tonsillitis
- Acute maxillary sinusitis (for Biaxin and Biaxin XL)
- Acute bacterial exacerbation of chronic bronchitis (for Biaxin and Biaxin XL)
- Community acquired pneumonia (for Biaxin and Biaxin XL)
- Otitis media
- Uncomplicated skin and skin structure infections
- Treatment of disseminated mycobacterial infections due to Mycobacterium avium
- Prophylaxis of Mycobacterium avium
- Treatment of active duodenal ulcer associated with H. pylori infection (in combination with omeprazole or ranitidine bismuth citrate)

USUAL ADULT DOSING: 250-500mg PO bid (immediate release formulation) or 1000mg PO qd w/food (XL formulation). MAC treatment and prophylaxis: 500mg PO bid.

Dosing Adjustments

GFR 50-80 mL/min: Usual dose

GFR 10-50 mL/min: Usual dose

GFR<10 mL/min: 0.25g-0.5g q24h

Hemodialysis: 500mg post-dialysis

Peritoneal Dialysis: No data, no supplemental dose

↓ *Hepatic Function:* No dose adjustment needed. May require dosage adjustment with concomitant renal dysfunction (Chu J Clin Pharmacol 1993;33:48)

ADVERSE DRUG REACTIONS: Occasional: GI intolerance (4%); diarrhea; metallic taste; transaminase elevation. Rare Headache; QTc prolongation; C. difficile colitis; reversible dose-related hearing loss.

DRUG INTERACTIONS

Clarithromycin is a substrate and inhibitor of CYP3A4

Contraindicated with: cisapride, ergot alkaloids, pimozide, cisapride, astemizole, terfenadine, midazolam and triazolam, lovastatin and simvastatin, fentanyl, rifampin, drugs that significantly prolong QTc interval.

Benzodiazepine (alprazolam, diazepam), carbamazepine, cyclosporine, tacrolimus, sirolimus, irinotecan, dofetilide, quinidine, digoxin, theophylline, warfarin, amiodarone, Ca channel blockers, itraconazole, ketoconazole, methadone, corticosteroid, drugs for impotence (sildenafil, tadalafil, and vardenafil), protease inhibitors (atazanavir, indinavir, ritonavir, saquinavir but dose adjustment recommended for atazanavir only) and other CYP3A4 substrates: clarithromycin may significantly increase serum level of the following drugs: Monitor closely with clarithromycin co-administration; may need to decrease dose of co-administered drug. **Rifabutin, rifapentine, carbamazepine, phenytoin, phenobarbital, nevirapine, and efavirenz:** clarithromycin levels may be decreased with the co-administration of these drugs. Consider switching to an alternative antimicrobial (i.e., azithromycin).

PREGNANCY RISK: C-Studies in monkeys show growth retardation. The teratogen information service in Philadelphia reported the outcome of 34 first or second trimester exposure were similar to those expected in nonexposed population.

BREAST FEEDING: Excreted into breast milk. The American Academy of Pediatrics consider erythromycin compatible with breast feeding. Risk to clarithromycin exposure is probably minimal.

COMMENTS: Oral macrolide with debated in vitro activity vs. H. influenzae. However, clinical trials showed elimination of this pathogen support the contention that it has in vivo activity against H. influenzae. An important component of treatment of H. pylori, M. avium complex and other MOTT infections. New XL formulation has comparable efficacy and toxicity to immediate release formulation.

FORMS

Brand name	Preparation	Mfr.	Route	Form	Strength	Cost (AWP)
Biaxin	Clar-ithromycin	Abbott	PO	suspension	125mg/5mL; 250mg/5mL	$2.09 per 5mL; $3.97 per 5mL
			PO	tablet	250mg; 500mg	$5.09; $5.09
Biaxin XL	Clar-ithromycin	Abbott	PO	XL tablet	500mg	$5.25

SELECTED READINGS

Dattwyler RJ; Grunwaldt E; Luft BJ. Clarithromycin in treatment of early Lyme disease: a pilot study. Antimicrob Agents Chemother 1996 Feb;40(2):468-9

Hamedani P; Ali J; Hafeez S et al. The safety and efficacy of clarithromycin in patients with Legionella pneumonia . Chest 1991 Dec;100(6):1503-6

Bradbury F. Comparison of azithromycin versus clarithromycin in the treatment of patients with lower respiratory tract infection. J Antimicrob Chemother 1993 Jun;31 Suppl E:153-62

Lam SK; Ching CK; Lai KC et al. Does treatment of Helicobacter pylori with antibiotics alone heal duodenal ulcer? A randomised double blind placebo controlled study . Gut 1997 Jul;41(1):43-8

Chaisson RE, Benson CA, Dube MP, et al. Clarithromycin therapy for bacteremic Mycobacterium avium complex disease. A randomized, double-blind, dose-ranging study in patients with AIDS. Ann Intern Med 1994 Dec 15;121(12):905-11

CLINDAMYCIN

FDA INDICATIONS

- Osteomyelitis
- Pelvic infections (endometritis, nongonococcal tubo-ovarian abscess, pelvic cellulitis, and postsurgical vaginal cuff infections)
- Streptococcal pneumonia (empyema, pneumonitis, and lung abscess)
- Septicemia
- Skin and soft tissue infections
- Actinomycosis
- Sinusitis

USUAL ADULT DOSING: Soft tissue infection: 300-450mg PO qid or 600mg IV q8h. PID: 900mg IV q8h. Bacterial vaginosis: 1 (100mg) application intravaginally qd x 7d. Acne: 1-2 topical application qd-bid.

Dosing Adjustments
GFR 50-80 mL/min: Usual dose
GFR 10-50 mL/min: Usual dose
GFR<10 mL/min: Usual dose
Hemodialysis: Usual regimen
Peritoneal Dialysis: Usual regimen
↓ *Hepatic Function:* Dose reduction recommended for severe hepatic failure

ANTI-INFECTIVES

ADVERSE DRUG REACTIONS: Frequent: Diarrhea (without C. difficile), GI intolerance (N/V). **Occasional:** Rash; C. difficile colitis (clindamycin is most common cause on a per patient basis)

DRUG INTERACTIONS

Aluminum salts (kaolin-pectin): Absorption of clindamycin may be delayed but total absorption is not altered. Administer kaolin-pectin suspension at least 2 hours before administration of clindamycin.

Nondepolarizing muscle relaxants (pancuronium, tubocurarine): Lincosamides may enhance the action of nondepolarizing muscle relaxant. Avoid combination, if concurrent administration is needed close monitoring of respiratory depression is indicated.

PREGNANCY RISK: B--In a surveillance study of Michigan Medicaid recipients, 647 exposures to clindamycin during the first trimester resulted in 4.8% birth defects. These data do not support an association between clindamycin and teratogenic effects.

BREAST FEEDING: Clindamycin is excreted into breast milk. The American Academy of Pediatrics considers clindamycin to be compatible with breast feeding.

COMMENTS: Oral and parenteral lincomycin with good in vitro and in vivo activity vs. anaerobes, but due to increasing resistance to B. fragilis it is no longer recommended for intra-abdominal infections. Metronidazole is preferred against B. fragilis. On a per patient basis clindamycin is the antimicrobial most likely to cause C. difficile colitis. QID dosing makes pt adherence a concern.

FORMS (♦ DENOTES AVAILABLE GENERICALLY)

Brand name	Preparation	Mfr.	Route	Form	Strength	Cost (AWP)
Cleocin phosphate	Clindamycin phosphate	Pharmacia	IV	vial	150mg/mL	$1.56 per mL
Cleocin Vaginal	Clindamycin phosphate	Pharmacia	vaginal	cre	2% (40g)	$54.68
Cleocin	Clindamycin HCl	♦ Pharmacia	PO	cap	75mg; 150mg	$1.49; $2.93
Cleocin phosphate	Clindamycin phosphate	Pharmacia	IV	vial	600mg/50mL	$11.12 per vial
Cleocin pediatric	Clindamycin palmitate	Pharmacia	PO	solution	75mg/5mL	$1.40 per 5mL
Cleocin vaginal ovules	Clindamycin phosphate	Pharmacia	vaginal	ovule suppository	100mg	$51.13 for 3
Cleocin	Clindamycin HCl	♦ Pharmacia	PO	cap	300mg	$5.95
Cleocin phosphate	Clindamycin phosphate	Pharmacia	IV	vial	900mg/50mL; 300mg/50mL	$13.62 per vial; $7.28 per vial

SELECTED READINGS

Gall SA; Kohan AP; Ayers OM et al. Intravenous metronidazole or clindamycin with tobramycin for therapy of pelvic infections. Obstet Gynecol 1998; 57(1):51-8

Safrin S; Finkelstein DM; Feinberg J et al. Comparison of three regimens for treatment of mild to moderate Pneumocystis carinii pneumonia in patients with AIDS. A double-blind, randomized, trial of oral TMP-SMX, dapsone-TMP & clinda-primaquine. Ann Intern Med 1996 May 1;124(9):792-802

Perlino CA. Metronidazole vs clindamycin treatment of anaerobic pulmonary infection. Failure of metronidazole therapy. Arch Intern Med 1981 Oct;141(11):1424-7

Stevens DL; Gibbons AE; Bergstrom R et al. The Eagle effect revisited: efficacy of clindamycin, erythromycin, and penicillin in the treatment of streptococcal myositis. J Infect Dis 1988 Jul;158 (1):23-8

Lennard ES; Minshew BH; Dellinger EP et al. Stratified outcome comparison of clindamycin-gentamicin vs chloramphenicol-gentamicin for treatment of intra-abdominal sepsis. Arch Surg 1985 Aug;120 (8):889-98

CLOTRIMAZOLE

FDA INDICATIONS
- Oral candidiasis
- Candidal vaginitis
- Dematomycosis

USUAL ADULT DOSING: Thrush: 10mg troche 5x/d (dissolved in mouth). Candida vaginitis: 100mg intravaginal tab bid x 3 days (preferred) or 100mg qd x 7 days or 500mg x1. Cutaneous candidiasis: apply cream, solution, or lotion to affected areas bid x 2-8 wks.

Dosing Adjustments
GFR 50-80 mL/min: Usual dose
GFR 10-50 mL/min: Usual dose
GFR<10 mL/min: Usual dose
Hemodialysis: Usual dose
Peritoneal Dialysis: Usual dose

ADVERSE DRUG REACTIONS: Occasional: Burning; itching; erythema (intravaginal and topical administration). Increase in liver enzymes; nausea and vomiting (lozenge)

DRUG INTERACTIONS
No significant interactions noted.

PREGNANCY RISK: C-Teratogenic in animal studies at high doses. No human data available with lozenge. No adverse effect seen with intravaginal administration during the 2nd and 3rd trimester.

BREAST FEEDING: No data.

COMMENTS: Oral and topical antifungal agent that is most commonly used for mucosal candida infections. Slightly less effective (measured as disease free period post-therapy) than fluconazole but preferred as 1st line due to the concern over azole-resistant candidiasis with long-term use of fluconazole.

FORMS (◆ DENOTES AVAILABLE GENERICALLY)

Brand name	Preparation	Mfr.	Route	Form	Strength	Cost (AWP)
Clotrimazole	Clotrimazole	◆ Ivax	vaginal	cre	1% (45g)	$8.99
Clotrimazole Troche	Clotrimazole	◆ Roxane	MM	loz	10mg	$1.61

SELECTED READINGS
Pons V, Greenspan D, Debruin M, et al. Therapy for oropharyngeal candidiasis in HIV-infected patients: a randomized, prospective multicenter study of oral fluconazole versus clotrimazole troches. The Multicenter Study Group. J Acquir Immune Defic Syndr. 1993;6:1311-6.

COLISTIMETHATE

FDA INDICATIONS
- Enteritis (caused by E. coli)
- External auditory canal infections (in combination with neomycin and hydrocortisone)
- Mastoidectomy infections (in combination with neomycin and hydrocortisone)
- Shigella gastroenteritis
- Acute or chronic infections due to sensitive strains of Pseudomonas aeruginosa

ANTI-INFECTIVES

USUAL ADULT DOSING: Otic drops q8-6h; IV: 2.5-5mg/kg/day divided q8h; inhalation: 75mg in 3mL NS via nebulizer 2x/day.

Dosing Adjustments
GFR 50-80 mL/min: 2.5-3.8 mg/kg/day divided in two doses
GFR 10-50 mL/min: 1.5-2.5 mg/kg q24h
GFR<10 mL/min: 1.5mg/kg q48h
Hemodialysis: No supplementation required, not removed in HD

ADVERSE DRUG REACTIONS: Occasional: Nephrotoxicity (20%; reversible and dose dependent); neurotoxicity-circumoral and peripheral paresthesia, dizziness, vertigo, ataxia, blurred vision, slurred speech with IM or IV use. **Rare:** Respiratory depression.

DRUG INTERACTIONS
Amikacin: may increase neuromuscular blockade.
Nondepolarizing muscle relaxants (atracurium, vecuronium, pancuronium, tubocurarine): Neuromuscular blockade may be enhanced with IM or IV use. Avoid co-administration, if concurrent administration is needed titrate the nondepolarizing muscle relaxant slowly and monitor neuromuscular function closely.

PREGNANCY RISK: B-No reports linking colistimethate with congenital defects have been located.

BREAST FEEDING: Colistimethate is excreted in breast milk. Milk:plasma ratio is 0.17.

COMMENTS: Parenteral & topical polymyxin rarely used as first line therapy due to earlier reports of nephrotoxicity and neurotoxicity, however a recent study did not support such findings (CID 2003;36: 1111). Inhaled use with CF. Active against virtually all P. aeruginosa and Acinetobacter strains but Proteus is usually resistant and may cause superinfection. An acceptable second line agent for VAP.

FORMS (♦ DENOTES AVAILABLE GENERICALLY)

Brand name	Preparation	Mfr.	Route	Form	Strength	Cost (AWP)
Coly-Mycin M	Colis-timethate sodium	♦ Monarch	IV	vial	150mg	$64.34

SELECTED READINGS

Garnacho-Montero J. et al. Treatment of Multidrug-Resistant Acinetobacter baumannii Ventilator-Associated Pneumonia with Intravenous Colistin: A Comparison with Imipenem-Susceptible VAP. CID 2003; 36:1111-8

Li J, Nation RL, Milne RW et al. Evaluation of colistin as an agent against multi-resistant Gram-negative bacteria. Int J Antimicrob Agents. 2005 Jan;25(1):11-25

Jensen T, et al. Cystic Fibrosis inhalation therapy. J Antimicrob Chemother 1987 Jun;19(6):831-8

DAPSONE

FDA INDICATIONS
- Leprosy
- Dermatitis herpetiformis

USUAL ADULT DOSING: 25-100mg PO qd. PCP prophylaxis: 100mg PO qd; PCP treatment: dapsone 100mg PO qd plus trimethoprim 5mg/kg q8h x 21 d.

Dosing Adjustments
GFR 50-80 mL/min: Usual dose
GFR 10-50 mL/min: Usual dose
GFR<10 mL/min: No data, metabolite excreted renally, may need adjustment

ADVERSE DRUG REACTIONS: Frequent: Rash, fever, nausea, anorexia, neutropenia.
Occasional: Blood dyscrasias (methemoglobinemia & sulfhemoglobinemia +/- G6PD def., sx - cyanosis & dark urine); nephrotic syndrome; blurred vision; photosensitivity; tinnitis; insomnia; irritability; headache.

DRUG INTERACTIONS

Antacids, H2 blockers, and **PPIs:** may decrease dapsone absorption.
Didanosine: Citrate phosphate buffer in didanosine renders dapsone insoluble therefore decreasing the absorption (no interactions with ddI EC). Dapsone must be administered at least 2 hours before didanosine administration (no interactions with ddI EC).
Rifampin: decreases dapsone serum levels. Avoid co-administration.
Trimethoprim: Increased serum level of both dapsone (40%) and trimethoprim (48%). Monitor of clinical toxicity (methemoglobinemia).

PREGNANCY RISK: C-No adverse effect reported with the use of dapsone.

BREAST FEEDING: Excreted in breast milk. The American Academy of Pediatrics considers dapsone compatible with breast feeding.

COMMENTS: Oral agent used for treatment and prevention of P. jiroveci and leprosy. Strong oxidizing agent, therefore G6PD deficiency screening is recommended. In addition to hemolytic anemia, may cause methemoglobinemia and bone marrow suppression.

FORMS

Brand name	Preparation	Mfr.	Route	Form	Strength	Cost (AWP)
Dapsone	Dapsone	Jacobus	PO	tab	25mg; 100mg	$0.20; $0.21

DAPTOMYCIN

FDA INDICATIONS

• Treatment of complicated skin and skin structure infections caused by susceptible strains of gram-positive microorganism (including MSSA and MRSA)

USUAL ADULT DOSING: 4mg/kg IV qd (FDA approved dose) 6mg/kg IV qd (ongoing trials for bacteremia and endocarditis, closer monitoring for myopathy recommended)

Dosing Adjustments
GFR 50-80 mL/min: 4mg/kg IV q24h
GFR 10-50 mL/min: Cr Clearance >30mL/min: 4mg/kg IV q24h Cr Clearance <30mL/min: 4mg/kg IV q48h
GFR<10 mL/min: 4mg/kg IV q48h
Hemodialysis: 4mg/kg IV q48h (minimal removal with HD 15% removal following 4hrs of HD)
Peritoneal Dialysis: 4mg/kg IV q48h (minimal removal with PD 11% removal following 48hrs of PD)
↓ *Hepatic Function:* 4mg/kg IV q24h (with moderate Child-Pugh Class B)

ADVERSE DRUG REACTIONS: Generally well tolerated. **Occasional:** LFTs elevation, dose dependent CPK elevation (reversible) with or without myopathy. Higher incidence of myopathy seen with 4mg/kg q12h (twice the recommended dose). **Rare:** neuropathy

DRUG INTERACTIONS

Daptomycin is not an inhibitor or inducer of human CYP450 isoform. Pharmacokinetic and pharmacodynamic interaction studies involving aztreonam, tobramycin, warfarin (single dose study), simvastatin, and probenecid did not result in interactions.

PREGNANCY RISK: B Animal data using 3-6 times the human dose did not result in teratogenicity. No human data.

BREAST FEEDING: No data.

COMMENTS: Daptomycin has a similar spectrum of activity to linezolid which includes virtually all gram-positive organisms including E. faecalis and E. faecium (including VRE) and S. aureus (including MRSA). Daptomycin should not be used for pneumonia due to high failure rates.

FORMS

Brand name	Preparation	Mfr.	Route	Form	Strength	Cost (AWP)
Cubicin	Daptomycin	Cubist	IV	vial	500mg	$171.07

SELECTED READINGS

Arbeit RD, Maki D, Tally FP et al. The safety and efficacy of daptomycin for the treatment of complicated skin and skin-structure infections. Clin Infect Dis. 2004;38(12):1673-81.

Personal communication. -. Cubist pharmaceuticals, Inc. Data on file.

DICLOXACILLIN

FDA INDICATIONS

- Respiratory tract infections (pharyngitis and pneumonia)
- Staphylococcal infections
- Streptococcal infections
- Skin and soft tissue infections

USUAL ADULT DOSING: Mild infections: 125 PO qid. Moderate to severe infections: 250-500mg PO qid.

Dosing Adjustments

GFR 50-80 mL/min: Usual dose
GFR 10-50 mL/min: Usual dose
GFR<10 mL/min: Usual dose
Hemodialysis: Usual regimen
Peritoneal Dialysis: Usual regimen

ADVERSE DRUG REACTIONS: Frequent: hypersensitivity reactions; rash; diarrhea. **Occasional:** GI intolerance; drug fever; Coombs' test positive; Jarisch-Herxheimer reaction. **Rare:** anaphylaxis.

DRUG INTERACTIONS

Tetracyclines: In vitro antagonism when co-administered. Bactericidal effect of penicillins may be diminished in vivo. Avoid concurrent administration. In two studies involving a total of 79 patients with pneumococcal meningitis treated with either penicillin plus tetracyclines or penicillin monotherapy there was a higher mortality rate (79-85%) in the combination therapy compared to penicillin monotherapy (30-33%). (Arch Intern Med 1951:88:489, Ann Intern Med 1961; 55:545). However there was not a difference in mortality between penicillin monotherapy and penicillin plus tetracycline in the treatment of pneumococcal pneumonia. (Arch Intern Med 1953; 91:197).

PREGNANCY RISK: B-Several collaborative perinatal project reports involving over 12,000 exposures to penicillin derivatives during the first trimester indicated no association between penicillin derivative drugs and birth defects.

BREAST FEEDING: Excreted in breast milk in low concentration. No adverse effects have been reported.

COMMENTS: Oral anti-staphylococcal penicillin with better bioavailability compared to cloxacillin. QID administration may decrease adherence for some patients.

FORMS (♦ DENOTES AVAILABLE GENERICALLY)

Brand name	Preparation	Mfr.	Route	Form	Strength	Cost (AWP)
Dicloxacillin sodium	Dicloxacillin sodium	♦ Sandoz	PO	cap	250mg; 500mg	$0.66; $1.20

SELECTED READINGS

Stevens DL, Smith LG, Bruss JB et al. Randomized comparison of linezolid (PNU-100766) versus oxacillin-dicloxacillin for treatment of complicated skin and soft tissue infections. AAC 2000;44 (12):3408-13.

DIDANOSINE (ddI)

FDA INDICATIONS

- HIV (in combination with other antiretrovirals)

USUAL ADULT DOSING: Wt >60kg dose: 400mg PO qd (tabs or EC caps) or 500mg PO qd (powder)on empty stomach. Wt <60kg dose: 250mg PO qd (tabs or ED caps) or 334mg PO qd (powder). Total daily dose may also be taken in two divided doses.

Dosing Adjustments

GFR 50-80 mL/min: Wt >60kg dose: 400mg PO qd (tabs) or 500mg PO qd (powder). Wt <60kg dose: 250mg PO qd (tabs) or 334mg PO qd (powder).

GFR 10-50 mL/min: 50% of usual dose qd

GFR<10 mL/min: 25% of usual dose qd

Hemodialysis: 25% of usual dose qd, on days of dialysis give post dialysis.

Peritoneal Dialysis: 25% of usual dose (little effec on removal with PD)[Clin Pharmacol Ther. 1996;60(5):535].

ADVERSE DRUG REACTIONS: GI intolerance (diarrhea, mouth sores), peripheral neuropathy in (5-12% of patients); PANCREATITIS (1-9% of patients, 6% cases fatal); transaminase elevation; rare cases of LACTIC ACIDOSIS and severe hepatomegaly with steatosis.

PREGNANCY RISK: B-Human studies demonstrated 35% (range 23-59%) placental passage. In 8 patients studied, no toxicities were observed in mothers, infants. (5th Conference Retroviral Oppor Infect 1998 Feb 1-5; 121 (Abst. No 226). Due to the small number of patients no firm conclusion can be made. PACTG 249 Phase I study showed that ddI was well tolerated by women and fetus when started at week 26-36. Pregnant patients may be at increased risk of lactic acidosis (FDA warns against its use in combination with d4T in pregnant patients).

BREAST FEEDING: Unknown breast milk excretion. Breast feeding is not recommended in the U.S in order to avoid post-natal transmission of HIV to the child, who may not yet be infected.

COMMENTS: GI intolerance may be bothersome in some patients. The enteric coated form (Videx EC) is now preferred as it is better tolerated, once daily and has fewer drug interactions. Both the buffered and EC formulations must be taken on an empty stomach. Major side effects are pancreatitis and peripheral neuropathy, especially if taken with d4T. Avoid ddI + d4T in pregnancy.

FORMS (♦ DENOTES AVAILABLE GENERICALLY)

Brand name	Preparation	Mfr.	Route	Form	Strength	Cost (AWP)
Videx	Didanosine (ddI)	♦ Bristol-Myers Squibb	PO	chew tab	25mg; 50mg; 100mg; 200mg; 150mg	$0.61; $1.23; $2.45; $4.91; $3.68
Videx EC	Didanosine (ddI)	♦ Bristol-Myers Squibb	PO	cap, EC	200mg; 250mg; 400mg	$5.56; $7.09; $11.07
			PO	Cap, EC	125mg	$3.48

(continued)

Brand name	Preparation	Mfr.	Route	Form	Strength	Cost (AWP)
Videx Pediatric	Didanosine (ddI)	Bristol-Myers Squibb	PO	susp	10mg/mL	$2.35 per 5mL

DIRITHROMYCIN

FDA INDICATIONS

- Acute bacterial bronchitis
- Legionnaires' disease
- Pharyngitis
- Community acquired pneumonia
- Skin and soft tissue infections

USUAL ADULT DOSING: 500mg PO qd

Dosing Adjustments

GFR 50-80 mL/min: Usual dose

GFR 10-50 mL/min: Usual dose

GFR<10 mL/min: Usual dose

Hemodialysis: Usual dose

Peritoneal Dialysis: Usual dose

↓ *Hepatic Function:* No dose adjustment (LaBreque JAC 1993; 32: 741)

ADVERSE DRUG REACTIONS: Frequent: GI intolerance abdominal pain and nausea. **Occasional:** dizziness; headache; weakness

DRUG INTERACTIONS

No significant interaction with CYP3A4.

Cyclosporin: Conflicting data, but may increase cyclosporin levels. With concurrent administration, close monitoring of cyclosporin level is indicated with dose adjustment when needed

Pimozide: Possible increase in pimozide concentration which may result in QT prolongation and cardiac arrhythmia. Contraindicated by manufacturer. Do not co-administer.

PREGNANCY RISK: C-Animal data shows significant increase in the incidence of fetal growth retardation and an increased occurrence of incomplete ossification. No human data is available.

BREAST FEEDING: No data available for dirithromycin, risk probably minimal based on data with erythromycin.

COMMENTS: An oral macrolide that shows no clear advantage over erythromycin. GI toxicity similar to erythromycin. Unlike erythromycin, no drug interactions with drug metabolized by the CYP 450 3A system. Should not be used for bacteremia due to inadequate serum concentration.

FORMS

Brand name	Preparation	Mfr.	Route	Form	Strength	Cost (AWP)
Dynabac	Dirithromycin	Muro	PO	tab	250mg	$4.25

SELECTED READINGS

Wasilewski MM; Johns D; Sides GD. Five-day dirithromycin therapy is as effective as seven-day erythromycin therapy for acute exacerbations of chronic bronchitis. J Antimicrob Chemother 1999 Apr;43(4):541-8

DOCOSANOL

FDA INDICATIONS

• Herpes labialis

USUAL ADULT DOSING: Apply topically 5 times per day as soon as possible during prodromal stage. Available over the counter

Dosing Adjustments

GFR 50-80 mL/min: No data: usual dose likely

GFR 10-50 mL/min: No data: usual dose likely

GFR<10 mL/min: No data: usual dose likely

Hemodialysis: No data: usual dose likely

Peritoneal Dialysis: No data: usual dose likely

↓ *Hepatic Function:* No data: usual dose likely

ADVERSE DRUG REACTIONS: Occasional: Burning/stinging with topical application. **Rare:** pruritis, rash.

DRUG INTERACTIONS

No significant interactions noted.

PREGNANCY RISK: C

BREAST FEEDING: No data.

COMMENTS: Topical docosanol may improve healing time by about 1 day if applied during the prodromal stage, but experimental animal study did not show a benefit (Arch Derm 2001; 137:1153). The inconvenience of 5x per day administration and its cost ($13.20) may limit the use of this over the counter (OTC) product.

FORMS

Brand name	Preparation	Mfr.	Route	Form	Strength	Cost (AWP)
Abreva	Docosanol	GlaxoSmithKline	topical	cream	10% (2g)	$13.20

SELECTED READINGS

McKeough MB, Spruance SL . Comparison of New Topical Treatments for Herpes Labialis: Efficacy of Penciclovir Cream, Acyclovir Cream, and n-Docosanol Cream Against Experimental Cutaneous Herpes Simplex Virus Type 1 Infection . Arch Derm 2001;137:1153

DOXYCYCLINE

FDA INDICATIONS

• Anthrax due to Bacillus anthracis, including inhalation anthrax (post-exposure). CDC recommends as first line agent + 1-2 additional agents with in vitro activity (for inhalation anthrax, see "Anthrax" in the Diagnoses section).

• Granuloma inguinale caused by Calymmatobacterium granulomatis.

• Lymphogranuloma venereum caused by chlamydia species.

• Psittacosis caused by Chlamydia psittaci.

• Q fever

• Rickettsial pox

• Rocky mountain spotted fever

• Typhus infections

• Nongonococcal urethritis

• Yaws caused by T. pertenue.

ANTI-INFECTIVES

USUAL ADULT DOSING: General dose: 100mg PO or IV q12h. Uncomplicated non-GC (urethral, endocervical, or rectal): 100mg PO bid x7d.

Dosing Adjustments
GFR 50-80 mL/min: Usual dose
GFR 10-50 mL/min: Usual dose
GFR<10 mL/min: Usual dose
Hemodialysis: Usual regimen
Peritoneal Dialysis: Usual regimen

ADVERSE DRUG REACTIONS: Frequent: Stains and deforms teeth in children up to 8 yrs old. **Occasional:** Esophagitis; hepatitis; GI intolerance; candidiasis; photosensitivity.

DRUG INTERACTIONS

Bismuth Salts (bismuth subsalicylate-Pepto-Bismol): Bismuth salts chelate tetracyclines resulting in a decreased absorption of tetracycline. Administer bismuth 2 hours after tetracycline.

Digoxin: May result in increased digoxin concentration (in about 10% of patients). May be due to tetracycline's alteration of bowel flora responsible for digoxin metabolism.

Penicillins: In vitro antagonism when co-administered. Bactericidal effect of penicillins may be diminished in vivo. Avoid co-administration.

Polyvalent metal cations (aluminum, zinc, magnesium, iron, calcium [milk"): Polyvalent metal cations form an insoluble chelate with tetracyclines resulting in decreased absorption and serum level of tetracyclines. Separate administration by 4 hours.

Urinary alkalinizers (sodium lactate, sodium bicarbonate): Increased urinary excretion of tetracyclines by 24-65%) resulting in lower serum concentration.

Warfarin: May increase hypoprothrombinemia. Monitor INR closely.

PREGNANCY RISK: D-Tetracyclines are contraindicated in pregnancy due to retardation of skeletal development and bone growth; enamel hypoplasia and discoloration of teeth of fetus. Maternal liver toxicity has also been reported.

BREAST FEEDING: Tetracyclines are excreted in breast milk at very low concentrations. There is theoretical possibility of dental staining and inhibition of bone growth, but infants exposed to tetracyclines have blood levels less than 0.05mcg/mL.

COMMENTS: Oral or parenteral twice daily tetracycline. Can be administered with or without food. Preferred tetracycline derivative in patients with renal failure. Agents of choice for rickettsial and vibrio infections.

FORMS (◆ DENOTES AVAILABLE GENERICALLY)

Brand name	Preparation	Mfr.	Route	Form	Strength	Cost (AWP)
Vibramycin	Doxycycline	◆ Pfizer	PO	cap	100mg	$5.10
			PO	susp	25mg/5mL	$1.30 per 5mL
			PO	syrup	50mg/5mL	$2.39 per 5mL
Adoxa	Doxycycline	Doak	PO	tab	50mg; 75mg; 100mg	$3.00; $3.58; $4.23
Monodox	Doxycycline	Watson	PO	cap	50mg; 100mg	$1.97; $3.07
Doryx	Doxycycline Hyclate	Warner Chilcott	PO	cap, EC	75mg; 100mg	$4.31; $5.07
Doxycycline Hyclate	Doxycycline	◆ Bedford	IV	vial	100mg	$14.16

SELECTED READINGS

Nadelman RB, et al. Prophylaxis With Single-Dose Doxycycline for the Prevention of Lyme Disease After an Ixodes Scapularis Tick Bite . NEJM 2001; 345: 79

DROTRECOGIN ALPHA

FDA INDICATIONS

- Reduction of mortality in adult patients with severe sepsis (sepsis associated with acute organ dysfunction) who have a high risk of death (e.g., as determined by APACHE II score [see Appendix II]). Not indicated in the pediatric population.

USUAL ADULT DOSING: 24mcg/kg/hr x 96 hours, if infusion is interrupted drotrecogin should be restarted at 24mcg/kg/hr (no bolus dose recommended).

Dosing Adjustments

GFR 50-80 mL/min: Limited data. Usual dose: 24 mcg/kg/hr x 96 hours

GFR 10-50 mL/min: See above

GFR<10 mL/min: See above.

Hemodialysis: See above

Peritoneal Dialysis: See above

↓ *Hepatic Function:* See above

ADVERSE DRUG REACTIONS: Bleeding reported in 25% of drotrecogin treated patients compared to 18% in placebo treated patients. Serious bleeding event reported in 3.5% of drotrecogin treated vs. 2% in placebo treated patients (P=0.06). Intracranial hemorrhage reported in 0.2-2.5%.

PREGNANCY RISK: C- No data.

BREAST FEEDING: No data.

COMMENTS: Due to the risk of severe bleeding and lack of demonstrable benefit in patients with APACHE II score of <25 (see Appendix II), the recommended criteria for use are: 1) patients with severe sepsis as determined by an APACHE II score of >25 with a suspected or proven source of infection, with three or more signs of systemic inflammation (see "Sepsis" in the Diagnoses section), and 2) sepsis-induced organ dysfunction of >1 organ. Drotrecogin showed no improvement over placebo in the primary endpoint of "Composite Time to Complete Organ Failure Resolution" in a interim analysis of a RCT. Risk of bleed may be higher.

FORMS

Brand name	Preparation	Mfr.	Route	Form	Strength	Cost (AWP)
Xigris	Drotrecogin alfa	Eli Lilly	IV	vial	5mg ; 20mg	$269.94; $1079.77

SELECTED READINGS

Gordon RB, Vincent JL, Laterre PF et al. Efficacy and Safety of Recombinant Human Activated Protein C For Severe Sepsis. NEJM 2001 344: 699.

Anon. Overview of Drotrecogin Product Development. www.fda.gov

EFAVIRENZ (EFV)

FDA INDICATIONS

- HIV infection treatment in combination with other antiretrovirals

USUAL ADULT DOSING: EFV 600mg PO qhs (avoid high fat meal, take on empty stomach). Dosing w/ PI: IDV 1000mg q8h with EFV 600mg qhs/ FPV 700mg/RTV 100mg with EFV 600mg qhs/ NFV 1200mg bid with EFV 600mg qhs, LPV 533mg (4caps) bid with EFV 600mg qhs.

Dosing Adjustments
GFR 50-80 mL/min: 600mg qhs
GFR 10-50 mL/min: usual dose likely
GFR<10 mL/min: usual dose likely
Hemodialysis: No data: 600mg qhs (unlikely to be dialysed out)

ADVERSE DRUG REACTIONS: Morbilliform rash in (15-27% of patients with 1-2% requiring discontinuation); one case of Stevens-Johnson syndrome reported; CNS effects (confusion, depersonalization, abnormal dreams) usually seen on day 1 (in up to 52% of patients); resolves in 2-4weeks

DRUG INTERACTIONS
Substrate of CYP3A4 and CYP2B6; inducer of CYP3A4 and CYP2B6; weak inhibitor of CYP3A4, 2B6, 2C9, and 2C19. Inducers of CYP3A4 and CYP2B6 may decrease EFV serum levels. EFV generally decreases serum levels of CYP3A4 and CYP2B6 substrates.
Contraindicated with: ergot alkaloids, midazolam, triazolam, terfenadine, astemizole, cisapride, rifapentine, and St Johns wort.

PREGNANCY RISK: C-Placental passage of 100% seen in cynomalgus monkeys, rats and rabbits. Teratogenicity demonstrated in cynomalgus monkeys resulting in anencephaly.

BREAST FEEDING: No human data, breast milk excretion in animal studies. Breast feeding is not recommended in the U.S. in order to avoid post-natal transmission of HIV to the child, who may not yet be infected.

COMMENTS: Potent non-nucleoside reverse transcriptase inhibitor. CNS side effects (confusion, depersonalization, abnormal dreams) seen in up to 52% of patients, but generally resolves within 2-4 weeks with continued treatment. Generally well tolerated with a convenient once a day dosing schedule.

FORMS

Brand name	Preparation	Mfr.	Route	Form	Strength	Cost (AWP)
Sustiva	Efavirenz (EFV)	Bristol-Myers Squibb	PO	cap	50mg; 100mg; 200mg	$1.33; $2.66; $5.33
			PO	tab	600mg	$15.98

EMTRICITABINE (FTC)

FDA INDICATIONS

• HIV-infection in adults in combination with other antiretroviral agents

USUAL ADULT DOSING: Emtricitabine (FTC) 200mg PO qd with or without meals. May be administered as combination product TDF300mg/FTC200mg (Truvada) 1 tablet PO QD with or without food.

Dosing Adjustments
GFR 50-80 mL/min: 200mg q24hrs
GFR 10-50 mL/min: 30-49mL/min: 200mg q48hrs. 15-29 mL/min: 200mg q72hrs.
GFR<10 mL/min: <15mK/min: 200mg q96 hrs.
Hemodialysis: 200mg q96hrs (30% of dose removed with 3-hr HD, on days of dialysis dose post-HD).
Peritoneal Dialysis: No data. 200mg q96hrs likely.
↓ *Hepatic Function:* No data. Usual dose likely

ADVERSE DRUG REACTIONS: Common: Generally well tolerated. Mild asymptomatic skin hyperpigmentation on the palm and/or soles. Asymptomatic and transient CPK elevation.
Occasional: Headache, diarrhea, nausea, asthenia, and rash that required discontinuation in approx. 1% of patients. Since emtricitabine has activity against hepatitis

B, hepatitis B exacerbation upon discontinuation of emtricitabine in pts coinfected with hepatitis B and HIV has been reported.

DRUG INTERACTIONS

Emtricitabine is not a substrate, inhibitor, or inducer of any CYP450 isoforms, likelihood of clinically significant drug interactions are low. Tenofovir Cmin was increased by 20% but AUC was unchanged.

PREGNANCY RISK: B-No human data. In animal studies, emtricitabine at 120-fold higher than human exposure did not result in fetal malformation.

BREAST FEEDING: No data. Breast feeding is not recommended for HIV-infected patients (in the US).

COMMENTS: Similar to lamivudine (3TC), emtricitabine (FTC) has activity against HBV, is well tolerated, and can be dosed once a day. FTC resistance profile is identical to that of 3TC; therefore, it offers really no clear advantage over 3TC. However, coformulatation of FTC with tenofovir, clinicians will be able to prescribe a simple, well-tolerated, and potent antiretroviral regimen.

FORMS

Brand name	Preparation	Mfr.	Route	Form	Strength	Cost (AWP)
Emtriva	Emtricitabine (FTC)	Gilead	PO	cap	200mg	$10.61
Truvada	tenofovir (TDF)/emtric-itabine (FTC)	Gilead	PO	tab	300mg/FTC 200mg	$26.03

SELECTED READINGS

. Study 301A submitted to the FDA . FDA briefing

Wakeford C et al. Study 303 was an open-label, active-controlled study comparing once daily emtricitabine (FTC) to twice daily lamivudine (3TC), in combination with d4T or AZT and a PI or NNRTI. CROI 2003, abstract 550

Molina et al. Once-daily Combination of FTC, ddI, and EFV vs. Continued PI-based HAART in HIV-infected Adults with Undetectable Plasma HIV-RNA: 48-week Results of a Prospective Randomized Multicenter Trial. 2003 CROI, abstract 551

ENFUVIRTIDE (ENF; T-20)

FDA INDICATIONS

- HIV-1 infection in treatment-experienced patients with evidence of HIV-1 replication despite ongoing antiretroviral therapy (in combination with other antiretroviral agents)

USUAL ADULT DOSING: 90mg (1mL) SQ q12h into upper arm, anterior thigh or abdomen with each injection given at a site different from the preceding injection site (prior to administration, reconstitute with 1.1mL of sterile water for injection giving a volume of 1.2mL).

Dosing Adjustments

GFR 50-80 mL/min: Estimated Clearance >35mL/min: 90mg SC q12h

GFR 10-50 mL/min: >35-50 mL/min: No significant change in PK parameters. Use usual dose

GFR<10 mL/min: <35mL/min: No data, usual dose likely.

Hemodialysis: No data, usual dose likely.

ADVERSE DRUG REACTIONS: Common ADR: local site reaction (grade 3 or 4) including pain (9%), erythema (32%), pruritus (4%), induration (57%), and nodules or cysts (26%)(with

3% requiring d/c). **Occasional:** Eosinophilia; bacterial pneumonia (in 4.68 events vs. 0.61 events per 100 pts-years

DRUG INTERACTIONS

No significant interactions noted. In vitro, enfuvirtide did not inhibit or induce the metabolism of CYP3A4, CYP2D6, CYP1A2, CYP2C19 or CYP2E1 substrates. Does not interact with SQV/r, RTV, or rifampin. (M. Boyd et al. 10th CROI 2003, Abstract 541).

PREGNANCY RISK: B Not teratogenic in animal studies. No human data.

BREAST FEEDING: Breastfeeding not recommended.

COMMENTS: Enfuvirtide offers clinicians an effective new antiretroviral class for the management of treatment-experienced patients. A clear advantage of enfuvirtide is the lack of cross-resistance with currently available antiretrovirals, however, as with other antiretrovirals and as seen in clinical trials, salvage therapy with enfuvirtide is only as good as the background regimen with which it is combined

FORMS

Brand name	Preparation	Mfr.	Route	Form	Strength	Cost (AWP)
Fuzeon	Enfuvirtide (T-20)	Roche	SC	kit	90mg	$2116.93 per box

SELECTED READINGS

Henry K et al./Clotet B et al. TORO 1 and TORO 2. 14th Int Conf AIDS 2002 Jul 7-12; 14: Abstract LbOr19A LbOr19B

ENTECAVIR

FDA INDICATIONS

- Chronic hepatitis B (HBV) infection in adult patients with evidence of active disease (active viral replication, elevated ALT or AST or histologic evidence)

USUAL ADULT DOSING: For nucleoside-na ve patients: 0.5mg PO qd on an empty stomach. For lamivudine (3TC) refractory patients: 1mg PO qd on an empty stomach (2hrs before or after food).

Dosing Adjustments

GFR 50-80 mL/min: usual dosing

GFR 10-50 mL/min: CrCl 30-49 mL/min, NRTI naïve: 0.25mg qd; 3TC-resist: 0.5mg qd. CrCl 10-29 mL/min, NRTI naïve: 0.15mg qd; 3TC-res. 0.25mg qd

GFR<10 mL/min: Cr Clearance <10mL/min: nucleoside naïve: 0.05mg qd; 3TC-refractory: 0.1mg qd.

Hemodialysis: Nucleoside naïve: 0.05mg qd (post HD); 3TC-refractory: 0.1mg qd (post HD).

Peritoneal Dialysis: Nucleoside naïve: 0.05mg qd; 3TC-refractory: 0.1mg qd.

↓ *Hepatic Function:* Usual dose

ADVERSE DRUG REACTIONS: Generally well tolerated with side effect profile comparable to lamivudine and placebo in clinical trials. **Rare:** headache, fatigue, nausea, diarrhea, and insomnia. Low likelihood of lactic acidosis.

DRUG INTERACTIONS

No significant interactions noted.

PREGNANCY RISK: C-Negative embryotoxicity and maternal toxicity in rat and rabbit studies at 28 and 212 times the levels achieved with the highest daily dose (1mg/day). Rat and rabbit embyo and fetal toxicities seen at 3,100 times the human drug levels. No studies in humans. Pregnancy registry for entecavir: 1-800-258-4263

BREAST FEEDING: No human data, breast milk excretion in animal studies. Breast feeding is not recommended.

COMMENTS: Entecavir is an effective and well tolerated treatment option for HBV-infected patient who are treatment naive or lamivudine-resistant. Unlike adefovir, entecavir has no activity against HIV, therefore may be a good option in co-infected patients with high CD4 count who only needs HBV treatment.

FORMS

Brand name	Preparation	Mfr.	Route	Form	Strength	Cost (AWP)
Baraclude	Entecavir	Bristol-Myers Squibb	PO	Oral solution	0.05mg/mL (210mL)	$518/200mL
			PO	tablets	0.5 mg, 1mg	$23.68

SELECTED READINGS

Wilkin Pessoa, B Gazzard, A Huang et al. Entecavir in HIV/HBV-co-infected Patients: Safety and Efficacy in a Phase II Study (ETV-038). 12th Conference on Retroviruses and Opportunistic Infection 2005, Boston MA, Feb 22-25; Abstract 123

Product Information. Study AI463022 (HIV-, HBeAg + patients) and AI463027 (HIV-, HBeAg- patients) . Baraclude package insert. Bristol-Myers Squibb Company: Princeton, NJ, March 2005.

Product Information. Study AI463026. Baraclude package insert. Bristol-Myers Squibb Company: Princeton, NJ, March 2005.

ERTAPENEM

FDA INDICATIONS
- Complicated intra-abdominal infections
- Complicated skin and skin structure infections
- Community-acquired pneumonia
- Complicated urinary tract infections (including Pyelonephritis)
- Acute pelvic infections (Postpartum endomyometritis, septic abortion, and postsurgical gynecologic infections)

USUAL ADULT DOSING: CAP, complicated UTI, complicated soft tissue infection, and intra-abdominal infection: 1g IV or IM qd x 10-14 days.

Dosing Adjustments
GFR 50-80 mL/min: Usual dose
GFR 10-50 mL/min: Usual dose
GFR<10 mL/min: <30 mL/min: 500mg qd
Hemodialysis: 500mg qd(150mg supplement post-HD if daily dose given 6 hours within HD)
↓ *Hepatic Function:* 1g qd (usual dose)

ADVERSE DRUG REACTIONS: Generally well tolerated. **Occasional:** diarrhea, n/v, phlebitis, headache. **Rare:** seizures (reported in 0.5% of patients; patients with renal insufficiency and/or CNS disorder are at increased risk).

DRUG INTERACTIONS
Does not interact with cytochrome p450 isoform (1A2, 2C9, 2C19, 2D6, 2E1, and 3A4) or P-glycoprotein.
Probenecid: Increases ertapenem AUC by 25%. Not compatible with dextrose (do not co-infuse with dextrose or other medications).

PREGNANCY RISK: B-Not teratogenic in animal studies. No human data.

BREAST FEEDING: Excreted in breast milk. Use only when clearly indicated.

ANTI-INFECTIVES

COMMENTS: Ertapenem has a spectrum of activity that includes all anaerobes and many gram-negative bacilli with the exception of P. aeruginosa and Acinetobacter. Risk of seizure is reported at 0.5% in clinical trials. T1/2 of 4-5h suggests caution in using q24h dosing for severely ill patients (i.e bacteremia and/or ICU). May be used as a convenient once-a-day outpatient IV antibiotic.

FORMS

Brand name	Preparation	Mfr.	Route	Form	Strength	Cost (AWP)
Invanz	Ertapenem sodium	Merck	IV	vial	1000mg	$53.86

SELECTED READINGS

Product Information. Ertapenem package insert.

Ortiz-Ruiz G et al. A Study Evaluating the Efficacy, Safety, and Tolerability of Ertapenem versus Ceftriaxone for the Treatment of Community-Acquired Pneumonia in Adults . CID 2002;34:1076

Graham DR, Lucasti C, Malafaia O et al. Ertapenem Once Daily Versus Pip/Tazo 4 Times per Day for Treatment of Complicated Skin and Skin-structure Infections in Adults: Results of a Prospective, Randomized, Double-Blind Multicenter Study. CID 2002; 34

ERYTHROMYCIN

FDA INDICATIONS

- Preoperative bowel preparation (with neomycin)
- Syphilis caused by Treponema pallidum (in patients allergic to the penicillins)
- Acute exacerbations of chronic bronchitis and sinusitis
- Acute otitis media and pharyngitis
- Diphtheria infections due to Corynebacterium diphtheriae, as an adjunct to antitoxin
- Intestinal amebiasis caused by Entamoeba histolytica
- Conjunctivitis in the newborn caused by Chlamydia trachomatis
- Legionnaires' disease
- Pertussis
- Rheumatic fever prophylaxis

USUAL ADULT DOSING: Erythromycin base 250-500mg PO tid-qid; erythromycin estolate 250-500mg PO qid; erythromycin ethylsuccinate 400-800mg PO qid; 0.5-1g IV q6h; bowel prep-1g PO 1pm, 2pm and 11pm prior to surgery.

Dosing Adjustments
GFR 50-80 mL/min: Usual dose
GFR 10-50 mL/min: Usual dose
GFR<10 mL/min: Usual dose
Hemodialysis: Usual regimen
Peritoneal Dialysis: Usual regimen
↓ *Hepatic Function:* No data. May require dose adjustment with severe hepatic insufficiency.

ADVERSE DRUG REACTIONS: Frequent: GI intolerance (oral-dose related); diarrhea; phlebitis with IV administration. **Occasional:** Stomatitis; cholestatic hepatitis (1:1000 especially with estolate salt formulation-reversible); generalized rash; prolonged QTc.

DRUG INTERACTIONS

Substrate of CYP3A4 and potent inhibitor CYP3A4 and CYP1A2. **Contraindicated with:** cisapride, ergot alkaloids, pimozide, cisapride, astemizole, terfenadine, midazolam and triazolam, lovastatin and simvastatin, fentanyl, drugs that significantly prolong QTc (type IA and III antiarrhythmic

Benzodiazepine (alprazolam, diazepam), carbamazepine, cyclosporine, tacrolimus, sirolimus, irinotecan, dofetilide, quinidine, digoxin, theophylline, olanzapine, warfarin, amiodarone, Ca channel blockers, itraconazole, ketoconazole, methadone, corticosteroid, drug for impotence (sildenafil, tadalafil, and vardenafil), and other CYP3A4 or CYP1A2 substrates: erythromycin may significantly increase serum level of the following drugs: Monitor closely with erythromycin co-administration; may need to decrease dose of co-administered drug.

Rifampin, rifabutin, rifapentine, carbamazepine, phenytoin, phenobarbital, nevirapine, and efavirenz: erythromycin levels may be decreased with the co-administration of these drugs. Consider switching to an alternative antimicrobial.

PREGNANCY RISK: B-In a surveillance study of Michigan Medicaid recipient, 6,972 patients were exposed to erythromycin during the first trimester, resulted in a 4.6% birth defect rate. This data does not support an association between erythromycin and congenital malformation. The CDC recommends the use of erythromycin for the treatment of chlamydia in pregnancy.

BREAST FEEDING: Erythromycin is excreted into breast milk. The American Academy of Pediatrics considers erythromycin compatible with breast feeding.

COMMENTS: Oral and parenteral macrolide that often causes GI distress especially with oral administration. It has decreasing activity against S. pneumoniae and it has multiple drug interactions with drugs metabolized by cytochrome P450. Other therapeutically equivalent and better tolerated drugs are azithromycin or clarithromycin, but they cost more.

FORMS (◆ DENOTES AVAILABLE GENERICALLY)

Brand name	Preparation	Mfr.	Route	Form	Strength	Cost (AWP)
Eryc	Erythromycin	◆ Warner Chilcott	PO	cap, EC	250mg	$0.64
PCE Dispertab	Erythromycin	◆ Abbott	PO	tab, EC	333mg; 500mg	$1.93; $2.55
Eryped	Erythromycin	◆ Abbott	PO	susp	100mg/2.5mL; 200mg/5mL; 400mg/5mL	$0.35 per 2.5mL; $0.41 per 5mL; $0.63 per 5mL
Erythrocin Lac-tobionate	Erythromycin	Hospira	IV	vial	500mg; 1000mg	$4.33 per vial; $7.73 per vial
Erythromycin stearate	Erythromycin	◆ Abbott	PO	tab	250mg; 500mg	$0.14; $0.27

SELECTED READINGS

Iannini PB. Cardiotoxicity of macrolides, ketolides and fluoroquinolones that prolong the QTc interval. Expert Opin Drug Saf. 2002 Jul;1(2):121-8

Ray WA, Murray KT, Meredith S et al. Oral erythromycin and the risk of sudden death from cardiac causes. N Engl J Med. 2004;351:1089-96.

ETHAMBUTOL

FDA INDICATIONS

• Tuberculosis (all forms), treatment in combination with other anti-tuberculosis medications.

USUAL ADULT DOSING: TB: 15-20mg/kg (max 2gm) qd; DOT regimen: 50mg/kg (max 4g) 2x/week or 25-30mg/kg (max 2gm) 3x/week. MAI: 15mg/kg qd (w/ macrolide).

Dosing Adjustments

GFR 50-80 mL/min: 15mg/kg/ q 24h (consider dose reduction with clearance less than 70mL/min.

GFR 10-50 mL/min: 15mg/kg/ q 24-36h

GFR<10 mL/min: 15mg/kg/ q 48h

ANTI-INFECTIVES

Hemodialysis: 15-20mg/kg/day post-dialysis 3x/week.
Peritoneal Dialysis: 15mg/kg/48 hours

ADVERSE DRUG REACTIONS: Occasional: Optic neuritis (decreased acuity, reduced color discrimination, constricted fields, scotomata-dose related [25mg/kg], >risk w/daily admin and renal failure); GI intolerance. **Rare:** Confusion; gout; skin rash; bone marrow suppression.

DRUG INTERACTIONS

Ethionamide: May increase adverse effect of ethambutol. Monitor for adverse effect of ethambutol (neuritis, hepatitis, GI distress).

PREGNANCY RISK: B-No congenital defects have been reported. The CDC considers ethambutol safe in pregnancy.

BREAST FEEDING: Ethambutol is excreted in breast milk. The American Academy of Pediatrics considers ethambutol compatible with breast feeding.

COMMENTS: Oral first line TB and MAI agent. Monitor for optic neuritis with loss of red-green color discrimination (esp. in patients receiving ethambutol 25mg/kg/d or more).

FORMS (♦ DENOTES AVAILABLE GENERICALLY)

Brand name	Preparation	Mfr.	Route	Form	Strength	Cost (AWP)
Myambutol	Ethambutol	♦ X-Gen	PO	tab	100mg; 400mg	$0.62; $1.80

SELECTED READINGS

American Thoracic Society, CDC, and Infectious Diseases Society of America. Official joint statement of the American Treatment of Tuberculosis . MMWR Recomm Rep. 2003;52(RR11):1-77

Ward TT, Rimland D, Kauffman C, et al. Randomized, open-label trial of azithromycin plus ethambutol vs. clarithromycin plus ethambutol as therapy for Mycobacterium avium complex bacteremia in patients with HIV. Clin Infect Dis. 1998;27:1278-85

FAMCICLOVIR

FDA INDICATIONS

• Recurrent herpes genitalis (suppression and treatment).
• Treatment of herpes zoster in immunocompetent host.

USUAL ADULT DOSING: Herpes zoster: 500mg PO q8h x 7-10 d. HSV (initial): 250mg PO q8h or 500mg PO bid x 7 d. Recurrent HSV: 125mg PO q8h or 250-500mg PO bid x 7d. Suppression of recurrent genital HSV: 250mg bid.

Dosing Adjustments

GFR 50-80 mL/min: Usual dose
GFR 10-50 mL/min: 125-500mg q12h-q24h
GFR<10 mL/min: 125-250mg q48h
Hemodialysis: 125-250mg q48h, on days of dialysis dose after dialysis

ADVERSE DRUG REACTIONS: Generally well tolerated with occasional headache, dizziness, and GI intolerance (nausea and diarrhea).

DRUG INTERACTIONS

Probenecid: Increase in penciclovir level due to competitive tubular secretion by probenecid. No dose adjustment needed.

PREGNANCY RISK: B- Carcinogenic, but not embryotoxic or teratogenic in animal studies. No human data.

BREAST FEEDING: No data: but due to the probable excretion into breast milk and the carcinogenicity potential in animal studies it is famciclovir is not recommended when breastfeeding.

COMMENTS: Oral antiviral agent for HSV and VZV with comparable efficacy to acyclovir and more convenient dosing.

FORMS

Brand name	Preparation	Mfr.	Route	Form	Strength	Cost (AWP)
Famvir	Famciclovir	Novartis	PO	tab	125mg; 250mg; 500mg	$4.28; $4.65; $10.33

SELECTED READINGS

Romanowski B, Aoki FY, Martel AY, et al. Efficacy and safety of famciclovir for treating mucocutaneous herpes simplex infection in HIV-infected individuals. Collaborative Famciclovir HIV Study Group. AIDS. 2000;14:1211-7

FLUCONAZOLE

FDA INDICATIONS

- Candidiasis prophylaxis (patients undergoing bone marrow transplant receiving cytotoxic chemotherapy and/or radiation therapy)
- Candidiasis oropharyngeal
- Disseminated candidiasis (including peritonitis, pneumonia, and urinary tract infections.)
- Chronic mucocutaneous candidiasis
- Vulvovaginal candidiasis
- Coccidioidomycosis (treatment, but itraconazole is preferred)
- Disseminated cryptococcosis
- Cryptococcal meningitis, treatment and suppression of

USUAL ADULT DOSING: 100-200mg PO or IV qd, up to 800mg per day.

Dosing Adjustments
GFR 50-80 mL/min: Usual
GFR 10-50 mL/min: 50% of dose
GFR<10 mL/min: 25%-50% of dose
Hemodialysis: 200mg post-dialysis
Peritoneal Dialysis: 25-50% of dose qd

ADVERSE DRUG REACTIONS: Frequent: GI intolerance w/bloating, nausea, vomiting, pain, anorexia, weight loss; reversible alopecia. **Occasional:** Transaminase elevation to >8x normal; prolonged PT time with warfarin.

DRUG INTERACTIONS

Fluconazole is a mild inhibitor of CYP2C8/9 and 3A4.

Benzodiazepines (alprazolam, diazepam, midazolam, triazolam): Azole antifungal decreases the metabolism of certain benzodiazepines, resulting in increased elimination half-life of certain benzodiazepines. Avoid concurrent administration. If used dose of benzodiazepine may need to be decreased. Use alternative benzodiazepines (lorazepam, oxazepam, temazepam) that will not likely interact with azole antifungal.

Cisapride: Inhibition of metabolism of cisapride resulting in increased concentration and cardiotoxicity. Contraindicated. Do not co-administer. metoclopramide may be used as an alternative pro-kinetic agent.

Cyclosporin: Coadministration may increase serum levels of this drug and other CYP3A4 substrates.

Lovastatin and **simvastatin:** Coadministration may increase serum levels of these drugs and other CYP3A4 substrates.

Nonsedating antihistamines (terfenadine, astemizole): Inhibition of metabolism of terfenadine and astemizole by azole antifungals resulting in QT interval prolongation and cardiotoxicity. Contraindicated. Do not co-administer. Alternative nonsedating antihistamines that may be used include Claritin, Allegra, and Zyrtec.

Phenytoin: Coadministration may increase serum levels of this drug and other CYP3A4 substrates.

Rifampin: Enzyme induction by rifampin resulting in increased metabolism and decreased serum concentration of fluconazole. Monitor therapeutic efficacy.

Tacrolimus and sirolimus: Coadministration may increase serum levels of these drugs and other CYP3A4 substrates.

Warfarin: Anticoagulant effect of warfarin is increased due to hepatic inhibition of warfarin by azole antifungals. Monitor INR closely with co-administration. The dose of warfarin may need to be decreased.

PREGNANCY RISK: C-Teratogenic in animal studies. Case reports of craniofacial, limb and cardiac defects have been reported in 3 infants with 1st trimester exposure to high dose fluconazole. The risk of low dose intermittent use has not been fully evaluated but appears to be low.

BREAST FEEDING: Fluconazole is excreted into breast milk w/ high concentration (up to 83% of plasma concentration). Since no drug-induced toxicity was encountered in infants during therapy with fluconazole, the likelihood of toxicity during breast feeding is low.

COMMENTS: Oral and parenteral azole with the best oral bioavailability. In general C. albicans, C. tropicalis and C. parapsilosis are susceptible. C. glabrata has variable susceptibility and likely requires higher dosing; C. krusei is intrinsically resistant.

FORMS (♦ DENOTES AVAILABLE GENERICALLY)

Brand name	Preparation	Mfr.	Route	Form	Strength	Cost (AWP)
Diflucan	Fluconazole	♦ Pfizer	IV	piggyback	200mg/100mL; 400mg/200mL	$116.52; $170.30
			PO	susp	50mg/5mL; 200mg/5mL	$5.76 per 5mL; $20.92 per 5mL
			PO	tab	50mg; 100mg; 150mg; 200mg	$6.27; $9.86; $15.69; $16.13

SELECTED READINGS

Tumbarello M, Caldarola G, Tacconelli E, et al. Analysis of the risk factors associated with the emergence of azole resistant oral candidosis in the course of HIV infection . J Antimicrob Chemother 1996 Oct;38 (4):691-9

P. Eggimann, et al. Fluconazole Prophylaxis Prevents Intra-Abdominal Candidiasis in High-Risk Surgical Patients . Crit Care Med 1999;27;1066

JD Sobel, et al. Practice Guidelines for the Treatment of Fungal Infections. CID 2000; 30: 652

D. J. Winston, et al. A Multicenter, Randomized Trial of Fluconazole versus Amphotericin B for Empiric Antifungal Therapy of Febrile Neutropenic Patients with Cancer. Am J Med 2000;108:282

Galgiani JN, et al. Comparison of Oral Fluconazole and Itraconazole for Progressive, Nonmeningeal Coccidioidomycosis: A Randomized, Double-Blind Trial. Ann Intern Med 2000;133:676

FLUCYTOSINE

FDA INDICATIONS

- Cryptococcal and candida endocarditis
- Cryptococcal meningitis (in addition with amphotericin B)
- Cryptococcal and candida pneumonia

- Cryptococcal and candida septicemia
- Candida and cryptococcus urinary tract infections

USUAL ADULT DOSING: Cryptococcal meningitis: 25mg/kg q6h (plus amphotericin). Candiduria: 12.5mg/kg q6h (azole generally preferred).

Dosing Adjustments

GFR 50-80 mL/min: 25mg/kg q12h (monitor levels)
GFR 10-50 mL/min: 25 mg/kg q16h (monitor levels)
GFR<10 mL/min: 25mg/kg q24h (monitor levels)
Hemodialysis: Dose post-dialysis
Peritoneal Dialysis: 0.5-1.0g q24h

ADVERSE DRUG REACTIONS: Frequent: GI intolerance-diarrhea, dyspepsia, abdominal pain, rash, taste perversion, hepatitis, pruritis; **Occasional:** Marrow suppression w/leukopenia or thrombocytopenia; confusion; rash; hepatitis; enterocolitis; headache; photosensitivity

DRUG INTERACTIONS

Drugs with bone marrow suppression (i.e., zidovudine, ganciclovir): additive bone marrow suppression.
Cytarabine: Antagonism. Avoid concurrent administration, monitor for therapeutic efficacy of flucytosine.

PREGNANCY RISK: C-Teratogenicity reported in animal studies. Three case reports of 2nd and 3rd trimester exposures found no defects in the infants

BREAST FEEDING: No data. Breast feeding during flucytosine therapy is not recommended

COMMENTS: Oral anti-fungal agent that may be used w/ AmB for Rx of cryptococcal meningitis. ACTG (NEJM 337:15,1997) demonstrated more rapid sterilization of the CSF, but clinical outcome was similar with or without flucytosine. Measure levels w/ goal peak of 50-100mcg/mL 2 hours post dose at steady state. USE WITH CAUTION IN PATIENTS WITH RENAL IMPAIRMENT. MONITOR RENAL, HEPATIC AND HEMATOLOGIC PARAMETERS.

FORMS

Brand name	Preparation	Mfr.	Route	Form	Strength	Cost (AWP)
Ancobon	Flucytosine	Valeant	PO	cap	250mg; 500mg	$4.89; $9.74

SELECTED READINGS

Van der Horst CM, et al. Treatment of cryptococcal meningitis associated with the acquired immunodeficiency syndrome. N Engl J Med 1997 Jul 3;337(1):15-21

FOSAMPRENAVIR (FPV)

FDA INDICATIONS

- HIV (in combination with other antiretrovirals)

USUAL ADULT DOSING: Fosamprenavir (FPV) 700mg PO bid plus ritonavir 100mg bid with or w/o food (author's preferred regimen) or FPV 1400mg PO bid with or w/o food or FPV 1400mg/ritonavir 200mg PO qd with or w/o food (QD for PI-naive pts only). FPV 700mg bid + RTV 100mg bid. with EFV co-administration: EFV 600 qhs.

Dosing Adjustments

GFR 50-80 mL/min: Usual dose
GFR 10-50 mL/min: No data. Usual dose likely.
GFR<10 mL/min: No data. Usual dose likely.
Hemodialysis: No data. Usual dose likely (on days of HD dose post HD)

↓ *Hepatic Function:* No clinical data. Based on PK data adjustment to 700mg bid with Child-Pugh score 5-8, and to avoid it with score >9.

ADVERSE DRUG REACTIONS: Adverse events (grades 2-4) from FPV were similar to comparator PIs (NFV and LPV/r). **Common:** rash 12-33% (severe in <1%). Severe GI intolerance in 5-10%. **Occasional:** elevated triglycerides (less common without RTV) and LDL, insulin resistance, hepatitis.

DRUG INTERACTIONS

Substrate, inhibitor, and likely an inducer of CYP3A4. CYP3A4 inhibitors may increase APV levels. CYP3A4 inducers may decrease APV levels. FPV may increase or decrease levels of CYP3A4 substrates.

Contraindicated with: terfenadine, astemizole, cisapride, ergot alkaloid, rifampin, bepridil, pimozide, flecainide, propafanone, St. Johns wort , midazolam and triazolam.

PREGNANCY RISK: C-Animal studies of FPV showed no embryo-fetal development abnormalities, however the rate of abortion was increased. No human data.

BREAST FEEDING: No data. Not recommended.

COMMENTS: Fosamprenavir (fosAPV) was formulated to contain 700mg fosamprenavir calcium (equivalent to 600mg amprenavir) per tab. Fosamprenavir is a prodrug of amprenavir. In PI-naive patients, daily fosAPV can be considered as an option, but FPV/r may not be similar in potency to LPV/r. FVP may have considerably less GI SE than APV.

FORMS

Brand name	Preparation	Mfr.	Route	Form	Strength	Cost (AWP)
Lexiva	Fosamprenavir calcium	GlaxoSmithKline	PO	tab	700mg	$10.54

SELECTED READINGS

Nadler J, et al. NEAT study . CROI 2003 Abstract No. 177

Shurmann D, et al . SOLO study . 6th ICDTHIV 2002 Abst. PL14.4

DeJesus E, et al. CONTEXT study . CROI 2003 Abst. 178

FOSCARNET

FDA INDICATIONS

- Cytomegalovirus retinitis
- Acyclovir-resistant mucocutaneous herpes simplex virus (HSV-1 and HSV-2) infections (e.g., orofacial, genital, digital) in immunocompromised pts

USUAL ADULT DOSING: CMV retinitis: induction 90mg/kg IV q12h x 14d over 1 hr; Maintenance 90-120 mg/kg IV qd over 2 hrs (120mg/kg IV qd after reinduction for a relapse). Acyclovir-resistant HSV and VZV: 60mg/kg x 3 wks

Dosing Adjustments

GFR 50-80 mL/min: 40-50 mg/kg q8h (Induction); 60-70mg/kg qd (maintenance)

GFR 10-50 mL/min: 20-30 mg/kg q8h (induction);65-80mg/kg q48h (maintenance)

GFR<10 mL/min: Contraindicated for CrCl <20mL/min

Hemodialysis: 38% removal, 60 mg/kg post HD (adjust to 500-800mcgM)

Peritoneal Dialysis: Dose for GFR <10mL/min

ADVERSE DRUG REACTIONS: Frequent: Renal insufficiency-often reversible; monitor 1-3x/wk & d/c if creatinine >2.9 mg/dL. Electrolyte imbalance: monitor electrolytes 1-2x/wk; monitor for paresthesias; seizures; fever. **Occasional:** GI intolerance, anemia, genital ulceration, neuropathy

DRUG INTERACTIONS

Nephrotoxic agents: amphoteracin B; aminoglycoside, cidofovir, pentamidine: Potential increased risk of nephrotoxicity. Avoid concurrent administration; if concurrent use needed monitor renal function closely and discontinue when indicated. Concurrent administration with pentamidine may also result in additive hypocalcemia and hypomagnesemia.

PREGNANCY RISK: C-Skeletal malformation or variation in animal studies. No human data available, however some experts feel that foscarnet should be used as first line agent for sight-threatening CMV retinitis in pregnant women (due to high incidence of nephrotoxicity antepartum testing of the fetus and close monitoring of the amniotic fluid to observe for fetal nephrotoxicity is recommended).

BREAST FEEDING: No data: Most likely excreted in human milk; excreted in breast milk in animal studies. Due to the potential for severe adverse reaction to foscarnet mother should avoid foscarnet when breast feeding.

COMMENTS: Parenteral antiviral agent with activity against HSV, VZV, and HHV8. Generally considered second line to ganciclovir for CMV infections due to unfavorable side effect profile (nephrotoxicity, electrolyte imbalance). Close monitoring of electrolytes and renal function needed. Active against ganciclovir-resistant CMV and acyclovir-resistant HSV, VZV.

FORMS

Brand name	Preparation	Mfr.	Route	Form	Strength	Cost (AWP)
Foscavir	Foscarnet sodium	Astra Zeneca	IV	vial	24mg/mL (500mL)	$169.09
			IV	vial	24mg/mL (250mL)	$84.91

SELECTED READINGS

Jacobson MA, Wulfsohn M, Feinberg JE, et al. ; Phase II dose-ranging trial of foscarnet salvage therapy for cytomegalovirus retinitis in AIDS patients intolerant of or resistant to ganciclovir AIDS Clinical Trials Group . AIDS. 1994;8:451-9

FOSFOMYCIN

FDA INDICATIONS

• Uncomplicated urinary tract infections due to E. coli and E. faecalis.

USUAL ADULT DOSING: 3g sachet x 1

Dosing Adjustments

GFR 50-80 mL/min: Usual dose

GFR 10-50 mL/min: no data, consider dose adjustment

GFR<10 mL/min: Half-life prolonged significantly. Use with caution; consider dose adjustment

Hemodialysis: Redose after dialysis, due to efficiently removed during HD

Peritoneal Dialysis: 1g q 36 hours

ADVERSE DRUG REACTIONS: Occasional: Diarrhea (10%), headache, vaginitis, nausea

DRUG INTERACTIONS

Antacids (Ca carbonate): Reduction of fosfomycin absorption. Separate administration time by 4 hours.

Food: Decreased absorption of fosfomycin. Administer fosfomycin on an empty stomach.

ANTI-INFECTIVES

PREGNANCY RISK: B-Animal data shows no teratogenic effects. Several published reports studied the efficacy and safety of oral fosfomycin in all stages of pregnancy. In these studies fosfomycin did not cause harm to the fetus.

BREAST FEEDING: No data, but expect excretion into breast milk due to fosfomycin's low molecular weight.

COMMENTS: Oral agent used only for uncomplicated UTI. Broad spectrum of activity includes all common uropathogenic bacteria. Single dose therapy (3g) has been equivalent to 7-day course of norfloxacin in randomized, blinded study. May be used for VRE in UTIs if renal function is good.

FORMS

Brand name	Preparation	Mfr.	Route	Form	Strength	Cost (AWP)
Monurol	Fosfomycin	Forest	PO	pds	3000mg	$39.47

SELECTED READINGS

Minassian MA; Lewis DA; Chattopadhyay D et al. A comparison between single-dose fosfomycin trometamol (Monuril) and a 5-day course of trimethoprim in the treatment of uncomplicated lower urinary tract infection in women. Int J Antimicrob Agents 1998 Apr;10(1):39-47

de Jong Z; Pontonnier F; Plante P. Single-dose fosfomycin trometamol (Monuril) versus multiple-dose norfloxacin: results of a multicenter study in females with uncomplicated lower urinary tract infections. Urol Int 1991;46(4):344-8

GANCICLOVIR

FDA INDICATIONS

- Cytomegalovirus retinitis (treatment and prophylaxis)
- Cytomegalovirus disease (prophylaxis)

USUAL ADULT DOSING: CMV retinitis: Induction 5mg/kg IV q12h x 2 weeks then maintenance 5 mg/kg IV qd (valganciclovir 900mg PO qd is a more convenient p.o alternative). Oral ganciclovir: 1g PO tid with food (for CMV maintenance only; valacyclovir is preferred).

Dosing Adjustments

GFR 50-80 mL/min: CrCL >80 mL/min-5mg/kg IV q12h; 1000mg PO tid. CrCL 50-79mL/min-2.5mg/kg q12h or 500mg PO tid.

GFR 10-50 mL/min: CrCL 25-49mL/min-2.5mg/kg IV q 24h or 1000mg PO qd. CrCL 10-25 mL/min-1.25 mg/kg IV q24h or 500mg PO qd

GFR<10 mL/min: 1.25mg/kg IV tiw

Hemodialysis: 50% of dose removed after 4 hours of HD. Dose 1.25 mg/kg IV tiw given post dialysis on dialysis days

Peritoneal Dialysis: No data, likely to be removed

↓ *Hepatic Function:* No data: Usual dose likely.

ADVERSE DRUG REACTIONS: Frequent: reversible neutropenia (consider G-CSF), thrombocytopenia. Monitor CBC 2-3/wk & d/c w/ANC <500-750 or platelets <25,000. **Occasional:** anemia, fever, rash, headache, seizures, confusion, change in mental status; abnormal liver functions.

DRUG INTERACTIONS

Class IA and Class III antirrythmics (quinidine, procainamide, amiodarone, sotalol): Avoid co-administration due to the potential for QTc prolongation.

ddI: Increases ddI serum levels.

Zidovudine, pyrimethamine, interferon: Increased risk for hematologic toxicity. Avoid concurrent administration; use alternative antiretroviral when possible or monitor for hematologic toxicity with adminstration of G-CSF when indicated.

PREGNANCY RISK: C-TERATOGENIC, CARCINOGENIC and embryogenic; growth retardation; aplastic organ and ASPERMATOGENESIS in animal studies. No human data, use only for life threatening CMV infection and warn patient of possible teratogenic effect

BREAST FEEDING: No data: due to the potential for serious toxicity, mother should avoid breast feeding.

COMMENTS: Most consider this the agent of choice for CMV infections due to better side effect profile compared to foscarnet and cidofovir. Generally, cross-resistance shown with acyclovir-resistant HSV. Oral ganciclovir is poorly absorbed and should not be used for severe CMV infections. Valganciclovir is the oral drug of choice for treatment and maintenance of CMV disease.

FORMS (♦ DENOTES AVAILABLE GENERICALLY)

Brand name	Preparation	Mfr.	Route	Form	Strength	Cost (AWP)
Cytovene	Ganciclovir	♦ Roche	IV	vial	500mg	$44.81 per vial
			PO	cap	250mg; 500mg	$4.81; $9.62
Vitrasert	Ganciclovir	Bausch & Lomb	ocular	ocular implant	4.5g	$5000 each

SELECTED READINGS

Drew WL; Ives D; Lalezari JP; Crumpacker C; Follansbee SE;. Oral ganciclovir as maintenance treatment for cytomegalovirus retinitis in patients with AIDS. N Engl J Med 1995 Sep 7;333(10):615-20

Martin DF; Parks DJ; Mellow SD; Ferris FL; Walton RC; Remaley. Treatment of cytomegalovirus retinitis with an intraocular sustained-release ganciclovir implant. A randomized controlled clinical trial . Arch Ophthalmol 1994 Dec;112(12):1531-9

GATIFLOXACIN

FDA INDICATIONS

- Acute bacterial exacerbation of chronic bronchitis
- Acute sinusitis
- Community-acquired pneumonia
- Uncomplicated and complicated urinary tract infection
- Pyelonephritis
- Uncomplicated urethral and cervical gonorrhea (note: increased fluoroquinolone resistance seen in California and Hawaii)
- Uncomplicated skin and skin structure infections.
- Bacterial conjunctivitis (as Zymar drops)

USUAL ADULT DOSING: CAP, uncomplicated SSTI, and complicated UTI: 400mg IV or PO qd x 7-14d. Uncomplicated GC: 400mg x1. Uncomplicated UTI: 400mg x1 or 200mg qd x 3d. Acute bacterial sinusitis: 400mg PO x 7-10d. AECB: 400mg PO x 5d.

Dosing Adjustments
GFR 50-80 mL/min: 400mg qd
GFR 10-50 mL/min: 200mg qd
GFR<10 mL/min: 200mg qd
Hemodialysis: 200mg qd
Peritoneal Dialysis: 200mg qd

ADVERSE DRUG REACTIONS: Occasional: GI intolerance; CNS-headache; malaise; insomnia; restlessness; dizziness; allergic reactions; diarrhea including C. difficile; photosensitivity; increased hepatic enzymes. **Rare:** Tendon rupture; QTc prolongation; hyper/hypoglycemia; seizure

Drug Interactions

Divalent and trivalent cations: Vitamins and minerals containing divalent and trivalent cation (i.e., calcium, zinc and iron), sucralfate, antacids (magnesium, aluminum, calcium) Formation of quinolone-ioncomplex results in decreased absorption of quinolones. If concurrent adminstration required, administer gatifloxacin 4 hours before cations.

Probenecid: Probenecid interferes with renal tubular secretion of gatifloxacin, this may result in increased serum level of gatifloxacin. Dose adjustment probably not needed due to the good safety profile of quinolones.

Pregnancy Risk: C-In a prospective follow-up study conducted by the European Network of Teratology Information Services (ENTIS), 666 cases of fluoroquinolone exposure (the majority of the exposures were during the first trimester) showed a congenital malformation rate of 4.8%. From previous epidemiologic data, the 4.8% did not exceed the background rate. Animal data demonstrated arthropathy in immature animals with erosions in joint cartilage. Fetoxicity and delay in skeletal ossification observed in animal data. The use of fluoroquinolone is not recommended in pregnancy.

Breast Feeding: No human data. Excreted in breast milk of rats. Fluoroquinolones are not recommended during breast feeding due to the potential for arthropathy.

Comments: Oral & parenteral fluoroquinolone w/ activity similar to levofloxacin w/ the exception of Pseudomonas. Enhanced activity against anaerobes, although there is minimal clinical experience w/ use in anaerobic infections. Therapeutically equivalent to levofloxacin & moxifloxacin for the tx of community-acquired pneumonia and other respiratory tract infections involving S. pneumoniae.

Forms

Brand name	Preparation	Mfr.	Route	Form	Strength	Cost (AWP)
Tequin	Gatifloxacin	Bristol-Myers Squibb	IV	vial	2mg/mL; 10mg/ mL	$0.95 per 5mL; $4.80 per 5mL
			PO	tab	200mg; 400mg	$9.85; $9.85
Zymar	Gatifloxacin	Allergan	oph-thalmic	gtt	0.3% (5mL)	$56.42 per 5 mL

Selected Readings

Mendonca JS, Yamaguti A, Correa JC et al. Gatifloxacin in the treatment of community-acquired pneumonias: a comparative trial of ceftriaxone, with or without macrolides, in hospitalized adult patients with mild to moderately severe pneumonia. Braz J Infect Dis. 2004;8(1):90-100.

Frothingham R. Gatifloxacin associated with a 56-fold higher rate of glucose homeostasis abnormalities than comparator quinolones in the FDA spontaneous reporting database. Program and abstracts of the 44th Interscience Conference on Antimicrobial Agents and Chemotherapy; October 30-November 2, 2004; Washington, DC. Abstract A-1092.

P. P. Gleason, et al. Associations Between Initial Antimicrobial Therapy and Medical Outcomes for Hospitalized Elderly Patients with Pneumonia . Arch Intern Med 1999;159:2562]

G-CSF

FDA Indications

- Neutropenia induced by chemotherapy
- Neutropenia post bone marrow transplantation
- Mobilization of hemapoietic progenitor cells for collection by leukopheresis.
- Neutropenia: severe chronic, cyclic, congenital or chronic idiopathic

Usual Adult Dosing: 5mcg/kg/dose to 10mcg/kg/dose qd. Dose should be titrated by 50%/ week to maintain ANC >1,000-2,000/mL. If unresponsive after 7 d at 10mcg/kg/day, treatment should be discontinued.

Dosing Adjustments

GFR 50-80 mL/min: Usual dose

GFR 10-50 mL/min: No data, usual dose likely.

GFR<10 mL/min: No data , usual dose likely.

Hemodialysis: HD: no data, usual dose administered post-HD on days of dialysis.

Peritoneal Dialysis: No data, usual dose likely

↓ *Hepatic Function:* No data, usual dose likely

ADVERSE DRUG REACTIONS: Common: bone pain, leukocytosis (if CBC not monitored properly) **Rare:** myelodysplastic syndrome or acute myeloid leukemia in patients with congenital neutropenia; pulmonary toxicity.

DRUG INTERACTIONS

Lithium: Possible increase in leukocytosis with G-CSF.

Vincristine: Additive peripheral neuropathy with G-CSF.

PREGNANCY RISK: C

BREAST FEEDING: No data

COMMENTS: 2002 USPHS/IDSA HIV guidelines for OI prophylaxis do not recommend routine use of G-CSF in neutropenic HIV-infected patients. Most authorities feel AIDS pts can tolerate low ANC better than cancer pts. Nevertheless, AIDS pts with low ANC (<500/mL) have a 2-3 fold increase in bacterial infection rates. Therefore, it is reasonable to use in neutropenic pts with active infections.

FORMS

Brand name	Preparation	Mfr.	Route	Form	Strength	Cost (AWP)
Neupogen	Filgrastim (G-CSF)	Amgen	SC	vial	300mcg/mL; 480mcg/0.8mL	$219.72; $384

SELECTED READINGS

Moore RD., Keruly JC, Chaisson RE et al. Neutropenia and Bacterial Infection in Acquired Immunodeficiency Syndrome . Arch Intern Med 1995; 155:1965

Kuritzkes DR., Parenti D, Ward DJ et al. Filgrastim prevents severe neutropenia and reduces infective morbidity in patients with advanced HIV infection: results of a randomized, multicenter, controlled trial. AIDS 1998,12:65-74

GEMIFLOXACIN

FDA INDICATIONS

- Community-acquired pneumonia
- Acute bacterial exacerbation of chronic bronchitis

USUAL ADULT DOSING: 320mg PO qd with or without food. Duration limited to 5 days for AECB and 7 days for CAP, due to potential for higher incidence of rash.

Dosing Adjustments

GFR 50-80 mL/min: >40mL/min = 320mg PO qd

GFR 10-50 mL/min: <40mL/min= 160mg PO qd

GFR<10 mL/min: 160mg PO qd

Hemodialysis: HD removes 20-30%. Dose: 160mg PO qd dose post HD on days of dialysis.

↓ *Hepatic Function:* 320mg PO qd (standard dose)

ADVERSE DRUG REACTIONS: Common: Maculopapular rash in 28% pts (risk factors: <40 years old, female, post-menopausal taking hormone replacement, and Rx >7d), 7% rash was severe involving >60% of the body. **Occasional:** LFT elevation. **Rare:** QTc prolongation, photosensitivity.

Anti-Infectives

Drug Interactions

Sucralfate, antacids/di-and trivalent cations: (give gemifloxacin >=2 hours). Class IA anti-arrhythmic (quinidine and procainamide) or Class III (amiodarone and sotalol) should be avoided due to the potential additive QTc prolongation with gemifloxacin.

Pregnancy Risk: C: No human data. High dose gemifloxacin (2- to 8-fold higher than usual dose) resulted in fetal growth retardation and fetal brain malformations in animal studies.

Breast Feeding: No data

Comments: Gemifloxacin has potent activity vs. S. pneumoniae (including PCN-resistant strains), H. influenzae, and atypicals (C. pneumoniae, M. pneumoniae, and Legionella). Higher incidence of macular papular rash w/ gemifloxacin may limit its use, especially when equally effective and better-tolerated fluoroquinolone are available (i.e., gati/levo/moxifloxacin). FDA recommends Rx limited to 5d AECB, 7d CAP.

Forms

Brand name	Preparation	Mfr.	Route	Form	Strength	Cost (AWP)
Factive	Gemifloxacin	Oscient	PO	tab	320mg	$18.78

Selected Readings

. . FDA briefing

Leophonte P, File T, Feldman C. Gemifloxacin once daily for 7 days compared to amoxicillin/clavulanic acid thrice daily for 10 days for the treatment of community-acquired pneumonia of suspected pneumococcal origin. Respir Med. 2004;98(8):708-20

Blondeau JM, Missaghi B. Gemifloxacin: a new fluoroquinolone. Expert Opin Pharmacother. 2004;5:1117-52.

GENTAMICIN

FDA Indications

- Serious infections caused by susceptible strains of organism causing:
- Bacterial neonatal sepsis
- Bacterial septicemia
- Meningitis
- Urinary tract
- Respiratory tract
- Gastrointestinal tract (including peritonitis)
- Skin, bone and soft tissue infections (including burns)

Usual Adult Dosing: QD dosing: 5-7mg/kg IV. Mild-mod infxn: 1.7mg/kg IV q8h (goal peak >6 mcg/mL). Severe infxn: 2mg/kg IV q8h (goal peak >8 mcg/mL). Synergy w/ beta-lactams for gram + infections: 1mg/kg IV q8h.

Dosing Adjustments

GFR 50-80 mL/min: 60-90% of usual dose q8-12h or 100% of usual dose q12-24 hrs. (monitor levels, redose <2mg/mL)

GFR 10-50 mL/min: 30-70% of usual dose q 12h or 100% of usual dose q24-48 hrs (monitor levels, redose <2mg/mL)

GFR<10 mL/min: 20-30% of usual dose q24-48 hrs or 100% q48-72 hrs

Hemodialysis: 1.0-1.7 mg/kg post-dialysis

Peritoneal Dialysis: 2-4mg per Liter of dialysate exchange per day. Aminoglycosides given for prolonged periods to patients receiving continuous peritoneal dialysis have been associated with high rates of ototoxicity. Monitor level after loading dose and follow for symptoms

ADVERSE DRUG REACTIONS: Frequent: renal failure (usually reversible). **Occasional:** vestibular and auditory damage (usually irreversible, genetic predisposition in some cases--check family for aminoglycoside ototoxicity). **Rare:** neuromuscular blockade.

DRUG INTERACTIONS

Cephalothin: Increased incidence of nephrotoxicity.
Loop diuretics(bumetanide, furosemide, ethacrynic acid, torsemide): Ototoxicity (auditory) may be increased (especially with ethacrynic acid); avoid co-administration.
Nephrotoxic agents (amphotericin B, foscarnet, cidofovir): Additive nephrotoxicity.
Nondepolarizing muscle relaxants (atracurium, pancuronium, tubocurarine, gallamine triethiodide): Possible enhanced action of nondepolarizing muscle relaxant resulting in possible respiratory depression.
Penicillins: In vitro inactivation.
Vancomycin: controversial but may increase risk of nephrotoxicity.

PREGNANCY RISK: C-Animal studies show dose-related nephrotoxicity. Reports of intra-amniotic instillations of gentamicin in patients (n=11) did not result in harm to the newborn. Ototoxicity has not been reported with in utero exposure, however eighth cranial nerve toxicity in the fetus is well known with exposure to other aminoglycosides (kanamycin and streptomycin) and can potentially occur with gentamicin.

BREAST FEEDING: Excreted in low concentration in breast milk.

COMMENTS: Gent appears more nephrotoxic but less ototoxic than tobramycin. Lower doses (1mg/kg q8h) used for synergy combined w/ betalactams to treat enterococcal or staphylococcal infections. Monitor renal function and watch for ototoxicity (auditory and vestibular). Don't use QD dosing in pts w/ unstable renal fxn, CrCl <60mL/min, endocarditis, meningitis, or increased Vd (e.g., pregnancy, ascites, edema, burns, shock).

FORMS (♦ DENOTES AVAILABLE GENERICALLY)

Brand name	Preparation	Mfr.	Route	Form	Strength	Cost (AWP)
Garamycin	Gentamicin sulfate	♦ Schering Plough	IV	vial	40mg/mL	$6.36 (2mL)
Gentamicin	Gentamicin sulfate	♦ Hospira	IV	vial	10mg/mL;40mg/mL	$2.59 (10mL); $0.81 (2mL)
			topical	cre	0.1% (15g)	$3.72
			topical	oint	0.1% (15g)	$3.72
Genoptic		♦ Allergan	ophth	oint	3mg/g (3.5g)	$18.03
			ophth	sol	3mg/mL (5mL)	$17.93

SELECTED READINGS

Sattler FR; Moyer JE; Schramm M et al. Aztreonam compared with gentamicin for treatment of serious urinary tract infections. Lancet 1984 Jun 16;1(8390):1315-8

Enderlin G; Morales L; Jacobs RF et al. Streptomycin and alternative agents for the treatment of tularemia: review of the literature. Clin Infect Dis 1994 Jul;19(1):42-7

Haffejee IE. A therapeutic trial of cefotaxime versus penicillin-gentamicin for severe infections in children. J Antimicrob Chemother 1984 Sep;14 Suppl B:147-52

Rice LB; Calderwood SB; Eliopoulos GM et al. Enterococcal endocarditis: a comparison of prosthetic and native valve disease. Rev Infect Dis 1991 Jan-Feb;13(1):1-7

Kelsey SM; Shaw E; Newland AC et al. Aztreonam plus vancomycin versus gentamicin plus piperacillin as empirical therapy for the treatment of fever in neutropenic patient: a randomised controlled study. J Chemother 1992 Apr;4(2):107-13

GRISEOFULVIN

FDA INDICATIONS

- Dermatomycosis
- Tinea capitis, T. corporis, T. pedis, T. unguium, T. cruris and T. barbae.

USUAL ADULT DOSING: Tinea: 500-1000mg (griseofulvin micronized) qd or 375-750mg (griseofulvin ultramicronized) qd x 4-6 weeks. Tinea unguium should be treated for at least 4 months.

Dosing Adjustments

GFR 50-80 mL/min: Usual dose

GFR 10-50 mL/min: Usual dose

GFR<10 mL/min: Usual dose

Hemodialysis: No data. Usual dose likely

Peritoneal Dialysis: No data. Usual dose likely

↓ *Hepatic Function:* May need dose reduction

ADVERSE DRUG REACTIONS: Occasional: GI side effects, disulfiram-like reaction and photosensitivity. **Rare:** Porphyria, hypersensitivity reaction (drug eruption, erythema multiforme, TEN and Stevens-Johnson syndrome).

DRUG INTERACTIONS

Barbiturates: May decrease griseofulvin levels.

Cyclosporin: May decrease cyclosporin levels.

Oral contraceptives: May decrease oral contraceptive efficacy.

Warfarin: May decrease anticoagulation effect.

PREGNANCY RISK: C Not recommended due to possible association with hypoplastic heart failure, conjoined twins, abortion and cleft palate.

BREAST FEEDING: No data

COMMENTS: Griseofulvin is an older antifungal agent that has been shown to be equivalent to azoles in the treatment of dermatomycosis caused by microsporum, epidermophytin and trichophyton (but not active against C. albicans).

FORMS (◆ DENOTES AVAILABLE GENERICALLY)

Brand name	Preparation	Mfr.	Route	Form	Strength	Cost (AWP)
Grifulvin	Griseofulvin (microcrys-talline)	◆ Ortho Neutro-gena	PO	tab	500mg	$2.40
Gris-PEG	Griseofulvin ultramicro-crystalline	◆ Pedinol	PO	tab	125mg; 250mg	$1.29; $2.02
Grifulvin	Griseofulvin (microcrys-talline)	◆ Ortho Neutro-gena	PO	susp	125mg/5mL (120mL)	$2.09 per 5mL

SELECTED READINGS

Wingfield AB, Fernandez-Obregon AC, Wignall FS et al. Treatment of tinea imbricata: a randomized clinical trial using griseofulvin, terbinafine, itraconazole and fluconazole. Br J Dermatol. 2004;150:119-26

Faergemann J, Mork NJ, Haglund A, et al. A multicentre (double-blind) comparative study to assess the safety and efficacy of fluconazole and griseofulvin in the treatment of tinea corporis and tinea cruris. Br J Dermatol. 1997;136(4):575-7.

HEPATITIS B HYPERIMMUNE GLOBULIN

FDA INDICATIONS
- Post-exposure prophylaxis (parenteral, sexual, mucocutaneous, and oral)

USUAL ADULT DOSING: 0.06 mL/kg IM as soon as possible after exposure if indicated (may be given up to 7 days after exposure)

Dosing Adjustments
GFR 50-80 mL/min: No data, usual dose likely
GFR 10-50 mL/min: No data, usual dose likely
GFR<10 mL/min: No data, usual dose likely
Hemodialysis: No data, usual dose likely

ADVERSE DRUG REACTIONS: Occasional: Pain, erythema, and tenderness at local injection site. **Rare:** Hypersensitivity reaction with urticaria and angioedema has been reported

PREGNANCY RISK: C- No risk to the fetus has been reported. When hepatitis B occurs during pregnancy, an increased rate of abortion and prematurity may be observed. The American College of Obstetricians and Gynecologists recommends its use in pregnancy for post exposure prophylaxis.

BREAST FEEDING: No data.

COMMENTS: Indication with HBV exposures in work place are: 1) unvaccinated HCW-HBIG +vaccine series; 2) vaccinated HCW with inadequate antiHBsAg response (<10 mIU/mL)- HBIG+vaccine series or HBIGx 2 doses (MMWR 2001; 50:RR-1)

FORMS

Brand name	Preparation	Mfr.	Route	Form	Strength	Cost (AWP)
BayHep B	Hep B Hyper-immune glob-ulin	Bayer	IM	syringe	0.5mL	$151.20
			IM	vial	5mL	$136.80
Nabi-HB	Hep B hyper-immune glob-ulin	Nabi	IM	vial	1mL; 5mL	$183.69; $804.44

SELECTED READINGS

Ballow M. Intravenous Immunoglobulins: Clinical Experience and Viral Safety. J Am Pharm Assoc 2002; 42:449

Quinti I, Pierdominice M, Marziali M et al. European Surveillance of Immunoglobulin Safety-Result of Initial Survey of 1243 Patients with Primary Immunodeficiencies in 16 Countries. Clininal Immunology 2002; 104:231

IMIPENEM/CILASTATIN

FDA INDICATIONS
- Bacterial endocarditis (caused by MSSA)
- Septicemia
- Bone and joint infections
- Community-acquired pneumonia.
- Noscomial pneumonia
- Endocarditis
- Intra-abdominal infections
- Osteomyelitis

- Skin and soft tissue infections
- Uncomplicated and complicated urinary tract infections (pyelonephritis)

USUAL ADULT DOSING: UTI: 250-500mg q6h. Mild to moderate infections: 500mg IV q6-8h. Severe infections: 1g IV q6-8h.

Dosing Adjustments
GFR 50-80 mL/min: 0.5g q6-8h
GFR 10-50 mL/min: 0.5g q8-12h
GFR<10 mL/min: 0.25g-0.5g q12h
Hemodialysis: 0.25g IV q12h with 0.25g post dialysis on dialysis days
Peritoneal Dialysis: 0.25g IV q12h

ADVERSE DRUG REACTIONS: Occasional: Phlebitis at infusion sites; allergic rxns (cross-allergy w/ PCN >50%); nausea, vomiting, diarrhea; eosinophilia; transient transaminitis. **Rare:** Drug fever; transient hypotension w/ infusion; seizures (more common w/ high dose & renal insuff.)

DRUG INTERACTIONS

Probenecid: Increase imipenem/cilastin level due to inhibition of tubular secretion by probenecid. Monitor for imipenem/cilastin toxicity.

PREGNANCY RISK: C-Animal studies (monkeys) show increase in embryogenic loss and intolerance to mother. No data in humans.

BREAST FEEDING: Excreted in breast milk.

COMMENTS: Parenteral carbapenem with very broad spectrum of activity that includes all anaerobes and most GNB, including P. aeruginosa & ESBL-producing organisms. The frequency of seizures range from 0.2% in patients without CNS or renal disease who were given the proper dose to 33% in those with CNS disease and renal insufficiency who were given a higher than recommended dose.

FORMS

Brand name	Preparation	Mfr.	Route	Form	Strength	Cost (AWP)
Primaxin	Imipenem/ Cilastatin sodium	Merck	IM	vial	500mg	$34.24
			IV	vial	250mg	$18.19

SELECTED READINGS

ATS and IDSA. Guidelines for the Management of Adults with Hospital-acquired, Ventilator-associated, and Healthcare-associated Pneumonia. Am J Respir Crit Care Med 2005;171:388

IMIQUIMOD

FDA INDICATIONS
- Condyloma acuminatum

USUAL ADULT DOSING: Topical administration 3 times per week to the wart (leave on for 6-10 hours). Treatment should be continued until total clearance of wart.

Dosing Adjustments
GFR 50-80 mL/min: no data-usual dose likely
GFR 10-50 mL/min: no data-usual dose likely
GFR<10 mL/min: no data-usual dose likely
Hemodialysis: no data-usual dose likely
Peritoneal Dialysis: no data-usual dose likely

ADVERSE DRUG REACTIONS: Frequent: burning or stinging of skin; edema of skin; mild erythema; flaking of skin; pain and soreness. **Occasional:** erosion or excoriation of skin (up to 30%); fungal infection at site of application; scabbing; ulceration or vesicles on skin

DRUG INTERACTIONS

No significant interactions noted.

PREGNANCY RISK: B-not teratogenic in animal studies.

BREAST FEEDING: Unknown

COMMENTS: An expensive topical therapy ($154/4 wks) for genital warts. Effective in immunocompetent host [J Infect 2000;41:148], however, efficacy in HIV-infected patients has been less impressive [AIDS 1999;13:2397]. Avoid occlusive dressing, such as bandages. More frequent administration did not result in improved efficacy. Effective for molluscum contagiosum in HIV-infected patients.

FORMS

Brand name	Preparation	Mfr.	Route	Form	Strength	Cost (AWP)
Aldara	Imiquimod	3M	topical	cream	5% (0.25g packet)	$15.17

SELECTED READINGS

Sauder DN, Skinner RB, Fox TL et al. Topical imiquimod 5% cream as an effective treatment for external genital and perianal warts in different patient populations. Sex Transm Dis. 2003;30(2):124-8.

INDINAVIR (IDV)

FDA INDICATIONS

• HIV infection treatment in combination with other antiretrovirals

USUAL ADULT DOSING: IDV 800mg q8h on an empty stomach. Combination dosing: IDV 800mg bid with RTV 100-200mg bid/ IDV 1200mg bid with NFV 1250mg bid/ EFV 600mg qhs with IDV 1000mg q8h or IDV 800mg/RTV 100mg bid.

Dosing Adjustments

GFR 50-80 mL/min: Usual dose

GFR 10-50 mL/min: Usual dose likely

GFR<10 mL/min: Usual dose likely (pharmacokinetic unchanged in renal failure)

Hemodialysis: Usual dose. Very small amount removed in dialysis.

Peritoneal Dialysis: No data: Usual dose likely

ADVERSE DRUG REACTIONS: Nephrolithiasis +/- hematuria in 5-20% of pts, interstitial nephritis; indirect hyperbilirubinemia (2.5mg/dL or over, clinically insignificant); lipodystrophy; hyperglycemia; incr. triglycerides and/or LDL; Incr. LFTs; leukocyturia (35% with incr. Scr)

DRUG INTERACTIONS

Substrate and inhibitor of CYP3A4 and weak inhibitor of CYP2D6. May increase levels of CYP3A4 (and possibly 2D6) substrates. CYP3A4 inhibitors and inducers may increase and decrease IDV levels, respectively.

Contraindicated with: terfenadine, astemizole, cisapride, ergot alkaloid, rifampin, midazolam, rifapentine, pimozide, simvastatin, St Johns wort, lovastatin, and triazolam.

PREGNANCY RISK: C-Placental passage is significant in rats, but low in rabbits. Not teratogenic in rodent studies (but extra ribs have been reported). Incidence of hyperbilirubinemia in neonatal Rhesus monkeys approximately fourfold above controls. No data on carcinogenicity.

BREAST FEEDING: Unknown breast milk excretion. Breast feeding is not recommended in the U.S. in order to avoid post-natal transmission of HIV to the child, who may not yet be infected.

COMMENTS: Indinavir as the only PI may be difficult due to q8h dosing plus the need for administration on an empty stomach. Taken with ritonavir, it may be taken bid without regard to meals (IDV 800mg bid + RTV 100mg bid), and has a better pharmacokinetic profile. Pts should drink 48oz of fluid qd to maintain urine output at >150/mL/h to prevent IDV kidney stones.

FORMS

Brand name	Preparation	Mfr.	Route	Form	Strength	Cost (AWP)
Crixivan	Indinavir sulfate (IDV)	Merck	PO	cap	100mg; 200mg; 333mg; 400mg	$0.76; $1.52; $2.54; $3.05

INTRAVENOUS IMMUNE GLOBULIN

FDA INDICATIONS

- BMT
- Immunoglobulin deficiency
- Idiopathic thrombocytopenic purpura
- CLL
- VZV post-exposure prophylaxis if varicella-zoster immune globulin is not available
- Non-FDA: Case series of sucessful treatment of anemia secondary to parvovirus B19. Most experts recommend IVIG 0.4g/kg x 5 days.
- Non-FDA approved indications with established efficacy: Kawasaki's syndrome; Guillain-Barre syndrome; steroid-resistant dermatomyositis; multifocal motor neuropathy.
- Non-FDA approved indication that is still controversial: IVIG had a mortality benefit for Strep TSS in an observational study.

USUAL ADULT DOSING: ITP: 400mg-1000mg per kg on days 1, 2, 14, then q2-3 weeks. Parvovirus B19: 0.4g/kg x 5 days (may require q month maintenance dose if anemia relapse in less than 6mos). STSS: 1g/kg day1, then 0.5gm/kg day 2 and 3 plus Abx (clinda/PCN)

Dosing Adjustments

GFR 50-80 mL/min: No data, usual dose likely

GFR 10-50 mL/min: No data, usual dose likely

GFR<10 mL/min: No data, usual dose likely

ADVERSE DRUG REACTIONS: Frequent: nonspecific infusion related side effects (hypotension, flushing, fever, chills, h/a, back pain, and chest tightness). **Rare:** Acute renal failure, hemolysis, transient neutropenia, aseptic meningitis, thrombosis, hyponatremia, and anaphylaxis

DRUG INTERACTIONS

Live vaccines: May affect immunogenicity of some live vaccines (i.e., rubella). It is recommended to separate administration time by 3 months.

PREGNANCY RISK: C- No risk to the fetus has been reported. The American College of Obstetricians and Gynecologists recommends its use in pregnancy.

BREAST FEEDING: No data.

COMMENTS: An effective Rx for ITP. The advantage over steroids and HAART is the quick onset of action. ARF secondary to the sucrose load in some preparations (Sandoglobulin, Panglobulin, Gammar-P.I.V, and Gammar-I.V.b.) has been reported. In pts with selective

IgA deficiency who may have circulating anti-IgA antibodies, the IVIG with the lowest IgA content should be used (GammagardSD and Venoglobulin).

FORMS

Brand name	Preparation	Mfr.	Route	Form	Strength	Cost (AWP)
Sandoglobulin	IVIG	Novartis	IV	vial	1gm; 12g	$95; $726
Gamimune-N 10%	IVIG	Bayer	IV	vial	1g; 5g; 10g; 20g	$101 per 1g
Gammagard SD	IVIG	Baxter	IV	vial	10g	$497

SELECTED READINGS

Ballow M. Intravenous Immunoglobulins: Clinical Experience and Viral Safety. J Am Pharm Assoc 2002; 42:449

Quinti I, Pierdominice M, Marziali M et al. European Surveillance of Immunoglobulin Safety-Result of Initial Survey of 1243 Patients with Primary Immunodeficiencies in 16 Countries. Clininal Immunology 2002; 104:231

Darenberg J, Ihendyane N, Sjolin J et al. IVIG therapy in STSS: A European Randomized, Double blind, Placebo-Controlled Trial. CID 2003; 37: 333

ISONIAZID

FDA INDICATIONS

• Tuberculosis (treatment and prevention)

USUAL ADULT DOSING: 5mg/kg (max 300mg) PO or IM qd. DOT regimen 15mg/kg (max 900mg) 2-3x/week (3x/week in the continuation phase for HIV patients with CD4<100).

Dosing Adjustments

GFR 50-80 mL/min: Usual dose

GFR 10-50 mL/min: Usual dose

GFR<10 mL/min: If slow acetylator use 150mg PO qd

Hemodialysis: 5 mg/kg post-dialysis

Peritoneal Dialysis: Daily dose post dialysis (50% of dose if slow acetylator)

↓ *Hepatic Function:* Use with caution in hepatic impairment; use is contraindicated if acute liver disease or history of INH-associated hepatitis.

ADVERSE DRUG REACTIONS: Occasional: diarrhea with liquid INH; + ANA in 20% of pts, but less than 1% w/ clinical lupus. Elevated ALT 10-20%. Clinical hepatitis 0.1-0.15% (fatal, 0.023%)age-related: < 20 yrs=nil; <35 yrs=0.1-2.0%; <45 yrs=0.2-3.0%; <55 yrs=0.3-3.5%. **Rare:** hypersensitivity; fever; dose-related peripheral neuropathy (<0.2%); monoamine poisoning; CNS toxicity.

DRUG INTERACTIONS

Carbamazepine: Increased carbamazepine concentration may be due to isoniazid inhibition of carbamazepine metabolism. Monitor for carbamazepine serum level and clinical signs of toxicity. Dose may need to be adjusted based on serum level and signs of toxicity.

Enflurane: In rapid acetylator of INH, high output renal failure may occur due to nephrotoxic concentration of inorganic fluoride secondary to high concentration of hyrazine (INH metabolite) that facilitate defluorination of enflurane. Monitor renal function closely with co-administration.

Phenytoin: Increased phenytoin level due to inhibition of phenytoins hepatic metabolism by isoniazid. Monitor phenytoin serum level and clinical signs of toxicity. Dose of phenytoin may need to be adjusted based on levels and signs of toxicity.

Rifampin: Possible additive hepatotoxicity due to the production of secondary pathway metabolite of isoniazid (hydrazine and isonicotinic acid). Monitor liver function test closely, INH and/or rifampin may need to be discontinued if liver enzymes increase 5 times above baseline.

PREGNANCY RISK: C-Animal studies show embryocidal effect, but not teratogenic. Retrospective analysis of more than 4,900 exposures to INH did not result in an increased rate of fetal malformation. The American Academy of Pediatrics recommends pregnant women with positive PPD should receive INH if HIV positive, have recent contact or X-ray showing old TB; begin after first trimester if possible.

BREAST FEEDING: Excreted in breast milk. The American Academy of Pediatrics considers isoniazid compatible with breast feeding.

COMMENTS: Oral and parenteral first line antituberculosis agent. Because of the high prevalence of resistance to isoniazid, treatment with a rifampin-containing regimen should be strongly considered for immigrants from Vietnam, Haiti, and the Philippines [NEJM 2002;347:1850]. Hepatitis is the major toxic effect and risk of hepatitis increases with age and alcohol.

FORMS (♦ DENOTES AVAILABLE GENERICALLY)

Brand name	Preparation	Mfr.	Route	Form	Strength	Cost (AWP)
Isoniazid	Isoniazid (INH)	♦ Barr	PO	tab	100mg; 300mg	$0.10; $0.21
Nydrazid	Isoniazid (INH)	Sandoz	IM	vial	100mg/mL (10mL)	$24.90
Rifamate	INH/Rifampin	Aventis	PO	cap	150mg/300mg	$2.76
Rifater	INH/Rifampin/PZA	Aventis	PO	cap	50mg/120mg/300mg	$2.04

SELECTED READINGS

Jasmer RM, et al. Twelve Months of Isoniazid Compared with Four Months of Isoniazid and Rifampin for persons with Radiographic Evidence of Previous Tuberculosis: An Outcome and Cost-Effectiveness Analysis. Am J Respir Crit Care Med 2000;162:1648

ATS/CDC/IDSA. Treatment of tuberculosis. Am J Respir Crit Care Med 2003;167:603-62

ITRACONAZOLE

FDA INDICATIONS

- Aspergillosis, treatment in pts intolerant or refractory to amphotericin B therapy (IV and oral capsule formulations)
- Pulmonary and extrapulmonary blastomycosis in immunocompromised and nonimmunocompromised patients (IV and oral capsule formulations)
- Oropharyngeal and esophageal candidiasis (oral liquid formulation)
- Histoplasmosis, including chronic cavitary pulmonary disease and disseminated disease (IV and oral capsule formulation)
- Empiric therapy of neutropenic fever in patients with a suspected fungal infection (IV and oral liquid formulation)
- Onychomycosis (oral capsule formulation)

USUAL ADULT DOSING: Oral capsules: 100-200mg PO qd to bid with food (usually 200-400mg/day); oral liquid: 100mg PO qd or bid on an empty stomach. IV: 200mg IV bid x 4 doses then 200mg IV qd.

Dosing Adjustments
GFR 50-80 mL/min: Usual
GFR 10-50 mL/min: Usual

GFR<10 mL/min: Usual; Some recommend decrease dose 50%

Hemodialysis: 100mg q12-24h

Peritoneal Dialysis: 100mg q12-24h

ADVERSE DRUG REACTIONS: Occasional: Headache; GI intolerance (nausea and vomiting), rash. High dose (>600mg) associated hypokalemia, adrenal insufficiency, impotence, gynecomastia, and leg edema. **Rare:** Clinical hepatitis (abnl LFT 4%), cardiotoxicity (negative inotrope).

DRUG INTERACTIONS

CYP3A4 substrate and inhibitor with many drug interactions.
Contraindicated with: cisapride, terfenadine, astemizole, pimozide and quinidine. Reduced absorption w/ any acid blocker. Increased serum level of CYP3A4 substrates **Benzodiazepine (alprazolam, diazepam), carbamazepine, cyclosporine, tacrolimus, sirolimus, irinotecan, dofetilide, quinidine, digoxin, warfarin, amiodarone, Ca channel blockers, methadone, corticosteroids, drugs for impotence (sildenafil, tadalafil, and vardenafil), and other CYP3A4 substrates:** May significantly increase serum level of these drugs. Monitor closely with Itraconazole co-administration; may need to decrease dose of co-administered drug.
Ergot alkaloids, pimozide, midazolam and triazolam, lovastatin and simvastatin, and fentanyl: may significantly increase these drugs. Avoid co-administration.

PREGNANCY RISK: C-Teratogenic in animal studies.

BREAST FEEDING: High breast milk excretion (up to 177% of plasma concentration). Because the safety of itraconazole has not been evaluated, the use of itraconazole during breast feeding should probably be avoided.

COMMENTS: Absorption of capsules is acid pH dependent. Avoid H-2 blockers, PPIs, and antacid co-administration. Measure serum levels (after 5 days). Goal should be > 1mcg/mL (Histoplasma Reference Lab 317-630-2515). Liquid formulation often preferred due to better absorption, especially in nonacidic environments.

FORMS

Brand name	Preparation	Mfr.	Route	Form	Strength	Cost (AWP)
Sporanox	Itraconazole	Janssen	PO	cap	100mg	$9.90
Sporanox	Itraconazole	Janssen	IV	vial	10mg/mL	$213.41 per 25mL
			PO	sol	10mg/mL	$4.70 per 5mL

SELECTED READINGS

Patterson TF, et al. Invasive Aspergillosis: Disease Spectrum, Treatment Practices, and Outcomes. Medicine 2000; 79: 250

Galgiani JN, et al. Comparison of Oral Fluconazole and Itraconazole for Progressive, Nonmeningeal Coccidioidomycosis: A Randomized, Double-Blind Trial. Ann Intern Med 2000;133:676

Boogaerts M et al. Intravenous and Oral Itraconazole versus Intravenous Amphotericin B Deoxycholate as Empirical Antifungal Therapy for Persistent Fever in Neutropenic Patients with Cancer Who Are Rec. Broad-Spect.abx. Ann Intern Med 2001;135:412

Lavrijsen AP, Balmus KJ, Nugteren-Huying WM, et al. Hepatic injury associated with itraconazole. Lancet. 1992 Jul 25;340(8813):251-2

IVERMECTIN

FDA INDICATIONS

- Onchocerciasis (river blindness)
- Strongyloidiasis (GI tract)

ANTI-INFECTIVES

USUAL ADULT DOSING: Strongyloidiasis: 200mcg/kg x 1 (70kg: 15mg or 2.5 x 6mg tabs). Onchocerciasis: 150 mcg/kg x1.

Dosing Adjustments
GFR 50-80 mL/min: Usual dose
GFR 10-50 mL/min: Usual dose
GFR<10 mL/min: Usual dose

ADVERSE DRUG REACTIONS: Mazzotti reaction in onchocerciasis with hypotension, fever, pruritis, bone and joint pain (mild in 10-15% in first time users but can be severe in 5%)

DRUG INTERACTIONS
No significant interactions noted.

PREGNANCY RISK: Animal data show risk of teratogenicity. In 203 exposures to ivermectin (85% during the first trimester), there was no association with congenital malformation found.

BREAST FEEDING: Excreted in breast milk

COMMENTS: Well-tolerated oral agent that is the preferred treatment for onchocerciasis, filariasis, strongyloidiasis, cutaneous larva migrans and may be helpful with severe scabies. When using ivermectin to treat onchocerciasis in a Loa loa-endemic area, it is recommended to screen for loiasis in order to prevent serious or even fatal encephalopathy.

FORMS

Brand name	Preparation	Mfr.	Route	Form	Strength	Cost (AWP)
Stromectol	Ivermectin	Merck	PO	tab	3mg	$5.44

SELECTED READINGS
Gann PH, Neva FA, Gam AA. A randomized trial of single- and two-dose ivermectin versus thiabendazole for treatment of strongyloidiasis. J Infect Dis. 1994;169(5):1076-9.

KETOCONAZOLE

FDA INDICATIONS
- Candidiasis, chronic mucocutaneous candidiasis, oral thrush, candiduria
- Blastomycosis
- Coccidioidomycosis
- Histoplasmosis
- Chromomycosis
- Paracoccidioidomycosis
- Severe recalcitrant cutaneous dermatophyte infections in pts who have not responded to topical therapy or oral griseofulvin, or who are unable to take griseofulvin.
- Dandruff (shampoo)
- Tinea versicolor, tinea cruris, tinea pedis, tinea corporis (cream)
- Seborrheic dermatitis (cream)

USUAL ADULT DOSING: 200-400mg/day PO q12h-24h (up to 1.6g per day); topical apply qd to bid.

Dosing Adjustments
GFR 50-80 mL/min: Usual
GFR 10-50 mL/min: Usual
GFR<10 mL/min: Usual
Hemodialysis: Not removed in hemodialysis, usual dose.
Peritoneal Dialysis: Not removed in peritoneal dialysis, usual dose.

ADVERSE DRUG REACTIONS: Frequent: GI upset; transient transaminitis. **Occasional:** decreased steroid & testosterone synthesis w/impotence, gynecomastia, oligospermia, reduced libido, abnl menses; H/A; somnolence; hepatitis, dizziness; asthenia; abd. pain; photophobia. **Rare:** Hepatic failure.

DRUG INTERACTIONS

CYP3A4 substrate and inhibitor with many drug interactions. Significantly increases CYP3A4 substrates.

Contraindicated with: cisapride, terfenadine, astemizole.

Benzodiazepine (alprazolam, diazepam), carbamazepine, cyclosporine, tacrolimus, sirolimus, irinotecan, dofetilide, quinidine, digoxin, warfarin, amiodarone, Ca channel blockers, itraconazole, ketoconazole, methadone, corticosteroids, drugs for impotence (sildenafil, tadalafil, and vardenafil), and other CYP3A4 substrates. May significantly increase serum level of these drugs; monitor closely with ketoconazole co-administration; may need to decrease dose of co-administered drug.

Ergot alkaloids, pimozide, midazolam and triazolam, lovastatin and simvastatin, and fentanyl: may significantly increase these drug levels. Avoid co-administration.

Rifampin, rifabutin, rifapentine, carbamazepine, phenytoin, phenobarbital, nevirapine, and efavirenz, H2 blockers, and PPIs (omeprazole, lansoprazole): decreases ketoconazole levels co-administration. Consider switch.

PREGNANCY RISK: C-Teratogenic in animal studies. In a surveillance study of Michigan Medicaid recipients, 20 newborns exposed to oral ketoconazole during the first trimester had no resulting birth defects. Since this study, however, the FDA has received six reports of limb defects.

BREAST FEEDING: Breast milk excretion likely. Effect on the fetus is unknown.

COMMENTS: Oral azole with absorption that is acid pH dependent. Avoid H-2 blockers, PPI, and antacid co-administration. Fluconazole is generally preferred due to more predictable absorption, better side effect profile, and fewer drug interactions. Ketoconazole is less expensive.

FORMS (◆ DENOTES AVAILABLE GENERICALLY)

Brand name	Preparation	Mfr.	Route	Form	Strength	Cost (AWP)
Nizoral	Ketoconazole	◆ Janssen	PO	tab	200mg	$4.55
Nizoral shampoo	Ketoconazole	◆ Janssen	topical	shampoo	2% (120mL)	$29.10
Ketoconazole	Ketoconazole	◆ Fougera	topical	cre	2% (30g; 60g)	$27.60;$42.04

SELECTED READINGS

Laine L, Dretler RH, Conteas CN et al. Fluconazole compared with ketoconazole for the treatment of Candida esophagitis in AIDS. A randomized trial. Ann Intern Med. 1992;117(8):655-60.

LAMIVUDINE (3TC)

FDA INDICATIONS

• HIV infection in combination with other antiretrovirals
• Chronic hepatitis B infection

USUAL ADULT DOSING: HIV: lamivudine 150mg PO q12h or 300mg PO qd, can also be administered as a combination product (Combivir: AZT/3TC 1 tab PO BID or Trizivir: ABC/ AZT/3TC 1 tab bid or Epzicom: ABC/3TC 1 tab QD). HBV: 100mg to 300mg qd x12months

Dosing Adjustments

GFR 50-80 mL/min: 150mg PO bid (HIV); 100mg qd (HBV)

GFR 10-50 mL/min: 150mg PO qd (HIV); 100mg x1 then 50mg PO qd (HBV)

GFR<10 mL/min: 150 mgx1 then 50mg qd (HIV); 35mg x1 then 15mg qd (HBV)

Hemodialysis: 25-50mg qd (post HD on days of HD)
Peritoneal Dialysis: 25-50mg qd (limited data)

ADVERSE DRUG REACTIONS: Occasional: headache, nausea, diarrhea, abdominal pain and insomnia. Rare cases of lactic acidosis. Tx of pts w/ HIV-HBV co-infection receiving 3TC may have a hepatitis flare if: 1) HBV develops resistance 2) 3TC is stopped or 3) by immune reconstitution

DRUG INTERACTIONS

No significant interactions noted.

PREGNANCY RISK: C-Negative carcinogenicity and teratogenicity studies in rodents. Placental passage ratio of 1.0 (newborn:mother). Well tolerated in pregnant patients.

BREAST FEEDING: No human data, breast milk excretion in animal studies. Breast feeding is not recommended in the U.S. in order to avoid post-natal transmission of HIV to the child, who may not yet be infected

COMMENTS: The best tolerated nucleoside analogue. Active against HBV. Mutation at codon 184 of HIV confers rapid high-grade resistance to 3TC but suppresses AZT resistance. Monotherapy for treatment of HBV is associated with high rates of resistance.

FORMS

Brand name	Preparation	Mfr.	Route	Form	Strength	Cost (AWP)
Epivir	Lamivudine (3TC)	GlaxoSmithKline	PO	sol	10mg/mL	$1.85 per 5mL
Epivir HBV	Lamivudine (3TC)	GlaxoSmithKline	PO	sol	5mg/mL	$1.85 per 5mL
			PO	tab	100mg	$7.36
Combivir	Lamivudine (3TC)/Zidovudine (AZT)	GlaxoSmithKline	PO	tab	150mg/300mg	$12.04
Epzicom	Abacavir/Lamivudine	GlaxoSmithKline	PO	tab	600mg/300mg	$26.03
Epivir	Lamivudine (3TC)	GlaxoSmithKline	PO	tab	150mg, 300mg	$5.55

SELECTED READINGS

Dienstag JL, et al. Lamivudine is tolerable, effective therapy for hepatitis B. NEJM 1999;341:1256.

LEVOFLOXACIN

FDA INDICATIONS

- Bacterial exacerbation of chronic bronchitis
- Community-acquired pneumonia (including those due to PCN-resistant S. pneumoniae).
- Sinusitis
- Uncomplicated and complicated skin and soft tissue infections
- Uncomplicated and complicated urinary tract infections (pyelonephritis)
- Bacterial conjunctivitis (opthalmic drops)
- Nosocomial pneumonia
- Inhalation Anthrax

USUAL ADULT DOSING: CAP (mild to moderate): 500mg IV or PO qd x 7-14 d. CAP (mild to severe): 750mg IV or PO qd x 5 d. Complicated skin and skin structure infections and nosocomial pneumonia: 750mg IV/PO qd x 7-14 d.

Dosing Adjustments

GFR 50-80 mL/min: 500-750mg q 24h

GFR 10-50 mL/min: 500-750mg, then 250mg q24h-750mg q48h

GFR<10 mL/min: 500-750mg, then 250-500mg q48 h

Hemodialysis: 500-750mg, then 250-500mg q48h

Peritoneal Dialysis: 500-750mg, then 250-500mg q48h

ADVERSE DRUG REACTIONS: Occasional: GI intolerance; CNS-headache; malaise; insomnia; restlessness; dizziness; allergic reactions; diarrhea including C. difficile; photosensitivity; increased hepatic enzymes. **Rare:** QTc prolongation; tendon rupture; peripheral neuropathy; seizure.

DRUG INTERACTIONS

Class IA and Class III antirrythmics (quinidine, procainamide, amiodarone, sotalol): Avoid co-administration due to the potential for QTc prolongation.

Sucralfate: Decreased oral absorption of fluoroquinolone due to chelation by the aluminum ions contained in the sucralfate. Avoid co-administration. If concurrent administration required, administer sucralfate at least 2 hours before or after quinolone antibiotics.

Vitamins and minerals containing divalent and trivalent cation (i.e., calcium, zinc and iron) and antacids (magnesium, aluminum, calcium): Formation of quinolone-ion complex results in decreased absorption of quinolones. Avoid co-administration, if concurrent administration required, administer cation at least 2 hours before or after quinolone antibiotics.

PREGNANCY RISK: C-In a prospective follow-up study conducted by the European Network of Teratology Information Services (ENTIS), 666 cases of fluoroquinolone exposure (the majority of the exposures were during the first trimester) showed a congenital malformation rate of 4.8%. From previous epidemiologic data, the 4.8% did not exceed the background rate. Animal data demonstrated arthropathy in immature animals with erosions in joint cartilage. Because of the animal data, and the availability of alternative antimicrobial agents, the use of fluoroquinolones during pregnancy is considered contraindicated.

BREAST FEEDING: Fluoroquinolones are not recommended during breast feeding due to the potential for arthropathy (based on animal data).

COMMENTS: Levofloxacin is the L-isomer of ofloxacin with good in vitro and clinical experience vs. S. pneumoniae. Used primarily for LRTI and FDA-approved for PCN-resistant S. pneumoniae and nosocomial pneumonia. Comparable to moxifloxacin and gatifloxacin for the treatment of CAP. Activity vs P. aeruginosa is comparable to ciprofloxacin, but less published clinical experience.

FORMS

Brand name	Preparation	Mfr.	Route	Form	Strength	Cost (AWP)
Levaquin	Levofloxacin	Ortho McNeil	IV	vial	5mg/mL; 25mg/mL	$0.39 per mL; $2 per mL
			PO	sol	25mg/mL	$3.50 per 5mL
			PO	tab	500mg; 250mg; 750mg	$11.31; $9.88; $21.05
Levaquin, Leva-Pak	Levofloxacin	Ortho McNeil	PO	tab	750mg	$105.24 per pack
Quixin	Levofloxacin	Vistakon	ophthalmic	sol	0.5% (5mL)	$52.14 per 5mL

SELECTED READINGS

ATS and IDSA. Guidelines for the Management of Adults with Hospital-acquired, Ventilator-associated, and Healthcare-associated Pneumonia. Am J Respir Crit Care Med 2005;171:388

Blazquez Garrido RM, Espinosa Parra FJ, Alemany Frances L et al. Antimicrobial chemotherapy for legionnaires disease: levofloxacin versus macrolides. Clin Infect Dis. 2005 ;40:800-6.

Adachi JA, et al. Empirical Antimicrobial Therapy for Traveler's Diarrhea . CID 2000;31:1079

P. P. Gleason, et al. Associations Between Initial Antimicrobial Therapy and Medical Outcomes for Hospitalized Elderly Patients with Pneumonia . Arch Intern Med 1999;159:2562]

File TM Jr, et al. A multicenter, randomized study comparing the efficacy and safety of intravenous and/or oral levofloxacin versus ceftriaxone and/or cefuroxime axetil in treatment of adults with CAP. Antimicrob Agents Chemother 1997 Sep;41(9):1965-72

LINDANE

FDA INDICATIONS
- Treatment of Sarcoptes scabiei (scabies) in patients who are intolerant or have failed first-line therapy with safer agents (i.e permethrin) for pediculosis or scabies.

USUAL ADULT DOSING: 1% shampoo apply to hair and scalp (for at least 4 min); 1% topical cream apply from head to toe (leave in place for 6-12 hours before rinsing). In epidemic setting or if live lice is still present after 2 weeks, a second application is recommended.

Dosing Adjustments
GFR 50-80 mL/min: Usual dose
GFR 10-50 mL/min: No data, usual dose likely
GFR<10 mL/min: No data, usual dose likely

ADVERSE DRUG REACTIONS: Pruritis; neurotoxicity (more common in pts <50kg, young children, and elderly patients): seizures, headache, lethargy, hallucinations, motor tics, paresthesias, myoclonic contractions. SEIZURES AND DEATHS reported with repeated and prolong use.

PREGNANCY RISK: B-No human data. Not teratogenic in animal studies. Due to the potential for neurotoxicity, permethrin is a safer alternative.

BREAST FEEDING: No data

COMMENTS: Permethrin is the preferred agent for scabies due to comparable efficacy with lower risk of neurotoxicity compared to lindane [Schultz et al. Arch Dermatol 1990;126:167-70]. Contraindicated in neonates, in patients with seizure disorder, and Norwegian scabies.

FORMS

Brand name	Preparation	Mfr.	Route	Form	Strength	Cost (AWP)
Lindane	Lindane	*Major, Alpharma	topical	lotion	1% (2 oz, 16oz)	$3.00, $7.00
			topical	shampoo	1% (16 oz)	$8.00

SELECTED READINGS
Schultz MW, Gomez M, Hansen RC et al. Comparative study of 5% permethrin cream and 1% lindane lotion for the treatment of scabies. Arch Dermatol. 1990;126(2):167-70.

LINEZOLID

FDA INDICATIONS
- Hospital- and community-acquired pneumonia
- Infections due to vancomycin-resistant Enterococcus faecium (VRE), with or without concurrent bacteremia
- Complicated and uncomplicated skin and skin structure infection

USUAL ADULT DOSING: 600mg bid IV or PO

Dosing Adjustments

GFR 50-80 mL/min: 600mg bid
GFR 10-50 mL/min: 600mg bid
GFR<10 mL/min: 600mg bid
Hemodialysis: 600mg bid (give dose post-hemodialysis on days of dialysis)
↓ *Hepatic Function:* No dose adjustment needed

ADVERSE DRUG REACTIONS: Occasional: Headache; nausea, diarrhea, vomiting; thrombocytopenia & anemia (dose dependent, reversible). **Rare:** Lactic acidosis; C. difficile; optic/peripheral neuropathy; serotonin syndrome reported with SSRI co-administration.

DRUG INTERACTIONS

Linezolid is a reversible, nonselective inhibitor of monoamineoxidase. Avoid tyramine rich foods, adrenergic drugs and serotonergic (SSRI) drugs due to the potential interactions. No interactions with CYP450 3A.

PREGNANCY RISK: C-not teratogenic in animal studies

BREAST FEEDING: Excreted in breast milk (concentration similar to maternal plasma)

COMMENTS: Linezolid is active against nearly all antibiotic resistant gram-positive bacteria & has a good short-term side effect profile. A retrospective study showed a significantly better survival and clinical cure rates compared to vancomycin in patients with nosocomial pneumonia due to MRSA [Chest. 2003; 124:1789-97]; prospective confirmation of these results is needed.

FORMS

Brand name	Preparation	Mfr.	Route	Form	Strength	Cost (AWP)
Zyvox	Linezolid	Pharmacia	IV	vial	200mg; 600mg	$41.03; $82.03
			PO	susp	100mg/5mL	$10.82 per 5mL
			PO	tab	600mg	$64.93

SELECTED READINGS

M.C Birmingham et al. Outcome with Linezolid from an Ongoing Compassionate Use Trial of Patients with Significant, Resistant Gram-Positive Infections. ICAAC 1999, Abstract 1098.

Wallace RJ, et al. Activities of Linezolid Against Rapidly Growing Mycobacteria . AAC 2001;45:764

Stevens DL, Smith LG, Bruss JB. Randomized Comparison of Linezolid vs. Oxacillin-Dicloxacillin for Treatment of Complicated Skin and Soft Tissue Infections. AAC 2000; 44: 3408.

Jones RN, et al. Multi-laboratory assessment of the linezold spectrum of activity using the Kirby-Bauer disk diffusion method: Report of the Zyvox Antimicrobial Potency Study (ZAPS) in the United States. Diag Microbiol Infect Dis 2001; 40: 59

Vergis EN et al. Determinants of Vancomycin Resistance and Mortality Rates in Enterococcal Bacteremia . Ann Intern Med 2001;135:484

LOMEFLOXACIN

FDA INDICATIONS

- Acute exacerbation of chronic bronchitis
- Prophylaxis for urinary tract infections (in transurethral surgical procedures)
- Complicated and uncomplicated urinary tract infections

USUAL ADULT DOSING: UTI: 400mg PO qd

Dosing Adjustments

GFR 50-80 mL/min: Usual dose

GFR 10-50 mL/min: 400mg x1 then 200mg qd
GFR<10 mL/min: 200mg qd
Hemodialysis: 200mg qd
Peritoneal Dialysis: 200mg qd

ADVERSE DRUG REACTIONS: **Frequent:** high rate (2.4%) photosensitivity reactions.
Occasional: GI intolerance; CNS-headache; malaise; insomnia; restlessness; dizziness;
allergic reactions; diarrhea; photosensitivity; increased hepatic enzymes; tendon rupture
(rare)

DRUG INTERACTIONS

**Vitamins and minerals containing divalent and trivalent cation (i.e., calcium, zinc and
iron). Antacid (magnesium, aluminum, calcium):** Formation of quinolone-ion complex
results in decreased absorption of quinolones. Avoid co-administration, if concurrent
administration needed separate administration time by at least 2 hours. Lomefloxacin may
be less affected.

PREGNANCY RISK: C-In a prospective follow-up study conducted by the European Network of
Teratology Information Services (ENTIS), 666 cases of fluoroquinolone exposure (the
majority of the exposures were during the first trimester) showed a congenital
malformation rate of 4.8%. From previous epidemiologic data, the 4.8% did not exceed the
background rate. Animal data demonstrated arthropathy in immature animals with
erosions in joint cartilage. Because of the animal data, and the availability of alternative
antimicrobial agents, the use of fluoroquinolones during pregnancy is considered
contraindicated.

BREAST FEEDING: Fluoroquinolones are not recommended during breast feeding due to the
potential for arthropathy (based on animal data).

COMMENTS: Oral fluoroquinolone that is not frequently used due to the high incidence of
photosensitivity and the availability of other alternative fluoroquinolones. Not a good agent
for respiratory infections due to poor S. pneumoniae activity.

FORMS

Brand name	Preparation	Mfr.	Route	Form	Strength	Cost (AWP)
Maxaquin	Lomefloxacin	Pharmacia	PO	tab	400mg	$7.28

SELECTED READINGS

Naber KG; European Lomefloxacin Prostatitis Study Group. Lomefloxacin versus ciprofloxacin in the
treatment of chronic bacterial prostatitis . Int J Antimicrob Agents 2002;20(1):18-27

LOPINAVIR (LPV)

FDA INDICATIONS

- HIV infection treatment in combination with other antiretrovirals
- LPV/r QD indicated in antiretroviral naive patients.

USUAL ADULT DOSING: LPV/r 400mg/100mg (3caps) bid w/ food. Combination dosing: LPV/r
533/133mg (4caps) bid w/ EFV 600mg qhs/ LPV/r 533/133mg (4caps) bid w/ NVP 200mg
bid/ LPV/r 3caps bid w/ IDV 600mg bid or SQV 1000mg bid. LPV/r 4 caps w/ FPV 1400mg
bid (limited data).

Dosing Adjustments

GFR 50-80 mL/min: Usual dose
GFR 10-50 mL/min: No data; usual dose likely
GFR<10 mL/min: No data; usual dose likely
Hemodialysis: Usual dose(not removed with HD)
Peritoneal Dialysis: No data; Usual dose likely

ADVERSE DRUG REACTIONS: Frequent: Diarrhea in 13.8% to 23.8% of patients .
Occasional: Nausea, vomiting, abdominal pain, asthenia, headache and rash have also
been reported. PI class adverse effect: hyperlipidemia, fat redistribution, hyperglycemia,
and hepatitis.

DRUG INTERACTIONS

Substrate inhibitor, and likely an inducer of CYP3A4 and glucoronyl transferase. May also
weakly induce CYP2C9 and CYP2C19 and weakly inhibit CYP2D6 (clinical significance
unknown). LPV/r generally increases serum levels of drugs that are substrates of CYP3A4
(but reduction in serum levels have also occurred). Drugs that are inducers of CYP3A4
may decrease serum levels of LPV/r. Drugs that are inhibitors of CYP3A4 may increase
serum levels of LPV/r: flecainide, propafenone, astemizole, terfenadine,
dihydroergotamine, ergonovine, ergotamine, methylergonovine, cisapride, pimozide,
midazolam, triazolam, rifampin, St Johns wort, lovastatin, simvastatin, alfuzosin,
bepridil, rifapentine

PREGNANCY RISK: C-No treatment-related malformation seen in animal studies. No embryonic
and fetal development toxicities seen in rabbits. No human data available.

BREAST FEEDING: No data

COMMENTS: Lopinavir (LPV) is the preferred PI for inital therapy due to long term efficacy.
LPV serum levels exceed the IC50 by over 25-fold throughout the dosing interval. This
enhanced pharmacokinetic profile will enable lopinavir to have activity against some PI
resistant strains and may have advantages for initial therapy.

FORMS

Brand name	Preparation	Mfr.	Route	Form	Strength	Cost (AWP)
Kaletra	Lopinavir (LPV)/Riton-avir (RTV)	Abbott	PO	cap	133.3mg/ 33.3mg	$3.91
			PO	sol	80mg/20mg/ mL	$11.00 per 5mL

LORACARBEF

FDA INDICATIONS

- Acute bronchitis
- Acute otitis media
- Acute bronchitis
- Maxillary sinusitis
- Pharyngitis
- Pharyngitis/tonsillitis
- Pneumonia, community-acquired (CAP)
- Sinusitis
- Skin and skin-structure infections (impetigo)

USUAL ADULT DOSING: CAP and sinusitis: 400mg PO bid. Sinusitis and tonsillitis: 200mg PO
bid. Uncomplicated soft tissue infection: 200-400mg PO bid. UTI: 200mg PO bid.

Dosing Adjustments
GFR 50-80 mL/min: Usual dose
GFR 10-50 mL/min: 0.2g-0.4g q24h
GFR<10 mL/min: 0.2g-0.4g q 3-5 days
Hemodialysis: Additional dose after HD
Peritoneal Dialysis: 0.2g-0.4g q 3-5 days

Anti-Infectives

ADVERSE DRUG REACTIONS: Occasional: allergic reactions (anaphylaxis rare); diarrhea and C. difficile colitis; eosinophilia; positive Coombs' test

DRUG INTERACTIONS

Probenecid: Increase in cephalosporin serum concentration due to inhibition of tubular secretion by probenecid. Monitor for potential cephalosporin toxicity, interaction may be beneficial if high serum concentration is desired

PREGNANCY RISK: B-Animal data shows no harm. Human data lacking, but closely related cephalosporins are generally considered compatible in pregnancy.

BREAST FEEDING: Loracarbef is excreted at low level in breast milk. The American Academy of Pediatrics classifies closely related cephalosporins as compatible with breast feeding

COMMENTS: Oral second-generation cephalosporin with relatively poor S. pneumoniae activity compared to cefpodoxime. Oral suspension is better absorbed than capsules.

FORMS

Brand name	Preparation	Mfr.	Route	Form	Strength	Cost (AWP)
Lorabid	Loracarbef	Monarch	PO	capsule	200mg; 400mg	$4.35; $6.38
			PO	suspension	100mg/5mL; 200mg/5mL	$2.38 per 5mL; $3.88 per 5mL

SELECTED READINGS

Hyslop DL, Jacobson K, Guerra FJ. Loracarbef (LY163892) versus amoxicillin/clavulanate in bronchopneumonia and lobar pneumonia. Clin Ther. 1992;14(2):254-67

MEBENDAZOLE

FDA INDICATIONS

- Ascariasis
- Enterobiasis
- Hookworm
- Intestinal roundworm
- Trichuriasis

USUAL ADULT DOSING: Hookworm: 100mg PO bid x 3 days or 500mg PO x1. Pinworm: 100mg PO x1 (may be repeated if infection persists for 3 weeks).

Dosing Adjustments
GFR 50-80 mL/min: Usual dose
GFR 10-50 mL/min: Usual dose
GFR<10 mL/min: Usual dose
Hemodialysis: Drug concentration not affected by dialysis

ADVERSE DRUG REACTIONS: Occasional: Diarrhea; abdominal pain

DRUG INTERACTIONS

Carbamazepine: Lowering of mebendazole serum concentration due to hepatic enzyme induction by carbamazepine. Avoid concurrent administration. Valproic acid may be substituted for carbamazepine.

PREGNANCY RISK: C-Embryotoxic and teratogenic in animal studies. One manufacturer reported 170 first trimester exposures which resulted in no identifiable teratogenic risk. In a Michigan Medicaid recipient surveillance study, 64 first trimester exposures did not result in a significant increase in teratogenicity risk.

BREAST FEEDING: Amount excreted in breast milk unknown.

COMMENTS: Well-tolerated oral agent with broad-spectrum antihelminthic.

FORMS

Brand name	Preparation	Mfr.	Route	Form	Strength	Cost (AWP)
Vermox	Mebendazole	McNeil	PO	chew tab	100mg	$5.91

SELECTED READINGS

Legesse M, Erko B, Medhin G. Efficacy of albendazole and mebendazole in the treatment of Ascaris and Trichuris infections. Ethiop Med J. 2002;40:335-43.

MEFLOQUINE

FDA INDICATIONS

- Malaria caused by chloroquine-resistant, chloroquine-susceptible and multiple drug-resistant (including sulfadoxine and pyrimethamine-resistant) strains of Plasmodium falciparum or P. vivax, prophylaxis and treatment
- Malaria prophylaxis

USUAL ADULT DOSING: 1250mg PO x 1 (malaria treatment); 250mg PO q week (malaria prophylaxis), start one wk prior to departure to an endemic area and continue for 4 wks after leaving endemic area.

Dosing Adjustments
GFR 50-80 mL/min: Usual dose
GFR 10-50 mL/min: Usual dose
GFR<10 mL/min: Usual dose
Hemodialysis: Usual dose, not removed in dialysis
Peritoneal Dialysis: No data, not removed in peritoneal dialysis

ADVERSE DRUG REACTIONS: Frequent: Vertigo; light-headedness; nausea; nightmares; H/A; visual disturbances (dose related); decreased fine motor function. **Occasional:** Psychosis & panic attacks; seizures; disorientation (dose related; rare at prophylaxis dose); GI intolerance; dizziness. **Rare:** QTc prolongation.

DRUG INTERACTIONS

Aurothioglucose (gold compound): Potential additive bloody scrasias. Contraindicated.
Class IA and Class III antirrythmics (quinidine, procainamide, amiodarone, sotalol): Avoid co-administration due to the potential for QTc prolongation.
Beta-blocker, quinine, quinidine: Additive depression of cardiac conduction. Contraindicated. Do not co-administer.

PREGNANCY RISK: C-Embryotoxic and teratogenic in animal studies. CDC accepts mefloquine as safe and effective in second and third trimester; advises contraception during prophylaxis and for 2 months after. A double-blind, placebo-controlled trial involving 360 pregnant patients (2nd trimester) found the incidence of stillbirth similar between mefloquine and placebo [Ann Trop Med Parasitol. 1998 Sep;92(6):643-53].

BREAST FEEDING: Excreted in small concentration in breast milk. Long term effects of mefloquine exposure via breast milk have not been studied.

COMMENTS: Oral antimalarial that is commonly used for prophylaxis where chloroquine-resistance is found. May cause vivid dreams, acute psychosis and seizures, therefore contraindicated in patients with psychiatric illness and epilepsy.

FORMS

Brand name	Preparation	Mfr.	Route	Form	Strength	Cost (AWP)
Lariam	Mefloquine	Roche	PO	tablet	250mg	$12.41
Mefloquine	Mefloquine	Barr	PO	tab	250mg	$10.59

MEROPENEM

FDA Indications
- Intra-abdominal infections (appendicitis and peritonitis)
- Meningitis (children 3 months of age and older.)

Usual Adult Dosing: 1g IV q8h. Severe and CNS infections: 2g IV q8h.

Dosing Adjustments
GFR 50-80 mL/min: Usual dose
GFR 10-50 mL/min: 26-50 mL/min: 1g IV q12h 10-25mL/min: 0.5g IV q12h
GFR<10 mL/min: 0.5g q24h
Hemodialysis: Dose after dialysis; or additional dose post dialysis
Peritoneal Dialysis: 0.5g IV q24h

Adverse Drug Reactions: Occasional: Diarrhea (5%); nausea; headache; rash; LFTs elevation. **Rare:** Seizure (decreased incidence of seizures in animal studies); hypersensitivity reaction.

Drug Interactions
Probenecid: Increase in meropenem level (56%) due to inhibition of tubular secretion by probenecid. Avoid concurrent administration, monitor for Meropenem toxicity.

Pregnancy Risk: B-Animal data shows no risk. No data in humans. Carbapenem antibiotic is considered safest to use during perinatal period (i.e., 28 weeks gestation or later) and most likely meropenem can be classified this way. The fetal risk of use before this period is unknown.

Breast Feeding: No data available

Comments: Similar spectrum of activity to imipenem that includes P. aeruginosa and ESBL producing organisms with comparable efficacy for intra-abdominal and soft tissue infections. May have an advantage over imipenem for the treatment of meningitis where up to 6g per day has been used with minimal seizure complications. More expensive compared to imipenem.

Forms

Brand name	Preparation	Mfr.	Route	Form	Strength	Cost (AWP)
Merrem	Meropenem	Astra Zeneca	IV	vial	500mg; 1000mg	$31.50; $63.00

Selected Readings
ATS and IDSA. Guidelines for the Management of Adults with Hospital-acquired, Ventilator-associated, and Healthcare-associated Pneumonia. Am J Respir Crit Care Med 2005;171:388

Schmutzhard E, et al. A randomised comparison of meropenem with cefotaxime or ceftriaxone for the treatment of bacterial meningitis in adults. J Antimicrob Chemother 1995 Jul;36 Suppl A:85-97

Odio CM, et al. Prospective, randomized, investigator-blinded study of the efficacy and safety of meropenem vs. cefotaxime therapy in bacterial meningitis in children. Pediatr Infect Dis J 1999 Jul;18 (7):581-90

Zanetti G, et al. Meropenem (1.5 g/day) is as effective as imipenem/cilastatin (2 g/day) for the treatment of moderately severe intra-abdominal infections. Int J Antimicrob Agents 1999 Feb;11(2):107-13

METRONIDAZOLE

FDA Indications
- Intra-abdominal infections
- Skin and skin structure infections

- Gynecologic infections (endometritis, endomyometritis, tubo-ovarian abscess, and postsurgical vaginal cuff infection)
- Bacterial septicemia
- Bone and joint infections
- Central nervous system infections (meningitis and brain abscess)
- Lower respiratory tract infections (in combination with another agent with activity against microaerophilic streptococcus)
- Endocarditis (caused by Bacteroides species)
- Elective colorectal surgery (classified as contaminated or potentially contaminated.)
- Bacterial vaginosis (Flagyl ER)

Usual Adult Dosing: 250-500mg PO tid or 500mg IV q6h (manufacturer's recommendation). Bacterial vaginosis: Flagyl ER 750mg PO qd x 7d. Consider 0.5-1g PO or IV q12h (based on PK data).

Dosing Adjustments
GFR 50-80 mL/min: Usual dose
GFR 10-50 mL/min: Usual dose
GFR<10 mL/min: Usual dose
Hemodialysis: Usual regimen
Peritoneal Dialysis: Usual regimen
↓ *Hepatic Function:* Consider decreasing dose in severe hepatic impairment.

Adverse Drug Reactions: Frequent: GI intolerance; metallic taste; headache; dark urine (harmless). **Occasional:** peripheral neuropathy (with prolonged use, usually reversible); phlebitis at injection sites; disulfiram-like reaction with alcohol; insomnia; stomatitis.

Drug Interactions
Barbiturates (phenobarbital): Decreased metronidazole blood concentration due to barbiturates enzyme induction leading to more rapid clearance of metronidazole. Monitor for antimicrobial efficacy. Dose of metronidazole may need to be increased.
Disulfiram: May cause nausea, vomiting, headache, abdominal cramps and flushing. Acute psychosis or confusional state may also result. Monitor for change in mental status. If change in mental status occurs one or both drugs needs to be discontinued.
Ethanol: Disulfiram-like reaction due to inhibition of alcohol dehydrogenase by metronidazole and increased levels of acetaldehyde. Avoid concomitant ethanol ingestion.
Phenytoin: The level of phenytoin may be increased possibly due to inhibition of hepatic metabolism. Monitor for toxicity and serum level of phenytoin. Adjust dose of phenytoin accordingly.
Warfarin: Anticoagulant effect of warfarin may be enhanced secondary to inhibition of S-warfarin metabolism by metronidazole. Closely monitor INR and sign of bleed. Dose of warfarin may need to be decreased.

Pregnancy Risk: B-Animal (rodents) data show risk of carcinogenicity. The use of metronidazole in pregnancy is controversial, reports in humans have arrived at conflicting data (but most studies show no risk). The manufacturer and CDC consider metronidazole to be contraindicated in the first trimester.

Breast Feeding: Excreted in breast milk. The American Academy of Pediatrics recommends using metronidazole with caution, discontinuation of breast feeding for 12-24 hours is recommended to allow excretion of the drug.

Comments: Oral and parenteral agent that is the gold standard anti-anaerobic. Active against virtually all anaerobes with the exception of actinomyces, Propionibacterium acnes, and lactobacillus species. Also not active against aerobic GPC such as S. milleri, which is the reason it is usually combined with a beta lactam for serious anaerobic infections such as brain or lung abscess. No aerobic activity. Warn patient against alcohol consumption due to disulfiram-like reaction. Nearly 100% oral bioavailability. Considered the preferred antibiotic for C. difficile associated diarrhea due to lower cost compared with PO vanco.

FORMS (♦ DENOTES AVAILABLE GENERICALLY)

Brand name	Preparation	Mfr.	Route	Form	Strength	Cost (AWP)
Flagyl	Metronida-zole	♦ Pharmacia	PO	cap	375mg	$3.91
			PO	tab	250mg; 500mg	$2.56; $4.57
			PO	tab, ER	750mg	$9.48
Metronidazole	Metronida-zole	♦ Baxter	IV	vial	500mg/100mL	$15.34
Metrocream	Metronida-zole	♦ Galderma	topical	cream	0.75% (45g)	$93.68
MetroGel-Vaginal	Metronida-zole	3M	vaginal	gel	0.75% (70g)	$72.72
MetroGel	Metronida-zole	Galderma	topical	gel	0.75% (45g)	$79.50
Metrolotion	Metronida-zole	Galderma	topical	lot	0.75% (59mL)	$93.68

SELECTED READINGS

Gall SA; Kohan AP; Ayers OM et al. Intravenous metronidazole in the treatment of pelvic infections. Obstet Gynecol 1981; 57(1):51-8.

Perlino CA. Metronidazole vs clindamycin treatment of anaerobic pulmonary infection. Failure of metronidazole therapy. Arch Intern Med 1981 Oct; 141(11):1424-7.

Joesoef MR; Schmid GP. Bacterial vaginosis review of treatment options and potential clinical indications for therapy. Clin Infect Dis 1995 Apr; 20 Suppl 1:S72-9

Sjolin J; Lilja A; Eriksson N et al. Treatment of brain abscess with cefotaxime and metronidazole: prospective study on 15 consecutive patients. Clin Infect Dis 1995 Apr;20 Suppl 1:S72-9.

Berglundh T; Krok L; Liljenberg B et al. The use of metronidazole and amoxicillin in the treatment of advanced periodontal disease. J Clin Periodontol 1998 May; 25(5):354-62.

MICAFUNGIN

FDA INDICATIONS

- Esophageal candidiasis (author's opinion: would reserve micafungin for azole-resistant cases)
- Prophylaxis of candida infections in hematopoietic stem cell transplantat pts (HSCT)

USUAL ADULT DOSING: Esophageal candidiasis: 150mg IV qd. Candida prophylaxis in HSCT: 50 mg IV qd.

Dosing Adjustments

GFR 50-80 mL/min: Usual dose

GFR 10-50 mL/min: Usual dose

GFR<10 mL/min: Usual dose

Hemodialysis: Usual dose. Not dialyzable, thus no supplemental doses needed post dialysis.

Peritoneal Dialysis: No data, usual dose likely.

↓ *Hepatic Function:* For Child-Pugh score of 7-9: No dose adjustment needed. No data for severe hepatic dysfunction.

ADVERSE DRUG REACTIONS: Well tolerated with ADR comparable to fluconazole. **Occasional:** Histamine-mediated sx including rash, facial swelling, pruritus & vasodilation; local phlebitis, fever, and LFTs elevation. **Rare:** Anaphylaxis and hemolytic anemia.

PREGNANCY RISK: C--No human data. Visceral abnormalities and abortion with high dose in animal studies.

BREAST FEEDING: Excreted in breast milk. Use with caution.

COMMENTS: Micafungin is an echinocandin antifungal with similar spectrum of activity to caspofungin, which includes all Candida spp and Aspergillus but randomized clinical trials are limited to esophageal candidiasis and Candida prophylaxis in hematopoietic stem cell transplant pts. Clinical data for the use of micafungin in the Rx of invasive fungal disease are limited. Cost may be lower than caspofungin.

FORMS

Brand name	Preparation	Mfr.	Route	Form	Strength	Cost (AWP)
Mycamine	micafungin sodium	Astellas Pharma	IV	vial	50mg	$112.20

SELECTED READINGS

Kohno S, Masaoka T, Yamaguchi H, et al. A multicenter, open-label clinical study of micafungin (FK463) in the treatment of deep-seated mycosis in Japan. Scand J Infect Dis. 2004; 36:372-9

. . Mycamine [package insert]. Deerfield, IL: Astellas Pharma, 2005.

. . Mycamine [package insert]. Deerfield, IL: Astellas Pharma, 2005.

MICONAZOLE

FDA INDICATIONS

- Cutaneous candidiasis
- Tinea cruris
- Tinea pedis
- Tinea corporis

USUAL ADULT DOSING: 100mg qhs intravaginalx7 days or 200mg intravaginal qhs x 3 days (Vulvovaginal candiasis); Apply topically bid x1-4 weeks (for cutaneous candidiasis)

Dosing Adjustments

GFR 50-80 mL/min: Usual dose

GFR 10-50 mL/min: Usual dose

GFR<10 mL/min: Usual dose

Hemodialysis: Usual dose

Peritoneal Dialysis: Usual dose

↓ Hepatic Function: Usual dose

ADVERSE DRUG REACTIONS: Occasional: Burning; itching; irritation

DRUG INTERACTIONS

No significant interactions noted with topical administration.

PREGNANCY RISK: Reports during which vaginal miconazole preparation was used up to 14 days in pregnant women have revealed no adverse effects. It is recommended to avoid first trimester administration.

BREAST FEEDING: No data.

COMMENTS: Topical antifungal agent that is effective forms of treatment for vaginal candidiasis. In the immunocompetent host, one time dose of fluconazole is equivalent and more cost effective.

FORMS

Brand name	Preparation	Mfr.	Route	Form	Strength	Cost (AWP)
Monistat-7	Miconazole	Personal Products	vaginal	cre	2% (35g; 45g)	$14.82; 12.08
			vaginal	sup	100mg	$12.08 for 7
Monistat-3	Miconazole	Ortho McNeil	vaginal	sup	200mg	$47.83 for 3
Monistat-3	Miconazole	Personal Products	vaginal	cre	4% (15g; 25g)	$14.38; $13.20

MINOCYCLINE

FDA INDICATIONS

- Acne vulgaris (adjunctive treatment) preferred agent
- Granuloma inguinale caused by Calymmatobacterium granulomatis
- Lymphogranuloma venereum caused by Chlamydia species
- Psittacosis caused by Chlamydia psittaci
- Q fever
- Rickettsial pox
- Rocky mountain spotted fever
- Typhus infections
- Nongonococcal urethritis
- Yaws caused by T. pertenue

USUAL ADULT DOSING: 100mg PO bid; 100mg IV bid

Dosing Adjustments
GFR 50-80 mL/min: Usual dose
GFR 10-50 mL/min: Usual dose
GFR<10 mL/min: Usual dose
Hemodialysis: Usual dose
Peritoneal Dialysis: Usual dose

ADVERSE DRUG REACTIONS: Frequent: Vertigo; ataxia; nausea; vomiting; GI intolerance (dose related); stains & deforms teeth in kids up to 8 yrs; increased azotemia w/ renal failure. **Occasional:** Hepatotoxicity; esophageal ulcerations; diarrhea; candidiasis; phlebitis; photosensitivity

DRUG INTERACTIONS

Bismuth salts (bismuth subsalicylate-Pepto-Bismol): Bismuth salts chelate tetracyclines resulting in a decreased absorption of tetracycline. Administer bismuth 2 hours after tetracycline.
Digoxin: May result in increased digoxin concentration (in about 10% of patients). May be due to tetracycline's alteration of bowel flora responsible for digoxin metabolism.
Penicillins: In vitro antagonism when co-administered. Bactericidal effect of penicillins may be diminished in vivo. Avoid co-administration.
Urinary alkalinizers (sodium lactate, sodium bicarbonate): Increased urinary excretion of tetracyclines by 24-65% resulting in lower serum concentration.
Polyvalent metal cations (aluminum, zinc, magnesium, iron, calcium [milk"): Polyvalent metal cations form an insoluble chelate with tetracyclines resulting in decreased absorption and serum level of tetracyclines. Separate administration by 4 hours.
Warfarin: May increased hypoprothrombinemia. Monitor INR closely.

PREGNANCY RISK: D-Tetracyclines are contraindicated in pregnancy due to retardation of skeletal development and bone growth; enamel hypoplasia and discoloration of teeth of fetus. Maternal liver toxicity have also been reported.

BREAST FEEDING: Tetracyclines are excreted in breast milk at very low concentrations. There is theoretical possibility of dental staining and inhibition of bone growth, but infants exposed to tetracyclines have blood levels less than 0.05mcg/mL.

COMMENTS: Oral and parenteral tetracycline that may be used in place of doxycycline, but dizziness may be very bothersome in some patients. Absorption is not significantly affected by food. Most active tetracycline against staphylococci. May be useful with rifampin as chronic suppressive treatment of infected bone and joint prosthesis.

FORMS

Brand name	Preparation	Mfr.	Route	Form	Strength	Cost (AWP)
Minocin	Minocycline	Lederle	PO	cap	50mg; 100mg	$2.39; $4.02
Dynacin	Minocycline	Medicis	PO	cap	50mg; 75mg; 100mg	$3.60; $5.35; $6.35
			PO	tab	50mg; 75mg; 100mg	$3.92; $5.35; $6.35
Myrac	Minocycline	Glades	PO	tab	50mg; 75mg; 100mg	$3.45; $5.06; $6.04

MOXIFLOXACIN

FDA INDICATIONS

- Bacterial exacerbation of chronic bronchitis
- sinusitis
- Community-acquired pneumonia (including those caused by multi-drug resistant Streptococcus pneumoniae)
- Complicated skin and skin structure infections
- Uncomplicated skin and skin structure infections
- Bacterial conjunctivitis (ophthalmic drops)

USUAL ADULT DOSING: 400 mg IV or PO qd

Dosing Adjustments

GFR 50-80 mL/min: Usual dose

GFR 10-50 mL/min: Usual dose

GFR<10 mL/min: Usual dose

Hemodialysis: Usual dose (no data)

Peritoneal Dialysis: Usual dose (no data)

ADVERSE DRUG REACTIONS: Occasional: GI intolerance; CNS-headache; malaise; insomnia; restlessness; dizziness; allergic reactions; diarrhea including C. difficile; photosensitivity; increased hepatic enzymes; QTc prolongation; tendon rupture (rare)

DRUG INTERACTIONS

Antacids (magnesium, aluminum, calcium): Formation of quinolone-ion complex results in decreased absorption of quinolones. Moxifloxacin should be taken 4 hours before or 8 hours after antacid administration.

Class IA and Class III antirrythmics (quinidine, procainamide, amiodarone, sotalol): Avoid co-administration due to the potential for QTc prolongation.

Sucralfate, iron, zinc: Decrease absorption of moxifloxacin. Moxifloxacin should be taken 4 hours before or 8 hours after sucralfate, iron or zinc administration.

Vitamins and minerals containing divalent and trivalent cation (i.e., calcium, zinc and iron

PREGNANCY RISK: C-No data for moxifloxacin. In a prospective follow-up study conducted by the European Network of Teratology Information Services (ENTIS), 666 cases of fluoroquinolone exposure (the majority of the exposures were during the first trimester) showed a congenital malformation rate of 4.8%. From previous epidemiologic data, the

4.8% did not exceed the background rate. Animal data demonstrated arthropathy in immature animals with erosions in joint cartilage. The use of fluoroquinolones is not recommended in pregnancy.

BREAST FEEDING: No data. Fluoroquinolones are not recommended during breast feeding due to the potential for arthropathy.

COMMENTS: Oral and parenteral fluoroquinolone with spectrum of activity similar to levofloxacin and gatifloxacin (this includes enhanced activity vs S. pneumoniae). Best anaerobic activity among quinolones, but clinical experience is limited. Poor Pseudomonas activity.

FORMS

Brand name	Preparation	Mfr.	Route	Form	Strength	Cost (AWP)
Avelox	Moxifloxacin	Bayer	IV	preml x bag	400mg/250mL	$43.75 per bag
			PO	tab	400mg	$10.69
Vigamox	Moxifloxacin	Alcon	oph-thalmic	sol	0.5%	$54.18 per 5mL

SELECTED READINGS

P. P. Gleason, et al. Associations Between Initial Antimicrobial Therapy and Medical Outcomes for Hospitalized Elderly Patients with Pneumonia . Arch Intern Med 1999;159:2562]

Petitpretz P. et al. Oral Moxifloxacin vs High-Dosage Amoxicillin in the Treatment of Mild-to-Moderate, Community-Acquired, Suspected Pneumococcal Pneumonia in Adults. Chest 2001; 119(1): 185-95.

MUPIROCIN

FDA INDICATIONS

- Eradication of nasal colonization with methicillin-resistant S. aureus
- Treatment of secondarily infected traumatic skin lesions due to susceptible strains of S. aureus and S. pyogenes.

USUAL ADULT DOSING: Staph nasal colonization: Topical apply bid to each nostril x 5 days.

Dosing Adjustments

GFR 50-80 mL/min: Usual dose
GFR 10-50 mL/min: Usual dose
GFR<10 mL/min: Usual dose
Hemodialysis: Usual dose
Peritoneal Dialysis: Usual dose

ADVERSE DRUG REACTIONS: Occasional: burning; stinging (irritation of mucous membrane), pain, pruritus, rash

DRUG INTERACTIONS

No significant interactions noted.

PREGNANCY RISK: Animal data show no risk. No human data available

BREAST FEEDING: No data available

COMMENTS: Topical agent that may be used for temporarily eradication of S. aureus (including MRSA) nasal carriage.

FORMS

Brand name	Preparation	Mfr.	Route	Form	Strength	Cost (AWP)
Bactroban	Mupirocin	GlaxoSmithKline	topical	cre	2% (15g)	$2.29 per gram
			topical	oint	2% (22g)	$2.27 per gram

SELECTED READINGS

Fernandez C; Gaspar C; Torrellas A et al. A double-blind, randomized, placebo-controlled clinical trial to evaluate the safety and efficacy of mupirocin calcium ointment for eliminating nasal carriage of S. aureus among hospital personnel. J Antimicrob Chemother 1995 Mar;35(3):399-408

Mupirocin Study Group. Nasal mupirocin prevents Staphylococcus aureus exit-site infection during peritoneal dialysis. J Am Soc Nephrol 1996 Nov;7(11):2403-8

Goldfarb J; Crenshaw D; O'Horo J et al. Mupirocin was equivalent to erythromycin in the treatment of impetigo. Antimicrob Agents Chemother 1988 Dec;32(12):1780-3

NAFCILLIN

FDA INDICATIONS

- Endocarditis
- Impetigo
- Staphylococcal infections (bone and joint infections, meningitis, septicemia, skin and soft tissue infections)

USUAL ADULT DOSING: MSSA endocarditis: 2g IV q4h. Soft tissue infections: 1-2g IV q6-4h (may be given IM)

Dosing Adjustments
GFR 50-80 mL/min: Usual dose
GFR 10-50 mL/min: Usual dose
GFR<10 mL/min: Usual dose
Hemodialysis: Usual dose
Peritoneal Dialysis: Usual dose
↓ *Hepatic Function:* Dose decrease needed only for severe hepatic and renal impairment

ADVERSE DRUG REACTIONS: Frequent: Phlebitis at IV sites. **Occasional:** Neutropenia; hypersensitivity reactions; rash; GI intolerance; drug fever; Coombs' test positive; sterile abscesses at IM sites; tissue necrosis with extravasation; Jarisch-Herxheimer reaction. **Rare:** Hepatitis

DRUG INTERACTIONS

No significant interactions noted.

PREGNANCY RISK: B-Several collaborative perinatal project reports involving over 12,000 exposures to penicillin derivatives during the first trimester indicated no association between penicillin derivative drugs and birth defects.

BREAST FEEDING: Excreted in breast milk in low concentration. No adverse effects have been reported.

COMMENTS: Parenteral anti-staphylococcal penicillin that is therapeutically equivalent to oxacillin. Incidence of hepatitis appears to be lower with nafcillin and may be used in patients developing oxacillin-induced hepatitis but may be associated with more neutropenia compared to oxacillin.

FORMS (♦ DENOTES AVAILABLE GENERICALLY)

Brand name	Preparation	Mfr.	Route	Form	Strength	Cost (AWP)
Nafcillin	Nafcillin	♦ Sandoz	IV	vial	1g; 2g; 10g	$7.85; $15.23; $74.63
Nafcillin	Nafcillin	♦ Samson	IV	vial	200g	$272.50

SELECTED READINGS

Maraqa NF et al. Higher Occurrence of Hepatotoxicity and Rash in Patients Treated with Oxacillin, Compared with Those Treated with Nafcillin and Other Commonly Used Antimicrobials. CID 2002;34:50

NELFINAVIR (NFV)

FDA INDICATIONS

- HIV infection, in combination with other antiretrovirals

USUAL ADULT DOSING: NFV 750mg PO tid or 1250mg PO bid with high fat meals. Most would avoid dual PI with NFV due to limited clinical data. NFV 1250mg bid with EFV 600mg qhs.

Dosing Adjustments

GFR 50-80 mL/min: Usual dose

GFR 10-50 mL/min: Usual dose likely

GFR<10 mL/min: Usual dose likely (pharmacokinetics unchanged in renal failure)

Hemodialysis: Usual dose. Removed with HD, must be given post-HD on days of dialysis (AIDS 2000; 14:89)

Peritoneal Dialysis: No data: usual dose likely

ADVERSE DRUG REACTIONS: Diarrhea (most respond to imodium and some respond to pancrealipase); lipodystrophy syndrome; hyperglycemia; increased triglycerides and/or cholesterol; LFTs elevation; urticaria (rare)

DRUG INTERACTIONS

Substrate of 2C19 (major) and CYP3A4 (minor), inducer and inhibitor at CYP 3A4, and inducer of glucuronosyl transferase. NFV active M8 metabolite is a substrate of CYP3A4 (major). Drugs that are inhibitors of CYP3A4 may increase levels of main NFV metabolite (N8). Drugs that are inducers of CYP2C19 may decrease NFV serum levels.

Contraindicated with: terfenadine, astemizole, cisapride, ergot alkaloid, rifampin, midazolam, rifapentine, pimozide, St Johns wort, and triazolam.

PREGNANCY RISK: B-Placental passage unknown. Not teratogenic in rodent studies. No data on carcinogenicity.

BREAST FEEDING: Unknown breast milk excretion. Breast feeding is not recommended in the U.S. in order to avoid post-natal transmission of HIV to the child, who may not yet be infected.

COMMENTS: High variability in absorption with dependence on fatty foods and lower potency at high viral load makes nelfinavir an unfavorable PI. Generally well tolerated but diarrhea can be bothersome. Diarrhea can usually be managed with loperamide and Metamucil.

FORMS

Brand name	Preparation	Mfr.	Route	Form	Strength	Cost (AWP)
Viracept	Nelfinavir (NFV)	Pfizer	PO	pow	50mg/g (144g)	$66.48
			PO	tab	625mg; 250mg	$6.05; $2.52

NEOMYCIN

FDA INDICATIONS

- Bladder irrigation
- Bowel preparation (w/ erythromycin for elective colon surgery)
- Minor dermal infection
- Ocular infections (keratoconjunctivitis, keratitis, conjunctivitis, blepharoconjunctivitis, blepharitis)
- Portal-systemic encephalopathy

USUAL ADULT DOSING: 1-4g PO tid

Dosing Adjustments

GFR 50-80 mL/min: Usual dose

GFR 10-50 mL/min: 1-4g q12-18 hours

GFR<10 mL/min: 1-4g q18-24 hours

Hemodialysis: No data, may require adjustment

ADVERSE DRUG REACTIONS: Occasional: Renal failure; vestibular and auditory damage may occur through systemic accumulation of oral doses in patients with decrease GFR.

DRUG INTERACTIONS

Digoxin: Increased serum digoxin level in about 10% of patients due to the alteration of microbial gut flora by oral neomycin resulting in decreased metabolism of digoxin in GI tract. Monitor serum level and clinical symptoms of digoxin toxicity (nausea, vomiting, blurred vision, yellow green halos around visual changes). Dose of digoxin may need to be decreased.

Loop diuretics (bumetanide, furosemide, ethacrynic acid, torsemide): May increase ototoxicity but less of an issue compared to systemically administered aminoglycosides.

Nephrotoxic agents (amphotericin B, foscarnet, cidofovir): May increase nephrotoxicity but less of an issue compared to systemically administered aminoglycosides.

PREGNANCY RISK: C-Ototoxicity has not been reported with in utero exposure, however eighth cranial nerve toxicity in the fetus is well known with exposure to other aminoglycosides (kanamycin and streptomycin) and can potentially occur with neomycin. A report of 30 exposures in the first trimester to neomycin found no association between neomycin and congenital defects.

BREAST FEEDING: No data available

COMMENTS: Cochlear toxicity precludes parenteral use. Main use is for treatment of hepatic encephalopathy and with erythromycin as the favored bowel prep in patients undergoing elective colon surgery. Though usually used only in a topical applications, systemic effects may occur when used in large volumes.

FORMS (♦ DENOTES AVAILABLE GENERICALLY)

Brand name	Preparation	Mfr.	Route	Form	Strength	Cost (AWP)
Neomycin sulfate	Neomycin sulfate	♦ Teva	PO	tab	500mg	$1.25
Neo-Fradin	Neomycin	X-Gen	PO	Sol	125mg/5mL	$0.40 per 5mL

NEVIRAPINE (NVP)

FDA INDICATIONS

• HIV infection, in combination with other antiretrovirals

USUAL ADULT DOSING: NVP 200mg PO qd for 14d then 200mg PO bid or 400mg PO qd (hepatotoxicity may be higher with qd dosing). Combination dosing: IDV 1000mg q8h with NVP 200mg bid/ NFV 1200mg bid with NVP 200mg bid, LPV 4 caps bid w/ NVP 200mg bid.

Dosing Adjustments

GFR 50-80 mL/min: 200mg qd x 14 days then 200mg bid

GFR 10-50 mL/min: 200mg qd x 14 days then 200mg bid

GFR<10 mL/min: 200mg qd x 14 days then 200mg bid

Hemodialysis: 200mg qd x 14 days then 200mg bid, on days of dialysis dose post dialysis.

↓ *Hepatic Function:* AUC may be increased up to 41%; may consider decreasing dose

ANTI-INFECTIVES

ADVERSE DRUG REACTIONS: Rash in 17% of patients (7% discontinued due to rash, many patient require hospitalization) Stevens-Johnson Syndrome and TEN reported; 5 deaths reported; LFTs elevation; SEVERE ACUTE HEPATITIS (higher CD4 and women are at increased risk); fever; nausea; h/a

DRUG INTERACTIONS

CYP3A4 substrate and inducer. May significantly decrease serum levels of other CYP3A4 substrates. CYP3A4 inducers may decrease NVP levels.

Co-administration not recommended with: ketoconazole, rifampin (but controversial), saquinavir (as a sole PI).

PREGNANCY RISK: C-Placental passage of 100% in humans. In HIVNET 006 trial (nevirapine 200mg given to 21 HIV-infected pregnant patients) nevirapine was well tolerated and no fetal defects were noted (AIDS; 1999 March 11; 13(4):479-486.).

BREAST FEEDING: Breast feeding is not recommended in the U.S. in order to avoid post-natal transmission of HIV to the child, who may not yet be infected.

COMMENTS: Potent non-nucleoside reverse transcriptase inhibitor that is equivalent to efavirenz. Incidence of lipodystrophy is low, but hepatotoxicity (esp. with 400mg qd dosing) and rash especially during the first 6-10 weeks is a concern. No longer advocated for post-exposure prophylaxis.

FORMS

Brand name	Preparation	Mfr.	Route	Form	Strength	Cost (AWP)
Viramune	Nevirapine (NVP)	Boehringer Ingle-heim	PO	susp	50mg/5mL	$1.92 per 5mL
			PO	tab	200mg	$7.08

NITAZOXANIDE

FDA INDICATIONS

- Diarrhea caused by Cryptosporidium and Giardia in children.
- Cryptosporidiosis in immunocompromised patients (orphan drug status)

USUAL ADULT DOSING: Immunocompetent Adult: 500mg PO q6-12h x 3d. Immunocompetent Peds 4-11y: 200mg q12h x3d. Immunocompetent Peds 1-3y: 100mg q12h x3d. Most experts would treat for 4-6 weeks in immunocompromised patients.

Dosing Adjustments

GFR 50-80 mL/min: No data; usual dose likely

GFR 10-50 mL/min: No data; usual dose likely

GFR<10 mL/min: No data; usual dose likely

ADVERSE DRUG REACTIONS: Occasional: abdominal pain (administer with food); headache. **Rare:** hypotension with tachycardia

DRUG INTERACTIONS

No significant interactions noted.

PREGNANCY RISK: No data

BREAST FEEDING: No data

COMMENTS: Nitazoxanide is effective in the treatment of diarrhea caused by Cryptosporidium parvum in immunocompetent host. Its efficacy in immunocompromised patients (i.e., HIV) remains to be determined. Avoid use in patients with hypersensitivity to aspirin or salicylates due to structural similarities.

FORMS

Brand name	Preparation	Mfr.	Route	Form	Strength	Cost (AWP)
Alinia	Nitazoxanide	Romark	PO	susp	100mg/5mL	$5.38 per 5mL
			PO	tab	500mg	$12.58

SELECTED READINGS

Rossignol J-F, et al. Treatment of diarrhea caused by Cryptosporidium parvum: a prospective randomized, double-blind, placebo-controlled study of nitazoxanide . JID 2001;184:103

Gilles HM et al. Treatment of intestinal parasitic infections: a review of nitazoxanide. Trends in Parasitology. 2002; 18:95-7.

NITROFURANTOIN

FDA INDICATIONS

- Uncomplicated urinary tract infections

USUAL ADULT DOSING: Treatment: 50-100mg PO q6h or Macrobid 100mg PO bid. UTI suppression: 50-100mg PO qd.

Dosing Adjustments

GFR 50-80 mL/min: Usual dose

GFR 10-50 mL/min: Avoid due to inadequate urinary level and potential for toxic serum level.

GFR<10 mL/min: See above

Hemodialysis: See above

Peritoneal Dialysis: See above

ADVERSE DRUG REACTIONS: Frequent: GI intolerance (macrocrystallin better tolerated). **Rare:** Hypersensitivity reactions; pulmonary infiltrates->fibrosis (acute pulmonary hypersensitivity: fever, cough, dyspnea w/ infiltrate & eosinophilia, occurs w/in hrs-wks); methemoglobinemia.

DRUG INTERACTIONS

Norfloxacin: May be antagonistic, avoid concurrent administration.

PREGNANCY RISK: B-In a surveillance study of Michigan Medicaid recipients, 1,292 exposures to nitrofurantoin resulted in a 4.0% birth defect rate. This data did not support an association between nitrofurantoin and congenital defects.

BREAST FEEDING: Excreted in breast milk. Theoretical chance of hemolytic anemia in G6PD deficiency. The American Academy of Pediatrics considers nitrofurantoin compatible with breast feeding.

COMMENTS: Antiseptic for uncomplicated UTI's. Caution when used in G6PD deficient pts. Avoid in pts w/ est. CrCl <40 mL/min since efficacy is decreased & side effects increased. Associated w/ acute allergic pneumonitis w/ short-term treatment & interstitial fibrosis w/ long-term use has been reported.

FORMS (♦ DENOTES AVAILABLE GENERICALLY)

Brand name	Preparation	Mfr.	Route	Form	Strength	Cost (AWP)
Macrodantin	Nitrofuran-toin macro-crystals	Procter&Gamble	PO	cap	25mg; 50mg; 100mg	$1.04; $1.37; $2.33
Macrobid	Nitrofuran-toin	Proctor&Gamble	PO	cap	100mg	$2.54
Furadantin	Nitrofuran-toin	♦ First Horizon	PO	susp	25mg/5mL	$3.08 per 5mL

SELECTED READINGS

Iravani A, Klimberg I, Briefer C et al. A trial comparing low-dose, short-course ciprofloxacin and standard 7 day therapy with co-trimoxazole or nitrofurantoin in the treatment of uncomplicated urinary tract infection. J Antimicrob Chemother. 1999;43 Suppl A:67-75.

NORFLOXACIN

FDA INDICATIONS

- Endocervical and urethral gonorrhea
- Prostatitis
- Uncomplicated and complicated urinary tract infections

USUAL ADULT DOSING: UTI, prostatitis, and prophylaxis in neutropenic pts: 400mg PO bid. Uncomplicated GC 800mg x1. SBP prophylaxis: 400mg PO qd.

Dosing Adjustments

GFR 50-80 mL/min: Usual dose

GFR 10-50 mL/min: 400mg qd

GFR<10 mL/min: 400mg qd

Hemodialysis: not removed in hemodialysis, dose 400mg qd

Peritoneal Dialysis: 400mg qd

↓ *Hepatic Function:* Serum level unchanged in hepatic insufficiency

ADVERSE DRUG REACTIONS: Generally well tolerated. **Occasional:** n/v/d, dyspepsia, flatulence, h/a, and dizziness. **Rare:** Photosensitivity; increased hepatic enzymes; myalgia; tendon rupture.

DRUG INTERACTIONS

Divalent and trivalent cations/sucralfate; nitrofurantoin: Avoid. May be antagonistic. Avoid concurrent administration.

Sucralfate: Decreased absorption of fluoroquinolone due to the complexation of the aluminum ions contained in the sucralfate. Avoid co-administration. If concurrent administration required, administer sucralfate at least 6 hours before or 2 hours after quinolone antibiotics.

Milk or dairy products: Decreased the GI absorption of norfloxacin by approximately 50% due to chelation by divalentcalcium ions. Avoid co-administration with milk or lengthen the interval between milk consumption a norfloxacin administration.

Vitamins and minerals containing divalent and trivalent cation (i.e., calcium, zinc and iron and antacids (magnesium, aluminum, calcium): Formation of quinolone-ion complex results in decreased absorption of quinolones. Avoid co-administration, if concurrent administration required, administer cation at least 6 hours before or 2 hours after quinolone antibiotics.

PREGNANCY RISK: C-In a prospective follow-up study conducted by the European Network of Teratology Information Services (ENTIS), 666 cases of fluoroquinolone exposure (the majority of the exposures were during the first trimester) showed a congenital malformation rate of 4.8%. From previous epidemiologic data, the 4.8% did not exceed the background rate. Animal data demonstrated arthropathy in immature animals with erosions in joint cartilage. Because of the animal data, and the availability of alternative antimicrobial agents, the use of fluoroquinolones during pregnancy is considered contraindicated.

BREAST FEEDING: Fluoroquinolones are not recommended during breast feeding due to the potential for arthropathy (based on animal data).

COMMENTS: Oral fluoroquinolone that is not well absorbed compared to most agents in this class. Main uses are as prophylaxis for spontaneous bacterial peritonitis (SBP) and prophylaxis in neutropenic patients.

FORMS

Brand name	Preparation	Mfr.	Route	Form	Strength	Cost (AWP)
Noroxin	Norfloxacin	Merck	PO	tab	400mg	$3.99

SELECTED READINGS

Orlandi E, et al. Norfloxacin versus cotrimoxazole for infection prophylaxis in granulocytopenic patients with acute leukemia. A prospective randomized study. Haematologica 1990 May-Jun;75(3):296-8

Grange JD, et al. Norfloxacin primary prophylaxis of bacterial infections in cirrhotic patients with ascites: a double-blind randomized trial . J Hepatol 1998 Sep;29(3):430-6

Thornton SA, et al. Norfloxacin compared to trimethoprim/sulfamethoxazole for the treatment of travelers' diarrhea among U.S. military personnel deployed to South America and West Africa. Mil Med 1992 Feb;157(2):55-8

NYSTATIN

FDA INDICATIONS

- Orapharyngeal candidiasis
- Vulvovaginal candidiasis
- Treatment of cutaneous or mucocutaneous mycotic infections caused by Candida albicans and other susceptible Candida species

USUAL ADULT DOSING: 500,000 to 1,000,000 Units (5-10mL) 3-5 times per day.

Dosing Adjustments

GFR 50-80 mL/min: Usual dose

GFR 10-50 mL/min: Usual dose

GFR<10 mL/min: Usual dose

Hemodialysis: Usual dose

Peritoneal Dialysis: Usual dose

↓ *Hepatic Function:* Usual dose

ADVERSE DRUG REACTIONS: Bad taste; diarrhea; GI distress (n/v/d); skin irritation with topical application

DRUG INTERACTIONS

No significant interactions noted.

PREGNANCY RISK: B-No fetal harm has been reported.

BREAST FEEDING: Compatible with breastfeeding.

COMMENTS: Nystatin has a bitter taste, causes GI side effects, must be given at least 4x/day, and may not work as well as clotrimazole. Clotrimazole lozenges preferred by most patients due to better taste.

FORMS (◆ DENOTES AVAILABLE GENERICALLY)

Brand name	Preparation	Mfr.	Route	Form	Strength	Cost (AWP)
Mycostatin	Nystatin	Westwood Squibb	topical	cre	100,000U/g	$28.52 per 30g
Nystatin	Nystatin	◆ Teva	PO	tab	500,000U	$0.68
Nystatin	Nystatin	◆ Alpharma	PO	susp	100,000U/mL	$16.94 per 60mL
Nystatin	Nystatin	Odyssey	vaginal	tab	100,00U	$42.23 for 15
Bio-statin	Nystatin	Bio-Tech	PO	cap	1,000,000U; 500,000U	$0.35; $0.24

OFLOXACIN
FDA INDICATIONS
- Acute exacerbation of chronic bronchitis
- Otitis media
- Community-acquired pneumonia
- Endocervical and urethral chlamydial infections
- Endocervical and urethral gonorrhea (Note: high resistance rates reported Hawaii and California)
- PID
- Prostatitis
- Skin and soft tissue infections
- Uncomplicated and complicated UTI
- Conjunctivitis, keratitis and corneal ulcers (ophthalmic solution)

USUAL ADULT DOSING: CAP, soft tissue infection, and URTI: 400mg PO bid. Uncomplicated GC: 400x1. Uncomplicated UTI: 200mg PO bid x 3-7d. NonGC Cervicitis/Urethritis: 300mg bid x 7d.

Dosing Adjustments
GFR 50-80 mL/min: Usual dose
GFR 10-50 mL/min: 0.2g-0.4g IV or PO q24h
GFR<10 mL/min: 0.1g-0.2g IV or PO q24h
Hemodialysis: 200 mg, then 100mg q24h
Peritoneal Dialysis: 100-200mg IV or PO q24h

ADVERSE DRUG REACTIONS: Occasional: GI intol; CNS-headache; malaise; insomnia; restlessness; dizziness; allergic rxn; diarrhea; photosensitivity; incr. LFTs; tendon rupture (incr. incidence seen in older men with concurrent use of corticosteroids Arch Intern Med 2003; 163:1801)

DRUG INTERACTIONS
Procainamide: Reduction of tubular secretion resulting in an increased level of procainamide. Monitor level of procainamide and clinical signs of toxicity.
Sucralfate: Decreased oral absorption of fluoroquinolone due to chelation by the aluminum ions contained in the sucralfate. Avoid co-administration. If concurrent administration required, administer sucralfate at least 6 hours before or 2 hours after quinolone antibiotics.
Vitamins and minerals containing divalent and trivalent cation (i.e., calcium, zinc and iron) and antacids (magnesium, aluminum, calcium): Formation of quinolone-ion complex results in decreased absorption of quinolones. Avoid co-administration, if concurrent administration required, administer cation at least 6 hours before or 2 hours after quinolone antibiotics.

PREGNANCY RISK: C-In a prospective follow-up study conducted by the European Network of Teratology Information Services (ENTIS), 666 cases of fluoroquinolone exposure (the majority of the exposures were during the first trimester) showed a congenital malformation rate of 4.8%. From previous epidemiologic data, the 4.8% did not exceed the background rate. Animal data demonstrated arthropathy in immature animals with erosions in joint cartilage. Because of the animal data, and the availability of alternative antimicrobial agents, the use of fluoroquinolones during pregnancy is considered contraindicated.

BREAST FEEDING: Fluoroquinolones are not recommended during breast feeding due to the potential for arthropathy (based on animal data).

COMMENTS: Oral FQ that has been largely supplanted by levofloxacin, its more active L-isomer. IV formulation is no longer available. Ofloxacin ophthalmic drops is equivalent to ciprofloxacin ophthalmic drops in the treatment of corneal ulcer. Ofloxacin is preferred over cipro due to a 20% incidence crystalline precipitate in the epithelial defect seen with ciprofloxacin drops.

FORMS

Brand name	Preparation	Mfr.	Route	Form	Strength	Cost (AWP)
Floxin	Ofloxacin	Ortho-McNeil	PO	tab	200mg; 300mg; 400mg	$5.40; $6.43; $6.78
Ocuflox	Ofloxacin	Allergan	oph-thalmic	gtt	0.3% (5mL); 0.3% (10mL)	$46.86; $93.59
Floxin	Ofloxacin	Daiichi	otic	gtt	0.3%(10mL); 0.3% (5mL)	$79.96; $48.21

SELECTED READINGS

Anon. Fluoroquinolone-Resistance in Neisseria gonorrhoeae, Hawaii, 1999, and Decreased Susceptibility to Azithromycin in N. gonorrhoeae, Missouri, 1999: [MMWR 2000;49:833]: . MMWR 2000;49:833

Adachi JA, et al. Empirical Antimicrobial Therapy for Traveler's Diarrhea . CID 2000;31:1079

Spencer RC et al. Ofloxacin versus trimethoprim and co-trimoxazole in the treatment of uncomplicated urinary tract infection in general practice. Br J Clin Pract 1992 Spring;46(1):30-3

Covino JM; Cummings M; Smith B et al. Comparison of ofloxacin and ceftriaxone in the treatment of uncomplicated gonorrhea caused by penicillinase-producing and non- penicillinase-producing strains. Antimicrob Agents Chemother 1990 Jan;34(1):148-9

DuPont HL; Ericsson CD; Mathewson JJ et al. Five versus three days of ofloxacin therapy for traveler's diarrhea: a placebo-controlled study. Antimicrob Agents Chemother 1992 Jan;36(1):87-91

OSELTAMIVIR

FDA INDICATIONS

- Uncomplicated acute illness due to influenza A and B infection in adults who have been symptomatic for no more than 2 days
- Prevention of influenza during an outbreak/epidemic

USUAL ADULT DOSING: Influenza treatment: 75mg PO q12h x 5 days (must be started within 48 hours of symptoms). Influenza prophylaxis: 75mg PO qd x at least 7 days following close contact or up to 6 weeks during a community outbreak, must be given within 48 hours.

Dosing Adjustments
GFR 50-80 mL/min: Usual dose
GFR 10-50 mL/min: 75mg q24h

ADVERSE DRUG REACTIONS: Frequent: nausea; vomiting; diarrhea

DRUG INTERACTIONS

Probenecid: Co-administration resulted in a twofold increase in oseltamivir. The clinical significance of this interaction is unknown.

PREGNANCY RISK: C-No data in human. Animal data using large dose resulted in maternal toxicity.

BREAST FEEDING: No data

COMMENTS: Oral anti-influenza agent that is active against influenza A and B. Treatment must be started within 48 hours of the onset of symptoms. Effective for prevention of influenza. More expensive compared to rimantidine or amantadine. GI side effects may be bothersome. Unlike rimantidine and amantadine, oseltamivir is active against influenza B and avian influenza.

FORMS

Brand name	Preparation	Mfr.	Route	Form	Strength	Cost (AWP)
Tamiflu	Oseltamivir	Roche	PO	cap	75mg	$7.35
			PO	susp	12mg/mL	$7.35 per 5mL

SELECTED READINGS

Welliver R, et al. Effectiveness of Oseltamivir in Preventing Influenza in Household Contacts: A Randomized Controlled Trial . JAMA 2001;285:748

F. G. Hayden, et al. Use of the Selective Oral Neuraminidase Inhibitor Oseltamivir to Prevent Influenza . NEJM 1999;341:1336

J. J. Treanor, et al. Efficacy and Safety of the Oral Neuraminidase Inhibitor Oseltamivir in Treating Acute Influenza: A Randomized Controlled Trial . JAMA 2000;283:1016

OXACILLIN

FDA INDICATIONS

- Endocarditis
- Staphylococcal infections
- Treatment of bacterial septicemia
- Skin and soft tissue infections

USUAL ADULT DOSING: MSSA endocarditis: 2g IV q4h (+/- aminoglycoside). Soft tissue infection: 1-2g IV q4-6h (may be given IM).

Dosing Adjustments
GFR 50-80 mL/min: Usual dose
GFR 10-50 mL/min: Usual dose
GFR<10 mL/min: Usual dose
Hemodialysis: Usual regimen
Peritoneal Dialysis: Usual regimen

ADVERSE DRUG REACTIONS: Frequent: Phlebitis at infusion site; hypersensitivity reactions; rash; hepatitis. **Occasional:** GI intolerance; drug fever; Coombs' test positive; Jarisch-Herxheimer reaction. **Rare:** Anaphylaxis; neutropenia

DRUG INTERACTIONS

Tetracyclines: In vitro antagonism when co-administered. Bactericidal effect of penicillins may be diminished in vivo. Avoid concurrent administration. In two studies involving a total of 79 patients with pneumococcal meningitis treated with either penicillin plus tetracyclines or penicillin monotherapy there was a higher mortality rate (79-85%) in the combination therapy compared to penicillin monotherapy (30-33%). (Arch Intern Med 1951:88:489, Ann Intern Med 1961; 55:545). However there was not a difference in mortality between penicillin monotherapy and penicillin plus tetracycline in the treatment of pneumococcal pneumonia. (Arch Intern Med 1953; 91:197).

PREGNANCY RISK: B-Several collaborative perinatal project reports involving over 12,000 exposures to penicillin derivatives during the first trimester indicated no association between penicillin derivative drugs and birth defects.

BREAST FEEDING: Excreted in breast milk in low concentration. No adverse effects have been reported.

COMMENTS: Anti-staphylococcal penicillin equivalent to nafcillin but more likely to cause reversible hepatitis.

Brand name	Preparation	Mfr.	Route	Form	Strength	Cost (AWP)
Oxacillin sodium	Oxacillin sodium	◆ Sandoz	IV	vial	1g; 2g; 10g	$7.85; $15.23; $74.63

SELECTED READINGS

Maraqa NF et al. Higher Occurrence of Hepatotoxicity and Rash in Patients Treated with Oxacillin, Compared with Those Treated with Nafcillin and Other Commonly Used Antimicrobials. CID 2002;34:50

PAROMOMYCIN

FDA INDICATIONS

- Intestinal amebiasis
- Hepatic coma

USUAL ADULT DOSING: 2-4g/day in four divided doses

Dosing Adjustments

GFR 50-80 mL/min: Usual dose

GFR 10-50 mL/min: Usual dose

GFR<10 mL/min: Usual dose

Hemodialysis: Usual dose

Peritoneal Dialysis: Usual dose

↓ *Hepatic Function:* Usual dose

ADVERSE DRUG REACTIONS: Anorexia; nausea; vomiting; cramps; epigastric burning pain.

DRUG INTERACTIONS

Digoxin: Decreased in digoxin serum concentration by 30 to 82%.

PREGNANCY RISK: C-Limited human data, due to poor systemic absorption risk of teratogenicity is low.

BREAST FEEDING: No data; not likely to be excreted in breast milk.

COMMENTS: Primary indication for cryptosporidiosis with only marginal efficacy. Immune reconstitution in HIV infected patients with Highly Active Antiretroviral Therapy (HAART) is the treatment of choice for cryptosporidiosis in patients with AIDS.

FORMS

Brand name	Preparation	Mfr.	Route	Form	Strength	Cost (AWP)
Humatin	Paromomycin	Monarch	PO	cap	250mg	$3.37

PEGINTERFERON ALFA

FDA INDICATIONS

- Peg-interferon alpha-2b (PegIntron): monotherapy for the treatment of chronic hepatitis C in patients not previously treated with interferon alpha who have compensated liver disease.
- Peg-interferon alpha-2a (Pegasys): monotherapy or in combination with ribavirin for the treatment of chronic hepatitis C virus infection who have compensated liver disease and have not previously treated with interferon alpha.
- Peg-interferon alpha-2a (Pegasys) plus ribavirin: treatment of HCV in patients who are coinfected with HIV.

USUAL ADULT DOSING: Peg-intron 1mcg/kg q week (monotherapy, but generally not recommended) or 1.5 mcg/kg q week (with ribavirin). [Dose reduction to 0.5 mcg/kg recommended for ANC<750 or plt<80k and D/C if ANC<500 or plt <50K]. Pegasys 180mcg SC qweek (w/ or w/o ribavirin)[dose reduce with heme toxicity].

Dosing Adjustments

GFR 50-80 mL/min: Usual dose

GFR 10-50 mL/min: Consider dose reduction to 0.5mcg/kg if the patient experiences ADRs (limited data).

GFR<10 mL/min: Consider dose reduction to 0.5mcg/kg if the patient experiences an ADRs (limited data).

↓ *Hepatic Function:* Usual dose

ADVERSE DRUG REACTIONS: Common: flu-like sxs, headache, dizziness, fatigue, fever, rigor, injection site inflamation, DEPRESSION (29%), insomnia, alopecia, GI (abd. pain, anorexia, n/v/d. **Occasional:** thrombocytopenia, neutropenia, hypo- & hyperthyroidism, LFTs elevation.

DRUG INTERACTIONS

No significant interactions noted. Does not appear to inhibit CYP 3A4,1A2, 2C8, 2C9, 2D6 or N-acetyltransferase.

Monitor closely with any drug that can suppress bone marrow.

PREGNANCY RISK: C- Abortifacient in rhesus monkeys. No human data. Recommend that patients use an effective form of contraception during treatment with interferon.

BREAST FEEDING: No data

COMMENTS: Peg interferon, due to an improved pharmacokinetic profile, offers patients a more effective and convenient once weekly administration (at higher cost). Clinical trials between the two peg-INF products have not been conducted, but most experts agree that they are clinically equivalent. Peg-intron may be preferred in pts who are >75kg since fixed dose Pegasys did not perform as well in this group.

FORMS

Brand name	Preparation	Mfr.	Route	Form	Strength	Cost (AWP)
Peg-Intron	Peginterferon alfa-2b	Schering	SC	kit	50mcg; 120mcg; 150mcg	$354.35; $390.66; $410.18
Pegasys	Peginterferon alfa-2a	Roche	SC	kit	180mcg/mL	$404.24

SELECTED READINGS

Fried MW, et al. Peginterferon alfa-2a plus ribavirin for chronic hepatitis C virus infection. NEJM 2002; 347:975-982

Chan HL, Leung NW, Hui AY, Wong VW, et al. A randomized, controlled trial of combination therapy for chronic hepatitis B: comparing pegylated interferon-alpha2b and lamivudine with lamivudine alone. Ann Intern Med. 2005;142:240-50

Strader B, et al. Diagnosis, Management, and Treatment of Hepatitis C. Hepatology 2005;39(4);1147-71

PENCICLOVIR

FDA INDICATIONS

• Herpes labialis

USUAL ADULT DOSING: Apply to affected area every 2 hours while awake for 4 days.

Dosing Adjustments

GFR 50-80 mL/min: Usual dose

GFR 10-50 mL/min: Usual dose
GFR<10 mL/min: Usual dose
Hemodialysis: Usual dose
Peritoneal Dialysis: Usual dose

ADVERSE DRUG REACTIONS: Occasional: Headache; hypoesthesia, skin rash

DRUG INTERACTIONS
No significant interactions noted.

PREGNANCY RISK: B- Animal data did not demonstrate teratogenicity. No human data

BREAST FEEDING: No data

COMMENTS: Topical antiviral agent for herpes labialis. Frequent administration (q2h) and minimal benefit even when started within 24 hours of symptoms make penciclovir somewhat impractical.

FORMS

Brand name	Preparation	Mfr.	Route	Form	Strength	Cost (AWP)
Denavir	Penciclovir	Novartis	topical	cre	1% (1.5g)	$16.93

SELECTED READINGS
McKeough MB, Spruance SL. Comparison of New Topical Treatments for Herpes Labialis: Efficacy of Penciclovir Cream, Acyclovir Cream, and n-Docosanol Cream Against Experimental Cutaneous Herpes Simplex Virus Type 1 Infection . Arch Derm 2001;137:1153

PENICILLIN

FDA INDICATIONS

- PCN procaine: Anthrax due to Bacillus anthracis, including inhalation anthrax (post-exposure). However, CDC does not recommend as first line agent due to betalactamase production (see "Anthrax" in the Diagnoses section).
- Endocarditis (see Tables 1a-1b in Appendix I)
- Skin and soft tissue infection (erysipelas, erysipeloid)
- Rat-bite fever
- Syphilis
- Vincent's infection fusospirochetosis (Vincent's gingivitis and pharyngitis)
- Actinomycosis
- Empyema
- Pasteurella infections
- Pneumonia

USUAL ADULT DOSING: PCN 2-4 MU IV q4h. PCN VK 250-500mg PO qid. Primary, secondary, and latent: PCN benzathine 2.4mU x 1. Late (latent): PCN benzathine: 2.4mU x 3 at 7-day intervals. Neurosyphilis: PCN4 mU IV q4h.

Dosing Adjustments
GFR 50-80 mL/min: Usual dose
GFR 10-50 mL/min: Usual dose
GFR<10 mL/min: 0.5-2mU IV q4-6h; No dose adjustment needed for sustained released preparations
Hemodialysis: 0.5-2mU IV q4-6h plus 500,000 units post-dialysis
Peritoneal Dialysis: 0.5-2mU IV q4-6h
↓ *Hepatic Function:* Dose decrease needed only for severe hepatic and renal impairment

ADVERSE DRUG REACTIONS: Frequent: Hypersensitivity reactions; rash. **Occasional:** GI intolerance; drug fever; Coombs' test positive; phlebitis at infusion sites and sterile abscesses at IM sites; Jarisch-Herxheimer reaction. **Rare:** Hemolytic anemia; anaphylaxis; thrombocytopenia

DRUG INTERACTIONS

Probenecid: Increased PCN concentration beneficial interaction when increased or high serum level needed.

Tetracyclines: Antagonism. Avoid co-administration.

PREGNANCY RISK: B-Several collaborative perinatal project reports involving over 12,000 exposure to penicillin derivatives during the first trimester indicated no association between penicillin derivative drugs and birth defects.

BREAST FEEDING: Excreted in breast milk in low concentration. No adverse effects have been reported.

COMMENTS: PCN is the gold standard for treating Group A strep infections and syphilis. Generic substitution of PCN G benzathine injection is not recommended.

FORMS (♦ DENOTES AVAILABLE GENERICALLY)

Brand name	Preparation	Mfr.	Route	Form	Strength	Cost (AWP)
Veetids	Penicillin V Potassium	♦ Sandoz	PO	Susp	125mg/5mL; 250mg/5mL	$0.21 per 5mL; $0.23 per 5mL
			PO	tab	250mg; 500mg	$0.22; $0.38
Bicillin L-A	PCN G Benzathine	♦ Monarch	IM	syringe	0.6mU/mL	$23.73 per mL
Pfizerpen	PCN G Potassium	♦ Pfizer	IV	vial	5mU; 20mU;	$3.44; 10.09
Penicillin G Potassium	PCN G Potassium	♦ Baxter	IV	vial	1mU/50mL; 2mU/50mL; 3mU/50mL	$12.67; 13.19; $13.69
Bicillin C-R	PCN G Benzathine; PCN G Procaine	Monarch	IM	syringe	0.30mU-0.30U/mL	$16.69 per mL
Bicillin C-R 900/300	PCN G Benzathine; PCN G Procaine	Monarch	IM	syringe	0.9mU-0.30mU/2mL	$17.05 per mL
Penicillin G Procaine	PCN G Procaine	♦ Monarch	IV	vial	0.6mU/mL	$11.87 per mL

SELECTED READINGS

Adam D, et al. Short-Course Antibiotic Treatment of 4,782 Culture-Proven Cases of Group A Streptococcal Tonsillopharyngitis and Incidence of Poststreptococcal Sequelae . JID 2000; 182: 509

Lan AJ, et al. Twice-Daily Dosing of Penicillin V is as Effective as More Frequent Dosing for Streptococcal Tonsillopharyngitis . Pediatrics. 2000;105:E19

PENTAMIDINE

FDA INDICATIONS

- Pneumocystis jiroveci pneumonia, treatment and prophylaxis

USUAL ADULT DOSING: PCP treatment: 4mg/kg IV q24h. PCP prophylaxis: 300mg aerosolize q month.

Dosing Adjustments

GFR 50-80 mL/min: Usual

GFR 10-50 mL/min: 4mg/kg q24-36h

GFR<10 mL/min: 4mg/kg q48h

Hemodialysis: Nonsignificant increase in elimination half-life during hemodialysis. No dosage adjustment needed

Peritoneal Dialysis: No data, no supplemental dose needed

ADVERSE DRUG REACTIONS: Frequent: Nephrotoxicity - usually reversible w/dc; cough (w/ aerosolized form). **Occasional:** Hypotension (give IV over 60 min to dc risk); hypoglycemia; marrow suppression; GI intolerance w/nausea, vomiting, decreased Ca, Mg and K. **Rare:** Pancreatitis and torsades

DRUG INTERACTIONS

Ampho B and **Foscarnet:** Increased risk of severe hypocalemia.

Didanosine: Potential for additive risk of pancreatitis.

Nephrotoxic agents (aminoglycoside, foscarnet, cidofovir, amphotericin B, cyclosporin): Additive nephrotoxicity. Monitor renal function closely. Drugs may need to be discontinued if nephrotoxicity occurs.

PREGNANCY RISK: C-Both manufacturer and CDC advise against the use of pentamidine in pregnancy. Spontaneous abortion reported, however causal relationship has not been established.

BREAST FEEDING: No data

COMMENTS: Parenteral agent that is used for treatment of severe PCP in patients who fail or are intolerant to TMP/SMX or clinda/primaquine. Toxicity such as hypotension, hypoglycemia and renal failure limit its use. Close monitoring of vital signs and blood sugar with infusion recommended. Avoid concurrent administration of nephrotoxic drugs due to additive nephrotoxicity. Monitor electrolytes.

FORMS (◆ DENOTES AVAILABLE GENERICALLY)

Brand name	Preparation	Mfr.	Route	Form	Strength	Cost (AWP)
Pentam	Pentamidine	◆ American Pharma	IV	vial	300mg	$98.75
NebuPent	Pentamidine	◆ American Pharma	inhalation	powder	300mg	$98.75

SELECTED READINGS

Klein NC, Duncanson FP, Lenox TH, et al. Trimethoprim-sulfamethoxazole versus pentamidine for Pneumocystis carinii pneumonia in AIDS patients: results of a large prospective randomized treatment trial. AIDS. 1992;6:301-5

PERMETHRIN

FDA INDICATIONS

- Pediculosis
- Scabies

USUAL ADULT DOSING: 1% cream rinse apply to hair and scalp (for at least 10 min); 5% topical cream apply from head to toe (leave in place for 8-12 hours before rinse). In epidemic setting or if live lice are present after 2 weeks, a second application is recommended.

Dosing Adjustments

GFR 50-80 mL/min: Usual dose

GFR 10-50 mL/min: Usual dose

GFR<10 mL/min: Usual dose

Hemodialysis: Usual dose

Peritoneal Dialysis: Usual dose

ADVERSE DRUG REACTIONS: Pruritis; burning or stinging

DRUG INTERACTIONS

No significant interactions noted.

PREGNANCY RISK: B-No human data. Not teratogenic in animal studies. CDC considers permethrin the drug of choice in pregnancy.

BREAST FEEDING: No human data; breast milk excretion in animal studies. CDC considers permethrin the drug of choice in breastfeeding women.

COMMENTS: Permethrin is the prefered agent for scabies due to comparable efficacy with lower risk of neurotoxicity compared to lindane [Schultz et al. Arch Dermatol 1990;126:167-70]

FORMS (◆ DENOTES AVAILABLE GENERICALLY)

Brand name	Preparation	Mfr.	Route	Form	Strength	Cost (AWP)
Elimite	Permethrin	◆ Allergan	topical	cre	5% (60g)	$41.42
Permethrin	Permethrin	◆ Clay-Park	topical	cre	5% (60g)	$29.25
Permethrin	Permethrin	◆ Alpharma	topical	lotion	1% (60mL)	$8.19

PIPERACILLIN

FDA INDICATIONS

- Bone and joint infections
- Gonococcal infections
- Gynecologic infections
- Intra-abdominal infections
- Lower respiratory tract infections
- Septicemia
- Skin and skin structure infections
- Surgical prophylaxis (intra-abdominal procedure, vaginal hysterectomy, abdominal hysterectomy, C-section)
- Urinary tract infections

USUAL ADULT DOSING: Moderate to severe infections: 3g IV q4-6h (up to 24g a day). Pneumonia and Pseudomonal infections: 3g IV q4h.

Dosing Adjustments

GFR 50-80 mL/min: Usual dose

GFR 10-50 mL/min: 3g q8h; for severe infection 3g q6h

GFR<10 mL/min: 3g q12h; for severe infx 3g q8h

Hemodialysis: 2g q8h plus 1g post-dialysis; for severe infection 3g q8h plus 1g post dialysis

Peritoneal Dialysis: 2g q8h; for severe infection 3g q8h

ADVERSE DRUG REACTIONS: Frequent: Hypersensitivity reactions; rash. **Occasional:** GI intolerance; drug fever; Coombs' test positive; phlebitis at infusion sites; Jarisch-Herxheimer reaction. **Rare:** Anaphylaxis; hemolytic anemia.

DRUG INTERACTIONS

Tetracyclines: In vitro antagonism when co-administered. Bactericidal effect of penicillins may be diminished in vivo. Avoid concurrent administration. In two studies involving a total of 79 patients with pneumococcal meningitis treated with either penicillin plus tetracyclines or penicillin monotherapy there was a higher mortality rate (79-85%) in the combination therapy compared to penicillin monotherapy (30-33%). (Arch Intern Med 1951:88:489, Ann Intern Med 1961; 55:545). However there was not a difference in mortality between penicillin monotherapy and penicillin plus tetracycline in the treatment of pneumococcal pneumonia. (Arch Intern Med 1953; 91:197).

PREGNANCY RISK: B-Several collaborative perinatal project reports involving over 12,000 exposures to penicillin derivatives during the first trimester indicated no association between penicillin derivative drugs and birth defects.

BREAST FEEDING: Excreted in breast milk in low concentration. No adverse effects have been reported.

COMMENTS: Parenteral anti-pseudomonal penicillin with improved enterococcal coverage compared to ticarcillin.

FORMS (♦ DENOTES AVAILABLE GENERICALLY)

Brand name	Preparation	Mfr.	Route	Form	Strength	Cost (AWP)
Piperacillin	Piperacillin	♦ American Pharm Partners	IV	vial	3g; 4g; 40g; 2g	$12.53; $16.70; $161.25; $8.35

SELECTED READINGS

Mattoes HM, Capitano B, Kim MK et al. Comparative pharmacokinetic and pharmacodynamic profile of piperacillin/tazobactam 3.375G Q4H and 4.5G Q6H. Chemotherapy. 2002;48(2):59-63.

PIPERACILLIN + TAZOBACTAM

FDA INDICATIONS

- Gynecologic infections (pelvic inflammatory disease, post-partum endometritis)
- Intra-abdominal infections (peritonitis, appendicitis)
- Skin and skin structure infections (including diabetic foot infections)
- Community-acquired pneumonia
- Nosocomial pneumonia

USUAL ADULT DOSING: 3.375g IV 6h. Nosocomial pneumonia, pseudomonal infection, or severe infection: 3.375g IV q4h or 4.5g q6h.

Dosing Adjustments

GFR 50-80 mL/min: Usual dose

GFR 10-50 mL/min: 2/0.25g q6h; for severe infections, dose 4/0.5g q8h

GFR<10 mL/min: 2/0.25g q8h; for severe infx, dose 4/0.5g q12h

Hemodialysis: 2.25g q8h plus 0.75g post-dialysis; for severe infections, 3.375 IV q8h plus 0.75g post dialysis

Peritoneal Dialysis: 2.25g q8h; for severe infection 3.375g q8h

ADVERSE DRUG REACTIONS: Occasional: hypersensitivity reactions; rash; GI intolerance; phlebitis at infusion sites and sterile abscesses at IM sites. **Rare:** drug fever; Coombs' test positive w/ hemolytic anemia; Jarisch-Herxheimer reaction

DRUG INTERACTIONS

Methotrexate: MTX serum level may be increased.

Probenecid: Prolongs Pip/Tazo T1/2.

Tetracyclines: May result in antagonism. In vitro antagonism when co-administered. Bactericidal effect of penicillins may be diminished in vivo. Avoid concurrent administration. In two studies involving a total of 79 patients with pneumococcal meningitis treated with either penicillin plus tetracyclines or penicillin monotherapy there was a higher mortality rate (79-85%) in the combination therapy compared to penicillin monotherapy (30-33%). (Arch Intern Med 1951:88:489, Ann Intern Med 1961; 55:545). However there was not a difference in mortality between penicillin monotherapy and penicillin plus tetracycline in the treatment of pneumococcal pneumonia. (Arch

ANTI-INFECTIVES

Intern Med 1953; 91:197).

Vecuronium: May prolong neuromuscular blockade.

PREGNANCY RISK: B-animal data shows no risk. Human data lacking.

BREAST FEEDING: Piperacillin is excreted in breast milk in low concentrations. Tazobactam excretion is not known.

COMMENTS: Parenteral betalactam-betalactamase inhibitor with broad-spectrum activity that includes most P. aeruginosa strains, Enterobacteriaceae, Enterococci and all anaerobes. More frequent dosing interval (3.375g IV q4h) or higher doses (4.5g IV q6h) are recommended for serious pseudomonal pulmonary infections.

FORMS

Brand name	Preparation	Mfr.	Route	Form	Strength	Cost (AWP)
Zosyn	Piperacillin/ Tazobactam	Lederle	IV	vial	2g-0.25g; 3g-0.375g; 4g-0.5g; 36g-4.5g; 40mg-5mg/mL; 60mg-7.5mg/mL; 4g-0.5g/100mL	$11.32; $17.56; $22.14; $206.70; $13 per 50mL vial; $19.51 per 50mL vial; $24.71

SELECTED READINGS

Polk HC Jr; Fink MP; Laverdiere M et al. Prospective randomized study of piperacillin/tazobactam therapy of surgically treated intra-abdominal infection. Am Surg 1993 Sep;59(9):598-605

Tan JS; Wishnow RM; Talan DA et al. Treatment of hospitalized patients with complicated skin and skin structure infections: double-blind, randomized, multicenter study of piperacillin-tazobactam versus ticarcillin-clavulanate. Antimicrob Agents Chemother 1993 Aug;37(8):1580-6.

Cometta A; Zinner S; de Bock R et al. Piperacillin-tazobactam plus amikacin versus ceftazidime plus amikacin as empiric therapy for fever in granulocytopenic patients with cancer. Antimicrob Agents Chemother 1995 Feb;39(2):445-52

Sweet RL; Roy S; Faro S et al. Piperacillin and tazobactam versus clindamycin and gentamicin in the treatment of hospitalized women with pelvic infection. Obstet Gynecol 1994 Feb;83(2):280-6

ATS and IDSA. Guidelines for the Management of Adults with Hospital-acquired, Ventilator-associated, and Healthcare-associated Pneumonia. Am J Respir Crit Care Med 2005;171:388

POLYMYXIN B

FDA INDICATIONS

- Prophylaxis of superficial skin infections
- Ocular infections (with or without steroids)

USUAL ADULT DOSING: Systemic: 0.75-1.25 mg/kg IM or IV q12h. Topical application (dermatologic or ophthalmic).

Dosing Adjustments

GFR 50-80 mL/min: 7500-12,500 u/kg/d divide dose q12h

GFR 10-50 mL/min: 5625-12,500 u/kg/d divide dose q12h

GFR<10 mL/min: 3750-6250 u/kg/d divide dose q12h

Hemodialysis: little data, some removal

Peritoneal Dialysis: little data, some removal

ADVERSE DRUG REACTIONS: Occasional: with IM or IV use = nephrotoxicity; neurotoxicity: circumoral and peripheral paresthesia, dizziness, vertigo, ataxia, blurred vision, slurred speech.

DRUG INTERACTIONS

Nondepolarizing muscle relaxants (atracurium, vecuronium, pancuronium, tubocurarine): Neuromuscular blockade may be enhanced w/ systemic administration. Avoid co-administration, if concurrent administration is needed titrate the nondepolarizing muscle relaxant slowly and monitor neuromuscular function closely. Nondepolarizing muscle relaxant with IM or IV use.

PREGNANCY RISK: B-A report of 7 exposures during the first trimester found no association with congenital defects.

BREAST FEEDING: No data available

COMMENTS: Topical agent in the polymyxin class thus active against Pseudomonas aeruginosa and other gram-negative bacilli. Rarely used systemically but may be a last resort for resistant pseudomonal infections (1mg=10,000u).

FORMS (♦ DENOTES AVAILABLE GENERICALLY)

Brand name	Preparation	Mfr.	Route	Form	Strength	Cost (AWP)
Polymyxin B sulfate	Polymyxin B sulfate	Bedford	IV	vial	500,000U	$13.80
Polytrim	polymyxin B sulfate plus trimethoprim	♦ Allergan	Oph-thalmic	sol	10,000U-1mg/mL	$34.55 per 10mL

PRIMAQUINE

FDA INDICATIONS

• Malaria, prevention of relapses (radical cure/liver stage Plasmodium vivax)

USUAL ADULT DOSING: 15-30mg (base) qd. PCP treatment: primaquine 15-30mg (base) + clindamycin.

Dosing Adjustments
GFR 50-80 mL/min: Usual dose
GFR 10-50 mL/min: Usual dose
GFR<10 mL/min: Usual dose
Hemodialysis: No data, dose post-HD

ADVERSE DRUG REACTIONS: Occasional: Hemolytic anemia (G6PD deficiency); warn patient to observe for dark urine and cyanosis; should screen for G6PD deficiency before use; GI intolerance; neutropenia (dose dependent).

DRUG INTERACTIONS
No significant interactions noted.

PREGNANCY RISK: C-No studies available. Theoretical concern is hemolytic anemia in G6PD deficient fetus.

BREAST FEEDING: No data available.

COMMENTS: Oral agent used in combination with clindamycin as second line treatment for P. jiroveci pneumonia. Oxidizing agent; therefore G6PD deficiency screening is recommended. In addition to hemolytic anemia, may cause methemoglobinemia and bone marrow suppression.

FORMS

Brand name	Preparation	Mfr.	Route	Form	Strength	Cost (AWP)
Primaquine phosphate	Primaquine phosphate	Sanofi syntholabo	PO	tab	26.3mg	$1.04

PYRAZINAMIDE

FDA INDICATIONS

- Mycobacterium tuberculosis treatment

USUAL ADULT DOSING: 20-25mg/kg (max 2g) PO qd. DOT regimen: 50-70mg/kg (max 3.5g) PO 2x/week or 50-70mg/kg (max 2.5g) PO 3x/week.

Dosing Adjustments

GFR 50-80 mL/min: Usual dose

GFR 10-50 mL/min: Usual dose, Risk of hyperuricemia is increased.

GFR<10 mL/min: 12-20mg/kg/day

Hemodialysis: Usual dose post-HD on days of HD. Risk of hyperuricemia is increased.

Peritoneal Dialysis: No data, avoid

↓ *Hepatic Function:* No data. Close monitoring if used highly recommended.

ADVERSE DRUG REACTIONS: Frequent: non-gouty polyarthralgia (up to 40%, Rx with ASA); asymptomatic hyperuricemia. **Occasional:** hepatitis (dose related--1% at 25mg/kg), monitor LFTs closely with RIF x 2mos); GI intolerance. **Rare:** gout (Rx w/ allopurinol and probenecid).

DRUG INTERACTIONS

Ethionamide: Increase in hepatotoxicity. Monitor serum transaminase enzymes. Co-administer only in patients with normal baseline liver function test.

PREGNANCY RISK: C-No animal data available. No human data available. PZA is not recommended for pregnancy with TB in the US due to lack of safety data; it is accepted in the WHO guidelines.

BREAST FEEDING: Excreted in breast milk.

COMMENTS: First-line agent in combination for TB. Monitor LFTs closely with rifampin co-administration x 2mos; PZA/rifampin 2 mos prophylaxis regimen is generally contraindicated due to high incidence of hepatotoxicity. Use with caution in patients with gout due to the potential for PZA to induce hyperuricemia.

FORMS (◆ DENOTES AVAILABLE GENERICALLY)

Brand name	Preparation	Mfr.	Route	Form	Strength	Cost (AWP)
Pyrazinamide	Pyrazinamide	◆ Stada	PO	tab	500mg	$1.21
Rifater	PZA/INH/ri-fampin	Aventis	PO	tab	300mg/50mg/120mg	$2.04

SELECTED READINGS

ATS/CDC/IDSA. Treatment of tuberculosis . Am J Respir Crit Care Med 2003;167:603-62

Jasmer RM, Saukkonen JJ, Blumberg HM. Short-course rifampin and pyrazinamide compared with isoniazid for latent tuberculosis infection: a multicenter clinical trial. Ann Intern Med. 2002 Oct 15;137 (8):640-7

PYRIMETHAMINE

FDA INDICATIONS

- Malaria (in combination with sulfadoxine and quinine in the treatment of chloroquine-resistant Plasmodium falciparum malaria)
- Toxoplasmosis (in combination with a sulfapyrimidine-type sulfonamide)

USUAL ADULT DOSING: Toxoplasmosis treatment: 200mg x1, then 50-75mg/d (plus folinic acid 10-20mg/d plus sulfadiazine or clindamycin). Presumptive Rx of chloroquine-resistant P. falciparum: 2 to 3 Fansidar tablets as a single dose.

Dosing Adjustments
GFR 50-80 mL/min: Usual dose
GFR 10-50 mL/min: Usual dose
GFR<10 mL/min: Usual dose
Peritoneal Dialysis: 47% removed after PD

ADVERSE DRUG REACTIONS: Occasional: folate deficiency with megaloblastic anemia and pancytopenia (dose related and reversed with leucovorin); allergic reactions; GI intolerance (nausea, anorexia, vomiting)

DRUG INTERACTIONS

Cotrimoxazole, trimethoprim, sulfamethoxazole, dapsone: Additive hematologic toxicities due to folic acid antagonism. Monitor for hematologic toxicity. Leucovorin (folinic acid) may be given to decrease the incidence of hematologic toxicities.

PREGNANCY RISK: C-Teratogenic in animal studies. No adverse fetal effects were reported in two reviews of treatment of toxoplasmosis in pregnancy. If pyrimethamine is used during pregnancy, folinic acid 5mg/day supplementation is recommended, especially during the 1st trimester, to prevent folate deficiency.

BREAST FEEDING: Excreted in breast milk. The American Academy of Pediatrics considers pyrimethamine compatible with breast feeding.

COMMENTS: Treatment of choice (with sulfadiazine) for CNS toxoplasmosis. Co-administration of folinic acid helps prevent bone marrow suppression.

FORMS

Brand name	Preparation	Mfr.	Route	Form	Strength	Cost (AWP)
Daraprim	Pyrimethami ne	GlaxoSmithKline	PO	tab	25mg	$0.58
Fansidar	Pyrimethami ne/Sulfadox-ine	Roche	PO	tab	25mg/500mg	$4.14

PYRIMETHAMINE + SULFADOXINE
FDA INDICATIONS
• Prophylaxis and treatment of chloroquine-resistant malaria

USUAL ADULT DOSING: Prophylaxis: 1 tablet once a week 1 or 2 days before entering the endemic area and continued during the time of residence, and then for 4 to 6 weeks after leaving the area. Treatment: 2-3 tablets as a single dose.

Dosing Adjustments
GFR 50-80 mL/min: Usual dose
Hemodialysis: No data: Sulfadoxine likely to be removed (may need to supplement)
Peritoneal Dialysis: No data: 47% of pyrimethamine is excreted by PD (may need to supplement)

ADVERSE DRUG REACTIONS: Occasional: Folic acid deficiency w/ megaloblastic anemia and pancytopenia; hemolytic anemia; leukopenia; thrombocytopenia; allergic reaction [incl. severe cutaneous-eg Stevens Johnson]; transaminase elevation; GI intolerance (nausea, anorexia, vomiting)

DRUG INTERACTIONS

Aurothioglucose: Contraindicated.

Dapsone, trimethoprim and **sulfa drugs:** Use with caution; additive bone marrow suppression.

PREGNANCY RISK: C- not recommended to be administered near term.

BREAST FEEDING: Both pyrimethamine and sulfadoxine are excreted in breast milk. Breast feeding not recommended.

COMMENTS: Fansidar is no longer the agent of choice for malaria prophylaxis due to the risk of severe cutaneous reactions (EM, TEN, and Stevens-Johnsons syndrome). However, for the treatment of uncomplicated malaria, Fansidar is recommended as a single dose (3 tabs on the last day of quinine therapy) to prevent recrudescence 3-4 weeks later.

FORMS

Brand name	Preparation	Mfr.	Route	Form	Strength	Cost (AWP)
Fansidar	Pyrimethamine/Sulfadoxine	Roche	PO	tab	25mg-500mg	$4.14

SELECTED READINGS

Djimde AA, Dolo A, Ouattara A, Diakite S, Plowe CV, Doumbo OK. Molecular Diagnosis of Resistance to Antimalarial Drugs during Epidemics and in War Zones. J Infect Dis. 2004;190:853-5

Alloueche A, Bailey W, Barton S et al. Comparison of chlorproguanil-dapsone with sulfadoxine-pyrimethamine for the treatment of uncomplicated falciparum malaria in young African children: double-blind randomised controlled trial. Lancet. 2004 Jun 5;363(9424):1843-8

QUINIDINE

FDA INDICATIONS

- Serious P. falciparum malaria treatment.
- Non-ID indications: atrial and ventricular arrhythmias

USUAL ADULT DOSING: Loading dose: 10mg/km over 1 to 2 hours followed by a maintenance dose of 0.02mg/km/min for up to 72 hours or until parasitemia decreases to less than 1% or oral therapy can be started.

Dosing Adjustments

GFR 50-80 mL/min: Usual dose

GFR 10-50 mL/min: Usual dose

GFR<10 mL/min: 75% of dose (levels may be higher with renal failure). Dose based on clinical response. Levels may be useful.

Hemodialysis: Removed with HD. Supplement with 100-200mg post dialysis. Levels may be useful

Peritoneal Dialysis: No data: Unlikely to be removed. Dose based on clinical response. Levels may be useful

↓ *Hepatic Function:* May need to be decreased with severe hepatic dysfunction.

ADVERSE DRUG REACTIONS: EKG changes (e.g., prolongation of the QT interval and QRS widening), arrhythmias and hypotension with infusion (close cardiac monitoring in the ICU recommended). Thrombocytopenia, hemolytic anemia, drug-induced SLE, transaminase elevation and rash.

DRUG INTERACTIONS

CYP3A4 inhibitor (i.e., macrolide, azole, protease inhibitors and cimetidine): May increase quinidine levels.

CYP3A4 inducer (i.e., rifamycin, nevirapine, phenobarbital, carbamezepine):May decrease quinidine levels.

Digoxin: May decrease digoxin levels.

PREGNANCY RISK: C

BREAST FEEDING: Excreted in breast milk.

COMMENTS: IV quinidine (plus doxycycline) is the agent of choice for treatment of complicated P. falciparum. Close monitoring with telemetry recommended (QT prolongation, hypotension, and hypoglycemia). In the event that pharmacy does not have drug in stock, call Eli Lilly Customer Service at: 1-800-821-0538.

FORMS

Brand name	Preparation	Mfr.	Route	Form	Strength	Cost (AWP)
Quinidine gluconate	Quinidine gluconate	Eli Lilly	IV	vial	80mg/mL	$21.56 per 10mL

SELECTED READINGS

Stauffer W, Fischer PR. Diagnosis and treatment of malaria in children. Clin Infect Dis. 2003 Nov 15;37 (10):1340-8

QUININE

FDA INDICATIONS

- Malaria (concurrently with tetracycline, doxycycline, clindamycin, or pyrimethamine plus sulfadiazine, or pyrimethamine plus sulfadoxine in the treatment of chloroquine-resistant malaria caused by Plasmodium falciparum.)

USUAL ADULT DOSING: Malaria: 650mg PO q8h x 3-7 days (plus doxycycline or pyrimethamine/sulfadoxine); quinine dihydrochloride 600mg IV q8h (IV not commercially available in the U.S.)

Dosing Adjustments

GFR 50-80 mL/min: Usual dose

GFR 10-50 mL/min: Usual dose

GFR<10 mL/min: Usual dose; some recommend increasing dosing interval to q24h

Hemodialysis: Usual dose; days of dialysis dose post dialysis

Peritoneal Dialysis: 650mg q24h

ADVERSE DRUG REACTIONS: Occasional: GI intolerance; cinchonism (tinnitus, headache, nausea, abdominal pain, visual disturbances); hemolytic anemia (G6PD deficiency)

DRUG INTERACTIONS

CYP3A4 inducers (i.e., rifampin, phenytoin, phenobarbital): Quinine serum level may be decreased.

PREGNANCY RISK: X-Animal data show teratogenic effects. Human data reports stillbirths and congenital malformation with large doses used for attempted abortions. CDC recommends quinidine gluconate for the treatment of malaria.

BREAST FEEDING: Excreted in breast milk. The American Academy of Pediatrics considers quinine compatible with breast feeding.

COMMENTS: IV quinine (not available in the U.S.) is the drug of choice for complicated Plasmodium falciprum malaria. Monitor blood levels in patients with renal or hepatic dysfunction. For parenteral therapy, IV quinidine may be substituted for quinine (see "Quinidine").

FORMS (♦ DENOTES AVAILABLE GENERICALLY)

Brand name	Preparation	Mfr.	Route	Form	Strength	Cost (AWP)
Quinine sulfate	Quinine sulfate	♦ Ivax	PO	cap	325mg	$0.78
			PO	tab	260mg	$0.87

QUINUPRISTIN + DALFOPRISTIN

FDA INDICATIONS

- Serious or life-threatening infections associated with vancomycin-resistant Enterococcus faecium (VREF) bacteremia
- Complicated skin and skin structure infections caused by Staphylococcus aureus (methicillin susceptible) or Streptococcus pyogenes.

USUAL ADULT DOSING: Complicated skin and skin structure infection 7.5mg/kg IV 12h. VRE (faecium) infection: 7.5mg/kg IV q8h.

Dosing Adjustments

GFR 50-80 mL/min: Usual dose
GFR 10-50 mL/min: Usual dose

ADVERSE DRUG REACTIONS: Frequent: Dose-dependent infusion related reaction at injection site (10% w/ 5mg/kg; 68% w/ 10-15mg/kg such as pain, itching, burning. Arthralgia/myalgia (15%); body pain. **Occasional:** Thrombophebitis (5%); asymptomatic hyperbilirubinemia (up to 25%).

DRUG INTERACTIONS

CYP3A4 inhibitor: Cyclosporin serum level may be increased (monitor level closely).
CYP3A4 substrate: Potential increase in serum level of CYP3A4 substrate (i.e., fentanyl, dofetilide, quinidine, irinotecan, tacrolimus, sirolimus, midazolam, triazolam, nifedipine, ergotamine, amiodarone, some HMG-CoA reductase inhibitors).

PREGNANCY RISK: No data. Manufacturer currently does not recommend the use in pregnancy.

BREAST FEEDING: No data

COMMENTS: Parenteral agent with activity against most gram-positive cocci including penicillin-resistant S. pneumoniae, Vancomycin intermediate resistant S. aureus and S. epidermidis and Vancomycin resistant-E faecium. It does not have activity against E. faecalis. Expensive at approximately $320.00 per day. May cause disabling myalgias that precludes continued use. Must be infused by central line.

FORMS

Brand name	Preparation	Mfr.	Route	Form	Strength	Cost (AWP)
Synercid	Quinupristin + Dalfopristin	Monarch	IV	vial	150mg-350mg; 180mg-420mg	$127; $151.25

SELECTED READINGS

Werner G, et al. Methicillin-Resistant, Quinupristin-Dalfopristin-Resistant Staphylococcus aureus with Reduced Sensitivity to Glycopeptides. J Clin Micro 2001;39:3586

Linden PK et al. Treatment of Vancomycin-Resistant Enterococcus faecium Infections with Quinupristin/Dalfopristin. CID 2001;33:1816

Vergis EN, et al. Determinants of Vancomycin Resistance and Mortality Rates in Enterococcal Bacteremia. Ann Intern Med 2001;135:484

RABIES HYPERIMMUNE GLOBULIN

FDA INDICATIONS

• Rabies, post exposure passive immunization

USUAL ADULT DOSING: 20 International units/kg IM (1/2 of total dose given in around the wound and the other 1/2 given in the gluteal area) post rabies exposure. 40IU/kg dose has been associated with interference with active immunization.

Dosing Adjustments

GFR 50-80 mL/min: No data, usual dose likely

GFR 10-50 mL/min: No data, usual dose likely

GFR<10 mL/min: No data, usual dose likely

Hemodialysis: No data, usual dose likely

ADVERSE DRUG REACTIONS: Common: Local tenderness, soreness, and induration at administration site. **Rare:** Hypersensitivity reaction in patients allergic to avian protein or chicken eggs.

PREGNANCY RISK: C- No risk to the fetus has been reported. The American College of Obstetricians and Gynecologists recommends the use of rabies immune globulin and vaccine for post-exposure prophylaxis.

BREAST FEEDING: No data.

COMMENTS: Rabies vaccine can be administered concurrently at a different site, but repeated doses of rabies-immune globulin are not recommended after rabies vaccine since immunogenicity may be decreased.

FORMS

Brand name	Preparation	Mfr.	Route	Form	Strength	Cost (AWP)
BayRab	Rabies hyper-immune glob-ulin	Bayer	IM	vial	150IU/mL	$168 per 2mL vial
Imogam Ra-bies-HT	Rabies Hyper-immune glob-ulin	Aventis Pasteur	IM	vial	150IU/mL	$162.60 per 2mL vial

RIBAVIRIN

FDA INDICATIONS

• Respiratory syncytial virus (RSV) infection (including bronchiolitis and pneumonia)

• Hepatitis C (in combination with alpha interferon or peginterferon alpha-2a)

USUAL ADULT DOSING: HCV infection (in combination with interferon or PEG-interferon): 600mg PO bid for >75kg; 400mg qam and 600mg qpm for <75 kg. RSV: mist w/190 mcg/L via SPAG-2 at 12.5 L/min.

Dosing Adjustments

GFR 50-80 mL/min: Usual dose

GFR 10-50 mL/min: Not recommended per manufacturer.

GFR<10 mL/min: Not recommended per manufacturer.

Hemodialysis: Small amount removed in dialysis; not recommended per manufacturer.

↓ *Hepatic Function:* Usual dose

ADVERSE DRUG REACTIONS: Frequent: Dose-related hemolytic anemia, not seen w/ aerosolized ribavirin. **Occasional:** Cough, dyspnea, fatigue, headache, insomnia (higher dose);

anorexia, nausea; bronchospasm with aerosolized ribavirin. Hypocalcemia with IV ribavirin

DRUG INTERACTIONS

AZT, d4t, 3TC: In vitro antagonism but not in vivo.

ddI: Increases intracellular concentration of ddI, may increase risk of pancreatitis (13 case reports to date, avoid co-administration).

PREGNANCY RISK: X-Embryotoxic and teratogenic in all animal species. CONTRAINDICATED IN PREGNANT WOMEN AND IN MALE PARTNERS OF PREGNANT WOMEN per manufacturer and CDC. Per CDC, healthcare workers who are pregnant should use caution when caring for patient on ribavirin inhalation therapy. WOMEN OF CHILBEARING AGE MUST USE EFFECTIVE FORM OF CONTRACEPTION DURING TREATMENT AND 6 MONTHS POST-TREATMENT.

BREAST FEEDING: No data available.

COMMENTS: Oral agent for hepatitis C infection when combined with alpha interferon or pegylated alpha interferon. Monitor for hemolytic anemia. Contraindicated in pregnancy. IV formulation available from ICN pharmaceutical for emergency use in hemorrhagic fever.

FORMS (♦ DENOTES AVAILABLE GENERICALLY)

Brand name	Preparation	Mfr.	Route	Form	Strength	Cost (AWP)
Rebetol	Ribavirin	Schering	PO	cap	200mg	$10.60
Virazole	Ribavirin	Valeant	inhalation	vial	6g	$1573.80
Rebetron	Ribavirin + Interferon alfa-2b	Schering	PO/SC	kit	600;1000;1200	$658.70; $804.32; $888.76
Copegus	Ribavirin	Roche	PO	tab	200mg	$8.03
Ribavirin	ribavirin	♦ Sandoz	PO	cap	200 mg	$9.93

SELECTED READINGS

Cummings KJ, et al. Interferon and Ribavirin vs. Interferon Alone in the Re-Treatment of Chronic Hepatitis C Previously Nonresponsive to Interferon: A Meta-analysis of Randomized Trials. JAMA 2001;285:193

Hadziyannis SJ, Sette H Jr, Morgan TR, et al. Peginterferon-alpha2a and ribavirin combination therapy in chronic hepatitis C: a randomized study of treatment duration and ribavirin dose. Ann Intern Med. 2004;140: 346-55

Strader D, et al. Diagnosis, Management, and Treatment of Hepatitis C. Hepatology 2005;39(4);1147-71

RIFABUTIN

FDA INDICATIONS

• Prophylaxis of mycobacterium avium complex (MAC aka MAI) disease

USUAL ADULT DOSING: 5mg/kg (300mg) PO qd or 2-3x/week; 450mg PO qd (with EFV co-administration); 150mg PO qd (with IDV, FPV, NFV, APV co-administration); 150mg PO qod (with RTV and LPV/r co-administration).

Dosing Adjustments

GFR 50-80 mL/min: Usual dose

GFR 10-50 mL/min: Usual dose

GFR<10 mL/min: Usual dose

Hemodialysis: No data, but usual dose suggested; no supplementation needed.

↓ *Hepatic Function:* Dose reduction may be necessary with severe liver dysfunction.

ADVERSE DRUG REACTIONS: Frequent: Orange discoloration of urine, tears, sweat; uveitis seen w/high doses (600mg/d or concurrent use of fluconazole or clarithromycin). **Rare:** Neutropenia in HIV-infected pts; hepatotoxity (<1%); pseudojaundice (w/ nl bilirubin).

DRUG INTERACTIONS

Rifabutin is a moderate inducer of CYP3A4. Serum level of CYP3A4 substrates (i.e., sirolimus, tacrolimus, cyclosporin, HIV protease inhibitors) may be decreased. **Decreases serum concentration of all of the following drugs:** Close monitoring of serum level and therapeutic efficacy is needed. Dose of affected drug may need to be increased: Warfarin; levothyroxine; oral contraceptives and estrogens; doxycycline; theophylline; diazepam, triazolam, midazolam; beta-blockers (bisoprolol, metoprolol, propranolol); azole antifungals (fluconazole, ketoconazole, itraconazole); corticosteroids (cortisone, fludrocortisone, hydrocortisone, methylprednisolone, prednisolone, prednisone); quinidine/quinine; cyclosporine; dapsone; protease inhibitors (dose modification needed); methadone and other narcotics, digoxin, digitoxin; oral hypoglycemic agents (glyburide, chlorpropamide, tolbutamide); amiodarone, dofetilide, disopyramide, mexiletine, calcium channel blockers, tocainide, sirolimus, tacrolimus, opiate agonist, lovastatin, simvastatin; phenobarbital, phenytoin, carbamazepine; irinotecan, and other CYP3A4 substrates). **CYP3A4 inhibitors** (i.e., HIV protease inhibitors, macrolide, azole antifungals): increases rifabutin serum level. Reduce rifabutin dose with PI co-administration.

PREGNANCY RISK: B-Animal data show skeletal abnormalities. No human data available.

BREAST FEEDING: No data available

COMMENTS: Oral rifamycin active against MAI and MTB. A good alternative to rifampin for MTB when needed for concurrent use with protease inhibitor or when non-nucleoside reverse transcriptase inhibitor is contraindicated. When used in combination with INH, PZA, and EMB for the treatment of TB, must be given daily for at least 8 weeks (induction) then daily or 3x/week x 6-9 months [MMWR 2002;51:214].

FORMS

Brand name	Preparation	Mfr.	Route	Form	Strength	Cost (AWP)
Mycobutin	Rifabutin	Pharmacia	PO	cap	150mg	$7.19

RIFAMIXIN

FDA INDICATIONS

- Traveler's diarrhea due to noninvasive E. coli

USUAL ADULT DOSING: Traveler's diarrhea: 200mg PO tid with or without food x 3 d

Dosing Adjustments
GFR 50-80 mL/min: Usual dose
GFR 10-50 mL/min: Usual dose likely
GFR<10 mL/min: Usual dose likely
Hemodialysis: Usual dose likely
Peritoneal Dialysis: Usual dose likely
↓ Hepatic Function: Usual dose

ADVERSE DRUG REACTIONS: Occasional: Flatulence, nausea and vomiting (comparable to placebo). **Rare:** Rash

DRUG INTERACTIONS

No significant interactions noted.

PREGNANCY RISK: C-No human data. Risk likely to be low since rifaximin is not systemically absorbed. Rifaximin was teratogenic in rats at doses 2- to 33-fold higher than human doses.

Anti-Infectives

BREAST FEEDING: No data.

COMMENTS: Rifaximin is effective and well tolerated in the treatment of uncomplicated traveler's diarrhea caused by E. coli. Rifaximin is not effective in diarrhea caused by invasive C. jejuni and has not been well studied in diarrhea caused by Shigella spp. or Salmonella spp. Since rifaximin is not systemically absorbed, it should not be used in complicated cases of traveler's diarrhea.

FORMS

Brand name	Preparation	Mfr.	Route	Form	Strength	Cost (AWP)
Xifaxan	Rifamixin	Salix	PO	tab	200mg	$3.75

SELECTED READINGS

DuPont HL et al. A randomized, double-blind, placebo-controlled trial of rifaximin to prevent travelers' diarrhea. Ann Intern Med 2005; May 17;142(10):805-812

DuPont HL, Jiang ZD, Ericsson CD et al. Rifaximin versus ciprofloxacin for the treatment of traveler's diarrhea: a randomized, double-blind clinical trial. Clin Infect Dis. 2001;33(11):1807-15

Huang DB, DuPont HL. Rifaximin--a novel antimicrobial for enteric infections. J Infect. 2005;50:97-106.

RIFAMPIN

FDA INDICATIONS

- Tuberculosis
- Meningococcal prophylaxis

USUAL ADULT DOSING: 600mg PO or IV qd; DOT TB regimen: 10mg/kg (max 600mg) 2-3x/week (3x/week with multi-lobar involvement). Staph nasal carrier: 600mg bid x 2d.

Dosing Adjustments

GFR 50-80 mL/min: Usual dose

GFR 10-50 mL/min: Usual dose

GFR<10 mL/min: Usual dose; some recommend a 50% decrease in dose.

Hemodialysis: 300-600mg qd

Peritoneal Dialysis: 300-600mg qd

↓ *Hepatic Function:* Clearance may be impaired, but should be given with close monitoring.

ADVERSE DRUG REACTIONS: Frequent: Orange discoloration of urine, tears, sweat. **Occasional:** Hepatitis (2.7% w/other TB Rx)-cholestatic changes in first month; jaundice; GI intolerance; pruritis (6%); hypersensitivity rxn (in 0.07-0.3%), flu-like syndrome (0.4-0.7%) when taking RIF 2x/wk.

DRUG INTERACTIONS

Potent CYP3A4, 1A2, 2C9, and 2E1 inducer w/ large decrease in serum level of CYP3A4 substrates (i.e., sirolimus, tacrolimus, cyclosporine). **Contraindicatedwith:** HIV protease inhibitors.

Aluminum containing antacids: Decreased oral absorption of rifampin. Separate oral administration.

Aminosalicylic acid granules: Absorption of rifampin may be impaired by the bentonite excipient. Separate the two drug administration time by 8-12 hours intervals.

Rifamycin: Warfarin; levothyroxine; oral contraceptives and estrogens; doxycycline; theophylline; diazepam, triazolam, midazolam; beta-blockers (bisoprolol, metoprolol, propranolol); azole antifungals (fluconazole, ketoconazole, itraconazole); corticosteroids (cortisone, fludrocortisone, hydrocortisone, methylprednisolone, prednisolone, prednisone); quinidine/quinine; cyclosporine; dapsone; protease inhibitors (dose modification needed); methadone and other narcotics, digoxin, digitoxin; oral hypoglycemic agents (glyburide, chlorpropamide, tolbutamide); amiodarone, dofetilide, disopyramide, mexiletine, calcium channel blockers, tocainide; sirolimus, tacrolimus, opiate agonists, lovastatin, simvastatin; phenobarbital, phenytoin, carbamazepine; irinotecan, and other CYP3A4 substrates)

PREGNANCY RISK: C-Considered safe in pregnancy. Animal data show congenital malformation-cleft palate, spina bifida, embryotoxicity. Administration in last weeks of pregnancy may cause postnatal hemorrhage. Several reviews have evaluated treatment of TB in pregnancy. All concluded that rifampin was not a proven teratogen and recommended use of the drug with INH and ethambutol if necessary.

BREAST FEEDING: Excreted in breast milk. The American Academy of Pediatrics considers rifampin compatible with breast feeding.

COMMENTS: Oral and parenteral rifamycin that is used for treatment and prophylaxis of TB, other mycobacterial infections, meningococcal prophylaxis and occasional infections involving Staphylococcus spp. When used in combination with INH, PZA, and EMB for the treatment of TB must be given daily for at least 8 weeks (induction) then daily or 3x/week x 6-9 months [MMWR 2002;51:214]. Many drug interactions.

FORMS

Brand name	Preparation	Mfr.	Route	Form	Strength	Cost (AWP)
Rifadin	Rifampin	Aventis	IV	vial	600mg	$92.84 per vial
			PO	cap	150mg; 300mg	$1.69; $2.40
Rifamate	Rifampin/INH	Aventis	PO	cap	300mg/150mg	$2.58
Rifater	Rifampin/INH/PZA	Aventis	PO	cap	120mg/50mg/300mg	$1.92

SELECTED READINGS

Jasmer RM, et al. Twelve Months of Isoniazid Compared with Four Months of Isoniazid and Rifampin for persons with Radiographic Evidence of Previous Tuberculosis: An Outcome and Cost-Effectiveness Analysis. Am J Respir Crit Care Med 2000;162:1648

Zimmerli W, Widmer A, Blatter M, et al. Role of Rifampin for treatment of Orthopedic Implant-Related Staphylococcal Infections. JAMA 1998; 279:1537

ATS/CDC/IDSA. Guidelines for the treatment of TB . Am J Respir Crit Care Med 2003;167:603-62

RIFAPENTINE

FDA INDICATIONS

• Tuberculosis, in combination with other anti-tubercular drugs

USUAL ADULT DOSING: 10mg/kg (600mg)q week (w/ INH as part of the continuation phase) or 600mg PO 2x/week.

Dosing Adjustments

GFR 50-80 mL/min: Usual dose

GFR 10-50 mL/min: Usual dose likely (only 17% excreted via kidneys)

GFR<10 mL/min: Usual dose likely(only 17% excreted via kidneys).

Hemodialysis: Usual dose, not removed in HD.

Peritoneal Dialysis: No data, Usual dose likely

ADVERSE DRUG REACTIONS: Frequent: Orange discoloration of urine, tears (contact lens), sweat. **Occasional:** Hepatitis.

DRUG INTERACTIONS

Major drug interactions with CYP3A4, 2C8, 2C9 substrates resulting in dramatic reduction of serum level of co-administered drug (i.e., protease inhibitors, cyclosporin, tacrolimus, sirolimus).

Aluminum containing antacids: Decreased oral absorption of rifampin. Separate oral administration.

Aminosalicylic acid granules: Absorption of rifampin may be impaired by the bentonite excipient. Separate the two drug administration time by 8-12 hours intervals.

Rifamycin: Warfarin; levothyroxine; oral contraceptives and estrogens; doxycycline; theophylline; diazepam, triazolam, midazolam; beta-blockers (bisoprolol, metoprolol, propranolol); azole antifungals (fluconazole, ketoconazole, itraconazole); corticosteroids (cortisone, fludrocortisone, hydrocortisone, methylprednisolone, prednisolone, prednisone); quinidine/quinine; cyclosporine; dapsone; protease inhibitors and NNRTIs (dose modification needed); methadone and other narcotics, digoxin, digitoxin; oral hypoglycemic agents (glyburide, chlorpropamide, tolbutamide); amiodarone, dofetilide, disopyramide, mexiletine, calcium channel blockers, tocainide; sirolimus, tacrolimus, opiate agonists, lovastatin, simvastatin; phenobarbital, phenytoin, carbamazepine; irinotecan, and other CYP3A4 substrates).

PREGNANCY RISK: C-Animal data demonstrated teratogenicity. No adequate data is available in humans. Administration in last weeks of pregnancy may cause postnatal hemorrhage. Most experts feel that rifamycins have not proven teratogenic, and recommend use of the drug with INH and ethambutol if necessary.

BREAST FEEDING: No data.

COMMENTS: Oral rifamycin with a prolonged half-life. May be used once weekly w/ INH in the continuation phase treatment in HIV-negative patients with noncavitary, drug-susceptible pulmonary TB who have negative sputum smears at completion of the initial phase of Rx. Once weekly dosing should not be used in HIV-infected patients. Many drug interactions.

FORMS

Brand name	Preparation	Mfr.	Route	Form	Strength	Cost (AWP)
Priftin	Rifapentine	Aventis	PO	tab	150mg	$3.12

SELECTED READINGS

The Tuberculosis Clinical Consortium. Rifapentine and Isoniazid Once a Week Versus Rifampicin and Isoniazid Twice a Week for Treatment of Drug-Susceptible Pulmonary Tuberculosis in HIV-Negative Patients: A Randomised Clinical Trial . Lancet 2002;360:528

RIMANTADINE

FDA INDICATIONS

• Influenza A, prophylaxis and treatment

USUAL ADULT DOSING: Prophylaxis: 100mg PO bid. Treatment: 100mg PO bid within 48 hours of symptoms x 7 days. Consider dose reduction in severe hepatic dysfunction, renal failure and in elderly

Dosing Adjustments

GFR 50-80 mL/min: 100mg bid

GFR 10-50 mL/min: 100mg bid

GFR<10 mL/min: 100mg qd

Hemodialysis: Not removed; dose at 100mg PO qd

↓ *Hepatic Function:* In severe hepatic insufficiency: 100mg PO qd

ADVERSE DRUG REACTIONS: Occasional: GI intolerance; light headedness, insomnia, reduced ability to concentrate, nervousness

Drug Interactions
No significant interactions noted.

Pregnancy Risk: C

Breast Feeding: No data

Comments: Oral agent for influenza A that is more expensive compared to amantadine, but CNS side effects are less bothersome. Less expensive than zanamivir or oseltamivir.

Forms

Brand name	Preparation	Mfr.	Route	Form	Strength	Cost (AWP)
Flumadine	Rimantadine	Forest	PO	syrup	50mg/5mL	$1.03 per 5mL
			PO	tab	100mg	$2.43

Selected Readings
T. O. Jefferson, et al. Amantadine and rimantadine for influenza. ACP Journal Club, 1999;131:68

RITONAVIR (RTV)

FDA Indications
- HIV infection (in combination with other antiretrovirals)

Usual Adult Dosing: RTV 600mg PO bid/ RTV often used in combination: RTV 400mg bid with IDV 400mg bid/ RTV 100-200mg bid with IDV 800mg bid/ RTV 400mg with SQV 400mg bid/ RTV 200-400mg bid with AMP 600mg bid/ RTV 400mg bid with NFV 500-750mg bid.

Dosing Adjustments
GFR 50-80 mL/min: 600mg bid
GFR 10-50 mL/min: 600mg bid
GFR<10 mL/min: 600mg bid
Hemodialysis: Usual dose, dose post-HD (small amount removed in HD)
Peritoneal Dialysis: No data: Usual dose likely, dose post

Adverse Drug Reactions: Severe GI intolerance (n/v/d; abdominal pain, common w/ 600mg bid dosing); taste perversion; asthenia; circumoral and peripheral paresthesias; lipodystrophy syndrome; hyperglycemia; increased triglycerides and/or cholesterol; transaminase elevation.

Drug Interactions
Substrate, potent inhibitor, and inducer of CYP3A4, CYP1A2, possibly CYP2C19 and, phase II glucuronidation and a mild CYP2D inhibitor. Generally increases serum levels of drugs that are CYP3A4 substrates although in some cases its inducing effects may also decrease serum levels of drugs that are substrate of CYP3A4, CYP1A2 and possibly CYP2C19. RTV may increase serum levels of drugs that are CYP2D6 substrates.
Contraindicated with: terfenadine, astemizole, cisapride, ergot alkaloid, midazolam, triazolam, propafenone, quinidine, flecainide, amiodarone, bepridil, pimozide simvastatin, lovastatin, alfuzosin, and St. Johns Wort

Pregnancy Risk: B-Placental passage of 115% midterm and 15-64% late-term demonstrated in rodent studies. In human placental perfusion model, ritonavir showed little accumulation in the fetal compartment and no accumulation in placental tissue. Not teratogenic but cryptochidism reported in rodents studies. No data on carcinogenicity.

Breast Feeding: Unknown breast milk excretion. Breast feeding is not recommended in the U.S in order to avoid post-natal transmission of HIV to the child, who may not yet be infected.

ANTI-INFECTIVES

COMMENTS: Monitor for drug interactions. Generally not well tolerated at full dose (600mg bid) secondary to GI side effects. Usually used in combination w/ second protease inhibitor at a lower dose for improved drug levels of the companion PI. Many drug interactions.

FORMS

Brand name	Preparation	Mfr.	Route	Form	Strength	Cost (AWP)
Norvir	Ritonavir (RTV)	Abbott	PO	cap	100mg	$10.29
			PO	sol	80mg/mL	$7.20 per mL

SAQUINAVIR (SQV)

FDA INDICATIONS
• HIV infection treatment in combination with other antiretrovirals

USUAL ADULT DOSING: SQV (Invirase or Fortovase, but Invirase prefered)1000mg bid plus RTV 100mg bid) Or Fortovase 1200mg PO tid. Invirase 600mg PO tid is not recommended as sole PI except in combination with ritonavir.

Dosing Adjustments
GFR 50-80 mL/min: Usual dose likely
GFR 10-50 mL/min: Usual dose likely
GFR<10 mL/min: Usual dose likely
Hemodialysis: Usual dose (not removed in HD)
Peritoneal Dialysis: No data: Usual dose likely (Unlikely to be removed in dialysis due to high protein binding and large volume of distribution.)

ADVERSE DRUG REACTIONS: GI intolerance (nausea, diarrhea, abdominal pain); lipodystrophy syndrome; hyperglycemia; increased triglycerides and/or cholesterol; transaminase elevation

DRUG INTERACTIONS
Substrate and weak inhibitor of CYP3A4. May modestly increase serum level of other substrates of CYP3A4. Drugs that are inducers of CYP3A4 may decrease SQV levels.
Contraindicated with: terfenadine, astemizole, cisapride, ergot alkaloid, rifampin, rifapentine, simvastatin, lovastatin, pimozide, rifabutin (when SQV used as sole-PI), , St. Johns Wort , midazolam and triazolam.

PREGNANCY RISK: B-Placental passage in humans unknown. Placental passage in rat and rabbit is minimal. No teratogenicity reported in rodent studies. No data on carcinogenicity.

BREAST FEEDING: Unknown breast milk excretion. Breast feeding is not recommended in the U.S. in order to avoid post-natal transmission of HIV to the child, who may not yet be infected.

COMMENTS: Invirase formulation is preferred (and now the only one available) in combination with ritonavir (INV 1000mg bid plus RTV 100mg bid) due to better pharmacokinetic profile, better tolerance, and less pill burden.

FORMS

Brand name	Preparation	Mfr.	Route	Form	Strength	Cost (AWP)
Invirase	Saquinavir	Roche	PO	cap	200mg	$2.40

STAVUDINE (d4T)

FDA INDICATIONS
- HIV infection treatment in combination with other antiretrovirals

USUAL ADULT DOSING: Wt >60kg dose: 40mg PO bid. Wt <60kg dose: 30mg PO bid.

Dosing Adjustments
GFR 50-80 mL/min: Wt >60kg dose: 40mg bid. Wt <60kg dose: 30mg bid
GFR 10-50 mL/min: Wt >60kg dose: 20mg q12-24h. Wt <60kg dose: 15mg q12-24
GFR<10 mL/min: Wt >60kg dose: 20mg q24h. Wt <60kg dose: 15mg q24h
Hemodialysis: Wt >60kg dose: 20mg q24h. Wt <60kg dose: 15mg q24h, on days of dialysis dose post dialysis. (Likely to be dialysed out)
Peritoneal Dialysis: Wt >60kg dose: 20mg q24h. Wt <60kg dose: 15mg q24h, on days of dialysis dose post dialysis. (Likely to be dialysed out)

ADVERSE DRUG REACTIONS: P. neuropathy (in 5-15% of pts); transaminase elevation (in 8% of pts; elevated triglyceride; rare cases of LACTIC ACIDOSIS and severe hepatomegaly with steatosis and ascending neuromuscular weakness. Pancreatitis. Macrocytosis (not assoc. with anemia).

DRUG INTERACTIONS
ddI: Increased risk of lactic acidosis. Avoid long-term co-administration.
Zidovudine: Antagonism (Co-administration contraindicated). ddC, ddI, INH, cisplatin, disulfiram, vincristine, gold (potential for additive peripheral neuropathy. Monitor for peripheral neuropathy).

PREGNANCY RISK: C-Studies in rhesus monkeys demonstrated 76% placental passage. Not teratogenic in rodent studies (but sternal bone calcium decreases seen). Carcinogenic studies not completed. Pregnant patients may be at increase risk of lactic acidosis (FDA warns against its use in pregnancy).

BREAST FEEDING: No human data, breast milk excretion in animal studies. Breast feeding is not recommended in the U.S. in order to avoid post-natal transmission of HIV to the child, who may not yet be infected.

COMMENTS: Generally a well-tolerated antiretroviral. Monitor for signs of peripheral neuropathy especially when combined with ddI. Associated with the highest risk of lactic acidosis which is rare but fatal in severe cases. Pregnant patients receiving d4T + ddI may be at increased risk of lactic acidosis (FDA warns against the combination in pregnancy). Lipoatrophy may complicate long-term use.

FORMS

Brand name	Preparation	Mfr.	Route	Form	Strength	Cost (AWP)
Zerit	Stavudine (d4T)	Bristol-Myers Squibb	PO	capsule	15mg; 20mg; 30mg; 40mg	$5.49; $5.71; $6.06; $6.17
			PO	solution	1mg/mL (200mL)	$1.70 per 5mL

STREPTOMYCIN

FDA INDICATIONS
- Mycobacterium tuberculosis
- Yersinia pestis (plague)
- Francisella tularensis (tularemia)
- Brucella

Anti-Infectives

- Calymmatobacterium granulomatis (Donovanosis, granuloma inguinale),
- Haemophilus ducreyi (chancroid)
- Urinary tract infections
- Endocarditis caused by Streptococcus viridans, Enterococcus faecalis (use with penicillin)
- Gram-negative bacillary bacteremia (concomitantly with another antibacterial agent)

USUAL ADULT DOSING: TB: 15mg/kg/d (max 1g) IM qd. TB DOT regimen:25-30mg/kg 2-3x/wk. Enterococcal endocarditis (synergy with ampicillin if sensitive to streptomycin w/ <2000 mcg/mL): 7.5mg/kg IM q12h (max dose per day is 2g)(target peak 1hour after IM dose is 20mcg/mL)

Dosing Adjustments

GFR 50-80 mL/min: 15 mg/kg q24-72h

GFR 10-50 mL/min: 15mg/kg q72-96h

GFR<10 mL/min: 7.5mg/kg q72-96h

Hemodialysis: HD:12-15mg/kg 2-3x/week

Peritoneal Dialysis: 20-40mg/L of dialysate per day

ADVERSE DRUG REACTIONS: Occasional: Renal failure, oto/vestibular damage, optic nerve dysfunction, peripheral neuritis, arachnoiditis, neuromuscular blockade, encephalopathy reported. The most ototoxic of all aminoglycosides. PEAK SHOULD NOT EXCEED 20-25 mcg/mL.

DRUG INTERACTIONS

Avoid concurrent use of nephrotoxic, ototoxic and neurotoxic drugs.

Loop diuretics (bumetanide, furosemide, (especially with ethacrynic acid), torsemide): Ototoxicity may be increased. The co-administration of aminoglycoside with loop diuretics may have an additive or synergistic ototoxic effect. Ototoxicity appears to be dose dependent and may be increased with renal dysfunction. Irreversible ototoxicity has been reported. Avoid concomitant administration, if used together careful dose adjustments needed in patients with renal failure and close monitoring for ototoxicity required. Volume depletion secondary to diuresis may increase risk of nephrotoxicity.

Nondepolarizing muscle relaxants (atracurium, pancuronium, tubocurarine, gallamine triethiodide): Enhanced action of nondepolarizing muscle relaxant resulting in respiratory depression. Avoid co-administration, if concurrent administration is needed titrate the nondepolarizing muscle relaxant slowly and monitor neuromuscular function closely.

PREGNANCY RISK: D-Eighth cranial nerve damage has been reported following in utero exposure to streptomycin.

BREAST FEEDING: Excreted in breast milk. The American Academy of Pediatrics considers streptomycin compatible with breast feeding.

COMMENTS: Parenteral aminoglycoside with the most ototoxicity potential. Use is generally limited to treatment of multiple-drug resistant tuberculosis (MDRTB), but high rate of SM resistance has been described in high-incidence countries. Also used for unusual infections: plague, tularemia and brucellosis. May be synergistic with ampicillin in cases of gentamicin resistant enterococcus endocarditis.

FORMS

Brand name	Preparation	Mfr.	Route	Form	Strength	Cost (AWP)
Streptomycin sulfate	Streptomycin sulfate	X-Gen	IM	vial	1g	$9.75

SELECTED READINGS

Doganay M; Bakir M; Dokmetas I et al. Treatment of tuberculous meningitis in adults with a combination of isoniazid, rifampicin and streptomycin: a prospective study. Scand J Infect Dis 1989;21(1):81-5

Enderlin G; Morales L; Jacobs RF et al. Streptomycin and alternative agents for the treatment of tularemia: review of the literature. Clin Infect Dis 1994 Jul;19(1):42-7

Ariza J; Gudiol F; Pallares R et al. Treatment of human brucellosis with doxycycline plus rifampin or doxycycline plus streptomycin. A randomized, double-blind study. Ann Intern Med 1992 Jul 1;117 (1):25-30

SULFADIAZINE

FDA INDICATIONS
• Toxoplasmosis

USUAL ADULT DOSING: CNS toxoplasmosis (in combination with pyrimethamine and leucovorin): 1-2g PO q6h x 6-8 weeks (then 1/2 of dose for maintenance).

Dosing Adjustments
GFR 50-80 mL/min: 0.5-1.5g q4-6h
GFR 10-50 mL/min: 0.5-1.5g q8-12h (half dose)
GFR<10 mL/min: 0.5-1.5g q12h-24h (1/3 dose)
Hemodialysis: No data, dose post-HD

ADVERSE DRUG REACTIONS: Frequent: Allergic reactions-rash, pruritus. **Occasional:** Fever; periarteritis nodosa, hypersensitivity; serum sickness; crystalluria w/ azotemia, urolithiasis and oliguria; GI intolerance;photosentivity; hepatitis. **Rare:** Stevens-Johnson syndrome and TEN.

DRUG INTERACTIONS
Cyclosporin: Decreased cyclosporine serum level. Monitor serum level closely.
Para-aminobenzoic acid (PABA) derivative (such as benzocaine, procaine, tetracaine): Possible antagonism of antimicrobial effect of sulfonamide. Avoid concurrent administration.
Phenytoin: May inhibit the hepatic metabolism or displace PTN from albumin-binding site of phenytoin. When administering these drugs concurrently, one should be alert for possible excessive phenytoin effect.
Porfimer: Additive photosensitivity reaction. Counsel patients on avoidance of sunlight for 30 days after the last porfimer dose.
Sulfonylureas: Increased hypoglycemic effects of sulfonylureas, due to protein displacement of sulfonylurea from protein binding site by sulfonamides. Monitor blood sugar closely with co-administration suffonamide.
Warfarin: Increased anticoagulant effect due to displacement of warfarin from albumin binding site. Monitor INR closely with co-administration.

PREGNANCY RISK: C-Contraindicated near term. Due to the potential of kernicterus in the newborn, sulfa drugs should be avoided near term.

BREAST FEEDING: Excreted in breast milk. Generally, breast feeding is not recommended.

COMMENTS: Oral sulfonamide with higher incidence of crystalluria compared to other sulfa agents. Agent of choice for toxoplasmosis (with pyrimethamine) due to superior CNS penetration.

FORMS

Brand name	Preparation	Mfr.	Route	Form	Strength	Cost (AWP)
Sulfadiazine	Sulfadiazine	Eon	PO	tab	500mg	$1.44

SELECTED READINGS
Dannemann B, et al. Treatment of toxoplasmic encephalitis in patients with AIDS. A randomized trial comparing pyrimethamine plus clindamycin to pyrimethamine plus sulfadiazine. Ann Intern Med 1992 Jan 1;116(1):33-43

SULFISOXAZOLE

FDA INDICATIONS
- Urinary tract infection
- Nocardia
- Plasmodium falciparum resistant to chloroquine
- Toxoplasmosis in combination with pyrimethamine (sulfadiazine preferred)
- Otitis media (peds)

USUAL ADULT DOSING: UTI: 1g PO q6h

Dosing Adjustments
GFR 50-80 mL/min: 1g q6h
GFR 10-50 mL/min: 1g q8h
GFR<10 mL/min: 1g q12h
Hemodialysis: 1g q12h; supplement 2g post dialysis
Peritoneal Dialysis: 1g q8h

ADVERSE DRUG REACTIONS: **Frequent:** Allergic reactions-rash, pruritus. **Occasional:** Fever; periarteritis nodosa, hypersensitivity, serum sickness; GI intolerance; photosentivity; hepatitis. **Rare:** Stevens-Johnson syndrome, TEN, crystalluria.

DRUG INTERACTIONS
Cyclosporin: Decreased cyclosporine serum levels Monitor serum level closely.
Para-aminobenzoic acid (PABA) derivative (such as benzocaine, procaine, tetracaine): Possible antagonism of antimicrobial effect of sulfonamide. Avoid concurrent administration.
Phenytoin: May inhibit the hepatic metabolism or displace PTN from albumin-binding site of phenytoin. When administering these drugs concurrently, one should be alert for possible excessive phenytoin effect.
Porfimer: Additive photosensitivity reaction. Counsel patients on avoidance of sunlight for 30 days after the last porfimer dose.
Sulfonylureas: Increased hypoglycemic effects of sulfonylureas, due to protein displacement of sulfonylurea from protein binding site by sulfonamides. Monitor blood sugar closely with co-administration suffonamide.
Warfarin: Increased anticoagulant effect due to displacement of warfarin from albumin binding site. Monitor INR closely with co-administration.

PREGNANCY RISK: C-Due to the potential of kernicterus in the newborn, sulfa drugs should be avoided near term.

BREAST FEEDING: Excreted in breast milk. The American Academy of Pediatrics considers sulfapyridine, sulfisoxazole, and sulfamethoxazole compatible with breast feeding. Avoid in hyperbilirubinemia and in G6PD deficiency.

COMMENTS: Oral sulfa antimicrobial with high solubility with little risk of crystalluria. Use primarily for uncomplicated UTI.

FORMS (♦ DENOTES AVAILABLE GENERICALLY)

Brand name	Preparation	Mfr.	Route	Form	Strength	Cost (AWP)
Gantrisin	Sulfisoxazole	Roche	PO	susp	500mg/5mL (16oz)	$50.58
Sulfisoxazole	Sulfisoxazole	♦ Ivax	PO	tab	500mg	$0.52

TELITHROMYCIN

FDA INDICATIONS

- Acute bacterial exacerbation of chronic bronchitis (AECB) due to S. pneumoniae, H. influenzae, or M. catarrhalis
- Acute bacterial sinusitis due to S. pneumoniae, H. influenzae, M. catarrhalis, or S. aureus
- Mild to moderate severe community-acquired pneumonia due to S. pneumoniae (including multi-drug resistant isolates), H. influenzae, M. catarrhalis, C. pneumoniae, or M. pneumoniae

USUAL ADULT DOSING: 800mg PO QD with or without food. AECB and acute bacterial sinusistis treat for 5d. Community-acquired pneumonia treat for 7-10 d.

Dosing Adjustments

GFR 50-80 mL/min: Usual dose

GFR 10-50 mL/min: Usual dose

GFR<10 mL/min: AUC increased by 1.9x in severe renal insufficiency. Consider dose reduction in patients with concurrent hepatic failure.

Hemodialysis: Usual dose (800mg PO QD, limited data)

Peritoneal Dialysis: No data (consider 800mg PO QD)

↓ *Hepatic Function:* (Child-Pugh Class A, B and C) Standard dose: 800mg PO QD

ADVERSE DRUG REACTIONS: Nausea/diarrhea 7-10% of pts. **Occasional:** H/A, dizziness, vomiting, reversible LFTs elevation & hepatitis. Reversible blurring, difficulty focusing, & diplopia observed in 1.1% of pts in phase 3 trials; females < 40 at incr. risk. **Rare:** QTc prolongation.

DRUG INTERACTIONS

Substrate and inhibitor of CYP 3A4. May significantly increase midazolam, triazolam, simvastatin, lovastatin and other CYP3A4 substrates.

Cisapride; pimozide; quinidine; procainamide; dofetilide; rifampin; ergot alkaloids: Contraindicated in use with telithromycin.

Statins: Should be avoided. If using telithromycin, hold statins for duration of therapy (exceptions are pravastatin and fluvastatin).

PREGNANCY RISK: C-No treatment related malformation seen in animal studies. No human data.

BREAST FEEDING: No data

COMMENTS: Advantages: active against nearly all likely bacterial pathogens of resp tract; FDA approved for infections involving penicillin-resistant S. pneumoniae; once daily therapy. Disadvantages: Available only in oral formulation; relatively high rate of GI intolerance; reversible visual disturbance in a small number of patients. Many drug interactions with CYP3A4 substrate.

FORMS

Brand name	Preparation	Mfr.	Route	Form	Strength	Cost (AWP)
Ketek	telithromycin	Aventis	PO	tab	400mg	$5.54

SELECTED READINGS

Pullman J et al. Efficacy and tolerability of once-daily oral therapy with telithromycin compared with trovafloxacin for the treatment of community-acquired pneumonia in adults. Int J Clin Pract. 2003; 57 (5):377-84

Hagberg L et al. Efficacy and tolerability of once-daily telithromycin compared with high-dose amoxicillin for treatment of community-acquired pneumonia. Infection. 2002;30(6):378-86

Buchanan PP et al. A comparison of the efficacy of telithromycin versus cefuroxime axetil in the treatment of acute bacterial maxillary sinusitis. Am J Rhinol. 2003;17(6):369-77

Luterman M et al. Efficacy and tolerability of telithromycin for 5 or 10 days vs amoxicillin/clavulanic acid for 10 days in acute maxillary sinusitis. Ear Nose Throat J. 2003; 82(8):576-80

Quinn J et al. Efficacy and tolerability of 5-day, once-daily telithromycin compared with 10-day, twice-daily clarithromycin for the treatment of group A beta-hemolytic streptococcal tonsillitis/pharyngitis. Clin Ther. 2003; 25(2):422-43

TENOFOVIR (TDF)

FDA INDICATIONS
• HIV infection, in combination with other antiretroviral drugs

USUAL ADULT DOSING: Tenofovir (TDF) 300mg qd without regard to meals (but fatty meals improves absorption by 40%). May be administered as combination product TDF300mg/FTC200mg 1 tablet PO QD with or without food.

Dosing Adjustments
GFR 50-80 mL/min: Usual dose
GFR 10-50 mL/min: 30-49 mL/min 300mg q48h. <30mL/min: 300mg twice a week
GFR<10 mL/min: 300mg q 7 days (healthy volunteers PK data)
Hemodialysis: 300mg q 7 days following dialysis (may require more if more than three 4-hr HD session)
Peritoneal Dialysis: No data. Dose reduction likely.
↓ *Hepatic Function:* No data, usual dose likely

ADVERSE DRUG REACTIONS: Generally well tolerated. Most common side effects: Nausea and vomiting. Asymptomatic elevation of CPK and transaminase levels in 10% [AAC 2001;45:2733]. Neutropenia in 7% and increased amylase in 6%. **Rare:** ARF, Fanconi Syndrome, ATN.

DRUG INTERACTIONS
Does not interact with CYP50 pathway. Tenofovir AUC increases 34% with concurrent LPV/RTV; TDF increases ddI AUC 44-60% (reduce ddI dose to 250 mg po qd with TDF). TDF decreases ATV AUC by 25% (dose ATV 300mg/RTV 100mg with TDF).

PREGNANCY RISK: B-Gravid Rhesus Monkeys study showed normal fetal development, however reduction in body weight, insulin-like growth factor, and increased fetal bone porousness observed (JAIDS 2002; 29:207).

BREAST FEEDING: Not recommended.

COMMENTS: Advantages includes: once daily administration, good side effect profile, active against hep B, active against strains that are often resistant to nucleosides (except with the T69S, K65R, or 3 or more mutation that include 210, 41, and 65), and no evidence of lactic acidosis. Triple NRTI combination that includes TDF/ddI/3TC or TDF/ABC/3TC are not recommended due to early virologic failure.

FORMS

Brand name	Preparation	Mfr.	Route	Form	Strength	Cost (AWP)
Viread	Tenofovir disoproxil fumarate (TDF)	Gilead	PO	tab	300mg	$15.92
Truvada	tenofovir (TDF)/emtricitabine (FTC)	Gilead	PO	tab	300mg/200mg	$26

SELECTED READINGS

Cundy KC, Safrin S, Coleman R et al . Oral PMPA prodrug: relationship between clinical pharmacokinetics, safety and anti-HIV activity. 12th World AIDS Conference; June 28, 1998; 53. abstract GS-97-910

Product Information. Viread, Gilead corp. GS-98-902

Product Information. Viread, Gilead corp. GS-99-907

Deeks SG, Barditch-Crovo P, Lietman PS. Safety, pharmacokinetics, and antiretroviral activity of intravenous 9-[2-(R)-(Phosphonomethoxy)propyl]adenine, a novel anti-human immunodeficiency virus (HIV) therapy, in HIV-infected adults. AAC 1998;42:2280

TERBINAFINE

FDA INDICATIONS

- Onychomycosis
- Tinea capitis
- Tinea corporis
- Tinea cruris
- Tinea pedis

USUAL ADULT DOSING: 250mg PO qd. Liver function testing recommended for long-term therapy if pretreatment LFT's are not nml, and hx of liver disease or use of concurrent potential hepatotoxic drugs.

Dosing Adjustments
GFR 50-80 mL/min: 250mg qd
GFR 10-50 mL/min: No data; avoid

ADVERSE DRUG REACTIONS: Occasional: GI intolerance-diarrhea, dyspepsia, abdominal pain, rash, taste perversion, pruritis. **Rare:** SEVERE HEPATITIS

DRUG INTERACTIONS

Ethanol and other hepatotoxic drugs (e.g., INH, PIs, NNRTIs): Potential additive hepatotoxicity. Avoid concurrent administration, monitor liver enzymes.

PREGNANCY RISK: B

BREAST FEEDING: Considered unsafe during breastfeeding, not recommended by the manufacturer.

COMMENTS: Terbinafine is superior to pulse dose itraconazole in the management of onychomycosis. Monitoring of liver enzymes recommended with long-term therapy if abnl LFTs or liver disease is preexisting.

FORMS

Brand name	Preparation	Mfr.	Route	Form	Strength	Cost (AWP)
Lamisil	Terbinafine	Novartis	PO	tab	250mg	$11.22
			topical	cre	1% (12g); 1% (24g)	$6.79; $10.19
			topical	spray	1% (1oz)	$8.49

SELECTED READINGS

Sigurgeirsson B, Olafsson JH, Steinsson JB et al. Long-term effectiveness of treatment with terbinafine vs itraconazole in onychomycosis: a 5-year blinded prospective follow-up study. Arch Dermatol. 2002;138 (3):353-7.

TETANUS HYPERIMMUNE GLOBULIN

FDA INDICATIONS

- Treatment and prophylaxis of tetanus in unvaccinated patients or in patients with unknown immunity

USUAL ADULT DOSING: Prophylaxis: 250 units IM (for clean wound in early injury). 500 units IM (for contaminated wound or wound of more than 24 hours old). Treatment of active tetanus: 3,000 units IM (up to 10,000U)

Dosing Adjustments
GFR 50-80 mL/min: Usual dose
GFR 10-50 mL/min: No data, usual dose likely
GFR<10 mL/min: No data, usual dose likely
Hemodialysis: No data, usual dose likely

ADVERSE DRUG REACTIONS: Rare: Unlike equine tetanus antitoxin, tetanus immune globulin hypersensitivity is rare.

PREGNANCY RISK: B- No risk to the fetus has been reported. The American College of Obstetricians and Gynecologists recommends its use in pregnancy for post-exposure prophylaxis.

BREAST FEEDING: No data

COMMENTS: Tetanus toxoid can be administered concurrently at a different site.

FORMS

Brand name	Preparation	Mfr.	Route	Form	Strength	Cost (AWP)
BayTet	Tetanus immune globulin	Bayer	IM	syringe	250U	$126.00

SELECTED READINGS

Ballow M. Intravenous Immunoglobulins: Clinical Experience and Viral Safety. J Am Pharm Assoc 2002; 42:449

Quinti I, Pierdominice M, Marziali M et al. European Surveillance of Immunoglobulin Safety-Result of Initial Survey of 1243 Patients with Primary Immunodeficiencies in 16 Countries. Clininal Immunology 2002; 104:231

TETRACYCLINE

FDA INDICATIONS

- Lymphogranuloma venereum caused by Chlamydia species
- Psittacosis caused by Chlamydia psittaci
- Rickettsial and Q fever
- Typhus infections and Rocky Mountain Spotted Fever
- Syphilis and trachoma
- Urinary tract infections and nongonococcal urethritis
- Acne vulgaris
- Anthrax (in PCN allergic)
- Bartonellosis, Brucellosis, Chancroid

USUAL ADULT DOSING: 250-500mg PO qid on an empty stomach.

Dosing Adjustments
GFR 50-80 mL/min: Usual dose

GFR 10-50 mL/min: Use doxycycline; avoid tetracycline
GFR<10 mL/min: Use doxycycline; avoid tetracycline
Hemodialysis: Avoid tetracycline; use doxycycline
Peritoneal Dialysis: Avoid tetracycline; use doxycycline

ADVERSE DRUG REACTIONS: **Frequent:** GI upset; stains & deforms/stains teeth in children < 8 yrs; phlebitis with IV. **Occasional:** Hepatotoxicity; esophageal ulcerations; diarrhea; candidiasis; photosensitivity.

DRUG INTERACTIONS

Bismuth salts (bismuth subsalicylate-Pepto-Bismol): Bismuth salts chelate tetracyclines resulting in a decreased absorption of tetracycline. Administer bismuth 2 hours after tetracycline.

Digoxin: May result in increased digoxin concentration (in about 10% of patients). May be due to tetracycline's alteration of bowel flora responsible for of digoxin metabolism.

Penicillins: In vitro antagonism when co-administered. Bactericidal effect of penicillins may be diminished in vivo. Avoid co-administration.

Polyvalent metal cations (aluminum, zinc, magnesium, iron, calcium [milk"): Polyvalent metal cations form an insoluble chelate with tetracyclines resulting in decreased absorption and serum level of tetracyclines. Separate administration by 4 hours.

Urinary Alkalinizers (sodium lactate, sodium bicarbonate): Increased urinary excretion of tetracyclines by 24-65%) resulting in lower serum concentration.

Warfarin: May increase hypoprothrombinemia. Monitor INR closely with co-administration.

PREGNANCY RISK: D-Tetracyclines are contraindicated in pregnancy due to retardation of skeletal development and bone growth, enamel hypoplasia and discoloration of teeth of fetus. Maternal liver toxicity has also been reported.

BREAST FEEDING: Tetracyclines are excreted in breast milk at very low concentrations. There is theoretical possibility of dental staining and inhibition of bone growth, but infants exposed to tetracyclines have blood levels less than 0.05mcg/mL.

COMMENTS: Oral tetracycline has broad activity, but doxycycline is usually preferred due to twice-a-day dosing convenience without regard to meals.

FORMS (♦ DENOTES AVAILABLE GENERICALLY)

Brand name	Preparation	Mfr.	Route	Form	Strength	Cost (AWP)
Sumycin	Tetracycline HCL	♦ Par	PO	susp	125mg/5mL (16oz)	$87.86
			PO	tab	250mg; 500mg	$0.28; $0.54
Tetracycline HCl	Tetracycline HCl	♦ Ivax	PO	cap	250mg; 500mg	$0.08; $0.12

THIABENDAZOLE

FDA INDICATIONS

- Larva migrans
- Strongyloidiasis
- Trichinosis

USUAL ADULT DOSING: Strongyloidiasis: 50mg/kg/d x 2d. Cutaneous larva migrans: 50mg/kg/d x 2d. Visceral larva migrans: 50mg/kg/d x 7d. Trichinosis: 50mg/kg/d x 2-4d.

Dosing Adjustments

GFR 50-80 mL/min: Use with caution
GFR 10-50 mL/min: Use with caution, dose may need to be reduced

GFR<10 mL/min: Use with caution, dose may need to be reduced
↓ *Hepatic Function:* Use with caution.

ADVERSE DRUG REACTIONS: Occasional: Nausea, vomiting, vertigo, rash, headache, drowsiness. **Rare:** Hallucination; olfactory disturbances; leukopenia; hepatotoxicity (including intrahepatic cholestasis); TEN

DRUG INTERACTIONS

Theophyllines: Increase theophylline serum level. Monitor for signs of theophylline toxicity and serum level. Dose of theophylline may need to be decreased.

PREGNANCY RISK: C-Teratogenic in some animal species. Case reports in human showing no fetal adverse effect. Use in pregnant patients only if parasite (Strongyloides stercoralis) causes clinical disease or public health problems.

BREAST FEEDING: No data available.

COMMENTS: Potent antihelminthic. Most commonly employed against Strongyloides species, but also effective in the treatment of cutaneous and visceral larva migrans and trichinosis. Use caution in the setting of hepatic insufficiency.

FORMS

Brand name	Preparation	Mfr.	Route	Form	Strength	Cost (AWP)
Mintezol	Thiabenda-zole	Merck	PO	chew tab	500mg	$1.26
			PO	susp	500mg/5mL	$1.10 per 5mL

SELECTED READINGS

Pitisuttithum P, Supanaranond W, Chindanond D. A randomized comparative study of albendazole and thiabendazole in chronic strongyloidiasis. Southeast Asian J Trop Med Public Health. 1995;26(4):735-8.

TICARCILLIN

FDA INDICATIONS

- Gynecologic infections (endomyometritis)
- Intra-abdominal infections
- Lower respiratory infections
- Septicemia
- Skin and skin structure infections
- Urinary tract infections
- Bone and joint infections

USUAL ADULT DOSING: 3g IV q4-6h (up to 24 mL/day)

Dosing Adjustments

GFR 50-80 mL/min: Usual dose
GFR 10-50 mL/min: 2g-3g q6-8h
GFR<10 mL/min: 2g q12h
Hemodialysis: 2g q12h plus 3g post-dialysis
Peritoneal Dialysis: 3g q12h

ADVERSE DRUG REACTIONS: Frequent: Hypersensitivity reactions; rash. **Occasional:** GI intolerance; drug fever; Coombs' test positive; phlebitis at infusion sites and sterile abscesses at IM sites; Jarisch-Herxheimer reaction (for syphilis or other spirochetal infections)

DRUG INTERACTIONS

Tetracyclines: In vitro antagonism when co-administered. Bactericidal effect of penicillins may be diminished in vivo. Avoid concurrent administration. In two studies involving a total of 79 patients with pneumococcal meningitis treated with either penicillin plus tetracyclines or penicillin monotherapy there was a higher mortality rate (79-85%) in the combination therapy compared to penicillin monotherapy (30-33%). (Arch Intern Med 1951;88:489, Ann Intern Med 1961; 55:545). However there was not a difference in mortality between penicillin monotherapy and penicillin plus tetracycline in the treatment of pneumococcal pneumonia. (Arch Intern Med 1953; 91:197).

Warfarin -Ticarcillin-induced inhibition of ADP-mediated platelet aggregation in addition to warfarin-induced hypoprothrombinemia may prolong bleeding time. Monitor INR closely and adjust warfarin dose accordingly.

PREGNANCY RISK: B-Several collaborative perinatal project reports involving over 12,000 exposures to penicillin derivatives during the first trimester indicated no association between penicillin derivative drugs and birth defects.

BREAST FEEDING: Excreted in breast milk in low concentration. No adverse effects have been reported.

COMMENTS: Anti-pseudomonal penicillin. Contains 4.75 meq of sodium per gram of ticarcillin. Reduced enterococcal activity compared to piperacillin. Reduced activity vs. S. pneumoniae

FORMS

Brand name	Preparation	Mfr.	Route	Form	Strength	Cost (AWP)
Ticar	Ticarcillin	Abbott	IV	vial	20g	$82.50

SELECTED READINGS

Bosseray A, et al. P. Evaluation of three types of empirical antibiotherapy in patients with febrile neutropenia: imipenem-cilastatin versus ceftazidime-vancomycin versus ticarcillin-amikacin-vancomycin. Pathol Biol 1992 Oct;40(8):797-804

TICARCILLIN + CLAVULANIC ACID

FDA INDICATIONS

- Bone and joint infections
- Intra-abdominal infections
- Lower respiratory tract infections
- Obstetric/gynecologic infections
- Septicemia
- Skin and soft-tissue infections
- Urinary tract infections

USUAL ADULT DOSING: 3.1g IV q4-6h (up to 24g per day). Pulmonary, Pseudomonad, and serious infections: 3.1g IV q4h.

Dosing Adjustments

GFR 50-80 mL/min: 50-60mL/min: 2g q4h >60mL/min: standard dose
GFR 10-50 mL/min: <30mL/min: 2g q8h 30-60mL/min: 2g q4h
GFR<10 mL/min: 2g q12h
Hemodialysis: 2g q12h plus 3.1g post-dialysis
Peritoneal Dialysis: 3.1g q12h
↓ *Hepatic Function:* For patients with hepatic dysfunction and creatinine clearance <10mL/min, give 2g IV/day in one or two doses.

ANTI-INFECTIVES

ADVERSE DRUG REACTIONS: Occasional: Hypersensitivity reactions; rash; GI intolerance; drug fever; Coombs' test positive; phlebitis at infusion sites and sterile abscesses at IM sites; Jarisch-Herxheimer reaction (w/ syphilis or other spirochetal infections). **Rare:** anaphylaxis

DRUG INTERACTIONS

Tetracyclines: In vitro antagonism when co-administered. Bactericidal effect of penicillins may be diminished in vivo. Avoid concurrent administration. In two studies involving a total of 79 patients with pneumococcal meningitis treated with either penicillin plus tetracyclines or penicillin monotherapy there was a higher mortality rate (79-85%) in the combination therapy compared to penicillin monotherapy (30-33%). (Arch Intern Med 1951;88:489, Ann Intern Med 1961; 55:545). However there was not a difference in mortality between penicillin monotherapy and penicillin plus tetracycline in the treatment of pneumococcal pneumonia. (Arch Intern Med 1953; 91:197).

Warfarin -Ticarcillin-induced inhibition of ADP-mediated platelet aggregation in addition to warfarin-induced hypoprothrombinemia may prolong bleeding time. Monitor INR closely and adjust warfarin dose accordingly.

PREGNANCY RISK: B-In surveillance study of Michigan Medicaid recipients, 556 newborns were exposed to clavulanate/penicillins during the first trimester. There was no association between birth defects and clavulanate/penicillins.

BREAST FEEDING: No data available

COMMENTS: Parenteral betalactam-betalactamase inhibitor with spectrum similar to that of piperacillin/tazobactam but with less activity against enterococcus and S. pneumoniae. Contains 4.75 meq of sodium per gram of ticarcillin. More frequent dosing interval (every 4 hours) recommended for serious pseudomonal infections.

FORMS

Brand name	Preparation	Mfr.	Route	Form	Strength	Cost (AWP)
Timentin	Ticarcillin + Clavulanic Acid	GlaxoSmithKline	IV	vial	3g/100mg; 30g/1g; 3g-100mg/100mL	$15.37; $150.41 per vial; $17.45 per vial

SELECTED READINGS

Schwigon CD; Hulla FW; Schulze B et al. Timentin in the treatment of nosocomial bronchopulmonary infections in intensive care units. J Antimicrob Chemother 1986 May;17 Suppl C:115-22.

Dougherty SH; Sirinek KR; Schauer PR et al. Ticarcillin/clavulanate compared with clindamycin/gentamicin (with or without ampicillin) for the treatment of intra-abdominal infections in pediatric and adult patients. Am Surg 1995 Apr;61(4):297-303

File TM et al. Ticarcillin-clavulanate therapy for bacterial skin and soft tissue infections. Rev Infect Dis 1991 Jul-Aug;13 Suppl 9:S733-6

TIGECYCLINE

FDA INDICATIONS

- Complicated skin and skin structure infections (including those caused by MRSA and vancomycin-susceptible E. faecalis)
- Complicated intra-abdominal infections (as a single agent)

USUAL ADULT DOSING: 100mg IV x 1, then 50mg IV q12h x 5-14 days.

Dosing Adjustments
GFR 50-80 mL/min: Usual dose
GFR 10-50 mL/min: Usual dose
GFR<10 mL/min: Usual dose

Hemodialysis: Not removed with HD. No dose adjustment needed

Peritoneal Dialysis: No data, usual dose likely

↓ *Hepatic Function:* 100mg IV x1, then 25mg IV q12h (for Child Pugh C)

ADVERSE DRUG REACTIONS: Common: Nausea and vomiting in 20-30% of tygecycline treated patients. **Occasional:** Hyperbilirubinemia (2.3%), BUN increase (2.1%) respectively. **Rare:** C. difficile colitis. Due to structural similarity, tetracycline photosensitivity may occur.

DRUG INTERACTIONS

Warfarin: Prothrombin time or other suitable anticoagulation test should be monitored if tigecycline is administered with warfarin.

PREGNANCY RISK: D--No human data. Avoid in pregnancy. Reduction in fetal weight and increased incidence of minor skeletal anomalies in rats and rabbits studies.

BREAST FEEDING: Excreted in breast milk, but tigecycline has limited oral bioavailability. Use only when clearly indicated.

COMMENTS: Tigecycline has a spectrum of activity that includes anaerobes, many gram-positive cocci & gram-negative bacilli w/ the exception of P. aeruginosa. Tigecycline is effective in the treatment of intra-abdominal infections and complicated soft-tissue infections with a more convenient twice-a-day dosing compared to imipenem/cilastin and pip/tazo. Nausea & vomiting may occur in up to a third of pts.

FORMS

Brand name	Preparation	Mfr.	Route	Form	Strength	Cost (AWP)
Tygacil	Tigecycline	Wyeth	IV	vial	50mg	$56.50

SELECTED READINGS

Postier RG, Green SL, Klein SR, et al. Results of a multicenter, randomized, open-label efficacy and safety study of two doses of tigecycline for complicated skin and skin-structure infections in hospitalized patients. Clin Ther. 2004;26:704-14

Wyeth Pharmaceuticals. . Tygacil [Package Insert]. Wyeth Pharmaceuticals Inc. Philadelphia, PA 19101 2005

TINIDAZOLE

FDA INDICATIONS
- Trichomoniasis
- Giardiasis
- Intestinal and amebic liver abscess caused by E. histolytica

USUAL ADULT DOSING: Trichomoniasis: 2g p.o x 1 with food. Giardiasis: 2g p.o x 1 with food Intestinal Amebiasis: 2g p.o QD with food x 3 days. Liver Amebiais: 2g p.o QD with food x 3-5 days. children >3yrs 50mg/kg single dose for giardiasis, amebiasis

Dosing Adjustments

GFR 50-80 mL/min: Standard dose

GFR 10-50 mL/min: Standard dose

GFR<10 mL/min: Standard dose.

Hemodialysis: Dosing in HD: 43% removed with HD, supplement with 50% (1gm) post-HD.

↓ *Hepatic Function:* No data. Increased in serum level of tinidazole may occur; use standard dose with close monitoring.

Anti-Infectives

Adverse Drug Reactions: Occasional: Nausea (9%),vomiting (3%), metallic/bitter taste (10%), anorexia (4.5%) [note: GI intolerance was less than metronidazole in clinical trials]. Candidiasis. **Rare:** Seizure, peripheral neuropathy, leukopenia, and neutropenia.

Drug Interactions

Alcohol and propylene glycol: Potential for disulfiram reaction.

Cholestyramine: Decreased tinidazole absorption.

Cyclosporin: Increased cyclosporine serum level.

CYP3A4 Inducers (e.g., rifampin, NVP, phenytoin): Potential of decreasing tinidazole serum concentration.

CYP3A4 Inhibitors (e.g., macrolides, azoles, PIs): May increase tinidazole serum concentration.

Fluorouracil: Increased fluorouracil serum level and toxicity.

Fosphenytoin: Prolonged t1/2 of fosphenytoin.

Lithium: Increased lithium serum level.

Tacrolimus: Increased tacrolimus serum level (based on case reports).

Warfarin: Enhanced anitcoagulant effect.

Pregnancy Risk: C No human data. Animal studies did not find any embryo-fetal toxicity or malformation.

Breast Feeding: Excreted in breast milk. No safety data.

Comments: Tinidazole is an alternative to metronidazole and may be preferred for the treatment of E. histolytica and Giardiasis due to better GI tolerance and superior efficacy.

Forms

Brand name	Preparation	Mfr.	Route	Form	Strength	Cost (AWP)
Tindamax	Tinidazole	Presutti	PO	tab	250mg; 500mg	$2.28; $4.56

Selected Readings

Anon. . Package insert

Anjaeyulu R, Gupte SA, Desai DB. Single-dose treatment of trichomonal vaginitis: a comparison of tinidazole and metronidazole. J Int Med Res. 1977;5(6):438-41.

Gazder AJ, Banerjee M. Single-dose treatment of giardiasis in children: a comparison of tinidazole and metronidazole. Curr Med Res Opin. 1977;5(2):164-8.

Singh G, Kumar S. Short course of single daily dosage treatment with tinidazole and metronidazole in intestinal amoebiasis: a comparative study. Curr Med Res Opin. 1977;5(2):157-60.

TOBRAMYCIN

FDA Indications

- Septicemia
- Lower respiratory tract infections
- Serious central-nervous-system infections
- Intra-abdominal infections, including peritonitis
- Skin, bone, and skin structure infections
- Complicated urinary tract infections
- Treatment of ocular infections (ophthalmic solution)
- Management of cystic fibrosis, with P. aeruginosa (as Tobi inhalation)

Usual Adult Dosing: QD dosing: 5-7mg/kg IV. Mild-mod infxn: 1.7mg/kg IV q8h (goal peak >6 mcg/mL). Severe infxn: 2mg/kg IV q8h (goal peak >8 mcg/mL). Sepsis, Pseudomonas, or pneumonia: 2mg/kg IV q8h (goal peak: >8 mcg/mL). Tobra Nebs 80-300mg inh q12-24h.

Dosing Adjustments

GFR 50-80 mL/min: 60-90% of usual dose q8-12h or 100% of usual dose q12-24 hrs. (monitor levels)

GFR 10-50 mL/min: 30-70% of usual dose q 12h or 100% of usual dose q24-48 hrs (monitor levels)

GFR<10 mL/min: 20-30% of usual dose q24-48 hrs or 100% q48-72 hrs (monitor serum level)

Hemodialysis: 1.0-1.7mg/kg post-dialysis (monitor levels); redose for <2 mg/mL

Peritoneal Dialysis: 2-4 mg/L of dialysate exchange per day. Aminoglycosides given for prolonged periods to patients receiving continuous peritoneal dialysis have been associated with high rates of ototoxicity. Monitor level after loading dose and follow for symptoms.

ADVERSE DRUG REACTIONS: Frequent: Renal failure (usually reversible). **Occasional:** Vestibular and auditory damage (usually irreversible, genetic predisposition in some cases check family for aminoglycoside ototoxicity). **Rare:** Neuromuscular blockade.

DRUG INTERACTIONS

Loop diuretics (bumetanide, furosemide, (especially avoid co-administration with ethacrynic acid), torsemide): Increased ototoxicity and/or nephrotoxicity. Ototoxicity appears to be dose dependent and may be increased with renal dysfunction. Irreversible ototoxicity has been reported.

Nephrotoxic agents (amphotericin B, foscarnet, cidofovir): Additive nephrotoxicity. Avoid co-administration, if used together monitor renal function closely and discontinue if warranted.

Nondepolarizing muscle relaxants (atracurium, pancuronium, tubocurarine, gallamine triethiodide): Enhanced action of nondepolarizing muscle relaxant resulting in respiratory depression. Avoid co-administration, if concurrent administration is needed titrate the nondepolarizing muscle relaxant slowly and monitor neuromuscular function closely.

Penicillins: In vitro inactivation of aminoglycoside by acylation. Do not mix together before administration (i.e., running in the same line or concurrent intraperitoneal administration). May be clinically apparent only in patients with renal failure receiving antipseudomal penicillin in large doses. (In vivo patients with poor renal function where renal excretion of the drugs are delayed, where the ratio of penicillin to aminoglycoside is greater than 50 to 1 there is a potential for drug inactivation). Amikacin may be less affected by this interaction compared to gentamicin and tobramycin.

Vancomycin: Controversial, but may increase risk of nephrotoxicity.

PREGNANCY RISK: C-(but manufacturer rates it D) Animal studies did not demonstrate teratogenicity. Case reports exist of irreversible bilateral congenital deafness in children whose mothers received streptomycin. Can potentially occur with tobramycin.

BREAST FEEDING: Only trace amount of tobramycin was found in some nursing infants. Due to the poor absorption of aminoglycoside the systemic toxicity should not occur, but alteration in normal bowel flora may occur in nursing infants.

COMMENTS: Parenteral aminoglycoside with slightly better anti-pseudomonal activity compared to gentamicin. May also be less nephrotoxic, but more ototoxic compared to gentamicin. Once daily dosing should not be used in pts w/ unstable renal function, CrCl <60 mL/min, endocarditis, meningitis, and any pts with increased vol (pregnancy, burn, ascites, edema, shock).

FORMS (◆ DENOTES AVAILABLE GENERICALLY)

Brand name	Preparation	Mfr.	Route	Form	Strength	Cost (AWP)
Tobramycin sulfate	Tobramycin sulfate	◆ Hospira	IV	vial	10mg/mL; 40mg/mL	$0.83 per mL; $1.48 per mL

(continued)

Anti-Infectives

Brand name	Preparation	Mfr.	Route	Form	Strength	Cost (AWP)
Tobi	Tobramycin inhalation	Chiron	inhalation	ampule	300mg/5mL	$61.45 per 5mL

Selected Readings

Wiesemann HG; Steinkamp G; Ratjen F et al . Placebo-controlled, double-blind, randomized study of aerosolized tobramycin for early treatment of Pseudomonas aeruginosa colonization in cystic fibrosis . Pediatr Pulmonol 1998 Feb;25(2):88-92

Richard DA, Nousia-Arvanitakis S, Sollich V, et al. Oral ciprofloxacin vs. intravenous ceftazidime plus tobramycin in pediatric cystic fibrosis patients: comparison of antipseudomonas efficacy and assessment of safety. Pediatr Infect Dis J 1997 Jun;16(6):572-8

Rivera-Vazquez CR, Ramirez-Ronda, et al:. A comparative analysis of aztreonam + clindamycin versus tobramycin + clindamycin or amikacin + mezlocillin in the treatment of gram-negative lower respiratory tract infections. Chemotherapy 1989;35 Suppl 1:89-100

Parry MF; Neu HC. A comparative study of ticarcillin plus tobramycin versus carbenicillin plus gentamicin for the treatment of serious infections due to gram- negative bacilli . Am J Med 1978 Jun;64 (6):961-6

Bendush CL; Weber R et al. Tobramycin sulfate: a summary of worldwide experience from clinical trials. J Infect Dis 1976 Aug;134 Suppl:S219-34

TRIMETHOPRIM

FDA Indications
• Urinary tract infections

Usual Adult Dosing: 200mg/day PO in 1-2 doses. Mild-moderate PCP: TMP 5mg/kg PO q8h + Dapsone 100mg PO qd.

Dosing Adjustments
GFR 50-80 mL/min: Usual dose
GFR 10-50 mL/min: 100mg q24h
GFR<10 mL/min: manufacturer recommends avoiding, but for PCP:5-7.5mg/kg/day (1/2-1/3 standard dose).
Hemodialysis: 4-5 mg/kg post dialysis
Peritoneal Dialysis: 100-200mg q48h

Adverse Drug Reactions: Frequent: GI upset (dose related); rash; pruritis. **Occasional:** Megaloblastic anemia, neutropenia, thrombocytopenia; reversible hyperkalemia w/high dose; photosensitivity; renal failure; hemolytic anemia with G6PD deficiency;hepatitis including cholestatic jaundice

Drug Interactions
Dapsone: Increased serum level of both dapsone (40%) and trimethoprim (48%). Monitor for clinical toxicity (nausea, vomiting, irritability, dizziness, confusion, pancytopenia and methemoglobinemia).
Methotrexate: Plasma concentration of methotrexate may be increased due to decreased renal clearance. Monitor for pancytopenia with co-administration. Dose of methotrexate may need to be decreased.
Phenytoin: May inhibit the hepatic metabolism of phenytoin. When administering these drugs concurrently, one should be alert for possible excessive phenytoin effect.
Procainamide: Elevated procainamide and N-acetylprocainamide (NAPA) serum level secondary to competitive inhibition of renal tubular secretion between trimethoprim and procainamide. Monitor serum level of procainamide and N-acetylprocainamide and monitor EKG for QTc prolongation and arrythmia. Dose may need to be adjusted.

PREGNANCY RISK: C-Animal data show teratogenicity at 40 times the human dose. Should be avoided in the first 3 months of pregnancy during the formation of vital organs. This agent should only be used in pregnancy if the potential benefits outweigh the risk. If used, it should be administered with a supplemental multivitamin containing folic acid.

BREAST FEEDING: Excreted in breast milk. The American Academy of Pediatrics considers trimethoprim compatible with breast feeding.

COMMENTS: Generally used in combination with sulfamethoxazole. Only acceptable indication for monotherapy is acute uncomplicated UTI.

FORMS (♦ DENOTES AVAILABLE GENERICALLY)

Brand name	Preparation	Mfr.	Route	Form	Strength	Cost (AWP)
Proloprim	Trimethoprim	♦ Monarch	PO	tab	100mg	$1.11
Primsol	Trimethoprim HCl	Taro	PO	sol	50mg/5mL	$0.70

TRIMETHOPRIM + SULFAMETHOXAZOLE

FDA INDICATIONS

- Bronchitis
- Otitis media
- Pneumocystis jiroveci (PCP) infections, prophylaxis and treatment
- Respiratory tract infections
- Traveler's diarrhea
- Urinary tract infections
- Enterocolitis caused by Shigella species.

USUAL ADULT DOSING: UTI and traveler's diarrhea: 1DS PO bid. PCP pneumonia: 15mg/kg/day divided q8h PO or IV. PCP prophylaxis: 1SS or 1DS PO qd. Toxoplasmosis prophylaxis: 1DS PO qd. Nocardia: 10-15mg/kg/d divided q8h.

Dosing Adjustments

GFR 50-80 mL/min: Usual dose

GFR 10-50 mL/min: 3-5mg/kg IV q12-24h; oral 50% of dose

GFR<10 mL/min: Manufacturer recommends avoiding, but for PCP: 5-7.5mg/kg/day divided q8h (1/2-1/3 standard dose).

Hemodialysis: 5 mg/kg post dialysis

Peritoneal Dialysis: 0.16/0.8g q48h

ADVERSE DRUG REACTIONS: Frequent: Allergic reactions-rash, pruritus. **Occasional:** Fever; periarteritis nodosa; crystalluria, urolithiasis and oliguria; GI intolerance; photosentivity; hepatitis; marrow suppression; reversible hyperkalemia. **Rare:** Stevens-Johnson syndrome, TEN

DRUG INTERACTIONS

Bone-marrow suppressant drugs: May increase bone-marrow suppression.

Cyclosporin: Decreased cyclosporine serum levels Monitor serum level closely.

Methotrexate: Increased methotrexate serum concentration.

Para-aminobenzoic acid (PABA) derivative (such as benzocaine, procaine, tetracaine) : Possible antagonism of antimicrobial effect of sulfonamide. Avoid concurrent administration.

Phenytoin: Sulfonamides may displace PTN from albumin-binding sites resulting in increased free PTN levels. Monitor free (unbound) PTN levels and for signs of toxicity (drowsiness, nystagmus).

Porfimer: Additive photosensitivity reaction. Counsel patients on avoidance of sunlight for 30 days after the last porfimer dose.

Procainamide: Increased procainamide serum concentration.

Sulfonylureas: Increased hypoglycemic effects of sulfonylureas, due to protein displacement of sulfonylurea from protein binding site by sulfonamides. Monitor blood sugar closely with co-administration suffonamide.

Warfarin: Increased anticoagulant effect due to displacement of warfarin from albumin binding site. Monitor INR closely with co-administration.

PREGNANCY RISK: C-In a surveillance study of Michigan Medicaid recipients, 2,296 exposures to sulfamethoxazole/trimethoprim in the first trimester resulted in a 5.5% birth defect rate. This incidence is suggestive of an association between the drug and congenital defects (cardiovascular), however other factors such as mother's disease, concurrent drug used and chance, may be involved. Contraindicated near term.

BREAST FEEDING: Excreted in breast milk at low concentrations. The American Academy of Pediatrics considers trimethoprim-sulfamethoxazole to be compatible.

COMMENTS: Oral and parenteral combination that is commonly used for uncomplicated cystitis, treatment and prophylaxis of Pneumocystis jiroveci pneumonia and many other infections including second line use for S. aureus. In-vitro resistance does not always correlate with clinical failure for uncomplicated cystitis. Higher incidence of intolerance in HIV infected patients.

FORMS (◆ DENOTES AVAILABLE GENERICALLY)

Brand name	Preparation	Mfr.	Route	Form	Strength	Cost (AWP)
Septra DS	Sulfamethox-azole/Trimethoprim	◆ Monarch	PO	tab	800mg/160mg	$1.25
Septra	Sulfamethox-azole/Trimethoprim	◆ Monarch	PO	tab	400mg/80mg	$1.17
SMX-TMP	Sulfamethox-azole/Trimethoprim	◆ Sicor	IV	vial	80mg-16mg/mL	$19.49 per 30mL vial
Septra	Sulfamethox-azole/Trimethoprim	◆ Monarch	PO	susp	200mg-40mg/5mL (473mL)	$68.30

SELECTED READINGS

McCarty JM, et al. A randomized trial of short-course ciprofloxacin, ofloxacin, or trimethoprim/sulfamethoxazole for the treatment of acute urinary tract infection in women. Am J Med 1999 Mar;106 (3):292-9

Talan DA, et al. Comparison of ciprofloxacin (7 d) and trimethoprim-sulfamethoxazole (14 d) for acute uncomplicated pyelonephritis pyelonephritis in women: a randomized trial. JAMA 2000 Mar 22-29;283 (12):1583-90

Bozzette SA, et al. A randomized trial of three antipneumocystis agents in patients with advanced human immunodeficiency virus infection. NIAID AIDS Clinical Trials Group . N Engl J Med 1995 Mar 16;332(11):693-9

Klein NC, et al. Trimethoprim-sulfamethoxazole versus pentamidine for Pneumocystis carinii pneumonia in AIDS patients: results of a large prospective randomized treatment trial. AIDS 1992 Mar;6(3):301-5

VALACYCLOVIR

FDA INDICATIONS

- Herpes genitalis, treatment and suppression in immunocompetent adults
- Herpes genitalis, recurrent episodes suppression in HIV patients

- Herpes zoster treatment in immunocompetent adults
- Herpes labialis

USUAL ADULT DOSING: Zoster: 1000mg PO tid for zoster. HSV first episode: 1g bid x 7-10d. HSV recurrent: 500mg PO bid. HSV suppression: 500mg q12-24h. Herpes labialis: 2g q12h x 1 day.

Dosing Adjustments

GFR 50-80 mL/min: Usual dose

GFR 10-50 mL/min: 500-1000mg q12h-24h

GFR<10 mL/min: 500mg qd

Hemodialysis: 500mg qd, on days of dialysis dose after dialysis

Peritoneal Dialysis: 500mg qd, no supplemental dose needed

ADVERSE DRUG REACTIONS: Generally well tolerated. **Occasional:** Rash: nausea and vomiting; diarrhea.

DRUG INTERACTIONS

Probenecid: Increase in acyclovir levels due to competitive tubular secretion by probenecid. No dose adjustment needed.

PREGNANCY RISK: B- Not teratogenic in animal studies; no human data available but likely to be similar to acyclovir.

BREAST FEEDING: No data: most likely distributed into breast milk as acyclovir; acyclovir was not associated with any problems in the newborn.

COMMENTS: Pro-drug of acyclovir that shows better absorption, higher blood level and more convenient dosing schedule compared to oral acyclovir. Valacyclovir when used in the treatment of zoster has been shown to decrease more effectively post-herpetic neuralgia compared to acyclovir.

FORMS

Brand name	Preparation	Mfr.	Route	Form	Strength	Cost (AWP)
Valtrex	Valacyclovir	GlaxoSmithKline	PO	tab	500mg; 1000mg	$5.41; $9.24

SELECTED READINGS

Tyring SK, Beutner KR, Tucker BA et al. Antiviral therapy for herpes zoster: randomized, controlled clinical trial of valacyclovir and famciclovir therapy in immunocompetent patients 50 years and older. Arch Fam Med. 2000;9(9):863-9.

Beutner KR, Friedman DJ, Forszpaniak C et al. Valacyclovir compared with acyclovir for improved therapy for herpes zoster in immunocompetent adults. Antimicrob Agents Chemother. 1995;39:1546-53.

VALGANCICLOVIR

FDA INDICATIONS

- CMV retinitis in patients with AIDS.
- Prevention of CMV disease in kidney, heart, and kidney-pancreas transplant patients at high risk for CMV disease (D+/R-).

USUAL ADULT DOSING: 900mg bid with food x 3 weeks (induction phase), then 900mg qd with food (maintenance phase).

Dosing Adjustments

GFR 50-80 mL/min: >60mL/min: 900mg bid (induction); 900mg qd (maintenance)

GFR 10-50 mL/min: 40-59mL/min: 450mg bid(ind); 450mg qd(maint) 25-39mL/min: 450mg qd(i); 450mg qod(m) 10-24mL/min: 450mg qod(i); 450mg biw(m)

GFR<10 mL/min: Not recommended by manufacturer

Hemodialysis: Not recommended (HD removes approx. 50% of ganciclovir)

↓ *Hepatic Function:* No data. Usual dose likely

ADVERSE DRUG REACTIONS: Frequent: Diarrhea, nausea, vomiting, Neutropenia and anemia (comparable to IV ganciclovir). **Occasional:** Thrombocytopenia, headache, fever, rash, confusion, abnormal LFTs. Contraindicated if ANC<500/mm3, Plt <25,000/mL or hemoglobin <8g/dL.

DRUG INTERACTIONS

Didanosine: Potential increase in didanosine serum level.
Myelosuppressive drugs (i.e., zidovudine): Increased risk of hematologic toxicity.
Probenecid: Potential increase in ganciclovir serum level (monitor for ganciclovir toxicity).

PREGNANCY RISK: C-TERATOGENIC, CARCINOGENIC, embryogenic and causes ASPERMATOGENEIS; growth retardation; aplastic organ in animal studies. No human data, use only for life-threatening CMV infection and warn patient of possible teratogenic effect. Effective form of contraception is recommended.

BREAST FEEDING: No data. Due to potential for serious toxicity, mother should avoid breast feeding.

COMMENTS: Oral valganciclovir has a 10-fold improvement in absorption over oral ganciclovir. The AUC of oral valganciclovir 900mg is comparable to 5mg/kg IV ganciclovir. Oral valgancicovir is equivalent to IV ganciclovir for the treatment of CMV retinitis in HIV + pts. Valgan is equivalent to PO ganciclovir for the prevention of CMV disease in kidney, heart, and kidney/pancreas Tx, but NOT liver Transplant.

FORMS

Brand name	Preparation	Mfr.	Route	Form	Strength	Cost (AWP)
Valcyte	Valganciclovir	Roche	PO	tab	450mg	$31.73

VANCOMYCIN

FDA INDICATIONS

- Bone and joint infections
- Pneumonia
- Septicemia
- Bone and joint infections
- Endocarditis prophylaxis (in penicillin-allergic patients)
- Endocarditis treatment
- Oral: C. difficile colitis & enterocolitis caused by S. aureus (including MRSA)

USUAL ADULT DOSING: 15mg/kg IV q12h (usually 1g IV q12h for a 70kg pt). C. difficile colitis: 125mg PO qid. Higher doses only with ileus.

Dosing Adjustments

GFR 50-80 mL/min: 1g IV q12-24h (monitor serum level)
GFR 10-50 mL/min: 1g IV qd-q2days (monitor serum level, redose when Cmin <15-20mcg/mL)
GFR<10 mL/min: 1g IV q3 days (monitor serum level, redose when Cmin <15-20mcg/mL)
Hemodialysis: 1-2g/week, with high flux dialysis 2-3g/week is generally needed (redose when Cmin <15-20mcg/mL)
Peritoneal Dialysis: 0.5-1.0g/week (redose when Cmin <15-20mcg/mL)

ADVERSE DRUG REACTIONS: Frequent: phlebitis. **Occasional:** "Red man syndrome": flushing over chest/face; +/- hypotension & pruritis (infuse > 60 m, may reverse or prevent rxn, Rx w/ antihistamines). **Rare:** Neutropenia, fever, eosinophilia, allergic Rx w/rash.

DRUG INTERACTIONS

Aminoglycozide: Controversial, but may increase risk of nephrotoxicity.

Cholestyramine: Binds to oral vancomycin.

Nondepolarizing muscle relaxants (atracurium, vecuronium, pancuronium, tubocurarine): Neuromuscular blockade may be enhanced. Avoid co-administration, if concurrent administration is needed titrate the nondepolarizing muscle relaxant slowly and monitor neuromuscular function closely.

PREGNANCY RISK: C-The manufacturer has received reports on the use of vancomycin in pregnancy without adverse fetal effects.

BREAST FEEDING: Excreted in breast milk.

COMMENTS: IV glycopeptide used for infections involving resistant gram-positive bacteria including methicillin-resistant S. aureus and S. epidermidis, infections involving enterococci and infections caused by gram-positive bacteria resistant to beta-lactams or in patients with contraindication to betalactams. Use should be restricted to CDC guidelines since VRSA has been reported (MMWR 2002; 51:565).

FORMS (♦ DENOTES AVAILABLE GENERICALLY)

Brand name	Preparation	Mfr.	Route	Form	Strength	Cost (AWP)
Vancocin	Vancomycin HCl	♦ Viropharma	PO	cap	250mg; 125mg	$17.50; $9
Vancocin	Vancomycin HCl	♦ Baxter	IV	vial	500mg; 1000mg	$17.53 per vial; $34.56 per vial

SELECTED READINGS

Levine DP; Fromm BS; Reddy BR et al. Slow response to vancomycin or vancomycin plus rifampin in methicillin- resistant Staphylococcus aureus endocarditis. Ann Intern Med 1991 Nov 1;115(9):674-80

Lee CE, et al. Incidence of Antimicrobial Allergies in Hospitalized Patients. Arch Intern Med 2000;160:2919

Karchmer AW; Archer GL; Dismukes WE et al. Staphylococcus epidermidis causing prosthetic valve endocarditis: microbiologic and clinical observations as guides to therapy. Ann Intern Med 1983 Apr;98 (4):447-55

Viladrich PF; Gudiol F; Linares J et al. Evaluation of vancomycin for therapy of adult pneumococcal meningitis. Antimicrob Agents Chemother 1991 Dec;35(12):2467-72

Teasley DG; Gerding DN; Olson MM et al. Prospective randomised trial of metronidazole versus vancomycin for Clostridium-difficile-associated diarrhoea and colitis. Lancet 1983 Nov 5;2(8358):1043-6

VORICONAZOLE

FDA INDICATIONS

- Invasive aspergillosis
- P. boydii (S. apiospermum) and Fusarium spp. (including F. solani) infections in persons intolerant of, or refractory to, other therapy
- Esophageal candidiasis
- Treatment of candidemia in nonneutropenic patients

USUAL ADULT DOSING: 6mg/kg IV q12h x 2 doses (load), then 4mg/kg IV q12h infused over 1-2 hrs. Oral: >40kg 200mg PO q12h; 300mg PO q12h for severe infection. <40kg - 100mg PO q12h; use 150mg PO q12h for severe infection. Give on an empty stomach, avoid high fat foods.

Dosing Adjustments

GFR 50-80 mL/min: Standard dose

GFR 10-50 mL/min: Standard dosing of oral voriconazole. IV voriconazole is not recommended due to potential for toxicity of the SBECD carrier.

GFR<10 mL/min: Standard dosing of oral voriconazole. IV voriconazole is not recommended due to potential for toxicity of the SBECD vehicle.

Hemodialysis: Voriconazole is dialyzed. Standard dosing of oral voriconazole (dose after HD). IV voriconazole is not recommended.

Peritoneal Dialysis: No data. Standard dose likely. IV voriconazole is not recommended.

↓ *Hepatic Function:* Mild to moderate hepatic insufficiency (Child-Pugh Class A and B): 6mg/kg q12h x 2 doses (load), then 2mg/kg IV q12h.

Adverse Drug Reactions: Common: Reversible visual disturbances (warn pts of blurriness, color changes, and enhanced vision) seen in 20.6% of pts but less than <1% required d/c. **Occasional:** Nausea/vomiting; elevated LFTs (13%) required d/c in 4-8%. Hallucinations (4.3%), rash (6%).

Drug Interactions

In vitro a substrate of CYP2C19>> CYP2C9>CYP3A4, and inhibitor of CYP2C19, CYP2C9, and CYP3A4.

Contraindicated with: sirolimus, terfenadine, astemizole, cisapride, pimozide, quinidine, rifabutin, rifampin, carbamazepine, long-acting barbiturates and ergot alkaloids, ritonavir, and efavirenz.

Benzodiazepines (e.g., midazolam, triazolam, and alprazolam): serum concentrations may be increased. Avoid midazolam and triazolam; consider temazepam, lorazepam, or oxazepam.

Calcium channel blockers (e.g., felodipine): serum levels of calcium channel blockers may be increased. Monitor closely for ADR with co-administration.

Cyclosporin: cyclosporin AUC increased by 70%. With co-administration decrease cyclosporine dose by 1/2 with close therapeutic drug monitoring.

Methadone: increased R-methadone (active) AUC by 47%. May need to dose adjust methadone with co-administration.

HMG-CoA reductase inhibitors (statins such as simvastatin and lovastatin): statin levels may be increased. Consider pravastatin with co-administration.

Omeprazole: omeprazole AUC increased by 4-fold. With co-administration reduce omeprazole dose to one-half.

Phenytoin: voriconazole AUC decreased by 70%. Phenytoin AUC increased by 80%. With co-administration increase voriconazole dose to 400mg po q12h or 5mg/kg IV q12h and frequent monitoring of phenytoin serum level with appropriate dose adjustment.

Sulfonylureas: serum level of sulfonylureas may be increased. Monitor closely for ADR with co-administration.

Tacrolimus: tacrolimus AUC increased by 3-fold. Dose reduce tacrolimus dose by 1/3 with close therapeutic drug monitoring.

Vinca alkaloids (e.g., vincristine and vinblastine): serum level of vinca alkaloid may be increased. Monitor closely for ADR and consider dose adjustment.

Warfarin: may increase PT by 2-fold. Monitor PT or INR closely with co-administration with proper dose adjustment.

No clinically significant interaction with cimetidine, ranitidine, and macrolides (i.e., azithromycin and erythromycin), prednisolone, digoxin, and mycophenolic acid.

Pregnancy Risk: D. Avoid in pregnancy. No human data, but teratogenic in animal studies.

Breast Feeding: No data. Not recommended.

Comments: Voriconazole is active against P. boydii, Fusarium spp., Candia spp (incl. C. glabrata and C. krusei) and Aspergillosis. In the treatment of aspergillosis, voriconazole had better clinical response at 12 weeks compared to amphotericin. Generally well tolerated with reversible visual disturbances (blurriness, color changes, and enhanced vision) reported in 20.6% of patients. Many drug interactions.

FORMS

Brand name	Preparation	Mfr.	Route	Form	Strength	Cost (AWP)
VFEND	Voriconazole	Pfizer	IV	vial	200mg/20mL	$110.32
			PO	susp	40mg/mL	$42.90 per 5mL
			PO	tab	50mg; 200mg	$8.84; $35.37

SELECTED READINGS

Walsh TJ, Pappas P, Winston DJ et al. Voriconazole compared with liposomal amphotericin B for empirical antifungal therapy in patients with neutropenia and persistent fever. N Engl J Med 2002 Jan 24;346(4):225-34

Ally R, Schurmann D, Kreisel W et al. A randomized, double-blind, double-dummy, multicenter trial of voriconazole and fluconazole in the treatment of esophageal candidiasis in immunocompromised patients. Clin Infect Dis 2001 Nov 1;33(9):1447-54

Herbrecht R et al. Voriconazole vs. Amphotericin B for primary therapy of invasive aspergillosis. NEJM 2002; 347:408

Anon. FDA submission. FDA

Pfaller MA, Messer SA, Hollis RJ et al. In vitro activities of ravuconazole and voriconazole compared with those of four approved systemic antifungal agents against 6970 clinical isolates of Candida spp. AAC 2002; 46:1723

ZANAMIVIR

FDA INDICATIONS

- Uncomplicated acute illness due to influenza A and B infection in adults who have been symptomatic for no more than 2 days

USUAL ADULT DOSING: Treatment: Two 5mg inhalations twice a day x 5 days (must be administered within 2 days of symptoms). Prophylaxis one 5mg inhalation qd (not FDA approved for prevention, but effective).

Dosing Adjustments
GFR 50-80 mL/min: Limited data; Normal dose likely due to limited systemic absorption
GFR 10-50 mL/min: See above
GFR<10 mL/min: See above

ADVERSE DRUG REACTIONS: Occasional: Bronchospasm (caution in patients with COPD or asthma); cough; **Rare:** Headache; diarrhea; nausea; vomiting; dizziness; increase in liver enzyme and CPK; lymphopenia and neutropenia

DRUG INTERACTIONS
No significant interactions noted.

PREGNANCY RISK: B- no malformation, maternal toxicity, or embryotoxicity were observed in animal studies. No data available in humans.

BREAST FEEDING: No data in humans. Excreted in breast milk in animal data.

COMMENTS: Aerosolized anti-infuenza agent with activity against influenza A and B. Effective for treatment only if treatment is started within 48 hours of onset of symptoms. More expensive compared to rimantidine or amantidine. Requires manual dexterity for use. Caution in patients with COPD or asthma due to the risk of bronchospasm.

FORMS

Brand name	Preparation	Mfr.	Route	Form	Strength	Cost (AWP)
Relenza	Zanamivir	GlaxoSmithKline	inhala-tion	pow	5mg	$3.23 per 5mg

SELECTED READINGS

Kaiser L, et al. Impact of Zanamivir on Antibiotic Use for Respiratory Events Following Acute Influenza in Adolescents and Adults . Arch Intern Med 2000;160:3234

Lalezari J, et al. Zanamivir for the Treatment of Influenza A and B Infection in High-Risk Patients . Arch Intern Med 2001;161:212

ZIDOVUDINE (AZT)

FDA INDICATIONS

- HIV infection in combination with other antiretrovirals
- Prevention of maternal-fetal HIV transmission

USUAL ADULT DOSING: 300mg PO bid; 200mg PO tid or Combivir (300mg AZT with 150mg lamivudine) 1 tab PO bid. Trizivir (ABC 300mg/AZT 300mg/3TC 150mg) 1 tab PO bid.

Dosing Adjustments

GFR 50-80 mL/min: 300mg bid

GFR 10-50 mL/min: 300mg bid

GFR<10 mL/min: 300mg qd.

Hemodialysis: 300mg qd

Peritoneal Dialysis: 300mg qd

↓ *Hepatic Function:* 100mg tid

ADVERSE DRUG REACTIONS: Frequent: GI intolerance, malaise; headache (in 5-10%); bone marrow suppression (ANEMIA AND GRANULOCYTOPENIA (more common with late stage AIDS); MYOPATHY; transaminase elevation; fingernail discoloration. **Rare:** LACTIC ACIDOSIS +/- hepatic steatatosis.

DRUG INTERACTIONS

Ganciclovir: Additive bone marrow toxicity. May require decreased dose of AZT, switch to alternative antiretroviral or use concomitant G-CSF.

Ribavirin: additive anemia; monitor closely.

Stavudine: Antagonism. Co-administration contraindicated.

PREGNANCY RISK: 'C-Human studies demonstrated 85% placental passage. No maternal toxicities or fetal defects noted with AZT during pregnancy. Long-term toxicity data (up to 3.9 years) for infants exposed to AZT in utero and post partum did not show an increased risk of adverse effects or developmental abnormalities.

BREAST FEEDING: Mean concentration of zidovudine was similar in human milk and in serum. Breast feeding is not recommended in the U.S. in order to avoid post-natal transmission of HIV to the child, who may not yet be infected.

COMMENTS: Many patients have intolerance with GI sx, headaches and asthenia. Anemia or neutropenia are common late complications-- D/C or give EPO/G-CSF. AZT has documented efficacy in preventing perinatal tx and preventing HIV after occupational exposure, therefore should be used in those settings.

FORMS

Brand name	Preparation	Mfr.	Route	Form	Strength	Cost (AWP)
Retrovir	Zidovudine	GlaxoSmithKline	IV	vial	10mg/mL	$23.40 per 10mL vial
			PO	cap	100mg	$2.16
			PO	syrup	50mg/5mL	$1.08 per 5mL
			PO	tab	300mg	$6.49
Combivir	Zidovudine/ Lamivudine	GlaxoSmithKline	PO	tab	300mg/150mg	$12.04

(continued)

Brand name	Preparation	Mfr.	Route	Form	Strength	Cost (AWP)
Trizivir	Zidovudine/ Lamivudine/ Abacavir	GlaxoSmithKline	PO	tab	300mg/150mg/ 300mg	$19.51

VACCINES AND PROPHYLAXIS

Note: See Appendix I, Tables 10a and 10b, for comprehensive immunization recommendations.

ANTHRAX VACCINE ADSORBED (AVA)

Paul Pham, Pharm.D. and John G. Bartlett M.D.

DIAGNOSTIC CRITERIA

- Anthrax Vaccine (BIOTHRAX), killed vaccine made from the cell-free filtrate of nonencapsulated, attenuated strain of B. anthracis. A live attenuated vaccine was manufactured in the fomer USSR.
- Formulation: Produced by Bioport Corp, Lansing, Mich. Limited supply, currently available to US Department of Defense. Vials 0.5mL each (single dose).
- Efficacy: pre-exposure prophylaxis (FDA approved).
- Effective in a placebo-controlled human trial against cutaneous anthrax. Primate models showed that antibiotic prevented inhalation anthrax, but were not protected from rechallenge.
- However, all animals given vaccine PLUS antibiotic were protected with re-challenge (Friedlander et al. JID 1993;167:1239).

TREATMENT REGIMENS

Indications

- All US military: active- and reserve-duty personnel.
- Persons considered by public health authorities to have been at high risk for inhalation anthrax (aerosol exposure) as an adjunct to prolonged postexposure abx prophylaxis.

Administration

- Dose (pre-exposure prophylaxis): 0.5mL SQ x 6 doses (0, 2 and 4 wks followed by injections at 6, 12 & 18 mos).
- Onset of protection: antibody titer increased 3-4x approximately 7d after the second dose (3-4 wks from first dose), however clear minimum therapeutic antibody response has not been established.
- Response: relationship between immunity and quantitative antibody levels has not been evaluated.
- Revaccination: yearly booster dose (0.5mL) required to maintain immunity.
- Six dose regimen used, because this regimen won FDA approval during registration trials in the 1950's (Brachman).

Adverse reactions

- Very well tolerated. Occasional ADR: local injection site reactions reported in 3.6%.
- Most frequently reported local reaction: injection site nodule, more common in women for unexplained reasons (60% vs 30% in men).
- About 4% w/ extensive erythema and swelling; may extend to the antecubital fossa and often misdiagnosed as bacterial cellulitis. Most frequently reported systemic ADR: headache (0.4%).
- No long-term sequelae reported.
- Safety in Pregnancy: Category D.
- Earlier unpublished study of infants born to women in the U.S. military service worldwide in 1998 and 1999 suggest that the vaccine may be linked with an increase in the number of birth defects.
- However, recent published study found no effect on pregnancy or adverse birth outcomes in a cohort involving 4092 women [Wiesen AR et al. JAMA 2002;287: 1556].

Important Points

- Post-exposure prophylaxis (not FDA approved): AVA given as a sole agent was not effective in one primates study. AVA was effective if abx with activity against anthrax was given concurrently.
- Department of Defense has mandated all US military active- and reserve-duty personnel receive pre-exposure (vaccine) prophylaxis.
- Pre-exposure vaccination of some persons deemed to be in high-risk groups should also be considered.
- The Working Group on Civilian Biodefense continues to recommend vaccination of exposed persons following a biological attack in conjunction with abx administration for 60 days following exposure.
- Vaccine indicated only for risk of inhalation anthrax, but prevents cutaneous anthrax as well. Until ample reserve stockpiles of vaccine are available, reliance must be placed upon abx protection.

HEPATITIS A VACCINE

Paul Pham, Pharm.D. and John G. Bartlett, M.D.

Diagnostic Criteria

- Description: killed, formalin inactivated vaccine.
- Formulation/cost: Havrix (SKB) $59.45/dose; VAQTA (Merck) $62.94/dose; Twinrix (HBV+HAV vaccines) $92/dose.
- Response: 80% seroconvert in 15 days; >96% at 30 days. With booster (2nd) dose, 100% respond.
- See "Hepatitis A" in Pathogens section for details of HAV.

Treatment Regimens

Indications

- Gay men; injection drug users; persons with clotting disorders; persons with chronic liver disease (e.g., HCV); lab workers handling HAV; persons working with nonhuman primates.
- Travel: travelers to countries with endemic HAV. HAV vaccination not needed in northern and western Europe, New Zealand, Australia, Canada, and Japan.

Adverse reactions

- Common: local reactions in 20-50%. Occasional: fever in 4%. Rare: anaphylaxis, Guillain-Barre syndrome.
- Pregnancy: Category C

Administration

- 1440 ELISA units (1mL) (Havrix) OR 50 units/1mL (VAQTA) x 1, or x 2 (separated by >6 mos). Twinrix 1mL (720 units HAV vaccine/20 mcg HBV vaccine) at 0, 1, and 6 mos.
- Onset of protection: 15-30 d.
- Duration of protection: 10 yr minimum (no booster recommendations exist beyond initial dosing)

Important Points

- Immunosuppressed patients may be unable to develop antibodies or may require additional boosters.
- For adequate protection, Hepatitis A Vaccine must be administered at least 2 wks before expected exposure. For travelers expecting high-risk exposure w/in 2 wks, pooled immunoglobulin suggest instead.

HEPATITIS B VACCINE

Paul Pham, Pharm.D. and John G. Bartlett, M.D.

DIAGNOSTIC CRITERIA

- Recombivax HB [Merck]: recombinant vaccine produced by Saccharomyces cerevisiae (baker's yeast).
- Engerix-B [GSK]: recombinant vaccine, also produced by Saccharomyces cerevisiae.
- Twinrix [GSK]: bivalent vaccine with HAV (720 ELISA units/mL) and HBV(20mcg HBsAg/mL).
- Formulation/cost: recombivax HB - 10 and 40 mcg HBsAg/mL ($71.00/10 mcg). Engerix 20mcg HBsAg/mL ($55.10/20mcg). Twinrix HAV (720 ELISA units/mL) and HBV (20mcg HBsAg/mL) ($92.00/mL).
- See "Hepatitis B virus" in the Pathogens section for more details.

TREATMENT REGIMENS

Indications

- All infants and children by the age of 18 yrs.
- Persons w/ vocational risks (e.g., healthcare workers); persons w/ lifestyle risks (e.g., IVDU, hx of STDs, homosexual and bisexual men, and those w/ multiple sex partners).
- Hemodialysis patients.
- Hemophiliac persons.
- Environmental risk factors : close contact of HBV carriers or persons from areas where HBV is highly endemic.
- HBV and pregnancy: 1) all pregnant women should be tested for HBsAg.
- 2) If infant born to HBsAg-positive mother, should receive HBIG (0.5mL) IM x1 (w/in 12 hrs of delivery) and HB vaccine (0.5mL) IM x 3 (5 mcg Recombivax or 10 mcg Engerix-B) at 0, 1, 6 mos.
- 3) Routine HB vaccination for infants of HBsAg-negative mothers.
- Travelers: consider in those who plan to reside x 6 mos or longer in areas with HBV surface antigen [HbsAg] prevalence >2%, and who will have high risk contact with the local population.

Administration

- Recombivax HB 10mcg/mL at 0, 1, and 6 mos. Recombivax HB 40mcg/mL at 0, 1, and 6 mos for patients on HD (and possibly other immunocompromised patients).
- Engerix-B 20 mcg (1mL) at 0, 1, and 6 mos (or 0, 1, 2, and 12 mo for more rapid induction of immunity).
- Note: if schedule is interrupted, may resume with good result providing that the second and third dose are separated by > 2 mos.
- Onset of protection: one month after 3rd dose.
- Revaccination: controversial, since Ab levels do not measure immunologic memory; immunologic protection proven to last > 12 yrs regardless of antibody levels. If done, response in 30-50% w/ 3 doses.
- Response: > 95% for young and healthy adults. Response rate lower if > 40 yrs (86%), certain HLA haplotypes, smoking history, obesity, diabetics (70-80%), HIV (50-70%), HD, renal & liver dz (60-70%).
- Post-vaccination serologic testing recommended for pts w/ lower response rates (e.g., HIV pts) and whose subsequent management depends on this knowledge (i.e health care workers and HD pts).
- Response defined as HBsAb level > 10 mIU/mL, checked > 1 mo after the 3rd dose.

- Efficacy: 80-95% for preventing HBV infection in gay men and virtually 100% if protective antibody response (>10 mIU/mL) is achieved.

Adverse reactions

- Common: injection site reactions, up to 20%. Occasional: fever (1-6%). Rare: anaphylaxis. NO role in the etiology or relapse of MS.
- Safety in pregnancy: Category C. Unless patient is at high risk for becoming infected during pregnancy, most experts recommend that HBV be deferred until after delivery.

IMPORTANT POINTS

- HBV deposited into fat rather than muscle results in lower seroconversion rates, so needle length is important.
- 60-90kg women and men: 2.5 cm needle length. >90kg women: 3.8cm needle length. <60kg women: 1.6 cm needle length.

INFLUENZA IMMUNIZATION AND PROPHYLAXIS
John G. Bartlett, M.D.

DIAGNOSTIC CRITERIA

- Vaccine efficacy: young adults or healthy elderly, appx. 70%.
- Vaccine efficacy: elderly in nursing homes, 30-40%; reduces influenza mortality by 80%.
- Vaccine efficacy depends on match of epidemic & vaccine strains - good in 14 of 16 past yrs.
- Trivalent vaccine for 2004-5: A H/3 N/2 (Fijian strain), A-H1N1, + B strain.
- Cost AWP: $4/dose for inactivated vaccine, $27/dose live attenuated (FluMist).

COMMON PATHOGENS: Influenza

TREATMENT REGIMENS

Vaccine indications

- High risk: >50 yrs, residents of chronic care homes, chronic pulmonary/cardiac disease, chronic illness (diabetes, renal failure, immunosuppression, sickle cell).
- 2004-05 season: due to shortage, given initially to high risk pts only; this recommendation later relaxed.
- Pregnancy: if during influenza season, give during 2nd/3rd trimesters.
- Transmission risk to high risk pts: medical personnel who serve high risk pts, household member of high risk pts.
- "Consider" category: HIV, anyone who wants it, or who provide essential services.
- Travelers: high risk pts to tropics (all yr), or to southern hemisphere in April-September.
- Contraindications to IM vaccine: allergy to eggs or prior severe allergic reaction, or fever > 40C; no contraindication if only prior local reaction.

Vaccine administration

- What: 0.5mL IM in deltoid, or FluMist by nasal administration.
- When: mid Oct - Nov best.
- Protection: starts in 2 wks, lasts 4-6 mos; usually 70-90% effective, if good match vaccine/ circulating strains.
- FluMist: limit to immunocompetent pts, ages 5-49 yrs. Not known to be protective in those >50 yrs.
- Pneumovax: may be given at same time, use different injection site.
- Info - products: Connaught http://www.sanofipasteur.us/; Wyeth 800-934-5556; Parke Davis 800-543-2111.

- Info - epidemiology: http://www.cdc.gov/flu/weekly
- Alternative prevention: amantadine 100-200 PO mg/d; rimantadine 100-200 PO mg/d; oseltamivir 75mg PO qd.

Vaccine adverse reactions

- Soreness at injection site, usually > 2 days in ~30%.
- Fever and malaise: infrequent.
- Allergy: hives, angioedema, asthma--all rare.
- Guillain-Barre: not associated with flu vaccine since 1993-94 season.
- FluMist: live attenuated virus; don't use if immunocompromised, or <5 or >49 yrs. HCW: do not work with severely immunocompromised pts x 7d. No reports of transmission person-person.

IMPORTANT POINTS

- CDC guidelines (MMWR2003;52:RR-8). Indications for vaccine now include about half of US citizens.
- Influenza - major infectious cause of death in US; nearly all are elderly, in nursing homes, or have chronic diseases.
- Vaccine efficacy depends on match between epidemiology, vaccine strains & host responses (decreased in elderly, advanced AIDS).
- Vaccine to healthy adults appears to generally reduce URIs & employee absenteeism; conflicting data on cost effectiveness.
- Health care workers - vaccination indicated to protect pts and infected health care workers; must avoid pt contact w/ FluMist x 7d post-administration.

SELECTED READINGS

Center for Disease Control. Prevention and Control of Influenza. MMWR 2003;52RR-8:1-36

Armstrong BG, et al. Effect of influenza vaccination on excess deaths occurring during periods of high circulation of influenza: cohort study in elderly people. BMJ. 2004;329(7467):660

Cooper NJ, et al. Effectiveness of neuraminidase inhibitors in treatment and prevention of influenza A & B: systematic review and meta-analysis of randomized controlled trials. BMJ 2003;326:1235

CDC. Avain Influenza. www.cdc.gov/flu/about/avianflu.htm accessed 9/10/04

CDC. Vaccine Recommendations. MMWR 2002;51RR-2:8

Nichol KL, et al. Influenza vaccination and reduction in hospitalization for cardiac disease and stroke among the elderly. NEJM 2003;348:1322

Zambon M. The inexact science of influenza prediction. Lancet 2004;363:582

Webby RJ, et al. Responsiveness to a pandemic alert. Lancet 2004;363:1099

Ault A. Shifting tactics in the battle against influenza. Science 2004;303:1280

CDC. Influenza Activity-US and Worldwide, 2003-2004 season and composition of the 2004-05 vaccine . MMWR 2004;53:547

MENINGOCOCCAL VACCINE

Paul Pham, Pharm.D. and John G. Bartlett, M.D.

DIAGNOSTIC CRITERIA

- Bacterial polysaccharides of serotype A/C/Y/W-135.
- Response: seroconversion rates for these polysaccharides are >90%. Seroconversion of group A and C is lower in children < 2-4 yrs of age.
- Efficacy: varies based on serogroup and patient population; 87% reduction of meningococcal meningitis from serogoup C in adult military recruits. Lower efficacy in children (<30% in children <4 yrs).

- Cost: $81/dose (manufacturer: Aventis).

TREATMENT REGIMENS

Indications

- Outbreaks of N. meningitidis serotype C disease; offer to college freshman living in dormitories.
- Travel: indicated if travel to epidemic area, most frequently sub-Saharan Africa during epidemics (Dec-June). Saudi Arabia requires certificate of vaccination for pilgrims to Mecca or Medina.

Administration

- Meningococcal vaccine: 0.5mL SC x 1.
- Onset of protection: Protective antibody levels at 7-10d. Antibody level declines over 2-3 year period.
- Revaccination: 2-3 yrs after initial immunization may be indicated for individuals at high-risk for infection, especially children who were first vaccinated at less than 4 years.

Adverse reactions

- Generally well tolerated. Occasional: Erythema at the site of injection (4%); irritability in young children (6%). Rare: Paresthesias; seizure; fever; allergic reaction +/- anaphylaxis.
- Contraindications: hypersensitivity to thimerosal.
- Pregnancy: Category C. No teratogenicity or growth abnormalities were observed among the 34 infants born to mothers immunized while pregnant [Letson GW et al. Pediatr Infect Dis J 1998; 17:261].

IMPORTANT POINTS

- Due to the poor immunogenicity in children < 2 yrs old & lack vaccine to serogroup B, chemoprophylaxis is recommended in lieu of vaccine for prevention of secondary cases in daycare centers.
- Meningococcal vaccine should not be administered concomitantly with whole-cell pertussis or whole-cell typhoid vaccines, but may be administered with other vaccines.
- Meningococcal B vaccine available, but not licensed in U.S.
- Menactra is a new Meningococcal (Group A, C, Y and W-135) polysaccharide diphtheria toxoid conjugate vaccine. Menactra produces a greater than four-fold rise in antibody titers for serogroups A, C, Y and W-135 in 82%-97% of adolescents (11-18 years old).

PNEUMOCOCCAL PROPHYLAXIS (PNEUMOVAX)

John G. Bartlett, M.D.

DIAGNOSTIC CRITERIA

- 23 valent vaccine w/ serotype antigens covering 87% bacteremic cases & most PCN-resistant serotypes.
- Response: most adults have 2x rise in type specific Ab at 2-3 wks; less if immunosuppressed.
- Cost: $16/dose (AWP).
- Efficacy: best data show prevention of pneumococcal bacteremia, but not pneumonia.

TREATMENT REGIMENS

Administration

- Vaccine: 0.5mL IM or SC

- When: best 2 wks before splenectomy or as long as possible before planned immunosuppression.
- Revaccination (at 5yrs): if > 5 yrs & immunosuppression, asplenia, turned >65 yrs, CD4 increased to >200 (for HIV pts).
- Protection: starts w/in 2 wks; lasts > 9 yrs; degree of protection - controversial.
- Influenza vaccine may be given together with Pneumovax; give at separate injection sites.

Adverse reactions
- Pain/erythema - injection site, rates ~50%.
- Fever, myalgia, severe local reaction in < 4%.
- Anaphylactoid reaction: 5 per/million
- Revaccination: local reaction increased 3.3x; severe reactions not increased.

Indications
- Age: >65 yrs
- Chronic diesase: pulmonary/cardiac disease, alcoholism, cirrhosis, diabetes, renal failure, nephrosis.
- Compromised host: HIV, asplenia/splenectomy, lymphoma, organ transplant, iatrogenic immune suppression.
- Hospitalized pts w/indications: ideal time to vaccinate.
- Specific populations: Native Americans, homeless, CSF leak.
- HIV: best response w/ CD4 > 200.
- Revaccination: HIV if CD4 < 200 -> CD4 > 200 or > 5yrs; dialysis q 5 yrs.
- Travel: no indication.
- Pregnancy: not contraindicated.
- Contraindications: Pneumovax for those < 13 mos of age (reactions increased).

IMPORTANT POINTS
- Guidelines from ACIP/CDC MMWR 1997; 46:RR-8
- Benefit: good evidence Pneumovax reduces pneumococcal bacteremia.
- No good evidence that Pneumovax reduces pneumonia or pneumococcal infections.
- Highest priority: asplenia, CSF leak, renal failure; possibly those at high risk of bacteremia - e.g., smokers (author opinion).
- Protein conjugated vaccine (Prevnar) works well in pediatric populations, no evidence of benefit in adults.

SELECTED READINGS

Centers for Disease Control and Prevention. Prevention of pneumococcal disease: Recommendations of ACIP. MMWR 1997;46:1

Butler JC, Breiman RF, Campbell JF, et al. Pneumococcal polysaccharide vaccine efficacy. JAMA 1993;270:1826

Jackson LA, Benson P, Sneller V-P, et al. Safety of revaccination with pneumococcal polysaccharide vaccine . JAMA 1999; 281:243

Metersky ML, et al. Lack of effect of a pneumonia clinical pathway on hospital - based pneumococcal vaccination rates. Am J Med 2001;110:141

Moore RA, Wiffen PJ, Lipsky BA. Are pneumococcal polysaccharide vaccines effective? Meta-analysis of the prospective studies. BMC Family Practice 2000;1:1

Ejstrud P, Kristensen B, Hansen JB, et al. Risk and patterns of bacteremia after splenectomy: a population - based study . Scandinavian Journal of Infectious Diseases 2000;32:521

French N, et al. 23 valent pneumococcal polysaccharide vaccine in HIV-1 infected Ugandan adults. Lancet 2000;355:2106

Jefferson T, Demicheli V. Polysaccharide pneumococcal vaccine. Brit Med J 2002;325:292

Jackson LA, et al. Effectiveness of pneumococcal polysaccharide vaccine in older adults. N Engl J Med 2003;348:1747

Sisk JE, et al. Cost-effectiveness of vaccination against invasive pneumococcal disease among people 50 through 64 years of age: Role of comorbid conditions and race. Ann Intern Med 2003;138:960

RABIES
John G. Bartlett, M.D.

Diagnostic Criteria
- Major risk: bats in US and Europe, dog bites in developing countries. Risk with bite from rabid dog and no prophylaxis: 36-57%.
- 32/35 rabies cases in US 1958-2000 were bat associated; 26/32 had no hx of bat bite.
- Dog/cat bites (US): quarantine x 10 days then if pet gets sx rabies, start prophylaxis & necropsy animal; escaped pet - consult health department but low risk in US.
- Skunks, raccoons, fox bite: consider rabid unless negative necropsy; consider immediate prophylaxis, but rare cause of human rabies.
- Livestock, rodents (gerbils, mice, rats, guinea pigs), rabbits, beavers, etc - almost never cause rabies, but consult public health official.

Common Pathogens: Rabies

Treatment Regimens

Administration
- 3 vaccine suppliers: human diploid cell (HDCV), (Imorax 800-822-2463), rabies vaccine absorbed (RVA 517-327-1500), purified chick embryo (PCEVC, RabAbert 800-244-7668).
- Combine with rabies immune globulin for severe exposures (RIG): 800-822-2463 or 800-288-8370.
- Cost: vaccine $700, RIG $700.
- Wound: immediately clean with soap; irrigate with viricidal agent, e.g., povidone, iodine, etc.
- RIG: 20 IU/kg at wound site & also IM (distant from vaccine administration site).
- Vaccine: 1mL IM deltoid day 0, 3, 7, 14 & 28d; PCEC, given intradermally.
- Pregnancy or HIV: no differences, routine recommendations.
- HIV: vaccine response is poor with low CD4; double dose or use intradermal route.
- Response to vaccine: neutralizing Ab in 7-10d, persists >2yrs.

Pre-exposure prophylaxis
- Consider with high-risk exposure (vet, labworker) or travel to area with endemic region and poor/slow access to rabies prophylaxis Rx.
- Use three 1-mL IM HDVC d0, 7 , 21 or 28; or PCEC intradermal d0, 7, and 21 or 28.
- Do not administer RIG.
- Monitor antibody levels (q 2yrs), if become undetectable then boost.

Important Points
- Guidelines are from ACIP/CDC (MMWR 1999; 48 RR-1).
- Most important: immediate cleansing of wound with viricidal reduces risk by 50%.
- Main concern in U.S.: bats, many exposures unwittingly while asleep.
- Main concern with travelers: dog bite in endemic area (developing countries).
- Rabies prophylaxis guidelines: conservative, expensive ($1,500), demanding (5 injections), and w/ side effects. Consider for occupational reasons (vets, animal handlers).

SELECTED READINGS

CDC. Human Rabies Prevention - US, 1999 Recommendations of the Advisory Committee on Immunization Practices (ACIP). MMWR 1999; 48 no. RR-1

Warrell MJ and Warrell DA. Rabies and other lyssavirus diseases. Lancet 2004;363:959

CDC. Investigation of rabies infections in organ donor and transplant recipients-Alabama, Arkansas, Oklahoma & Texas 2004. MMWR 2004;53:686-9

CDC. Human rabies. MMWR 1999; 49:1111

CDC. Human rabies. MMWR 2002;51:828

CDC. Human rabies. MMWR 2002;51:686

Messenger SL, et al. Emerging epidemiology of bat-associated cryptic cases of rabies in humans in the US. Clin Infect Dis 2002;35:738

Strady A, et al. Antibody persistence following postexposure regimens of cell-culture rabies vaccine. J Infect Dis 1998;177:1290-95

Kaplan MM, Cohen D. Studies on the local treatment of wounds for the prevention of rabies. Bull WHO 1962;765-75

Warrell, MJ. Rabies encephalitis and its prophylaxis. Pract Neurol:2001;1:14-29

SMALLPOX VACCINE (VACCINIA)

Khalil G. Ghanem, M.D.

DIAGNOSTIC CRITERIA

- Resistant to drying agents & many disinfectants; sensitive to chlorine, autoclaving, heat (60C x 10mins), formaldehyde, iodophores and ammonium compounds. Infective: months at rm temp, yrs at -20C.
- DNA virus; "cowpox"; Poxviridae family; broad host range; rarely isolated outside lab; multiple strains w/ different virulence; often used for recombinant viruses or engineered w/foreign DNA.
- Vaccinia and variola (smallpox) share common antigens. Neutralizing Abs are cross-protective (also to monkeypox). Adequate Abs persist for < 5 yrs post vaccine; waning immunity > 10 yrs noted.
- Transmission: exposure to vaccine or contaminated dressing (mostly in household w/ children); no reports of transmission to health care workers published; lab personnel at higher risk.
- Virus used in "smallpox (SP) vaccine". Enabled global eradication of smallpox virus.
- Vaccine currently recommended for lab workers w/exposure to nonhighly attenuated orthopoxviruses. Revaccination q 10yrs. Ab levels after revaccination remain higher for longer periods.
- Vaccinia vaccine: lyophilized, live-virus; administered by multiple puncture technique w/ bifurcated needle. Reformulated vaccine now being developed (using cell culture).
- Vaccination voluntary without attack - NOT recommended if contraindications; WITH ATTACK, VACCINATE ALL EXPOSED EVEN THOSE WITH CONTRAINDICATIONS.
- Efficacy: probability of SP w/contact + no vaccination = 70%; if infected, SP mortality = 30%. Vaccine efficacy = 98% if vaccinated within 5-10 yrs; no prior vaccination: 98% efficacy.

TREATMENT REGIMENS

Treatment of vaccine complications

- Vaccinia Immune Globulin (VIG): Rx eczema vaccinatum, progressive vaccinia (pt ill or underlying dz); ocular autoinoculation (not vaccinial keratitis; may exacerbate), generalized vaccinia (consider).
- VIG not to be used for encephalitis or smallpox.
- Dose: 0.6mL/kg IM ASAP after symptom onset; given in divided doses over 24-36h. Repeat doses q2-3 days until no new lesions.
- The CDC has very limited supplies of VIG. Report vaccine complications to 800-822-7967.
- Other antiviral agents with in vitro activity against poxviruses (e.g. cidofovir) are not currently recommended for use.

Prevention of contact transmission

- Hand hygiene (soap/water); cover vaccine site w/porous bandage until scab has separated; change dressing q1-2 days; place contaminated bandages in sealed bags.
- Use occlusive dressing (e.g., polyurethane dressing such as Opsite) for vaccinees who come in contact with susceptible pts. Apply dry gauze below dressing to avoid accumulated secretions.
- Thorough hand hygeine mandatory after any manipulation of vaccine site or bandages.

IMPORTANT POINTS

- Contact transmission to nonvaccinees: 27 cases/million vaccine; 44% in kids<5y; usually eczema vaccinatum but also encephalitis and vaccinia necrosum reported.
- Contraindications: h/o eczema or skin dz (even if inactive); pregnant/breast feed, HIV; immunodeficient (malignancy, txp, chemo, prednisone >20mg/d >2wks); <12mos age; moderate or severe short term dz
- In emergency (if available) VIG (0.3mg/kg IM) can be given WITH vaccine in pts w/ contraindications.[currently not enough supply available at CDC].
- www.cdc.gov\smallpox can be accessed for up to date recommendations, info on vaccine delivery, AND pictures of all complications. Call CDC at (404) 639-3670 for questions.
- Vaccine is protective 3-4 d after known EXPOSURE to smallpox (NOT first sign of illness). Benefit may be seen up to 7 days after exposure.

SELECTED READINGS

Talbot TR, Bredenberg HK, Smith M, et al. Focal and generalized folliculitis following smallpox vaccination among vaccinia-naive recipients . JAMA. 2003 Jun 25;289(24):3290-4

Halsell JS, Riddle JR, Atwood JE, et al. Myopericarditis following smallpox vaccination among vaccinia-naive US military personnel. JAMA. 2003 Jun 25;289(24):3283-9

Talbot TR, Stapleton JT, Brady RC, et al. Vaccination success rate and reaction profile with diluted and undiluted smallpox vaccine: a randomized controlled trial . JAMA. 2004 Sep 8;292(10):1205-12

Eckart RE, Love SS, Atwood JE, et al. Incidence and follow-up of inflammatory cardiac complications after smallpox vaccination . J Am Coll Cardiol. 2004 Jul 7;44(1):201-5

Hepburn MJ, Dooley DP, Murray CK, et al. Frequency of vaccinia virus isolation on semipermeable versus nonocclusive dressings covering smallpox vaccination sites in hospital personnel . Am J Infect Control. 2004 May;32(3):126-30

Garde V, Harper D, Fairchok MP. Tertiary contact vaccinia in a breastfeeding infant . JAMA. 2004 Feb 11;291(6):725-7

Talbot TR, Ziel E, Doersam JK, et al. Risk of vaccinia transfer to the hands of vaccinated persons after smallpox immunization . Clin Infect Dis. 2004 Feb 15;38(4):536-41

Suarez VR, Hankins GD. Smallpox and pregnancy. Obstet Gynec 2002;100:87

el-Ad B, Roth Y, Winder A, et al. The persistence of neutralizing antibodies after revaccination against smallpox. J Infect Dis 1990 Mar;161(3):446-8

Neff JM, Lane JM, Fulginiti VA,, et al. Contact vaccinia--transmission of vaccinia from smallpox vaccination. JAMA 2002 Oct 16;288(15):1901-5

TETANUS-DIPHTHERIA

John G. Bartlett, M.D.

DIAGNOSTIC CRITERIA

- Product: Td absorbed (tetanus + diphtheria toxoids).
- Cost: $5 US
- Tetanus: 1999, total US - 40 cases; diphtheria: 1999 total US - 0 cases.
- Efficacy: Ag response usually good, but reduced in elderly.
- Need: about 25% of US adults > 70 yrs to have protective tetanus ab titers.

TREATMENT REGIMENS

Administration

- What: Td preferred for adults (less local reactions).
- Primary series (3): 0.5mL IM then at 1-2mos & again at 6-12mos; do not repeat if schedule delay.
- Boosters: 0.5mL IM q 10 yrs
- Wounds, minor: < 3 prior Td doses or unknown - give Td; > 3 doses - Td if >10 yrs since last booster.
- Wounds, severe or contaminated: < 3 prior Td doses, give Td + TIG; if > 3 doses - give Td if > 5yrs since last Td booster.
- TIG: tetanus immune globulin, if < 3 doses Td or unknown + contaminated wound (dirt, stool, saliva, soil), crush, burn or frostbite.
- Contraindication: anaphylactic or neurologic, neurologic reaction to prior Td if after 1938.
- DT: Pediatric preparation, contraindicated in persons >7 yrs.
- Product information: Aventis-Pasteur, 800-822-2463.
- TIG: tetanus Immune globulin 500 units IM (prophylaxis), or 3,000-10,000 units (active tetanus).

Indications

- Guidelines ACIP/CDC (MMWR 1991;40:RR-10).
- Travelers: give if diphtheria risk high
- Tetanus prophylaxis in wound care: < 3 prior doses, unknown, >10 yrs post Td or severe injury + >5 yrs post Td.
- Pregnant women without Td for 10 yrs.
- Booster doses q 10yrs.

Adverse reactions

- Anaphylaxis, arthragia, fever: rare.
- Pain & tenderness at injection site; rate incrases with more doses.

IMPORTANT POINTS

- Td supply shortage 2001-2003. Supplies now adequate for routine q 10 year boosters.
- Most cases in US occur in elderly population; presumed underimmunized, waning or no immunity.

SELECTED READINGS

Center for Disease Control. Deferral of routine booster doses of tetanus and diphtheria toxoids for adolescents and adults. MMWR 2001;50:418

Gergen P, et al. A population-based serologic survey of immunity to tetanus in the US. NEJM 1995;332:761

TYPHOID VACCINE

Paul Pham, Pharm.D. and John G. Bartlett M.D.

DIAGNOSTIC CRITERIA

- Two forms: live oral attenuated bacterial vaccine (Ty 21a, Vivotif), and polysaccharide IM vaccine (Typhim Vi).
- An older, heat-phenol inactivated vaccine is no longer commercially available.
- Efficacy 67% in US military recruits while in endemic areas if immunized w/ the enteric coated oral typhoid vaccine. Protective efficacy of 77.4% seen with polysaccharide IM vaccine.
- Cost: Vivotif (manufacturer: Berna) $38.50/vaccination. Typhim Vi (manufacturer: Aventis Pasteur) $49.11/vaccination.

TREATMENT REGIMENS

Indications

- Travelers to endemic areas; laboratory microbiologists with expected frequent contact with Salmonella typhi.
- Travel: rural areas of countries where typhoid fever is endemic (especially Peru, India, Pakistan, and Chile) or in areas with outbreaks.

Administration

- Vivotif 1 cap qod (empty stomach) x 4 doses for children > 6 and adults (starting at least 2 weeks before travel). Do not take antimalarials or antibiotics for two weeks as may decrease efficacy.
- Typhim Vi 0.5mL (25mcg) IM x 1 (children > 2 and adults).
- Onset of protection: within 1 week from the last dose.
- Revaccination: recommended every 2 years for the Typhim Vi vaccine and every 5 years for the Vivotif oral vaccine in individuals with continued exposure risks to Salmonella typhi.

Adverse reactions

- Heat-phenol inactivated vaccine (no longer commercially available) has a high incidence of systemic side effects (fever, headache, and local pain at injection site).
- Fever and headache reported in less than 6% with live oral vaccine or polysaccharide IM vaccine (new formulation).
- Rare: nausea, vomiting, and abdominal discomfort (oral) and local reaction at injection site in less than 7% (IM polysaccharide).
- Patients with hypersensitivity to parenteral vaccine may tolerate oral vaccine.
- Pregnancy: Category C for both oral & IM polysaccharide vaccine. No data. ACOG (Bulletin No. 160) recommends vaccination during pregnancy only for close continued exposure or travel to endemic areas.
- Contraindications: oral typhoid vaccine - acute febrile, respiratory, or gastrointestinal illness; immunodeficiency; concurrent antibiotic use (esp. sulfa abx) may impair adequate immune response.
- Use with caution: IM vaccine - immunosuppressed individuals (may decreased immune response) and individuals with thrombocytopenia or coagulation disorders.

IMPORTANT POINTS

- Oral typhoid vaccine is preferred over the parenteral killed bacterial vaccine because of comparable efficacy, longer protection (5 yrs vs 2 years) [Lancet 1990; 336:891].
- Many travel clinics suggest IM vaccine for simplicity, as many travelers do not complete appropriately four pill oral vaccine dosing.
- Oral vaccine heat intolerant, keep in cool location. Excessive heat (e.g., car trunk in the summer) may reduce potency of vaccine.

VARICELLA (VARIVAX)

Paul Pham, Pharm.D. and John G. Bartlett M.D.

DIAGNOSTIC CRITERIA

- Live attenuated virus vaccine.
- Response: seroconversion rate in adults is 78% with one dose; 99% with two doses. Protection at 7-10 yr is 70-90% against infection and 95% against severe disease.
- Efficacy: rate of zoster in vaccine recipients was 2.6/100,000 person-yr in vaccine recipients compared with 68/100,000 person-yr in a general population of persons age <20 yr.
- In a recent report involving an outbreak in a day-care center, the effectiveness of the vaccine was only 44 percent [Galil K, et al. NEJM 2002;347:1909].
- Formulation/cost: Varivax $65.40/dose (Merck).

TREATMENT REGIMENS

Indications

- Susceptible health care workers
- Susceptible household contacts of immunosuppressed persons
- Susceptible persons living or working in areas where transmission of VZV is likely (e.g., teachers of young children, day care employees, staff members in institutional settings).
- Susceptible young adults in closed or semiclosed populations (military personnel, college students, inmates, and staff of prisons and jails).
- Susceptible nonpregnant women of childbearing potential; international travelers; adolescents or adults living in households with children.
- Travel: not a requirement for entry into any country (including the US), people traveling or living abroad should be advised to ensure that they are immune.
- Contraindications: pregnancy or this possibility within 1 mo; immunosuppressed pts; active TB; persons who have received blood products within 6 mo; anaphylaxis to gelatin or neomycin.

Adverse reactions

- Common: local reaction at injection site (30% in 0-2 d).
- Occ: fever >100 F (10%); varicella-like rash at injection site (3%); generalized varicella rash: 10% in 7-21 d (usually consists of <10 lesions and lasting >3 d and may be source of VZV transmission).
- Rare: transmission of the vaccine strain reported in three cases out of 15 million vaccinees (MMWR 48(RR-6), 1999).

Administration

- Adult-0.5mL SC x 2, separated by 4-8 wks.
- After one dose of varicella vaccine, 97% of infants and children 1-12 yrs of age develop detectable antibody titers. Vaccine-induced immunity is believed to be long-lasting.

- Vaccine efficacy estimated 90% against VZV infection, and 95% against severe disease.
- Among healthy adolescents and adults, ~78% develop antibody after one dose and 99% develop antibody after a second dose given 4-8 wks later.

Important Points

- Vaccine must be stored frozen < -15C to maintain potency. Once reconstituted it must be used within 30 min.
- 90% current adults likely infected as children (pre-vaccine era), and therefore will not require varicella vaccine.
- 10% > 15 yrs susceptible to infection. Adult clinical hx of chickenpox often unreliable; varicella serology may wane by adult yrs. If pt thought susceptible, check serology [if negative, immunize].

YELLOW FEVER VACCINE

Paul Pham, Pharm.D. and John G. Bartlett M.D.

Diagnostic Criteria

- Live, attenuated virus preparation made from 17D yellow fever virus strain.
- Response: immunity in more than 95% of recipients. Less immunogenic in pregnant women (39%), asymptomatic HIV-infected adults (77%), and HIV-infected infants (17%).
- Cost: FY-VAX $62/dose (Aventis-Pasteur). Available only in designated U.S. yellow fever vaccination centers.

Treatment Regimens

Indications

- Recommended with travel to endemic areas: tropical South America and most of Africa between 15°North and 15° South latitudes.

Administration

- Yellow fever vaccine 0.5 milliliter SC x 1 (for adults and children > 9 months).
- Consider in children between 4-9 mos with exposure risk.
- Onset of protection: 10 days.
- Revaccination: booster q 10 yrs if still at risk.

Adverse reactions

- Occasional: headache and myalgia. Rare: allergy with anaphylaxis in 1:116,000 (desensitization protocol available); encephalitis; hepatitis.
- ACIP recently reported 7 cases of multiple organ failure in recipients of 17D derived yellow fever vaccine; all became ill within 2-5 days of vaccination and six died (MMWR 2001; 50-643).
- Pregnancy: Category C. Contraindicated unless exposure to YF can not be avoided. The yellow fever vaccine was not apparently harmful effects to the fetuses of 101 women who received YF vaccine.

Important Points

- Contraindications: known hypersensitivity to egg, chicken protein, or gelatin; infants less than 4 months of age (increased risk of encephalitis); immunocompromised host; pregnant women and HIV+ pts.
- If exposure cannot be avoided, vaccination should be offered to pregnant women and HIV-infected patients-in small studies no adverse events have been reported.

DIAGNOSES

ABSCESS, BRAIN

Paul Auwaerter, M.D.

DIAGNOSTIC CRITERIA

- Clinical symptoms of mass lesion: headache, nausea and vomiting, seizures, mental status changes; fever (50% only). Focal neurologic signs; fever in only half.
- CT or MRI: hypodense lesion(s) with diffuse (cerebritis) or peripheral/ring (abscess) enhancement +/- surrounding edema. Often occur at grey/white matter junction. Confusion w/neoplasia not uncommon.
- Lumbar puncture contraindicated, yields little specific data.
- Dx: gold standard is aspiration/surgery with examination of contents and gram-stain/culture. Putative dx with compatible clinical picture/imaging +/- positive blood cx or known source.
- Ddx includes tumor, rarely hemorrhage. Though bacterial etiology most common, if AIDS or immune-suppressed or immigrant need to also consider TB, fungi, parasitic causes

COMMON PATHOGENS: Streptococcus most common (30-50%), anaerobic or aerobic; In 80-90% of abscesses, multiple organisms are found; Gram negatives are more common in infants; FUNGAL CAUSES include Candida spp., Aspergillus, Zygomycetes; Most series of pyogenic abscess appx. 25% unknown source (cryptogenic); Microbiology of brain abscess by source; PARANASAL SINUSITIS: microaerophilic (S. intermedius group) and anaerobic strep, Haemophilus species, Bacteroides sp, Fusobacterium sp, Prevotella sp; OTOGENIC infection: aerobic and anaerobic streptococci, Enterobacteriaceae, Pseudomonas aeruginosa, Prevotella sp, B. fragilis; ODONTOGENIC infection: S. viridans and anaerobic streptococci, Bacteroides sp, Fusobacterium sp, Prevotella sp, Actinomyces sp; ENDOCARDITIS: Staphylococcus aureus, S. viridans streptococci, Enterococcus; LUNG ABSCESS: microaerophilic and anaerobic streptococci, Actinomyces species, Fusobacterium species, Nocardia species, Prevotella; Penetrating TRAUMA: Staphylococcus aureus, aerobic streptococci, Clostridium species, Enterobacteriaceae; POSTOPERATIVE: Staphylococcus epidermidis, S. aureus, Enterobacteriaceae, Pseudomonas aeruginosa; Right to left SHUNT (congenital heart disease): microaerophilic and aerobic strep; Compromised host (AIDS, cancer CHEMOTHERAPY, chronic steroids, lymphoma): toxoplasmosis, Nocardia, EBV lymphoma, TB, fungal; IMMIGRANT: cysticercosis, echinococcus, TB (tuberculoma)

TREATMENT REGIMENS

Empiric antimicrobial therapy

- May be based on predisposing condition. Efforts should be made to aspirate or drain to help guide therapy. Exceptions: multiple abscesses, difficult locations, (+) blood culture, poor surgical risk.
- Unknown: cefotaxime 2g IV q6h or ceftriaxone 2g IV q12h + metronidazole 500mg IV q6h
- Odontogenic infection: penicillin G 4mU IV q4h + Metronidazole 500mg IV q6h
- Sinusitis: cefotaxime 2g IV q4-6h or ceftriaxone 2g IV q12h + metronidazole 500mg IV q6h
- Otitis/mastoiditis: cefotaxime 2g IV q4-6h or ceftriaxone 2g IV q12h or cefepime 2g IV q12h + Metronidazole 500mg IV q6h
- Endocarditis: nafcillin or oxacillin 2g IV q4h + gentamicin 1-1.5 mg/kg IV q8h
- Lung abscess/empyema: penicillin G 4mU IV q4h + metronidazole 500mg IV q6h
- Trauma/post-neurosurgical: vancomycin 1g IV q8-12h + ceftazidime 2g IV q8h or cefepime 2g IV q12h
- Nocardia suspected: add trimethoprim/sulfamethoxazole 5-6mg/kg IV q6-8h

- Duration of therapy unclear. Common course is 4-8 wks, longer times esp. if not drained. Treat until sufficient response by neuroimaging (note time to mean resolution 4 mos, but may take up to a year)

Pathogen-directed therapy (may combine)
- Strep: penicillin G 4mU or ampicillin 2g IV q4h
- S. aureus: nafcillin or oxacillin 2 g IV q4h
- MRSA: vancomycin 1g IV q8-12h
- Strep, GNB, H. influ: cefotaxime 2g IV q4-6h or ceftriaxone 2g IV q12h or ceftazidime 2g IV q8h or cefepime 2g IV q12h
- Anaerobes: metronidazole 500mg IV every 6 hours and clindamycin 600-1200mg IV q6-8h
- GNB, anaerobes: meropenem 2g IV q8h
- H. flu, GNB, strep: ciprofloxacin 400mg IV q12h or levofloxacin 500mg IV q24h
- GNB: aztreonam 2g IV q6-8h
- Nocardia: trimethoprim/sulfamethoxazole 10-20 mg/kg IV divided every 6-8 hours (highest dosage for nocardiosis). See Nocardia pathogen module for other alternatives.
- Cysticercosis: albendazole 400mg PO bid 8-30d or praziquantil 15mg/kg tid PO x 15d

Adjunctive and surgical therapy
- Dexamethasone (10mg IV load, then 4mg q6h) may be needed if there is significant mass effect (increased ICP) and/or neurological decline.
- Sz risk is 35-80%. Phenytoin or other anticonvulsant may be required to prevent seizures.
- Lesions <2.5-3.0cm may respond to medical therapy alone.
- Surgical options: generally either stereotactic aspiration of abscess by burr hole placement OR surgical drainage by craniotomy.
- No clear data exist showing superiority of aspiration vs. excision.

DRUG-SPECIFIC COMMENTS

Ampicillin + Sulbactam: A second-line agent, primarily because of limited clinical experience. Although variation in abscess levels were observed, therapeutic success was achieved for 11 patients in one series. Active against all strep and anaerobes.

Aztreonam: A second-line agent for use in treatment combinations. This monolactam has good CSF penetration, but activity is limited to gram-negative organisms, including some Pseudomonas. Very little clinical experience treating brain abscess. Useful in beta-lactam allergic patient.

Cefepime: Like ceftazidime, this agent's broad spectrum of activity, particularly against Pseudomonas, makes it a good choice for empiric treatment of nosocomial or iatrogenic infections.

Ceftazidime: The treatment of choice for CNS infections suspected of or involving Pseudomonas aeruginosa. Good penetration into abscess cavities established.

Ceftriaxone: Drug has been reported extensively in brain abscess and meningitis series with excellent CSF penetration. High dose (2g IV q12h) recommended. With empirical treatment need to combine with metronidazole for anerobic coverage. Cefotaxime is equivalent. 3rd generation cephalosporins should be adequate for good MSSA (but not MRSA) coverage.

Imipenem/Cilastatin: Broad-spectrum agent with activity against streptococci, gram-negative bacilli, anaerobes, and nocardia would seem to make this an ideal drug. Use somewhat controversial since there is a potential for reducing the seizure threshold. However, most seizures reported in setting of renal insufficiency perhaps suggesting that

Imipenem was not dose-adjusted for CrCl. Meropenem said to have similar efficacy with fewer adverse events.

Meropenem: Broad-spectrum agent with activity against streptococci, gram-negative bacilli, anaerobes, and nocardia. Limited clinical experience with this agent, but it has been used with success extensively for meningitis.

Metronidazole: This is a favored drug for cerebral abscesses due to substantial clinical experience, activity against all anaerobes and excellent penetration into brain abscesses. No activity against aerobes so it is combined with a second drug.

Sulfadiazine: Treatment for nocardial infections of the CNS because of its exceptional CNS penetration among sulfonamides. No comparative trials exist, but clear treatment failures have been documented with sulfadiazine or trimethoprim/sulfamethoxazole. Combinations of sulfonamides with other agents (imipenem, cefotaxime, AG) have been more effective than sulfadiazine or TMP/SMX alone in animal models. Therefore, consideration should be given to combination or alternative combination treatment for the highly immunocompromised patient or the patient failing therapy with sulfonamides alone.

IMPORTANT POINTS

- Guidelines are author's opinion.
- Patients with cerebritis small abscess (<3cm), multiple abscesses often treated empirically.
- Indications for surgery for dx/drainage - large abscess, abscess refractory to empiric therapy, immunocompromised host.
- Coma at presentation bodes for poor outcome regardless of treatment.
- Complications include rupture (ventriculitis/meningitis), coma, neurologic sequelae (25-45%), death. Recurrence ~8%.
- Unusual pathogens should be suspected in patients from Latin America (Cysticercosis - check serology) or in compromised hosts with AIDS, chronic steroids, cancer chemotherapy etc - toxoplasmosis, Nocardia, TB, crypto etc - See AIDS)
- HIV testing should be performed, as a positive result will change the differential diagnosis.

SELECTED READINGS

Jansson AK, Enblad P, Sjolin J. Efficacy and safety of cefotaxime in combination with metronidazole for empirical treatment of brain abscess in clinical practice: a retrospective study of 66 consecutive cases. Eur J Clin Microbiol Infect Dis. 2004 Jan;23(1):7-14

Wispelwey B, Dacey RG, Scheld WM. Brain abscess. In: Scheld WM, Whitley RJ, Durack DT, eds. Infections of the Central Nervous System. 2nd ed. Philadelphia: Lippincott-Raven, 1997, pp.463-493

Mathisen GE, Johnson JP. Brain abscess. Clin Infect Dis 1997;25:763

Heilpern KL, Lorber B. Focal intracranial infections. Infect Dis Clin North Am 1996;10:879

Shahzadi S, Lozquo AM, Bernstein M et al. Stereotactic management of bacterial brain abscesses. Can J Neurol Sci 1996; 23:24

Mamelak AN, Mampalam TJ, Obana WG, Rosenblum ML. Improved management of multiple brain abscesses: A combined surgical and medical approach. Neurosurgery 1995;36:76

Sjolin J, Lilja A, Eriksson N, et al. Treatment of brain abscess with cefotaxime and metronidazole: Prospective study on 15 consecutive patients. Clin Infect Dis 1993;17:857

Leys D, Christiaens JL, Derambure PH, et al. Management of focal intracranial infections: Is medical treatment better than surgery?. J Neurol Neurosurg Psychiatry 1990;53:472

Britt RH, Enzmann DR. Clinical stages of human brain abscesses on serial CT scans after contrast infusion. Computerized tomographic, neuropathological, and clinical correlations. Neurosurg. 1983 Dec;59(6):972-89

Ingram HR, Selkon JB, Roxby CM et al. Bacteriologic Study of Otogenic Cerebral Abscesses. Brit Med J 1977; 2:991

ABSCESS, EPIDURAL   Eric Nuermberger, M.D.

Diagnostic Criteria

- Sx: Fever (60-80%), focal vertebral pain, tenderness to percussion, radicular pain or paresthesias along involved nerve roots
- Evidence of spinal cord compression: motor weakness, bowel or bladder dysfunction, sensory changes, paralysis (poss. depressed respiratory function if cervical cord involved)
- Dx: Radiographic evidence (usually MRI) of inflammation in the epidural space (frequently accompanied by diskitis or vertebral osteomyelitis)
- Obtain blood culture, CT-guided aspiration of abscess or operative gram-stain and culture (preferably before abx)

Common Pathogens: S.aureus ; Streptococcus species ; Mycobacterium tuberculosis ; Enterobacteriaceae

Treatment Regimens

Drug regimens (for suspected pathogens)

- Staph/Strep: nafcillin or oxacillin 2g IV q4h; or cefazolin 2g IV q8h
- Staph/Strep: clindamycin 600mg IV q6h
- MRSA, coag-neg Staph: vancomycin 15mg/kg IV q12h
- Strep/Enterococci: penicillin 3-4 mU IV q4h or ampicillin 2g IV q4h
- Enterobacteriaceae: ceftriaxone 1-2g IV q12h or cefotaxime 2g IV q6-8h
- Gram-negatives: ceftazidime 2g IV q8h or cefepime 2g IV q12h
- Gram-negatives: ciprofloxacin 400mg IV q12h or levofloxacin 750mg IV qd or gatifloxacin or moxifloxacin 400mg IV qd (early conversion to oral possible)
- Anaerobes: metronidazole 500mg IV q6h (early conversion to oral possible)
- Staph/Gram-negatives/Anaerobes: ampicillin/sulbactam 3g IV q6h or ticarcillin/clavulanate 3.1g IV q4h or piperacillin/tazobactam 3.375g IV q4-6h
- Staph/Gram-negatives/Anaerobes: imipenem 500-1000mg IV q6h or meropenem 1-2g IV q8h

Drainage

- Urgent surgical drainage together with IV antibiotics remains the treatment of choice
- The surgical standard is decompressive laminectomy with complete debridement
- Drainage must be performed emergently for eligible patients with neurological (esp. motor) deficit
- CT-guided aspiration and/or drainage has been used successfully in absence of neurologic deficits

Antimicrobial therapy

- Antimicrobial therapy alone may be attempted in the absence of neurologic deficit with close monitoring if the infectious etiology is known (e.g., + blood culture)
- Initial empiric therapy may be guided by concomitant or recent infection elsewhere (e.g., bacteremia/line sepsis, skin/soft tissue infection/decubitus, dental infection, UTI)
- Minimal empiric coverage must cover S. aureus (incl. vancomycin if MRSA expected)

- Expand coverage for aerobic gram-negative bacilli in patients with recent spinal surgery or intravenous drug use
- Empiric therapy should be modified by culture results
- Duration of therapy typically 2-4 wks IV, then orally to complete 6-8 wks or until CRP normal

DRUG-SPECIFIC COMMENTS

Ampicillin + Sulbactam: Like other beta-lactam/lactamase inhibitor combinations, it provides broad coverage. A good choice for polymicrobial infections or infections with resistant nosocomial organisms.

Aztreonam: Broad activity against gram-negative bacilli, but no gram-positive or anaerobic activity. An alternative for resistant nosocomial pathogens.

Ceftriaxone: Ceftriaxone, like cefotaxime, broad-spectrum activity and excellent tissue penetration make it a good choice for susceptible organisms. Pharmacokinetics may allow once-daily dosing for convenient outpatient parenteral therapy when appropriate.

Ciprofloxacin: Remains the fluoroquinolone of choice for infections with Pseudomonas aeruginosa and Enterobacteriaceae. Rapid resistance may develop among staphylococci. No reliable anaerobic activity. May allow early conversion to oral therapy (750mg PO twice daily for severe infections).

Imipenem/Cilastatin: Broad-spectrum, including anaerobes, make this agent an attractive alternative for polymicrobial infections or infections with resistant organisms.

Linezolid: Spectrum includes MRSA. Excellent bioavailability offers early IV to oral conversion, but little experience with bone/joint infections. Hematologic toxicity may be problematic with long-term administration.

Meropenem: Broad-spectrum, including anaerobes, make this agent an attractive alternative for polymicrobial infections or infections with resistant organisms.

Metronidazole: Broad-spectrum antianaerobic agent. Exceptional tissue penetration makes it an excellent choice for treatment of abscess. May allow early conversion to oral therapy.

Penicillin: The drug of choice for infections with susceptible streptococci.

Piperacillin + Tazobactam: Like other beta-lactam/lactamase inhibitor combinations, it provides broad coverage. A good choice for polymicrobial infections or infections with resistant nosocomial organisms.

Ticarcillin + Clavulanic Acid: Like other beta-lactam/lactamase inhibitor combinations, it provides broad coverage. A good choice for polymicrobial infections or infections with resistant nosocomial organisms.

IMPORTANT POINTS

- Infecting organism should always be sought! Abscess cultures positive in up to 90%. Blood cultures in 60-70%. Culture for anaerobes, mycobacteria, and fungi when suspected.
- Drainage must be performed emergently for eligible patients with neurologic deficit, as improvement is strongly related to the rapidity of surgical intervention.
- Likelihood of neurologic recovery very low if surgery delayed >24-36 hours after onset of paralysis.
- Antibiotic therapy alone may be considered if the patient is not a surgical candidate, has no neurologic deficit, and/or has interval improvement in pain, neurologic status, fever, leukocytosis.

- Paralysis of more than 2-3 days duration may be another indication for nonsurgical management.
- Progression to paralysis may occur over hrs. All pts must be monitored closely for new or worsening neurologic deficit indicating need for further drainage.

Selected Readings

Sorensen P. Spinal epidural abscesses: conservative treatment for selected subgroups of patients . Br J Neurosurgery 2003;17:513

Soehle M & Wallenfang T. Spinal epidural abscesses: clinical manifestations, prognostic factors, and outcomes. Neurosurgery 2002;51:79

Darouiche RO, Hamill RJ, Greenberg SB, et al. Bacterial spinal epidural abscess: Review of 43 cases and literature survey. Medicine. 1992;71:369-85

Wheeler D, Keiser P, Rigamonti D, et al. Medical management of spinal epidural abscesses: Case report and review. Clin Infect Dis. 1992;15:22-7

Curling OD, Gower W, McWhorter JM. Changing concepts in spinal epidural abscess: A report of 29 cases. Neurosurgery 1990;27:185

Hlavin ML, Kaminski HJ, Ross JC, et al. Spinal epidural abscess: A ten-year perspective. Neurosurgery 1990;27:177

Danner RL and Hartman BJ. Update of spinal epidural abscess: 35 cases and review of the literature. Rev Infect Dis 1987;9:265

ABSCESS, HEPATIC

Pamela A. Lipsett, M.D.; Chris Carpenter, M.D.

Diagnostic Criteria

- Signs and sx: fever +/- RUQ pain, tenderness w/hepatomegaly; some may only have fever (60%) and presentation may be subacute/chronic.
- Positive blood cultures up to 50%, with alkaline phosphatase and WBC counts frequently elevated. Hyperbilirubinemia with or without jaundice occurs in < 50% of patients.
- Although dx may be suggested on plain films (e.g., gas within the abscess); CT, US, and MRI are the imaging modalities of choice in suspected liver abscess or FUO.
- CT or US-guided percutaneous or surgical drainage should be considered in all cases of hepatic abscess for diagnostic confirmation and cx.
- Positive amebic or echinococcal serology helps differentiate parasitic liver abscess from pyogenic, especially in nonendemic areas.
- Diaphragmatic irritation may refer pain to the right shoulder +/or cough or pleural rub.
- Source: most commonly biliary w/ direct infection via a contiguous structure (e.g., the gall bladder), hematologic (either via the hepatic artery and systemic circulation or via the portal vein and intestinal sources), traumatic, or cryptogenic (approximately 20%).
- Uncomplicated small abscesses due to Entamoeba histolytica in endemic areas may not require aspiration; ?empiric Rx.
- Amebic hepatic abscesses are typically solitary right lobe lesions.

Common Pathogens: Enterobacteriaceae ; Gram-positive streptococci and enterococcus; Anaerobes ; Candida species ; Yersinia enterocolitica ; Entamoeba histolytica ; Echinococcus spp.

TREATMENT REGIMENS

Drainage

- Authors opinion based on Surgical Infection Society guidelines. Abscess drainage is the optimal therapy.
- CT or US-guided percutaneous needle aspiration +/- catheter drainage initial method of choice; if drainage inadequate, surgical drainage may be required.
- Hepatotomy generally successful approach, but improvements in percutaneous techniques make it secondary management in most cases.
- Surgical drainage may be primary treatment if a complex abscess, multiple abscesses, percutaneously unreachable abscess, or additional surgical problem is present; may be done laparoscopically.
- General recommendations are for at least one week of drainage with CT follow-up.
- Underlying disease typically is the primary determinant of outcome

Adjunctive antibiotic treatment

- Empiric coverage should include Enterobacteriaceae, enterococci, anaerobes, and in certain situations staphylococci and streptococci. In stable patient may defer abx until post-aspiration/drainage.
- In patients who have received adequate drainage, duration of treatment depends on resolution of fever and leukocytosis (often 7-28 days)
- Longer courses (up to several months) may be required in the patient who is inadequately drained or treated solely medically.
- Follow-up imaging studies should be performed to determine resolution, CT and/or US.
- Consider empiric antifungal Rx in immunosuppressed patients at risk for chronic disseminated candidiasis (hepatosplenic candidiasis, see C. albicans module).
- Culture results may help narrow coverage, but for pyogenic abscess do not trim anaerobic coverage given difficulty cx these organisms.
- Empiric Rx: ampicillin 2.0g IV q6h plus gentamicin 1.7g IV q8h plus metronidazole 0.5g IV q8h
- Alt: cefotaxime 2.0g IV q8h or ceftriaxone 2.0g IV qd plus metronidazole 0.5g IV q8h
- B-lactam/B-lactamase inhibitors are reasonable alternatives; metronidazole should be included if amebic abscess is in the differential.
- Fluoroquinolone plus metronidazole an alternative; often used as an oral regimen for prolonged therapy.

Amebic hepatic abscess

- Metronidazole (750mg PO tid x 10 days) followed by paromomycin (500mg tid x 7d) or iodoquinol (650mg tid x 20d) or diloxanide furoate (500mg tid x 10d).
- Alt: tinidazole 800mg tid or 2g qd x 3-5d followed by paromomycin (500mg tid x 7d) or iodoquinol (650mg tid x 20d) or diloxanide furoate (500mg tid x 10d)
- Percutaneous aspiration has no clear role in therapy, but consider for diagnosis.
- MORE TREATMENT DETAILS: Echinococcus species:
- Surgical resection is first choice.
- If inoperable or surgery unfeasible because of the patient's condition, Rx w/ albendazole or mebendazole.
- Must avoid closed aspiration due to risk of anaphylaxis or secondary cysts.

DRUG-SPECIFIC COMMENTS

Ampicillin + Sulbactam: Good coverage of gram-positive, gram-negative, and anaerobic pathogens; lacks Pseudomonas aeruginosa coverage but good Enterococcus species coverage.

Diagnosis

Aztreonam: Excellent gram-negative coverage; use in combination with anaerobic agent and agent covering gram-positives for empiric therapy; would reserve for seriously ill patients with B-lactam allergies and no other reasonable alternatives.

Cefepime: Excellent coverage of gram negative w/ some gram positive pathogens; use in combination with anaerobic agent for empiric therapy.

Daptomycin: New agent for resistant gram-positive infections

Ertapenem: Newer carbapenem with excellent broad-spectrum coverage except P. aeruginosa, Acinetobacter spp., and Enterococci.

Gatifloxacin: Excellent broad spectrum coverage but clinical data limited on anaerobe coverage; would use other agents first while clinical data accumulates on its use in serious infections.

Imipenem/Cilastatin: Excellent broad spectrum (gram-positive, gram-negative, and anaerobe) coverage; would reserve for seriously ill patients.

Linezolid: Excellent coverage of resistant GPC infections; marrow suppression a concern with prolonged use

Meropenem: Excellent broad spectrum (gram-positive, gram-negative, and anaerobe) coverage; would reserve for seriously ill patients.

Moxifloxacin: Excellent broad-spectrum coverage

Piperacillin + Tazobactam: Excellent broad spectrum coverage including gram-positive coverage, gram-negative coverage (including Pseudomonas aeruginosa and B-lactamase producing pathogens) and anaerobic coverage.

Ticarcillin + Clavulanic Acid: Broad spectrum coverage including gram-positive coverage, gram-negative coverage (including Pseudomonas aeruginosa and B-lactamase producing pathogens) and anaerobic coverage.

Important Points

- Frequently polymicrobial; single/multiple lesions occur in approximately a 1:1 ratio, with the majority in the right lobe (especially when solitary); cryptogenic abscesses are generally solitary.
- Untreated, the mortality rate associated with pyogenic hepatic abscess approaches 100%, with treatment in some series it is below 15%; the latter mortality is dependent upon underlying disease.
- Recurrence is more frequent after simple percutaneous aspiration without placement of a temporary drain, or in patients in whom drains are removed too early.
- Abscesses are frequently associated with chronic medical conditions (e.g., diabetes mellitus) hematologic disease (e.g., leukemia), and chronic granulomatous disease (Staphylococcus aureus).
- Chronic disseminated candidiasis (CDC, a.k.a. hepatosplenic candidiasis) occurs in immunosuppressed patients, e.g., bone marrow transplant recipients.

Selected Readings

Solomkin et al. Guidelines for the Selection of Anti-infective Agents for Complicated Intra-abdominal Infections. Clin Infect Diseases 2003 October 15;37:997-1005.

Mazuski JE, Sawyer RG, Mathans AB et al. The Surgical Infection Society Guidelines on Antimicrobial Therapy for Intra-Abdominal Infections: An Executive Summary. Surgical Infections, 2002, Vol 3

Balci N, SIrvanci. MR imaging of infective liver lesions. Magn Reson Imaging Clin N Am 2002; 10:121-35

Lambertucci JR , Rayes AA, Serufo JC, Nobre V. Pyogenic abscess and parasitic diseases. Rev Inst Med Trop Sao Paulo 2001;43: 67-74

Hansen P, Ludemann R, Swanstrom LL. Minimally invasive approaches to hepatic surgery. Hepatogastroenterology 2001;48:37-40

Liew KV, Lau TC. Cheng TK et al. Pyogenic liver abscess-a tropical centre's experience in management with review of the current literature. Singapore Med J 2000 ;41:489-92

Huang C, Pitt HA,Lipsett PA, Osterman F, Lillemore KD, Cameron JLC, Zuidema G. Pyogenic hepatic abscesses: Changing trends over 42 years. Ann Surg;1996;223:600-609

Koneru S, Peskin GW, and Sreenivas V. Pyogenic Hepatic Abscess in a Community Hospital. The American Surgeon. April 1994, Vol. 60(4);278-81

Robert JH, Mirescu D, Ambrosetti P, Khoury G, Greenstein AJ, and Rohner A. Critical Review of the treatment of pyogenic hepatic abscess. Surgery, Gynecology and Obstetrics February 1992, vol. 174(2): 97-102

Branum GD, Tyson GS, Branum MA, and Meyers WC. Hepatic Abscess: changes in Etiology, Diagnosis, and Management. Annals of Surgery 1990 Dec;212(6):655-62

ABSCESS, INTRA-ABDOMINAL

Pamela A. Lipsett, M.D.; Chris Carpenter, M.D.

DIAGNOSTIC CRITERIA

- Sx: Fever, pain, local tenderness, possible palpable mass
- Lab: Elevated WBC, direct aspiration +, blood cultures positive ~25% depending on site
- CT most helpful. US and MRI used occasionally. MRI not used for drainage guidance
- CT or US-guided percutaneous or surgical drainage should be considered in all cases for diagnostic confirmation, microbiologic evaluation, and therapy.
- Postoperative assessment for abscess confounded by analgesics and incisional pain; over half present within 10 days of initial operation.

TREATMENT REGIMENS

Primary therapy: abscess drainage

- All recommendations are the authors' opinion based on Surgical Infection Society guidelines.
- CT or US-guided percutaneous needle aspiration with subsequent catheter drainage is considered by many as the first line of therapy; if drainage is inadequate surgery may be required.
- Surgery used primarily after percutaneous therapy has failed, has stabilized condition for primary surgical therapy, or when concurrent surgical source control needed.
- Infected pancreatic necrosis not well suited to percutaneous therapy because of cellular debris
- If an enteric abscess unrelated to a surgical procedure is encountered, must consider the possibility of an underlying necrotic cancer
- Follow up CT scan/US and/or sinograms needed to show resolution of source and abscess

Adjunctive antibiotic treatment

- Empiric coverage (i.e., when the microbiologic source of infection is unknown) should include coverage of Enterobacteriaceae, Enterococci, and anaerobes.
- After adequate drainage, at least 5-10 days of antibiotic coverage is indicated, with duration in part based on resolution of fever and leukocytosis, severity of infection, and clinical response.
- Duration of therapy has not been subjected to rigorous study. If the underlying surgical problem has been controlled (source) short course of antibiotics maybe appropriate. Clincial studies ongoing.

- Empiric coverage may be broadened or cautiously narrowed on the basis of the abscess and blood cultures results
- Cefoxitin 1-2.0g IV q6h
- Ticarcillin-clavulanate 3.1g IV q6h or piperacillin-tazobactam 3.375g IV q6h or 4.5g IV q8h or ampicillin-sulbactam 3.0g IV q6h
- Ciprofloxacin 400mg IV q12h or gatifloxacin 400mg IV qd or levofloxacin 500mg IV qd plus metronidazole 1.0g IV loading dose, then 500mg IV q6h or clindamycin 450-900mg IV q6h
- Imipenem 0.5g IV q6h or meropenem 1.0g IV q8h
- Cefotaxime 2.0g IV q8h or ceftriaxone 2.0g IV qd or cefepime 2.0g IV q12h plus metronidazole 1.0g IV loading dose, then 500mg IV q6h or clindamycin 450-900mg IV q6h
- Ampicillin 2.0g IV q6h plus gentamicin 1.7mg/kg IV q6h plus metronidazole 1.0g IV loading dose, then 500mg IV q6h or clindamycin 450-900mg IV q6h

Drug-Specific Comments

Ampicillin + Sulbactam: Good coverage of gram-positive, gram-negative, and anaerobic pathogens - lacks Pseudomonas aeruginosa coverage but good Enterococcus species coverage.

Aztreonam: Excellent gram-negative coverage; use in combination with anaerobic agent plus/minus an agent covering Enterococcus species for empiric therapy; would reserve for seriously ill patients with B-lactam allergies and no other reasonable alternatives.

Cefepime: excellent coverage of gram-negative and gram-positive pathogens; use in combination with anaerobic agent (plus/minus an agent covering Enterococcus species) for empiric therapy.

Gatifloxacin: Excellent broad spectrum coverage but clinical data limited on anaerobe coverage; would use other agents first while clinical data accumulates on its use in serous infections.

Imipenem/Cilastatin: Excellent broad spectrum (gram-positive, gram-negative, and anaerobe) coverage; would reserve for seriously ill patients.

Meropenem: Excellent broad spectrum (gram-positive, gram-negative, and anaerobe) coverage; would reserve for seriously ill patients.

Piperacillin + Tazobactam: Excellent broad spectrum coverage including gram-positive coverage, gram-negative coverage (including Pseudomonas aeruginosa and B-lactamase producing pathogens) and anaerobic coverage.

Ticarcillin + Clavulanic Acid: Excellent broad spectrum coverage including gram-positive coverage, gram-negative coverage (including Pseudomonas aeruginosa and B-lactamase producing pathogens) and anaerobic coverage.

Important Points

- Non-visceral intra-abdominal abscesses should be considered polymicrobial in nearly all cases.
- Local susceptibility patterns (e.g., for Pseudomonas spp., etc.) should be considered in the decision for empiric coverage.
- Multiple factors, including severity of illness, bacteremia, multiple abscesses, and location of abscess are predictive of mortality (with treatment may still approach 30% depending on the population)
- Percutaneous drainage should be utilized IF possible and surgical source is controlled
- Rate of recovery of yeast from intraoperative specimens of a perforated viscus was >30% and was associated with death and complications

- On-demand relaparotomy rather than a planned relaparotomy may be associated with better results in selected cases
- Source control is essential. The open abdomen approach is occasionally necessary to control the source of infection.

SELECTED READINGS

Mazuskil JE, Sawyer RG, Nathans AB et al. The Surgical Infection Society Guidelines on Antimicrobial Therapy for Intra-Abdominal Infections: An Executive Summary . Surgical Infections 2002 Vol 3

Buijk SE, Bruining. Future directions inthe management of tertiary peritonitis. Intensive Care Med 2002;28:1024-1029

Sandven P, Qvist H, Skovlund E et al. Signficance of Candida recovered from intraoperative specimens in patients with intra-abdominal perforations. Crit Care Med 2002;30:541-7

Lamme B,Boermeester MA, Reisma JB, et al. Meta-analysis of relaparotomy for secondary peritonitis. Br J Surg 2002;89,1516-1524

vanSonneberg E, Wittch GR, Goodacre BW et al. Percutaneous Abscess Drainage: An update . World J SUrg 2001;25:362-372

Stinner B. Invited Commentary to: Percutaneous Drainage an Update. World J Surg 2001:25:370-372

Barie PS. Management of complicated intra-abdominal infections. J Chemother 1999;11:464-77

ABSCESS, LUNG

John G. Bartlett, M.D.

DIAGNOSTIC CRITERIA

- Clinical: cough, fever, sputum that is often putrid, +/- weight loss, chronic course, night sweats, predisposition to aspiration, &/or pleurisy
- PE: fever & signs of pneumonia +/- pleural effusion +/- gingivitis
- Studies: XR or CT scan showing parenchymal infiltrate with cavity; leukocytosis and anemia
- Differential of air fluid level on xray: TB, MAC, empyema, CA, cyst, fungi, nocardia
- Bronchoscopy for refractory & atypical cases only.

COMMON PATHOGENS: Streptococcus milleri ; Anaerobes ; S.aureus ; Aerobic & microaerophilic strep including S. anginosus complex; Other: Gram-negative bacteria; Legionella; Nocardia; Actinomyces; Group A strep; Type B H. influenzae; Mycobacteria: M. tuberculosis, MAI, M. kansasii; Fungi: aspergillus, cryptococcus, cocci, histo, blasto

TREATMENT REGIMENS

Antibiotics: anaerobic lung abscess

- Principles: Dx - x-ray/CT shows cavity; main cause- anaerobes; R/O TB, Ca, etc; Usual Rx - clind (esp if putrid); Bronch if atypical or failure to respond
- Clindamycin 600mg IV q8h, then clindamycin 300mg PO qid x 3 months or until XR shows small stable lesion or is clear
- Ampicillin-sulbactam (Unasyn) 1.5-3g IV q6h, then amoxicillin-clavulanate (Augmentin) 875mg PO bid or clind 300mg PO qid
- Alternative: piperacillin-tazobactam (Zosyn) 3.375g IV q6h, then amoxicillin-clavulanate (Augmentin) 875mg PO bid or clind 300mg PO qid
- Alternative: imipenem (Primaxin) 0.5-1g PO q6-8h, then clindamycin 300mg PO qid or amoxicillin-clavulanate (Augmentin) 875mg PO bid
- Most "non-specific" lung abscesses are treated empirically with clindamycin & respond, but require 3 mo. or longer course.

DIAGNOSIS

- Most patients are treated with IV antibiotics until clinical improvement, then receive oral antibiotics x 2-3 mos. or until a f/u XR is clear or shows a small, stable residual lesion.

Drainage and surgery

- Most pts have already drained abscess via bronchus & need only abx.
- Bronchoscopic drainage--not generally useful.
- Percutaneous transthoracic drainage--indicated in refractory lung abscess cases.
- Postural drainage--often done but probably plays no role in treatment and may be dangerous.
- Resectional surgery--usually a lobectomy or pneumonectomy
- Resection Indications (rare): failure to respond to abx treatment usually due to abscess cavity >6cm diameter, complicated/serious associated diseases, or caused by GNB.

Antibiotics: special hosts, settings

- Compromised host, e.g., AIDS: TB, P. aeruginosa, nocardia, cryptococcus, aspergillus, PCP, Rhodococcus equi, MAC, M. kansasii, lymphoma
- Nosocomial: GNB, esp. Klebsiella; S. aureus
- Post-influenza: S.aureus-including MRSA and/or toxic shock
- Nursing home: anaerobes, GNB, S.aureus
- Injection drug user: aspiration-anaerobes & strep; septic emboli-S. aureus & Strep. viridans

DRUG-SPECIFIC COMMENTS

Amoxicillin + Clavulanate: (Augmentin) Good alternative to clindamycin for oral treatment. Active against virtually all anaerobes. Use the 875mg dose form.

Ampicillin + Sulbactam: (Unasyn) Active against virtually all anaerobes. Expands spectrum to other bacterial causes of lung abscess.

Chloramphenicol: Active vs. all anaerobes, but usually other agents are preferred due to greater experience and concern for chloramphenicol toxicity.

Doxycycline: No longer regarded as a dependable drug for oral anaerobes.

Gatifloxacin: (Tequin) Good in vitro activity vs. anaerobes and many other bacteria that cause lung abscess. Oral or parenteral. Clinical experience is nil.

Imipenem/Cilastatin: (Primaxin) Active against virtually all anaerobes. Expands spectrum to other bacterial causes of lung abscess including most GNB.

Metronidazole: Excellent activity vs anaerobes but poor track record in anaerobic lung abscesses, presumably due to lack of activity vs aerobes esp microaerophilic and aerobic strep. Add penicillin if used.

Moxifloxacin: (Avelox) Oral and IV agent with good anti-anaerobic activity in vitro, but clinical experience is nil.

Piperacillin + Tazobactam: (Zosyn) Active against virtually all anaerobes. Expands spectrum to other bacterial causes of lung abscess, especially GNB.

Ticarcillin + Clavulanic Acid: (Timentin) Active against virtually all anaerobes. Expands spectrum to other bacterial causes of lung abscess.

IMPORTANT POINTS

- Guidelines from IDSA (CID 2000;31:34) and author's opinion
- Most common cause is anaerobes due to aspiration
- Must R/O mycobacteria (esp. TB), fungi (histo, cocci, blasto, crypt), cancer, infected cyst
- Clues to anaerobes: putrid discharge, chronic course, predisposition to aspiration (decreased consciousness, dysphagia, or gingivitis)

• Abx Rx duration--until XR clear or small stable residual scar (arbitrary)

SELECTED READINGS

Kanamori S., et al. The role of the capsule of the streptococcus milleri group in it's pathogenicity. J Infect Chemother 2004;10:105-9

Allewelt M, Schuler P, Boleskei PL, et al. Ampicillin and sulbactam vs. clindamycin +/- cephalosporin for the treatment of aspiration pneumonia and primary lunch abscess. Clin. Microbial Infect 2004;10:163

Fernandez-Sabe, N, et al. Efficacy and safety of sequential amoxicillin- clavulanate in the treatment of anaerobic lung infections. Eur J Clin Microbial Infect Dis 2003;22-185

Gillet Y, et al. Association between Staphylococcus aureus strains carrying gene for Panton-Valentine leukocidin and highly lethal necrotizing pneumonia in young immunocompetent patients . Lancet 2002;359:753-9

Wali SO, et al. Percutaneous drainage of pyogenic lung abscess. Scand J Infect Dis 2002;34:673-9

Smith DT. Experimental aspiratory abscesses. Arch Surg 1927;14:23.

Bartlett JG, Gorbach SL, Tally FP, Finegold SM. Bacteriology and treatment of primary lung abscess. Am Rev Resp Dis 1974;109:510.

Landay MJ, Christensen EE, Bynum. Anaerobic pleural and pulmonary infections. Am J Roentgen 1980;134:233.

Levinson ME, Mangura CT, Lorber B. Clindamycin compared to penicillin for the treatment of anaerobic lung abscess. Ann Intern Med 1983;98:466.

Perlino CA. Metronidazole vs. clindamycin treatment of anaerobic pulmonary infection. Arch Intern Med 1981;141:1412.

ACNE VULGARIS

Ciro R. Martins, M.D.

DIAGNOSTIC CRITERIA

• Hx: insidious development of multiple follicular lesions with periods of clinical improvement and exacerbation. Peak prevalence: age 17, but may start as early as 8 yrs.
• Hx: most cases involute spontaneously and completely after a few years, but a small percentage remains active through adult life. Some patients first develop acne in their 3rd and 4th decades of life.
• PE: any combination of open and closed comedones, inflammatory papules, pustules, nodules and cysts, affecting the face, neck, upper chest, back and/or proximal extremities.
• PE (other associated findings): excessive oiliness of the skin, post-inflammatory hyper/hypo-pigmentation, atrophic or hypertrophic scars, excoriations, hirsutism and/or alopecia in women
• Lab: no dx test for acne vulgaris

COMMON PATHOGENS: Propionibacterium species

TREATMENT REGIMENS

Topical therapy

• Benzoyl peroxide 2.5-10% (Acne-Aid, Ambi 10, Benoxyl 10, Benzac, Brevoxyl, Desquam, PanOxyl) lotion, liquid soap, cream or gel qd-bid
• Erythromycin 2% (Akne-Mycin, A/T/S, Emgel, Erycette, EryDerm, Erythra-Derm, Erygel, Erymax, Staticin, Theramycin Z, T-Stat) lotion, solution, cream or gel qhs
• Benzoyl peroxide 5%/ erythromycin 3% gel (Benzamycin) qHS; Benzoyl peroxide 5%/ clindamycin 1% gel (Benzaclin, Duac) qHS
• Clindamycin solution, lotion or gel (Cleocin T, Clindagel, Clindets) qhs

- Sodium sulfacetamide 10% lotion (Avar, Clenia, Plexion, Rosula, Rosanil, Sulfacet-R, Klaron) qd-bid
- Azelaic acid 20% (Azelex, Finacea, Finevin) cream qd-bid
- Tretinoin 0.025-0.1% (Retin-A, Retin-A micro, Renova, Avita, Altinac) cream, gel, solution qhs
- Adapalene 0.1% (Differin) gel qhs
- Tazarotene 0.05%. 0.1% (Avage, Tazorac) cream or gel qhs
- Salicylic acid 3-5% or lactic acid 12% compounded in lotion or cream base qd-bid

Systemic therapy

- Tetracycline 250-500mg PO qd-bid and reassess in 1-2 mos
- Doxycycline 50-100mg PO qd-bid and reassess in 1-2 mos
- Minocycline 50-100mg PO qd-bid and reassess in 1-2 mos
- Erythromycin 250-500mg PO qid or 333mg PO tid x 1 mo
- TMP/SMX DS 1 tab PO qd-bid and reassess in 1 mo
- Azithromycin (Z-Pack) q 15d or q mo
- Dapsone 50-100mg PO qd
- Isotretinoin (Accutane) 0.5-1mg/kg/d x 20 wk
- Hormonal therapy: oral contraceptives, estrogen or anti-androgen agents (spironolactone, flutamide)
- Prednisone 20-40mg PO qd x 1-2 wks (in cases of acne fulminans, pyoderma faciale or in early association with isotretinoin)

Surgical therapy

- I+D of cysts and fistula tracts
- Intralesional injection of nodules and cysts with triamcinolone 2.5-5mg/cc
- Punch excision, punch elevation and punch grafting of depressed, "ice-pick" scars
- Collagen injections in depressed, rolled scars
- CO_2 LASER resurfacing
- Dermabrasion

DRUG-SPECIFIC COMMENTS

Dapsone: Second-line drug for severe nodulo-cystic acne where isotretinoin is not a therapeutic option. Signifcant potential hematologic side-effects.

Doxycycline: Excellent alternative to tetracycline as a first-line therapy for moderate acne, although more expensive. Best advantage is that it can be taken with food. Risk of photosensitivity (3-10%).

Minocycline: This is the most active drug against P. acnes and resistance develops rarely. Can be taken with food. Pigmentation of skin, nails and teeth may develop. Also photosensitizing, but not as much as doxycycline. Potentially serious reactions have been described, although rare. Dizziness may be bothersome in some patients.

Tetracycline: Excellent and very inexpensive first-line choice for moderate acne. It must be taken on an empty stomach, what makes scheduling more complicated. Can be photosensitizing, but not as much as doxycycline. Increased incidence of vaginal yeast infections in women.

IMPORTANT POINTS

- These guidelines are based on the guidelines of care of the American Academy of Dermatology
- Acne vulgaris is a condition where multiple factors contribute to its pathogenesis, including abnormal follicular keratinization and occlusion, excessive oil production and bacterial superinfection

- DDx: folliculitis, miliaria, acneiform drug eruptions, rosacea, perioral dermatitis, follicular mucinosis, papular urticaria, follicular eczema
- P. acnes secretes several extracellular products such as hyaluronidase, proteases, lipases and chemotactic factors that may play a significant role in the inflammatory reaction seen in acne
- Pregnancy: safety using erythromycin (PO or topical), benzoyl peroxide (topical), azeleic acid (topical), clindamycin (topical)

SELECTED READINGS

Webster G. Clinical Review: Acne Vulgaris. British Medical Journal 2002; 325:475-9.

Thiboutot DM. Acne and Rosacea: New and Emerging Therapies. Dermatologic Clinics, 18(1):63-71, January 2000

Burkhart CG, Burkhart CN, Lehmann PF. Acne: a review of immunologic and microbiologic factors. Postgrad Med J 75:328-331, 1999

White GM. Acne Therapy. Advances in Dermatology, 14:29-59, 1999.

ANTHRAX, CUTANEOUS

John G. Bartlett, M.D.

DIAGNOSTIC CRITERIA

- Suspected case: Compatible clinical illness plus one non-cult test or epidemiologic link
- Confirmed case: Compatible clinical illness plus positive culture or 2 non-cult tests (PCR, Immunohisto, serology)
- Sx: Papule (esp arms, face, chest); then vesicles/bullae, then black eschar + edema evolving over 3-5d
- Epid: Exposure time & place to environment w/B. anthracis (proven or suspect)
- Dx: Pre-treatment culture of lesion +/- blood culture; Bx - PCR, Immunohisto, silver stain (Formalin)

COMMON PATHOGENS: Bacillus anthracis

TREATMENT REGIMENS

Treatment

- Systemic sx, face/neck involved and/or extensive edema: IV cipro 400mg PO or IV q 12h or doxy 100mg q 12h IV or PO or levofloxacin 500mg IV or PO each, plus 1-2 other antibiotics
- Adjunctive IV abx: clind 600mg q 8h, imipenem 1g q 6h, pen 4 MU q 4h, vanco 1g q 12h, rifampin 300 q 12h
- Skin lesion, uncomplicated: cipro 500mg PO bid or doxy 100mg PO bid x 60d
- IV-PO switch when clinically stable plus at least 7-10 days; treat 60 days w/doxy 100 bid or cipro 500 bid
- Extensive edema: consider prednisone 60-80mg/d
- Notify public health and infection control

Treatment: special populations

- Pregnancy or lactation: cipro or doxy IV or PO as above consider amox 0.5-1g PO tid after Rx 7-10d + stable
- Peds - cipro: 10-15mg/kg q 12h IV not >1g/d
- Peds doxy: >8 yrs & >45kg: 100mg bid; >8yrs & <45kg or <8 yrs: 2.2mg/kg bid
- Immunosuppressed: standard

DIAGNOSIS

DRUG-SPECIFIC COMMENTS

Amoxicillin: Penicillin is FDA-approved for anthrax and shown to work in primate model; concerns with amoxicillin are levels achieved with oral administration and the inducible penicillinase often produced by B. anthracis. Amoxicillin is an option if there is low microbial load (post initial therapy or post initial prophylaxis) plus reason to avoid cipro & doxy (peds or pregnancy), even then some would not use it and some would use it only in high doses of 3-3.5g/d.

Amoxicillin + Clavulanate: Betalactamase inhibitor does not inactivate betalactamases of B. anthracis and may contribute to inducing betalactamase production.

Ampicillin + Sulbactam: Betalactamase inhibitor does not inactivate betalactamases of B. anthracis and may contribute to inducing betalactamase production.

Ceftazidime: This and other 3rd generation cephalosporins are not active vs. B. anthracis due to cephalosporinases. Bad choice.

Ciprofloxacin: FDA approved for anthrax, good record in the primate model and good record for prophylaxis in the 2001 anthrax attack.

Clarithromycin: Marginal in vitro activity vs. B. anthracis and no clinical experience. Not a good choice.

Doxycycline: Very active in vitro, FDA-approved for anthrax and effective in primate model. This plus cipro and levo are preferred drugs for treatment and prophylaxis.

Gatifloxacin: As active as cipro in vitro, but not FDA -approved for anthrax and untested in primate model. Most authorities think that cipro is preferred but that Gatifloxacin should work just as well.

Imipenem/Cilastatin: Highly active in vitro but not tested in animal model & not FDA-approved for anthrax. Rational adjunct to cipro or doxy with systemic disease.

Levofloxacin: FDA-approved for anthrax and good record in the primate model.

Moxifloxacin: As active as cipro in vitro, but not FDA-aproved for anthrax and untested in primate model. Most authorities think that cipro is preferred but that Moxifloxacin should work just as well.

Penicillin: Penicillin G FDA-approved for anthrax, reasonably effective in primate model, very active in vitro and extensive prior use with favorable outcomes with clinical anthrax. Concern is that B. anthracis makes an inducible penicillinase that makes penicillin possibly risky as single agent with high microbial load although it is sometimes advocated as adjunct to cipro or doxy with serious clinical disease esp with meningitis.

Piperacillin + Tazobactam: Betalactamase inhibitor does not inactivate betalactamases of B. anthracis and may contribute to inducing betalactamase production.

Ticarcillin + Clavulanic Acid: Betalactamase inhibitor does not inactivate betalactamases of B. anthracis and may contribute to inducing betalactamase production.

IMPORTANT POINTS

- Source document: CDC (MMWR 2001;50:909) and JAMA (2002;287:2236)
- Dx: Exposure + papule progressing to black eschar on exposed area in 3-4d +/- local edema
- Most patients are managed as outpts, but may be sick; mortality without antibiotics is reported as high as 20%
- Cutaneous anthrax can be treated in 7-10 days
- Cipro, levo & doxy are equivalent; all other abx less effective/not studied

SELECTED READINGS

Reissman DB, Whitney EA, Taylor TH Jr, et al. One-year health assessment of adult survivors of Bacillus anthracis infection. JAMA 2004;2004:291:1944-8

Meyerhoff A, Albrecht R, Meyer JM, et al. US Food and Drug Administration approval of ciprofloxacin hydrochloride for management of postexposure inhalational anthrax. Clin Infect Dis 2004;39:303-308

Blank S, Moskin LC, Zucker JR. An ounce of prevention is a ton of work: Mass antibiotic prophylaxis for anthrax, New York City, 2001. Emerg Infect Dis 2003;9:615.

Inglesby TV, et al. Anthrax as a biological weapon, 2002: Updated recommendations for management. JAMA 2002;287:2236

Freedman A, et al. Cutaneous anthrax associated with microangiopathic hemolytic anemia and coagulopathy in a 7 month old infant. JAMA 2002;287:869

Layton M, Weiss D. Rickettsialpox mimics cutaneous anthrax. NYC Dept Health Alert #6, Feb 21, 2002

Centers for Disease Control. Suspected cutaneous anthrax in a laboratory worker. MMWR 2002;51:279

Centers for Disease Control. Update: Investigation of bioterrorism - related anthrax and interim guidelines for clinical evaluation of persons with possible anthrax. MMWR 2001;50:941

Centers for Disease Control. Update: Investigation of bioterrorism - related anthrax & interim guidelines for exposure management and antimicrobial prophylaxis. MMWR 2001;50:909

Ringertz SH, Holby EA, Jensenius M. Injectional anthrax in a heroin skin popper. Lancet 2000;356:1574

ANTHRAX, INHALATION
John G. Bartlett, M.D.

DIAGNOSTIC CRITERIA
- Confirmed case (CDC): compatible clinical illness PLUS positive culture or 2 other tests (PCR, immunohistochemistry, serology)
- Suspected case: compatible illness PLUS one non-culture test OR epidemiological link
- Sx Stage 1 (first 3-4d): fever, chills, sweats, GI sx, cough, HA, malaise, chest pain, but no coryza; Stage 2: sepsis.
- Epidemiology: exposure in time & place to airspace of case/environment.
- Lab: pre-Rx blood (+); CXR: wide mediastinum & bloody pleural effusion; CT scan: hyperdense mediastinal nodes + edema

COMMON PATHOGENS: Bacillus anthracis

TREATMENT REGIMENS

Treatment
- Ciprofloxacin 400mg IV q8h or doxycycline 100mg IV q12h or levofloxacin 750mg IV qd; each plus 1-2 additional antibiotics
- Additional IV ABX: clindamycin 600mg q8h, imipenem 1gm q6h, chloramphenicol 1g q6h, rifampin 300mg q12h, pen G 4mU q4h--all IV.
- Drain pleural effusion: repeated thoracentesis or thoracotomy tube
- Meningitis (CNS penetration): add penicillin, chloramphenicol and/or rifampin.
- Mediastinal edema/meningitis: consider prednisone 60-80mg/d
- PO switch when stable & > or equal to 14-21 d IV: ciprofloxacin 750mg bid or doxy 100mg bid, levofloxacin 750mg qd; each +/- rifampin 300mg bid PO
- Duration: 60-100 d, then close follow-up

Treatment - special populations
- Pregnancy, lactation: doxy/cipro regimen; consider amoxicillin 0.5-1g PO tid +/- rifampin 300mg PO bid after >14-21d & stable to complete 60-100d
- Immunosuppressed: standard Rx

- Peds: cipro 10-15mg/kg IV q 12h, not to exceed 1gm/day OR doxy >8yrs >45kg: 100mg q 12h; >8 & <45kg or <8: 2.2mg/kg q 12h

Drug-Specific Comments

Amoxicillin: Penicillin is FDA-approved for anthrax and shown to work in primate model; amoxicillin is not FDA-approved for anthrax & not tested in primates. Other concerns are that levels achieved with oral administration and the inducable penicllinase produced by B. anthracis. Conclusion: amoxicillin is an option if there is low microbial load (post initial therapy or post initial prophylaxis) plus reason to avoid cipro & doxy (peds or pregnancy); even then some would not use it & some would use it only in high doses of 3-3.5gm/d.

Amoxicillin + Clavulanate: Beta-lactamase inhibitor does not inactivate beta-lactamases of B. anthracis and may contribute to inducing beta-lactamase production.

Ampicillin + Sulbactam: Beta-lactamase inhibitor does not inactivate beta-lactamases of B. anthracis and may contribute to inducing beta-lactamase production.

Ceftazidime: This and other 3rd generation cephalosporins are not active vs. B. anthracis due to cephalosporinases. Bad choice.

Ciprofloxacin: Ciprofloxacin is one of four FDA-approved drugs for inhalation anthrax. It was accepted based on the experience with the primate model at USAMRIID ten years ago. It is active against virtually all strains and performed well in the 2001 epidemic.

Clarithromycin: Marginal in vitro activity vs. B. anthracis and no clinical experience. Not a good choice.

Doxycycline: Very active in vitro, FDA-approved for anthrax and effective in primate model. This plus cipro and levo are preferred drugs for treatment and prophylaxis.

Gatifloxacin: As active as cipro in vitro, but not FDA-approved for anthrax and untested in primate model. Most authorities think that cipro is preferred but that gatifloxacin should work just as well.

Imipenem/Cilastatin: Highly active in vitro but not tested in animal model & not FDA-approved for anthrax. Rational adjunct to cipro or doxy with systemic disease.

Levofloxacin: FDA approved for inhalation anthrax and effective in the primate model.

Linezolid: Active in vitro, but no clinical or animal model experience. May be used as adjunct to cipro or doxy with systemic disease when IV therapy needed.

Moxifloxacin: As active as cipro in vitro, but not FDA-approved for anthrax and untested in primate model. Most authorities think that cipro is preferred but that moxifloxacin should work just as well.

Penicillin: Penicillin G: FDA-approved for anthrax, reasonably effective in primate model, very active in vitro & extensive prior use with clinical anthrax. Concern is that B. anthracis makes inducible penicillinase that makes penicillin risky as single agent with high microbial load. Sometimes advocated as adjunct to cipro, levo or doxy with serious clinical disease especially with meningitis.

Piperacillin + Tazobactam: Beta-lactamase inhibitor does not inactivate beta-lactamases of B. anthracis and may contribute to inducing beta-lactamase production.

Ticarcillin + Clavulanic Acid: Beta-lactamase inhibitor does not inactivate beta-lactamases of B. anthracis and may contribute to inducing beta-lactamase production.

Important Points

- Guidelines: CDC (MMWR 2001;50:909) & Hopkins Biodefense Center (JAMA 2002;287:2236)
- Keys to dx: exposure + CT chest, bloody pleural effusions & positive pretreatment blood cultures.

- Key Rx: early abx & drain pleural effusions
- Notify Infection Control & Public Health Dept. immediately; inhalation anthrax = bioterrorism.
- Rx 60-100 days because spores persist in vivo > 30 days. Rx required in primate model. Cipro, levo & doxycycline considered equal & superior to other abx.

Selected Readings

Meyerhoff A, Albrecht R, Meyer JM, et al. US Food and Drug Administration approval of ciprofloxacin hydrochloride for management of postexposure inhalational anthrax. Clin Infect Dis 2004;39:303-308

Reissman DB, Whitney FA, Taylor TH Jr, et al. One-year health assessment of adult survivors of Bacillus anthracis infection. JAMA 2004;291:1944-8

Keuhnert MJ, Doyle TJ, Hill HA, et al. Clinical features that discriminate inhalational anthrax from other acute respiratory illnesses. Clin Infect Dis 2003;36:328-36.

Blank S, Moskin LC, Zucker JR. An ounce of prevention is a ton of work: Mass antibiotic prophylaxis for anthrax, New York City, 2001. Emerg Infect Dis 2003;9:615

Barakat LA, et al. Fatal inhalation anthrax in a 94 year old Connecticut woman. JAMA 2002;287:863

Mina B, et al. Fatal inhalational anthrax with unknown source of exposure in a 61 year old woman in NYC. JAMA 2002;287:858

Inglesby TV, O'Toole T, Henderson DA, et al. Anthrax as a biological weapon, 2002: updated recommendations for management. JAMA 2002;287:2236

Baillie L, Read TD. Bacillus anthracis, a bug with an attitude. Curr Opinion Microbiol 2001;4:78

Centers for Disease Control. Considerations for distinguishing influenza - like illness from inhalation anthrax. MMWR 2001;50:984

Centers for Disease Control. Update: Investigation of bioterrorism - related anthrax and interim guidelines for clinical evaluation of persons with possible anthrax. MMWR 2001;50:941

ANTHRAX, PROPHYLAXIS
John G. Bartlett, M.D.

Diagnostic Criteria

- Goal is to prevent inhalation anthrax
- Risks: Particle size (<10 microns), airspace exposure w/cases, positive nasal cult, positive environmental culture
- High risk occurrence: Postal workers, media, politicians (2001 epidemic)
- Mail contact accounted for 20/22 anthrax cases in 2001

Common Pathogens: Bacillus anthracis

Treatment Regimens

Antibiotics

- Preferred: Doxycycline 100mg bid or ciprofloxacin 500mg bid or levofloxacin 500mg qd x 60-100d +/- anthrax vaccine
- Alternative (after doxy, levo or cipro x 14d
- Pregnancy: Cipro or levo regimen; consider amoxicillin after 14 days
- Immunosuppressed: Standard
- Peds: Cipro 10-15mg/kg q 12h x 60d
- Peds: Doxy >8yrs & >45kg - 100mg bid; <8 or >8 & <45kg - 2.2mg/kg bid x 60d
- Duration: 60 days or 100 days or vaccine at 60 days and then 40 more days

Prophylaxis candidates

- Goal - prevent inhalation anthrax via aerosolized spores from powder particle size <10 microns
- Risk assessment: Defined by public health officials

Diagnosis

- Environmental sampling: Best cultures - nasal, environ, surface and suspect powder
- Duration prophylaxis: exposure confirmed - 60-100 days; exposure excluded - D/C prophylaxis

Drug-Specific Comments

Amoxicillin: Penicillin is FDA-approved for anthrax and shown to work in primate model; amoxicillin is not FDA-approved for anthrax and not tested in primates. Other concerns are that levels achieved with oral administration and the inducible penicillinase produced by B. anthracis. Conclusion: Amoxicillin is consequently an option if there is low microbial load (post initial therapy or post initial prophylaxis) plus reason to avoid cipro & doxy (peds or pregnancy); even then some would not use it and some would use it only in high doses of 3-3.5g/d

Doxycycline: Very active in vitro, FDA-approved for anthrax and effective in primate model. This plus cipro and levo are preferred drugs for treatment and prophylaxis.

Gatifloxacin: As active as cipro in vitro, but not FDA-approved for anthrax and untested in primate model. Most authorities think that cipro is preferred but that Gatifloxacin should work just as well.

Levofloxacin: FDA approved for anthrax and effective in the primate model.

Moxifloxacin: As active as cipro in vitro, but not FDA-approved for anthrax and untested in primate model. Most authorities think that cipro is preferred but that gatifloxacin should work just as well.

Important Points

- Guidelines (treatment) from CDC (MMWR 2001;50:909; 987; 1008); MMWR 2002;50:1142)
- Purpose of prophylaxis is to prevent inhalation anthrax
- 60-100 days because this was required in primate model
- Doxy, levo & cipro are equivalent and preferred
- Must start prophylaxis based on suspected exposure, then D/C at 10-14 days if risk assessment neg
- Recommendations based on 2001 epidemic; next one, will need abx sensitivity.

Selected Readings

Manobee RJ, Stewart WD. The decontamination of Gruinard Island. Chem Br July 1988;690

Friedlander A, Welkos SL, Pitt ML, et al. Postexposure prophylaxis against experimental inhalation anthrax. JID 1993;167:1239

Cole LA. Bioterrorism threats: Learning from inappropriate responses. J Pub Health Manag Prat 2000;6:8

Kiel JL, Parker JE, Alls JL, et al. Rapid recovery and identification of anthrax bacteria from the environment. Ann NY Acad Sci 2000;916:240

Doganay M, Aydin N. Antimicrobial susceptibility of Bacillus anthracis. Scan J Infect Dis 1991;23:333

Inglesby T, Henderson DA, Bartlett JB, et al. Anthrax as a biological weapon. JAMA 1999;281:1735

Centers for Disease Control. Update: Investigation of bioterrorism - related anthrax, 2001. MMWR 2001;50:1008

Centers for Disease Control. Notice to Readers: Interim guidelines for investigation of and response to Bacillus anthracis exposures. MMWR 2001;50:987

Centers for Disease Control. Update: Interim recommendations for antimicrobial prophylaxis for children and breastfeeding mothers and treatment of children with anthrax. MMWR 2001;50:1014

Centers for Disease Control. Update: Investigations of bioterrorism - related anthrax and adverse events from antimicrobial prophylaxis. MMWR 2001;50:973

ANTIRETROVIRAL THERAPY (INITIAL REGIMEN)

John G. Bartlett, M.D.

DIAGNOSTIC CRITERIA
- Indications: definite: CD4 <200 or AIDS dx; indications for all guidelines in world.
- Indications: probably : CD4 200-350; influenced by VL, CD4 slope, pt readiness.
- Indications: usually not : CD4 >350 except pregnancy (to protect infant) and viral load (VL) >100,000 (no consensus).
- DHHS (federal) & IAS-USA are nearly identical for indications for ART.

COMMON PATHOGENS: HIV

TREATMENT REGIMENS

Regimens
- Preferred DHHS: EFV + (3TC or FTC) + (ZDV or TDF); or LPV/r + (3TC or FTC) + AZT.
- Preferred IAS-USA: 2 NRTI + EFV or boosted PI (ATV/r, SQV/r, LPV/r or IDV/r) + (ZDV or TDF) + (3TC or FTC).
- Alternatives (DHHS): 2NRTIs + ATV, FPV/r, FPV, IDV/r, LPV/r, NFV or SQV/r.
- NRTIs (DHHS): (3TC or FTC) + (ZDV, d4T, ABC, ddI, or TDF).
- Principles: start w/ 3 active drugs from 2 classes, emphasize adherence, warn of side effects and monitor VL as most important goal of Rx.

Doses (in mg/d)
- NRTI: ABC - 600mg/d; ddI - 400mg/d, FTC - 200mg/d, 3TC - 300mg/d, d4T 30 or 40mg bid, TDF 300mg/d, AZT 300mg bid.
- NNRTI: EFV 600mg qhs, NVP 200mg/d x 2 wks, then 200mg bid.
- PI: ATV/r 300/100 qd; LPV/r 3 tabs bid; FPV/r 700/100 bid; IDV/r 800/100 bid; SQV/r 1000/100 bid; NFV 1250 bid.
- Combinations: AZT/3TC (Combivir) bid; AZT/3TC/ABC (Trizivir) bid; TDF/FTC (Truvada) qd; 3TC/ABC (Epizicom) qd.
- Food: fasting - ddI, IDV. Food required: NFV, ATV, LPV.

Monitoring HAART
- Baseline: CBC, Chem, U/A, LFTs, fasting lipids, fasting glucose, viral load, CD4 count.
- Optional: pregnancy test, HIV resistance test.
- Virologic goals: VL decrease by 1 log at 1-4 wks, <500 by 16-24 wks, <50 by 48 wks.
- CD4 increase: expect increase of 100-150/yr if achieving viral load suppression goals
- Viral failure: caused by resistance or failure of drugs to reach target - adherence, food effect, drug interaction, metabolism.
- Adherence: need >95% adherence to get VL <500 in >80% pts.

DRUG-SPECIFIC COMMENTS

Abacavir (ABC): (Ziagen) Most potent of the NRTIs. Main concern is sparce studies with anything other than AZT +/- 3TC and hypersensitivity reactions that may be serious. The hypersensitivity reactions scare pts & physicians due to severity & result in many unnecessary discontinuations. Most have fever + GI sx +/- rash. If unclear - may wish to give under observation; this will always result in reaction if it is due to hypersensitivity. Cause is completely unknown. Gaining interest is ABC + 3TC for once daily admin.

Atazanavir (ATV): A potent, once daily PI without a lipid effect. Most use it with RTV. Be aware of drug interactions, especially anything that neutralizes gastric acid. (Need food and acid for optimal absorption)

Delavirdine (DLV): This NNRTI is not being used much, probably because it wasn't studied extensively, the pill burden was too high and no niche was defined.

Efavirenz (EFV): (Sustiva) An NNRTI that has an excellent track record including good results in pts with a VL >100,000 c/mL at baseline. Long half-life gives good pharmacologic barrier to resistance. Main problem is poorly understood CNS toxicity during the first 2-3 wks. This will be experienced with the first dose and usually resolve in 2-4wks. There is concern about using this drug in pts with addictions or major psychiatric illnesses, but the experience is too limited to know if the concern is justified.

Fosamprenavir (FPV): Now supplants amprenavir due to reduced pill burden. Potent PI that is usually boosted.

Indinavir (IDV): (Crixivan) A potent PI, but has some problems: Must be given at 8hr intervals due to close toxic-therapeutic ratio, must be taken in empty stomach and causes nephrolithiasis due to IDV kidney stones. Most HIV providers give IDV with RTV to eliminate the need for q8h administration and the pharmacology profile looks good. The main question is the dose - 400/400 bid or 800/100-200 bid. The 800mg dose of IDV increases the risk of kidney stones, but is better tolerated due to the lower dose of RTV. No good answer here.

Lamivudine (3TC): Best tolerated of the nucleosides. Also unique in the rapid development of high level resistance which is bad news (3TC resistance) and good news (reduced fitness and high activity of AZT, tenofovir, etc). Probably can be used once daily, but not FDA approved for this.

Lopinavir (LPV): (Kaletra) Combined with a small dose of RTV to give a really good pharmacologic profile. This is 1 of 2 agents showing superior activity vs other commonly used HAART regimens in pts w/ a baseline VL >100,000 c/mL (Efavirenz is the other). Main controversy here is whether LPV/RTV should be used 1st or should be saved for salvage. Resistance profile is interesting-no defined primary resistance mutations, but poor response when there are >/= 5 secondary PI mutation. Drug is well tolerated but high rates of diarrhea that are less severe than w/ nelfinavir, and easily controlled w/imodium.

Nelfinavir (NFV): A favored PI because of good clinical performance. It may have advantages in ease of salvage, and there is good pt tolerance. More recent studies now question its favored status compared to alternative regimens, esp. the PI-RTV combinations and these alternative regimens in the presence of a high baseline VL. Of the PIs, this is the one that gets the least boost with RTV. Main side effect is diarrhea which is secretory and usually controlled by Imodium or calcium. Mechanism is unclear. Dose is 750mg tid or 1250 bid; most now use 1250 bid.

Nevirapine (NVP): (Viramine) This NNRTI has performed reasonably well in clinical trials including use as part of a 3 drug regimen in chronically infected pts and as a single dose regimen to prevent perinatal transmission. There are two important side effects - rash in 15-20% that may be serious in 2-3% and hepatotoxicity in 16-18%. Both occur primarily in the first 6 wks of therapy and in women with CD4 counts of >250mm3.

Ritonavir (RTV): This drug is the most potent inhibitor of the p450 metabolic pathway which is the main mechanism of elimination of most PIs. RTV is commonly included with another PI as an "extender" to improve the pharmacology profile of the companion PI. When 100-200 doses are used, RTV is there only for its pharmacology properties; when 400mg are used, RTV may act as an antiretroviral agent as well. The main problem with RTV as a single PI is that few pts can tolerate the 500-600mg bid dose necessary to achieve anti-HIV activity.

Saquinavir (SQV): (Inviron, Fortovase) Two formulation: Invirase which is always combined with RTV and now preferred over Fortovase due to better GI tolerance.

Stavudine (d4T): A charmed NRTI until recently. This drug is well tolerated, easily taken, and commonly given with ddI or 3TC. More recently there is concern about lactic acidosis, peripheral neuropathy and pancreatitis, esp when combined with ddI. Nevertheless, lactic acidosis & pancreatitis are relatively rare and peripheral neuropathy is pretty easy to detect early enough to stop use.

Zidovudine (AZT): (Retrovir) First FDA approved antiretroviral agent - 1987. Established efficacy in preventing perinatal tx, preventing tx after occupational exposure, Rx of HIV-associated dementia and ITP. By itself, not very potent and resistance is common after prolonged use with incomplete viral suppression. Multiple side effects which are subjective (GI intol, asthemia, headache) and objective (neutropenia & anemia).

IMPORTANT POINTS

- Guidelines from Dept Health Human Services (www.hivatis.org) 4/7/2005
- Therapeutic goal: maximal viral suppression as long as possible, e.g., VL <50 or <500.
- Patient readiness for adherence to complex regimen is CRITICAL.
- Compliance with 95% of pills necessary for VL < 500 in > 50% pts; risk of noncompliance is HIV progression & viral resistance.
- About 50% pts change regimen within 2 yrs - half for ADR and half for virologic failure.

SELECTED READINGS

Yeni PG, Hammer SM, Hirsch M, et al. Treatment for adult HIV infection. JAMA 2004;292:251

Pau A, et al. Guidelines for the use of antiretroviral agents in HIV-1 infected adults and adolescents. October 29, 2004; http://AIDSinfo.nih.gov

Gallant JE, et al. Efficacy and safety to tenofovir vs. stavudine in combination therapy in antiretroviral-naive patients. JAMA 2004;292:191

Gulick RM, et al. Triple nucleoside regimens versus efavirenz - containing regimens for the initial treatment of HIV-1 infection. N Engl J Med 2004;350:1850

van Loth F, et al. Comparison of first-line antiretroviral therapy with regimens including nevirapine, efavirenz or both drugs, plus stavudine and lamivudine. Lancet 2004;363:1253

Kempf DJ, et al. Incidence of resistance in a double-blind study comparing lopinavir/ritonavir plus stavudine and lamivudine to nelfinavir plus stavudine and lamivudine. J Infect Dis 2004;189:51

Gulick RM, et al. Triple nucleoside regimens versus efavirenz-containing regimens for the initial treatment of HIV-1 infection. N Engl J Med 2004;350:1850

Palella FJ Jr, Delaney KM, Mooremar AC, et al. Declining mortality and morbidity among patients with advanced HIV. NEJM 1998;338:853

Moncroft A, Vella S, Benfield TL, et al. Changing patterns of mortality across Europe in patients infected with HIV-1. EuroSIDA Study Group. Lancet 1998;352:1725

Lucas GM, Chaisson RE, Moore RD. Highly active antiretroviral therapy in a large urban clinic. Ann Intern Med 1999;131:81

APPENDICITIS   Pamela A. Lipsett, M.D.; Chris Carpenter, M.D.

DIAGNOSTIC CRITERIA

- Despite advances in imaging and laboratory studies in recent years, patient history and physical exam (often serial exams) remain the basis for diagnosis.
- Hx/PE: Abdominal tenderness progressing to rigidity, right lower quadrant pain, and migration of pain from the periumbilical region to the right lower quadrant
- Lab: Leukocytosis with left shift and an elevated C-reactive protein are non-specific

Diagnosis

- Graded compression/color flow ultrasound and helical CT are useful adjuncts to clinical impression. Use in equivocal cases is of benefit
- A normal appendix seen in 15% of cases; perforation rates remain approximately 20%, higher in young (40-57%), and elderly (55-70%)

Treatment Regimens

Single agent prophylaxis or treatment

- Surgical removal of appendix is definitive therapy
- All treatment recommendations based on author's opinion according to Surgical Infection Society guidelines.
- Cefoxitin 1-2g IV q6
- Cefotetan 1-2g IV q12h
- Ticarcillin-clavulanate 3.1g IV q6h
- Ampicillin-sulbactam 3.0g IV q6h
- Piperacillin-tazobactam 3.375g IV q6h or 4.5g IV q8h
- Imipenem 0.5g IV q6h
- Meropenem 1.0g IV q8h

Combination prophylaxis or treatment

- Combination of either clindamycin (450-600mg IV q8h) or metronidazole (0.5g IV q6-8h)(load with 15/kg if life threatening) with one of the following:
- Cefuroxime 0.75g-1.5g IV q8h
- Ceftriaxone 2.0g IV q24h
- Cefotaxime 2.0g IV q6-8h
- Cefepime 2.0g IV q12h
- Ciprofloxacin 400mg IV q12h
- Levofloxacin 500mg IV q24h
- Gatifloxacin 400mg IV q24h
- Atreonam 1g IV q8hr - 2g IV q6h
- Gentamicin or tobramycin 2.0mg/kg loading dose then 1.7mg/kg q8h IV; once-a-day dosing may be considered

Drug-Specific Comments

Ampicillin + Sulbactam: Good single agent choice.

Aztreonam: Excellent gram negative coverage with no significant penicillin hypersensitivity cross-reaction; would reserve for seriously ill patients without good alternative coverage; use in combination with an antianaerobic agent.

Cefepime: Like ceftazidime, this agent's broad spectrum of activity, particularly against Pseudomonas, makes it an agent of choice for empiric treatment of nosocomial or iatrogenic infections.

Cefotetan: Good single agent coverage, drug currently not available in the U.S.

Gatifloxacin: Excellent gram-negative coverage with anaerobic activity; would combine with antianaerobic agent until further work suggests it can be used as a single agent.

Imipenem/Cilastatin: Good single agent choice, would consider reserving for seriously ill patients.

Meropenem: Good single agent choice, would consider reserving for seriously ill patients.

Piperacillin + Tazobactam: Good single agent choice.

Ticarcillin + Clavulanic Acid: Good single agent choice.

Tobramycin: Good gram negative coverage; use in combination with an antianaerobic agent; consider once-a-day dosing in appropriate patients.

IMPORTANT POINTS

- The differentiation between simple appendicitis and gangrenous appendicitis/ perforated appendicitis with peritonitis should determine the length of antibiotic administration.
- Simple appendicitis requires ONLY preoperative antibiotic prophylaxis.
- Gangrenous appendicitis and perforated appendicitis with peritonitis require a therapeutic course; 3 to 5 days is likely sufficient but longer courses may be indicated in complicated cases.
- Laparoscopy helpful with diagnostic accuracy esp in women ages 16-39, decreases unknown diagnosis
- Studies of non-operative management have not demonstrated comparable outcomes with surgery.
- Mortality 1/600; diagnostic accuracy varies by gender, male 78-92%, female 58-95%

SELECTED READINGS

Paulson EK,Kalady MF, Pappas TN. Suspected Appendicitis. N Engl J Med 2003;348:236-242

Mazuski JE. Sawyer, RG. Nathens AB et al. The Surgical Infection Society Guidelines on Antimicrobial Therapy for Intra-Abdominal Infections: An Executuve Summary. Surgical Infections, 2002, Vol 3

Andersen Br, Kallehave Fl, Anderson HR. Antibiotics vs. placebo for the prevention of Post Operative Infection after appendectomy. Coch Lib Issue 4 2002

Sauderland S, Leferang R, Neugebauer EAM: . Laparoscopic versus open surgery for suspected appendicitis. Coch Lib Issue 4, 2002

The Medical Letter, Inc. Antimicrobial Prophylaxis in Surgery. The Medical Letter,2001, October 29: Vol. 43 (1116-1117):92-97

PF Jones . Suspected acute appendicitis: Trends in management over 30 years. Br J Surgery 2001: 88;1570-1577

Birnbaum BA, Wilson SR. State of the Art. Appendicitis at the Millennium. Radiology 2000:215:337-348.

Hale DA, Molloy M, Pearl RH, Schutt DC, Jaques DP. Appendectomy: A Contemporary Appraisal. Annals of Surgery, Vol. 225(3), March 1997, 253-61

ARTHRITIS, COMMUNITY-ACQUIRED SEPTIC

Eric Nuermberger, M.D.

DIAGNOSTIC CRITERIA

- Hx: fever, chills, malaise, joint pain, swelling, decreased ROM
- Joint exam: tenderness, erythema, heat, swelling, decreased ROM (usually marked)
- Joint aspirate: + gram stain and/or Cx, neutrophilic leukocytosis (esp. >50,000/mm3), low glucose (<40 mg/dL), and/or no crystals
- Neg gram stain/Cx from joint, but + Cx from blood, cervix, urethra, throat, or rectum; positive nucleic acid test on urine or joint fluid; and/or typical skin lesions suggests gonococcal arthritis
- Ddx: Rheumatoid arthritis, gout, pseudogout, reactive arthritis (all cause PMN's in joint fluid); viral arthritis, Lyme disease; consider trauma or hemorrhage if bloody

COMMON PATHOGENS: Neisseria gonorrhoeae ; Staphylococcus aureus ; Streptococcus pyogenes (Group A) ; Enterobacteriaceae

TREATMENT REGIMENS

Empiric antimicrobial therapy

- nafcillin or oxacillin 2g IV q4h (GPC in clusters on Gram stain, IVDU, rheumatoid arthritis)

- Cefazolin 2 g IV q8h (GPC on gram stain)
- Vancomycin 1g IV q12h (suspected MRSA)
- Pen G 12-18mU/d or ampicillin 2mg IV q4h (GPC in chains on gram stain)
- Ceftriaxone 1-2g IV/IM q12-24h or cefotaxime 2g IV q8h (young adult, suspected gonorrhea or suggestive rash, gram-negative cocci on gram stain, concomitant meningitis)
- Ceftazidime 2g IV q8h or cefepime 2g IV q12h (GNR on gram stain, suspected Pseudomonas)
- Ampicillin/sulbactam 1.5-3g IV q4h (human, dog or cat bite)
- EMPIRIC THERAPY SHOULD ALWAYS BE MODIFIED BY CULTURE RESULTS

Pathogen-directed antimicrobial therapy

- Staph: nafcillin or oxacillin 2g IV q4h x 3wk
- Staph: cefazolin 2g IV q8h x 3wk
- Staph (MRSA): vancomycin 1g IV q12h x 3wk
- Strep (incl. PCN-sens S. pneumoniae [MIC<0.2 mg/L)]): PCN G 12-18 MU or ampicillin 2g IV q4h x 2wk
- Strep pneumoniae (PCN-resist): ceftriaxone 1-2g IV q12h or cefotaxime 2g IV q8h
- GNB: ceftriaxone 1-2g IV q12h or cefotaxime 2g IV q8h x 3wk
- GNB (P. aeruginosa): ceftazidime 2g IV q8h or cefepime 2g IV q12h, plus gentamicin or tobramycin 5 mg/kg IV q24h x 3wk
- GNB: ciprofloxacin 400mg IV or 750mg PO q12h or levofloxacin 500mg IV or 750mg PO qd x 3wk
- Staph/Anaerobes: ampicillin/sulbactam 1.5-3g IV q4h x 3wk
- Staph/Anaerobes: clindamycin 600mg IV q6-8h x 3wk

Therapy of gonococcal arthritis/disseminated infection

- Ceftriaxone 1g IV or IM q24h or cefotaxime 1g IV q8h or ceftizoxime 1g IV q8h
- Spectinomycin 2g IV or IM q12h (beta-lactam allergy) NO LONGER AVAILABLE IN U.S.
- CONTINUE PARENTERAL THERAPY UNTIL 24-48 HOURS AFTER IMPROVEMENT, THEN SWITCH TO ORAL AGENTS TO COMPLETE ONE WEEK (PURULENT ARTHRITIS MAY REQUIRE 2 WEEKS OF THERAPY)
- Cefixime 400mg PO bid
- Ciprofloxacin 500mg PO bid or levofloxacin 750mg PO qd
- Amoxicillin 500mg PO tid (if susceptibility established)
- All patients should also be empirically treated for concomitant chlamydia infection with doxycycline 100mg or ofloxacin 300mg PO bid x 7d or, if pregnant, azithromycin 1000mg PO once
- Sexual partners should receive ceftriaxone 125mg IM or cefixime 400mg PO once PLUS doxycycline 100mg PO bid x 7d
- Given rise of fluoroquinolone resistance in isolates from men who have sex with men and from Asia, Great Britain, Calif. and Hawaii, ceftriaxone is treatment of choice for these infections.

Drug-Specific Comments

Ampicillin + Sulbactam: The treatment of choice for infections which follow animal or human bites. Also a reliable alternative agent for staphylococcal infection.

Cefepime: Like ceftazidime, this agent's broad spectrum of activity, particularly against Pseudomonas, makes it an agent of choice for empiric treatment of nosocomial or iatrogenic infections.

Cefixime: Only CDC-recommended cephalosporin for oral stepdown therapy of disseminated gonococcal therapy. Empiric oral treatment of choice for men who have sex with men, infections acquired in Asia, England/Wales, Hawaii or California, where fluoroquinolone resistance has become prevalent. Only recently approved for manufacture again in the US--non-CDC-approved alternatives may include cefpodoxime 400mg or azithromycin 2g, possibly cefdinir 600mg.

Ceftazidime: Like cefepime, this agent's broad spectrum activity, particularly for Pseudomonas, makes it a favored agent for empiric coverage of nosocomial or iatrogenic infections

Ceftriaxone: 3rd generation cephalosporin is agent of choice for N. gonorrhoeae, Enterobacteriaceae and penicillin-non-susceptible Strep pneumoniae.

Ciprofloxacin: An alternative agent for Enterobacteriaceae and P. aeruginosa. Pro: early transition to oral therapy. Con: less clinical experience. No longer a recommended empiric regimen for gonococcal arthritis for patients at risk for infection with resistant isolate.

Daptomycin: Parenteral option for MRSA infections, though less experience with this drug than linezolid or quinupristin/dalfopristin.

Linezolid: Active against virtually all staphylococci. Excellent oral bioavailability offers early switch option to oral therapy, but it's expensive. Little experience treating septic arthritis.

Oxacillin: With nafcillin, the treatment of choice for methicillin-susceptible staphylococcal infections.

Spectinomycin: Alternative therapy for disseminated gonococcal infection as recommended by the CDC. Use for patients allergic to beta-lactams.

IMPORTANT POINTS

- Early treatment with IV abx and aspiration or surgical drainage reduces joint destruction.
- Suspect gonorrhoea in young adults, particularly if: sexually active, recent menses or childbirth, pustular skin lesions, tenosynovitis, if joint cultures are negative.
- When GC suspected, culture blood, urethra, cervix, rectum, pharynx, pustules & joint fluid. Notify microbiology laboratory to assure proper handling. Send urine nucleic acid test.
- Recommended treatment duration is 1 wk for GC; 2wk for streptococci, H. influenzae; 3wk for staph or GNB. Treatment must, however, be individualized.
- Pathogen Associations: rheumatoid arthritis--S. aureus; IVDU--S aureus, P. aeruginosa; dialysis-S. aureus; unpasteurized dairy products-Brucella; Sickle Cell Dz--Salmonella; diabetes-Grp B strep

SELECTED READINGS

Centers for Disease Control and Prevention. Increases in Fluoroquinolone-Resistant Neisseria gonorrhoeae Among Men Who Have Sex with Men --- United States, 2003, and Revised Recommendations for Gonorrhea Treatment, 2004 . MMWR 2004;53(16);335-338

Bardin T. Gonococcal arthritis. Best Pract Res Clin Rheumatol 2003;17:201-8

Centers for Disease Control and Prevention. Sexually transmitted diseases treatment guidelines 2002. MMWR Morb Mortal Wkly Rep 2002; 51(No. RR-6):1

Shirtliff ME, Mader JT. Acute Septic Arthritis. Clin. Microbiol. Rev. 2002;15 527-544

Donatto KC. Orthopedic management of septic arthritis. Rheum Dis Clin North Am 1998;24:275

Dubost J, Fis I, Denis P, et al. Polyarticular septic arthritis. Medicine 1993;72:296.

Ho G. How best to drain an infected joint. Will we ever know for certain?. J Rheumatol 1993;20:2001

ARTHRITIS, HARDWARE-ASSOCIATED SEPTIC

Eric Nuermberger, M.D.

DIAGNOSTIC CRITERIA

- Early-onset infections (within 2-3 mo. of surgery). Hx: joint pain (95%), fever (43%), swelling (38%), drainage (32%)
- PE: Erythema, induration, and edema at incision site +/- wound drainage
- Lab: Joint aspirate--cloudy fluid, WBC > 50,000 - 150,000 cells/mm3 predominantly neutrophilic, & pos gram-stain or culture.
- Late-onset infections. Hx: loosening of joint, progressive joint pain w/o fever or local signs of infections. PE: findings may be minimal.

COMMON PATHOGENS: Staphylococcus (coagulase-negative) ; S.aureus ; Streptococcus species ; Enterococcus ; Enterobacteriaceae

TREATMENT REGIMENS

Replacement arthroplasty (two-stage procedure)

- Stage 1: Remove prosthesis and debride infected tissue, replace prosthesis with abx-impregnated methylmethacrylate cement spacer
- IV abx for 6 weeks (see parenteral therapy below)
- Clinical monitoring for 2-4 weeks off abx then joint aspirate
- Stage 2: If aspirate negative, joint replacement with new prosthetic abx-impregnated cement. If positive, repeat irrigation/debridement, then IV antibiotics for 6 weeks, then aspirate
- One-stage replacements (removal and replacement of prosthesis during the same operation)--less successful; reserve for infx with highly-susceptible organisms (e.g., streptococci)
- Arthrodesis required when tissues inadequate for functional arthroplasty or for antibiotic-resistant organisms or prior failed replacement
- Amputation is last resort for intractable pain, incurable infection, or heavy bone loss that prevents arthrodesis
- Some early infections may respond to debridement and long course IV and oral abx if acted upon early (e.g., within 48 hours of onset of symptoms)

Parenteral therapy

- Staph (MSSA): nafcillin or oxacillin 2g IV q4-6h x 4-6 wks
- Staph (MSSA): cefazolin 2g IV q8h x 4-6 wks
- Staph (MRSA): vancomycin 30mg/kg/d IV divided q12h x 4-6 wks
- Staph: clindamycin 600-900mg IV q8h x 4-6 wks
- GNB: ceftriaxone 2 g IV qd or bid or cefotaxime 2g IV q6-8h x 4-6 wks
- GNB: ceftazidime 2g IV q8h or cefepime 2g IV q12h (+ gentamicin or tobramycin 1.7 mg/kg IV q8h >/= 2 wks) x 4-6 wks
- GNB: ciprofloxacin 400mg IV q12h or levofloxacin 750 mg IV q24h x 4-6 wks (may allow early conversion to orals)
- Candida: amphotericin B 0.5-1.0 mg/kg IV qd x 6-8 wks
- Candida (not krusei or glabrata): fluconazole 400mg PO or IV qd or bid x 6-8 wks
- Strep: penicillin G 4mU IV q4h x 4-6 wks

Oral therapy (consolidative or suppressive)

- Suppressive abx therapy appropriate if removal of prosthesis not possible and pathogen susceptible to oral abx

- Long-term oral abx rarely successful long term due to loosening of prosthesis, purulent arthritis and/or fistulization, or sepsis
- Suppressive oral therapy is most effective after induction with IV antibiotics
- Ciprofloxacin 750mg PO q12h or levofloxacin 750mg PO qd + rifampin 600mg PO qd (preferred for staphylococcal infections)
- Cephalexin 500mg PO q6h
- Dicloxacillin 500mg PO q6h
- Clindamycin 300-450mg PO q6-8h
- Amoxicillin/clavulanate 500mg PO q8h
- Minocycline 100mg PO q12h + rifampin 600mg PO qd
- Fluconazole 400mg PO q12-24h

DRUG-SPECIFIC COMMENTS

Cefepime: This 4th generation cephalosporin has broad coverage for a variety of gram-positive and -negative organisms, including S. aureus and P. aeruginosa. It is probably most helpful in empiric coverage when highly resistant gram-negatives are suspected or treatment of infections in which resistance to other agents is confirmed.

Ceftazidime: Enhanced activity against Pseudomonas aeruginosa over other cephalosporins makes this agent the treatment of choice when that organism is suspected or confirmed, including empiric treatment of post-operative joint infection when the Gram stain of the joint aspirate shows gram-negative bacilli or no organisms. This agent should be avoided in staphylococcal infections due to reduced activity in comparison to other cephalosporins.

Ciprofloxacin: Together with ofloxacin, these older-generation fluoroquinolones have demonstrated efficacy for infections of hardware, particularly when given with rifampin. Though untested, newer fluoroquinolones with more potent gram-positive activity would be expected to perform even better.

Linezolid: Broad gram-positive activity including S. epidermidis, MRSA and VRE. Use should be restricted to cases in which there are no alternative options. Available for oral and parenteral use; both are very expensive. Long-term use may be complicated by reversible thrombocytopenia and anemia.

Minocycline: A good choice for the chronic suppression of prosthetic joint infection with MRSA. Minocycline is the tetracycline with the greatest activity against staphylococci and beta-hemolytic streptococci. It is active against some strains of S. aureus which are resistant to tetracycline. Administration with rifampin may prevent the development of resistance to either agent during therapy.

IMPORTANT POINTS

- Must obtain joint aspirate when possible for micro dx to guide abx therapy
- When possible, AVOID ANTIBIOTICS (including perioperatively) before obtaining joint aspirate or intraoperative cultures
- Culture of S. epidermidis or other common contaminant more likely true infxn if: seen on Gram stain, grown on agar (not broth only) and >1 culture pos.
- Cultures may be falsely neg. in late-onset infections, requiring open bx of synovium and periprosthetic tissue.
- For cultures before elec. revision arthroplasty, send 3 or more specimens from different sites in operative space.
- Guidelines are authors' opinion.

SELECTED READINGS

Brandt CM, Sistrunk WW, Duffy MC, et al. Staphylococcus aureus prosthetic joint infection treated with debridement and prosthesis retention. Clin Infect Dis 1997;24:914

Zimmerli W, Widmer AF, Blatter M, et al. Role of rifampin for treatment of orthopedic implant-related staphylococcal infections. JAMA 1998;279:1537

Drancourt M, Stein A, Argenson JN, et al. Oral rifampin plus ofloxacin for treatment of Staphylococcus-infected implants. Antimicrob Agents Chemother 1993;37:1214

Ure KJ, Amstutz HC, Schmalzried TP. Direct-exchange arthroplasty for the treatment of infection after total hip replacement. J Bone Joint Surg Am 1998, 80-A:961

Wininger DA, Fass RJ. Antibiotic impregnated cement and beads for orthopedic infections. Antimicrob Agents Chemother 1996;40:2675

Garvin KL, Hanssen AD. Infection after total hip arthroplasty. J Bone Joint Surg Am 1995;77:1576

Goulet JA, Pellicci PM, Brause BD, et al. Prolonged suppression of infection in total hip arthroplasty. J Arthroplasty 1988;3:109

Segreti J, Nelson JA, Trenholme GM. Prolonged suppressive antibiotic therapy for infected orthopedic prostheses. Clin Infect Dis 1998;27:711

Steckelberg JM, Osmon DR . Prosthetic joint infections. In: Infections Associated with Indwelling Medical Devices, Bisno AL, Waldvogel FA (Eds.), Washington: ASM Press, 1994, pp259-290

Phelan DM, Osmon DR, Keating MR, Hanssen AD. Delayed reimplantation arthroplasty for candidal prosthetic joint infection: A report of 4 cases and review of the literature. Clin Infect Dis 2002;34:930-8

ARTHRITIS, LYME
Eric Nuermberger, M.D.

DIAGNOSTIC CRITERIA

- Suspect in pts with outdoor activity, history of tick bite in endemic region OR prior history of Lyme disease (e.g., erythema migrans).
- Late Lyme arthritis: Recurrent attacks (weeks or months) of objective joint swelling in one or few (<5) large joints, generally with intercurrent remission.
- Chronic (persistent) arthritis: at least one episode of continual joint inflammation lasting 1 year or longer
- Synovial fluid: WBC 10,000 - 100,000 with predominance of PMNs. Evidence of B. burgdorferi infection in synovial fluid: pos. culture (<20%), PCR (depending on lab, >90%) are definitive.
- Or typical arthritis and positive blood serology for B. burgdorferi by EIA with Western blot IgG (seronegative Lyme arthritis is distinctly rare).

COMMON PATHOGENS: Borrelia burgdorferi

TREATMENT REGIMENS

Initial therapy

- Doxycycline 100mg PO bid x 28d
- Amoxicillin 500mg PO tid x 28d
- Constant pain usually decreases within 2-3 weeks of antibiotic therapy although swelling and intermittent pain can take up to 8 wks to respond.
- If symptoms persist or relapse two months or more after completion of therapy, options include repeating an oral course or giving parenteral therapy (see below)

Parenteral therapy

- Parenteral therapy is given initially if arthritis is accompanied by neurologic manifestations or after failure of oral therapy
- Ceftriaxone 2g IV qd x 14-28d

- Cefotaxime 2g IV q8h x 14-28d
- Penicillin G 18-24 mU IV in 4 divided doses qd x 14-28d

Adjunctive therapy
- For patients with persistent/recurrent arthritis despite one month of appropriate parenteral therapy (mechanism is likely immune-mediated): Consider rheumatology evaluation.
- Non-steroidal anti-inflammatory drugs
- Intraarticular corticosteroid injections
- Hydroxychloroquine or methotrexate
- Arthroscopic synovectomy for persistent pain and functional limitation

DRUG-SPECIFIC COMMENTS

Amoxicillin: Recommended by IDSA guidelines and most experts as a first line therapy for Lyme arthritis. When used with probenecid, more patients developed later neuroborreliosis than after doxycycline therapy in a small study. Some have stated that probenecid may inhibit CNS penetration of amoxicillin. Dosing frequency may make this less attractive than doxycycline for initial therapy.

Ceftriaxone: Agent of choice if arthritis is accompanied by neurologic manifestations or following failure of oral therapy. No benefit to increasing daily dose from 2g to 4g. Biliary complications (incl. cholecystitis) may occur during 28-day course.

Doxycycline: First-line oral agent for Lyme arthritis according to IDSA guidelines and other expert recommendations. Lower cost and fewer serious adverse effects make initial oral therapy preferable to parenteral therapy.

Penicillin: Aqueous penicillin G is an alternative to the 3rd generation cephalosporins, although it appears less effective than ceftriaxone. Benzathine penicillin should not be used due to low achievable blood levels.

IMPORTANT POINTS

- Guidelines based on IDSA recommendations (Wormser GP, Nadelman RP, et al; Practice Guidelines for the Treatment of Lyme Disease; Clin Infect Dis 2000; 31 (Suppl 1)S1 - S14.)
- Because Lyme disease is primarily a clinical diagnosis, laboratory confirmation (serologic testing) is adjunctive. Seropositivity does not imply active disease or causality.
- Patients with late Lyme arthritis almost always have positive serology.
- Any associated neurologic or cognitive complaints should be pursued (MRI, lumbar puncture, neuropsychiatric testing) to evaluate for neuroborreliosis that would require parenteral therapy.
- Use objective clinical findings (inflamm. arthritis, neurologic signs), not non-specific symptoms to monitor treatment efficacy. Synovial fluid PCR may help differentiate lack of response.
- Post-Lyme disease syndromes following appropriate abx therapy (myalgia, fatigue etc.) do not respond to additional antibiotic therapy. We suggest trials of low impact aerobic exercise conditioning programs, NSAIDs, trials of venlafaxine XR (for those with significant somatic pain titrating up to 150-225mg qd) or SSRI's (esp. with anxiety) or tricyclics (for those with esp. disturbed sleep).
- Some patients will have persistent or recurrent joint swelling following one month of parenteral therapy. For patients with evidence of ongoing borrelial infection of the synovium (positive synovial fluid culture or PCR for B. burgdorferi DNA, increased synovial fluid concentrations of specific antibody to B. burgdorferi by ELISA or western

blot), another course of parenteral therapy may be efficacious. For those without evidence of persistent infection, further antibiotic therapy is not recommended. Use of long courses of parenteral antibiotics, antibiotic combinations or pulse therapy has not been rigorously studied and may lead to detrimental adverse effects. For patients with chronic symptoms after appropriate antibiotic therapy, adjunctive therapies (listed above) are recommended. Furthermore, the natural history of Lyme arthritis is such that the majority of cases resolve over a period of years with the exception of those suffering persistent inflammation (<10% likelihood).

SELECTED READINGS

Stanek G, Strle F. Lyme borreliosis. Lancet 2003;362:1639-47

Klempner MS, Hu LT, Evans J et al. Two controlled trials of antibiotic treatment in patients with persistent symptoms and a history of Lyme disease. N Engl J Med 2001;345:85-92.

Gary P. Wormser, Robert B. Nadelman, Raymond J. Dattwyler, et al. Practice Guidelines for the Treatment of Lyme Disease. Clin Inf Dis 2000;31:S1-14

Eckman MH, Steere AC, Kalish RA, et al. Cost effectiveness of oral as compared with intravenous antibiotic therapy for patients with early Lyme disease or Lyme arthritis. N Engl J Med 1997;337:357

Steere AC. Diagnosis and treatment of Lyme arthritis. Med Clin North Am 1997;81:179

Steere AC, Levin R, Molloy P, et al. Treatment of Lyme arthritis. Arthritis Rheum 1994;37:878

Nocton JJ, Dressler F, Rutledge BJ, et al. Detection of Borrelia burgdorferi DNA by polymerase chain reaction in synovial fluid from patients with Lyme arthritis. N Engl J Med 1994;330:229

Sigal LH. Persisting complaints attributed to chronic Lyme disease: Possible mechanisms and implications for management. Am J Med 1994;96:365

Lightfoot RW, Luft BJ, Rahn DW, et al. Empiric parenteral antibiotic treatment of patients with fibromyalgia/fatigue and a positive serologic result for Lyme disease: A cost-effectiveness analysis. Ann Intern Med 1993;119;503

Anonymous. Ceftriaxone-associated biliary complications of treatment of suspected disseminated Lyme disease--New Jersey, 1990-1992. M.M.W.R. 1993;42:39

ARTHRITIS, SEXUALLY ASSOCIATED REACTIVE (SARA)

Noreen A. Hynes, M.D., M.P.H.

DIAGNOSTIC CRITERIA

- Hx: Arthritis onset in last 30d; antecedent NGU/cervicitis 1 to 4 wks before onset or new sexual partner in last 90 days with NGU/cervicitis; family Hx of spondyloarthritis or iritis.
- Sx: arthritis in up to 6 joints (esp knees, feet); enthesopathy/fasciitis (20%); low back pain/stiffness; irritable eyes w/ or w/o redness; conjunctivitis (20-50%); iritis (2-11%); malaise (10%)
- Signs: urethritis in men or cervicitis in women seen at times concurrent with onset; asymmetric arthritis of 1-5 lower limb joints; tenosynovitis (30%); psoriasiform rash (12%); nail dystrophy (6-12%)
- Other findings: circinate balanitis or vulvitis (14-40%); geographical tongue (16%); keratoderma blennorrhagica (up to 30%); cardiac conduction delays (5-14%); fever and wt loss (10%).
- Essentials of Dx: (1) recognize clinical features of spondyloarthropathy, (2) full screening for STDs (3) ESR, CRP or plasma viscosity (4) CBC (5) urinalysis.

COMMON PATHOGENS: Chlamydia trachomatis ; Neisseria gonorrhoeae

Treatment Regimens

General approach
- Genital infection present: Abx for infection identified (see "Cervicitis" or "Urethritis")
- Constitutional sx: rest, NSAIDs
- Arthritis: rest with activity restriction esp weight bearing when leg joints involved; physical therapy; NSAIDs; ? intra-articular steroids (in consultation with rheumatologist)
- Ocular lesions: managed in consultation with an ophthalmologist. Slit lamp exam essential as missed anterior uveitis may rapidly lead to cataract formation and blindness.
- Skin/mucous membrane lesions: In consultation with a dermatologist.

Drug-Specific Comments

Cefixime: Single dose directly observed therapy is preferred for those patients for whom adherence is in question. Excellent single dose therapy for gonorrhea. Longer course antibiotic Rx has been considered in SARA. Most trials have been small and used ciprofloxacin, a drug with low efficacy against C. trachomatis, the prinicple microbe associated with SARA. Conflicting results obtained with some showing benefit to 3 mos of Rx and others showing no benefit. The role of long-term Abx in non-chlamydial SARA is not established.

Ceftizoxime: Ceftizoxime offers NO advantage in comparison to ceftriaxone.

Ceftriaxone: Ceftriaxone has been shown in clinical studies to be safe and highly effective against uncomplicated urogenital and anorectal gonococcal infections.

Doxycycline: Highly effective against C. trachomatis. Very inexpensive but must be taken for 7 days. Avoid this Rx if suspect pt will be non-adherent.

Gatifloxacin: Gatifloxacin appears to be safe and effective for the treatment of uncomplicated gonorrhea, but data regarding its use are limited. Fluoroquinolones (FQ) should not be used to Rx GC acquired in MA, CA, HI, New York City or the Pacific Basin due to the emergence of FQ-resistant GC.

Lomefloxacin: Lomefloxacin appears to be safe and effective for the treatment of uncomplicated gonorrhea, but data regarding its use are limited. Fluoroquinolones (FQ) should not be used to Rx GC acquired in MA, CA, HI, New York City or the Pacific Basin due to the emergence of FQ-resistant GC.

Norfloxacin: Norfloxacin appears to be safe and effective for the treatment of uncomplicated gonorrhea, but data regarding its use are limited. Fluoroquinolones (FQ) should not be used to Rx GC acquired in MA, CA, HI, New York City or the Pacific Basin due to the emergence of FQ-resistant GC.

Spectinomycin: Spectinomycin is expensive and must be injected. However, it has been effective in published clinical trials, curing 98.2% of uncomplicated urogenital and anorectal gonococcal infections. Its role is in the treatment of pts who cannot tolerate cephalosporins or quinolones.

Important Points

- Recommendations based on 2001 UK National Guideline on the Management of Sexually Acquired Reactive Arthritis [Clinical Effectiveness Group of AGM and MSSVD]
- SARA is probably best managed in consultation with a rheumatologist; HLA-B27 association; recurrences common; can also occur following certain GI infections.
- Constitutional symptoms: fatigue malaise, fever, weight loss. Must distinguish from disseminated gonococcal infection!

- HIV patients with SARA usually do not have conjunctivitis or arthritis, having only asymmetric oligoarthritis. Mucocutaneous manifestations often seen and more severe than in those w/o HIV infection.
- Classic Reiter's syndrome: is a subset of SARA occurring in men. Triad is urethritis, arthritis, and conjunctivitis.
- Microbiology: CT found in only 50% of SARA cases (up to 70% of cases where an organism is identified); there are a few case reports of SARA following successful Rx of GC. Can be caused by sexually and non-sexually acquired shigellosis, campylobacteriosis or salmonellosis.
- Rare findings: heart conduction defects, peripheral or central nervous system defects, aortic insufficiency, pulmonary infiltrates
- Lab findings: ESR elevated acutely, elevated WBCs, may have mild anemia, long-standing symptoms can lead to radiologically evident joint changes
- Treatment impact: Minimal evidence that treatment of the STD will abrogate the manifestations of SARA; most sx resolve in 4-6 months; 50% have at least 1 recurrence.
- Complications: More likely in those with HLA-B27 gene; 17% have sx persisting > 1 yr; erosive joint damage esp small joints of feet in 12%; persistent locomotor disability in 15%, due mostly to erosive damage of metatarsophalangeal, ankle, or knee joints or as consequence of sacroiliitis or spondylitis.

SELECTED READINGS

Bell C et al. Management of sexually acquired reactive arthritis in 19 North Thames GUM clinics. Int J STD AIDS 2004 15:195-198.

Centers for Disease Control and Prevention. Sexually transmitted diseases treatment guidelines 2002. MMWR 2002; 51 (RR-6).

Fendler C et al. Frequency of triggering bacteria in patients with reactive arthritis and undifferentiated oligoarthritis and the relative importance of the tests used for diagnosis. Ann Rheum Dis 2001; 60:337-43.

Barth WF and Segal K. Reactive arthritis (Reiter's syndrome). Am Fam Physician. 1999 60(2):499-503, 507

Lauhio A et al. Double-blind, placebo-controlled study of three-month treatment with lymecycline in reactive arthritis, with special reference to Chlamydia arthritis. Arthritis Rheum 1991;34:6-14

Rosenthal L et al. Aseptic arthritis after gonococcal infection. Ann Rheum Dis 1980;39:141-5

Kousa M et al. Frequent association of chlamydial infection with Reiter's syndrome. Sex Transm Dis 1978;5:57-9

Rice P and Handsfield HH, editors Holmes KK et al. Arthritis associated with sexually transmitted diseases. Sexually Transmitted Diseases, 3rd ed, McGraw-Hill pp 921-935

Clinical Effectiveness Group. 2001 National guideline on the management of sexually acquired reactive arthritis. http://www.mssvd.org.uk/PDF/CEG2001/Sara%200601.PDF

BACTERIAL VAGINOSIS   Noreen A. Hynes, M.D., M.P.H.

DIAGNOSTIC CRITERIA

- Lab Dx is required!!! BV is NOT an infection; it is a disruption of the normal vaginal ecology that results in signs and symptoms.
- Amsel criteria (3 of 4) = 1) thin, white, homogeneous discharge; 2) clue cells on microscopy; 3) pH of vag fluids >4.5, 4) release of fishy odor on adding 10% KOH (+ whiff test).
- Nugent criteria (on gram stain): Normal-Lactobacillus predominates; BV-Predominantly Gardnerella and/or Mobiluncus morphotypes; few or absent Lactobacilli. Training required to read slide.

- A DNA probe-based test for high concentrations of G. vaginalis may have some utility in diagnosis; cervical Pap smear of limited utility.
- Cultures for Gardnerella vaginalis are of little use in dx; G. vaginalis can be recovered from almost all women with BV and 58% without BV.
- PATHOGENESIS AND EPIDEMIOLOGY: BV is a clinical syndrome resulting from replacement of normal peroxide-producing Lactobacillus spp in the vagina with high concentrations of anaerobic bacterial (e.g., Mobiluncus sp and Prevotella spp), G. vaginalis, and Mycoplasma hominis.
- BV is the most common cause of vaginal discharge or malodor.
- The cause of this microbial alteration is not known.
- Women who have never been sexually active are rarely affected.
- Treatment of the male partner has never been shown to be effective in preventing relapse

COMMON PATHOGENS: Disruption of vaginal flora ecology

TREATMENT REGIMENS

Nonpregnant women (HIV neg or pos)
- Recommended: metronidazole (MTZ) 500mg PO bid X 7d
- Recommended: metronidazole gel 0.75%, one full applicator (5g) intravag bid x 5d
- Recommended: clindamycin cream 2%, one full applicator (5g) intravag hs x 7d
- Alternative: metronidazole 2g PO x 1
- Alternative: clindamycin 300mg PO bid x 7d
- Alternative: clindamycin ovules 100mg intravag HS x 3d

Preg w/Sx or no Sx but H/O previous preemie
- Recommended: metronidazole 250mg PO tid x 7d (preferred)
- Recommended: clindamycin 300mg PO bid x 7d

Allergy/intolerance to recommended Rx
- Preferred: clindamycin cream 2%, 1 full applicator (5g) intravag HS x 7d. NOT IN PREGNANCY.
- Systemic intolerance to metronidazole (not allergy):Metronidazole gel 0.75%, 1 full applicator (5 g) intravag qd x 5d

DRUG-SPECIFIC COMMENTS

Metronidazole: 1) Must abstain from alcohol during treatment and for 24 to 48 hours thereafter to avoid disulfiram-like effects; 2) Side effects much lower with gel form. A recent meta-anlaysis does NOT support teratogenicity in humans, hence this drug can be used to treat pregnant women, when indicated. Lower doses recommended, however, to minimize fetal exposure; 3) 2 g single dose Rx is an alternative regimen because of lower efficacy. 750mg daily dose FDA approved but clinical equivalency data is lacking; 4) Mean peak serum concentration after intravag admin is <2% of 500-mg dose level.

IMPORTANT POINTS
- Recommendations based on 2002 CDC STD Treatment Guidelines, MMWR 2002; 51 (No. RR-6); Rx only 80-90% efficacious w/ up to 30% recurrence.
- RX ALL preg women w/sx. BV assoc w/ adverse outcomes (PROM, postpartum endometritis, chorioamnionitis, preterm birth, post-cesarean wound infection). Consider Rx of asx preg women w/prev preterm birth
- Associated risks: douching, IUDs, multiple or new sex partners. Vinegar and water douches DO NOT treat BV!

- A true STD only in women-who-have-sex-with-women; partners require treatment. Sexually-associated in all other women; partners do not need treatment
- BV is the most prevalent cause of vaginal sx among childbearing aged women; may be seen in up to 50% of women seen in public STD clinics. Self-dx of vaginitis is usually INCORRECT.

SELECTED READINGS

Holley RL et al. A randomized, double-blind clinical trial of vaginal acidification versus placebo for the treatment of symptomatic bacterial vaginosis. Sex Transm Dis 2004 31:236-238.

Centers for Disease Control and Prevention. Sexually transmitted diseases treatment guidelines 2002. MMWR. 2002; 51 (RR-6).

Marrazzo JM et al. Characterization of vaginal flora and bacterial vaginosis in women who have sex with women. J Infect Dis 2002; 185(9):1307-13

Schwebke JR and Lawing LF. Prevalence of Mobiluncus spp among women with and without bacterial vaginosis as detected by polymerase chain reaction. Sex Transm Dis 2001;28:195-9.

Carey JC et al. Metronidazole to prevent preterm delivery in pregnant women with asymptomatic bacterial vaginosis. New Engl J Med 2000 342:534-40.

Guise J et al. Screening for bacterial vaginosis in pregnancy: a meta-analysis. 2000

Schmid G et al. Bacterial vaginosis and HIV infection;. Sex Transm Infect 2000, 76:3-4.

Sturm-Ramirez K et al. High levels of tumor necrosis factor-alpha and interleukin-1 beta in bacterial vaginosis may increase susceptibility to human immunodeficiency virus. J Infect Dis 2000; 182:467-73.

Schwebke JR. Bacterial vaginosis. Curr Infect Dis Reprts 2000 2(1):14-17.

Taha TE et al. Bacterial vaginosis and disturbances of vaginal flora: association with increased acquisition of HIV. AIDS 2000 12(13):1699-1706.

BALANITIS

Spyridon Marinopoulos, M.D.

DIAGNOSTIC CRITERIA

- Inflamed glans penis +/- prepuce. hx: tender glans, d/c, difficult to retract prepuce +/- impotence/difficult urination. PE: penile erythema/edema/ulcers/plaques +/- d/c +/- phimosis
- Various types: 1) Candidal: KOH prep/cx 2) Aerobic: cx - Strep/Staph/Gardnerella, r/o syphilis/trich/HSV. 3) Anaerobic: foul-smelling d/c, edema, + LN. GS-mixed flora, cx. 4) HPV: typical path
- 5) Circinate: manifestation of Reiter's. Bx - spongiform pustules, chlamydia probe. 6) Irritant/Allergic: ? sec condoms, diaphragms, lubricants/spermicides etc. Hx atopy. Patch testing. Bx nonspecific
- 7) Fixed drug eruptions: med hx (tetracycline, sulfa, pcn, salicylates, phenacetin, phenolphthalein, some hypnotics); + oral/ocular mucosa lesions. Rechallenge to confirm dx.
- 8) Lichen Sclerosus: dx by bx. 1% risk CA. Annual f/u.
- 9) Erythroplasia of Queyrat: Bx-SCC in situ.
- 10) ZOON'S (plasma cell): "Cayenne pepper spots." May resemble #9. Dx by bx.

COMMON PATHOGENS: Candida albicans ; Gardnerella vaginalis ; Trichomonas vaginalis ; Chlamydia trachomatis ; Neisseria gonorrhoeae ; Treponema pallidum (syphilis) ; Herpes Simplex Virus ; Human papillomavirus (HPV) ; Strep sp./Staph aureus

TREATMENT REGIMENS

Topical

- All cases: retract prepuce qd & soak in warm water/NS to clean glans penis & prepuce. If phimosis, refer urology to relieve surgically. Avoid soaps while inflammation present
- Candida balanitis: clotrimazole 1% OR miconazole 2% cream bid until resolved (recommended regimen). If marked inflammation, add 1% HC bid. If azole allergy/resistance, nystatin cream 100000 u bid
- Anerobic balanitis: clindamycin 2% cream bid until resolved (alternative to PO metronidazole)
- Aerobic balanitis: mupirocin 2% oint tid covers staph/strep
- HPV balanitis: 5FU 5% cream 1-2x/wk OR podophyllotoxin 0.15% gel/soln bid tiw. Reassess 1 mo
- Lichen sclerosus: clobetasol 0.05% OR betamethasone 0.05% qd until remission (recommended regimen). May need to cont qwk to maintain remission
- Zoons's (plasma cell) balanitis: topical steroids (i.e., clobetasol 0.05%) qd to bid
- Erythroplasia of Queyrat: 5FU 5% cream (alternative to surgery). note: annual follow up required (SCC in situ)
- Circinate balanitis: HC 1% bid for Sx relief + Rx underlying infxn (i.e., chlamydia etc.) use more potent topical steroid (i.e., clobetasol 0.05%) if ineffective
- Fixed drug eruption or irritant/allergic balanitis: 1% HC bid until resolved + avoid precipitant

Systemic

- Candida balanitis: fluconazole 150mg PO once very effective (use if severe/persistent or DM, but some prefer as primary regimen)
- Anaerobic balanitis: metronidazole 500mg PO bid x 7d (recommended regimen). Alternative: amoxicillin/clavulanate 500mg PO tid x 7d
- Aerobic balanitis: Cx and Rx by organism - strep, staph, HSV, trichomonas, syphilis, gonorrhea
- Staph/Strep: cephalexin 500mg PO qid OR erythromycin 500mg PO bid x 7d OR azithromycin 500mg, then 250mg x 5d (Z-Pak) OR clindamycin 300-450mg PO tid x 7d
- HSV initial episode: acyclovir 400mg PO tid OR valacyclovir 1g PO bid x 10d. HSV recurrence: acyclovir 400mg PO tid OR famciclovir 125mg PO x 5d OR valacyclovir 500mg PO bid x 3d
- Trichomonas vaginalis: metronidazole 2g PO x1 OR 500mg PO bid x 7d
- Syphilis (primary): benzathine pen G 2.4 mU IM x1 (preferred). Alternatives: doxy 100mg PO bid x 14d OR tetracycline 500mg PO qid x 14d OR ceftriaxone 1g IM/IV qd x 10d
- Gonorrhea: ceftriaxone 125mg IM x 1 OR (cefixime 400mg OR cipro 500mg OR oflox 400mg OR levo 250mg OR gati 400mg) PO x 1 + Rx chlamydia
- Circinate balanitis (chlamydia): doxy 100mg PO bid x 7d OR azithromycin 1g PO x1 + Rx gonorrhea
- Fixed drug eruption: (severe cases only) PO steroids - i.e., prednisone or medrol dosepack

Surgical

- Lichen Sclerosus (in addition to topical Rx): if phimosis, circumcise. If meatal stenosis, consider meatoplasty, urethroplasty or laser vaporization
- Zoon's (plama cell) Balanitis: Circumcision may lead to resolution of lesions. CO_2 laser used to Rx individual lesions

Diagnosis

- Erythroplasia of Queyrat: local excision adequate and effective (recommended regimen). Note: annual follow up required (premalignant condition). Alternatives: laser resection or cryotherapy

Drug-Specific Comments

Amoxicillin + Clavulanate: Alternative to metronidazole in anaerobic balanitis

Cephalexin: Good Staph (MSSA) and Strep coverage.

Clotrimazole: Candidal balanitis alternative to PO fluconazole

Fluconazole: One time dose may be more cost effective than topical preparations, but drug drug interactions an issue w/ PO

Metronidazole: Great choice for anaerobic balanitis. Avoid alcohol (Antabuse potential). P450 metabolism.

Miconazole: Topical antifungal effective for candidal balanitis. No drug interactions likely w/ topical administration

Nystatin: Topical alternative to azoles in fungal balanitis

Important Points

- Recommendations are from the 2002 national guidelines (www.guideline.gov & Beuchner reference) and author opinion
- Causes: infection, diabetes mellitus, poor hygiene (uncircumcised), chemical irritants (soap, petroleum jelly), anasarca, drugs, morbid obesity, penile CA
- Adult males: acceptable to assume and Rx empirically for probable candidal balanitis, then reassess. If no response/persistent cases: 1) cx d/c then Rx infxn w/ appropriate abx 2) bx then Rx accordingly
- Screen sexual partners in any type of balanitis caused by an STD, including Candida
- High rates of fluoroquinolone-resistant GC have been reported in MSM and Asia, Pacific Basin, Hawaii, & California. Use cefixime.

Selected Readings

Buechner SA. Common skin disorders of the penis. BJU Int. 2002 Sep;90(5):498-506

Weyers W, Ende Y, Schalla W, et al. Balanitis of Zoon: a clinicopathologic study of 45 cases. Am J Dermatopathol. 2002 Dec;24(6):459-67.

Edwards SK; European Branch of the International Union against Sexually Transmitted Infection. European guideline for the management of balanoposthitis. Int J STD AIDS. 2001 Oct;12 Suppl 3:68-72

Bunker CB. Topics in penile dermatology. Clin Exp Dermatol. 2001 Sep;26(6):469-79

Gatto-Weis C, Topolsky D, Sloane B, et al. Ulcerative balanoposthitis of the foreskin as a manifestation of chronic lymphocytic leukemia: case report and review of the literature. Urology. 2000 Oct 1;56(4):669

British Association of Sexual Health and HIV. 2002 national guideline on the management of balanitis. British Association of Sexual Health and HIV - Medical Specialty Society, 1999 Aug (revised 2002). Various pagings. NGC:002277

Mallon E, Hawkins D, Dinneen M, et al. Circumcision and genital dermatoses. Arch Dermatol. 2000 Mar;136(3):350-4

Mayser P. Mycotic infections of the penis. Andrologia. 1999;31 Suppl 1:13-6.

English JC 3rd, Laws RA, Keough GC, Wilde JL, Foley JP, Elston DM. Dermatoses of the glans penis and prepuce. J Am Acad Dermatol. 1997 Jul;37(1):1-24; quiz 25-6.

Edwards S. Balanitis and balanoposthitis: a review. Genitourin Med. 1996 Jun;72(3):155-9

BARTHOLINITIS

Noreen A. Hynes, M.D., M.P.H.

DIAGNOSTIC CRITERIA

- PE: Glands located bilateral & posterolateral to introitus at 5 and 7 o'clock are swollen and tender. The entire gland is palpable between the thumb & 1st finger.
- SX: Tender at introitus.
- Pus from ostium of gland may be diagnostic; putrid drainage and polymicrobial flora on gram stain indicate anaerobic infection. (NB: collect cervical specimens also for GC and chlamydia)

COMMON PATHOGENS: Chlamydia trachomatis ; Neisseria gonorrhoeae

TREATMENT REGIMENS

First-line treatment = drainage

- Word Catheter placement is preferred (consult surgery if not skilled in the procedure).
- Aspiration of abscess w/ or w/o 70% alcohol sclerotherapy (no RCT of sclerotherapy).
- Incision and drainage of abscess (associated with 13% recurrence rate; makes future Word catheter placement or marsupialization procedure more difficult, if needed).

Supportive treatment and follow-up

- Sitz baths BID to TID x 72h to promote healing and provide comfort
- Re-examination 72h after drainage; assess for overlying cellulitis; modify ABX (if given) based on culture and sensitivities
- Marsupialization procedure or Word catheter placement if problem recurs.
- Post-menopausal women: Evaluate for malignancy after acute problem has resolved.

Pathogen-specific therapy

- Anaerobes: Metronidazole 2g PO x 1 or 500mg PO bid x 7d
- Gonorrhea: See Cervicitis
- Chlamydia: See Cervicitis

DRUG-SPECIFIC COMMENTS

Cefixime: Does not attain adequate penetration of the Waldeyer's ring and should not be used to treat gonorrhea in anyone with orogenital exposure. Probenicid increases concentration.

Spectinomycin: Expensive, must be injected. Effective in curing 98.2% of uncomplicated urogenital and anorectal gonococcal infections. Test of cure required if used to treat patient with orogenital exposure. Use in patients with gonorrhea who cannot tolerate quinolones or cephalosporins.

IMPORTANT POINTS

- There is no U.S. published consensus guideline on the Rx of bartholinitis. These recommendations reflect common practice reported in the literature and the author's opinion.
- Gland abscess requires drainage unless ruptures spontaneously. I&D provides quick relief but 13% failure rate. Word catheter placement or aspiration preferred.
- If the inflammation recurs, a marsupialization or Word catheter placement may be necessary after antibiotic Rx.
- 2% risk of duct cyst or gland abscess during woman's life; less likely after 30 yrs. Consider malignancy in a postmenopausal woman who presents with a new Bartholin's cyst or abscess.
- ABX after drainage needed only for 1) proven associated STD (GC or CT); or 2) overlying cellulitis. Putrid drainage is diagnostic of an anaerobic infection.

DIAGNOSIS

- If incision and drainage is not undertaken at the time of presentation, follow-up within 72 hours is needed to assess the need for surgical intervention.
- A case report of non-menstrual toxic shock-like syndrome has been reported in which streptococcal enterotoxin elaborated by organisms infecting the Bartholins gland was implicated.

SELECTED READINGS

Kafali H et al. Aspiration and alcohol sclerotherapy: a novel method for management of Bartholin's cyst and abscess. Eur J Obstet Gynecol Repor Biol 2004 112:98-101.

Omole F et al. Management of Bartholin's cyst and gland abscess. Am Fam Physician 2003 68:135-140.

Centers for Disease Control and Prevention. The 1998 guidelines for treatment of sexually transmitted infections. MMWR 1998;47 (No. RR-1): pp 49-75. 1998.

Sing A et al. Bartholinitis due to Streptococcus pneumoniae: case report and review. Clin Infect Dis 1998;27:1324-5.

Black MM, McKay ME, Braude P. Obstetric and Gynecologic Dermatology. Mosby-Wolfe/Times Mirror Publishers Ltd, London, UK, pp 79-81, 148-9. 1995.

Lynch P and Edwards L. Genital Dermatology. Churchill Livingstone, Inc, New York, pp 141-2. 1994.

Shearin RS, Bochlke J, Karanth S. Toxic-shock-like syndrome associated with Bartholin's gland abscess: case report. Am J Obstet Gynecol 160(5 Pt 1):1073-4. 1989.

Cheetham DR. Bartholin's cyst: marsupialization or aspiration?. Am J Obstet Gynecol 152:569-70. 1985.

BITE WOUNDS

John G. Bartlett, M.D.

DIAGNOSTIC CRITERIA

- Dx: Wound >8h - signs infection: fever, cellulitis, purulent drainage, abscess
- Lab: gram stain & cult for aerobes & anaerobes; Xray for ? osteo
- Dx: Wound <8h - crush or puncture wound, scratches

COMMON PATHOGENS: Pasteurella multocida ; Capnocytophaga canimorsus ; Eikenella corrodens ; Streptococcus sp (all bites) ; Staph aureus (all bites) ; Staph intermedius (dog) ; Anaerobes (all bites)

TREATMENT REGIMENS

General care

- Principles: 1) clean & debride, 2) Abx (severe early or late & infected) usually amox/clav, 3) tetanus toxoid, 4) animal bite: rabies (rare except w/bat exposure in US)
- Clean wound: copious soap & water, alcohol, povidone-iodine; puncture wound - high pressure 20mL syringe with #18 needle
- Debride necrotic tissue; immobilize and elevation of extremity
- Wound closure - usually not sutured except early uninfected wound & face wound; use adhesive strips to approximate edges
- Tetanus vaccine hx - <3 doses or unknown & minor wound: Tetanus toxoid (Td) series 0.5mL at 0, 1-2 mo & 6-12 mo. Severe injury: Td series + Tetanus Immune Globulin

Antibiotic prophylaxis and treatment

- Prophylaxis Indications: Severe injury <8h, crush injury; bone or joint penetration; wound of face, hand or genitals; immunosuppressed host
- Preferred for prophylaxis: amoxicillin/clavulanate (Augmentin) 875/125mg PO bid x 7d
- Alternative: gatifloxacin (Tequin) 400mg qd or moxifloxacin (Avelox) 400mg qd x 7d
- Alternative: amoxicillin, doxycycline, cefuroxime (active vs. most oral flora of man & animals)

- Established infection hospitalized pts (preferred): ampicillin-sulbactam (Unasyn) 1-2g IV q6h or ticarcillin-clavulanate (Timentin) 3-6g IV q4-6h
- Hospitalized pts (alternative): cefoxitin 1-2g IV q6h or gatifloxacin 400mg IV qd
- Outpt treatment (preferred): Amox/clav (Augmentin) 875/125mg PO bid or 2000 (XR)/125mg bid. Outpt(alt): gatifloxacin 400mg PO qd; moxifloxacin 400mg PO qd; azithromycin 500mg PO, then 250mg qd.

Rabies prophylaxis

- Presumed exposure: Dog or cat with suspected rabies; presumed risk with bite from raccoon, skunk, bat, fox
- Reality issue: 1990-2003 record with 30 human cases in U.S., 28 had no prior hx of bite and most were bat-associated
- Rabies prophylaxis (see "Rabies" in the Vaccines and Prophylaxis section): 1) Wound cleansing ASAP w/ alcohol or iodine; 2) Vaccine x 5 IM doses; 3) RIG-expensive, scarce and only for severe bites
- Vaccine: Imovax (800-288-8370) or Rabipur (800-244-7668) 1mL IM days 0,3,7,14 and 28
- RIG (800-822-2463 or 800-288-8370) 20 IU/kg - 1/2 IM and 1/2 into wound
- No human-human transmission except 2004 cases with organ transplant

DRUG-SPECIFIC COMMENTS

Amoxicillin: Active against most anticipated pathogens from the mouth of dogs, cats & people: Pasteurella, Capnocytophaga & Eikenella. Some oral anaerobes are resistant and most S. aureus (from the skin) are resistant.

Amoxicillin + clavulanate: (Augmentin) The oral drug of choice for most bites due to activity against most of the likely pathogens and extensive experience. Main oral pathogens of people and pets are sensitive to amoxicillin. The addition of clavulanate adds S. aureus and anaerobes.

Cefuroxime and cefuroxime axetil: (Ceftin) Active vs Pasteurella, Capnocytophaga, Staph intermedius, Eikenella and MSSA. Probably adequate for oral anaerobes when used prophylactically. This drug is a reasonable option.

Doxycycline: Good activity vs Pasteurella, Capnocytophaga, Staph Intermedius and Eikenella. Variable activity against anaerobes and S. aureus. Resonable choice, esp for dog or cat bite, and at a very low price.

Gatifloxacin: This drug has the right spectrum but published experience is nil. The in vitro activity includes oral flora of most animals and people. It is also active against most meth-sensitive S. aureus.

Moxifloxacin: The same as gatifloxacin - the right spectrum but limited experience.

IMPORTANT POINTS

- Guidelines for bite (NEJM 1999;350:85); for rabies (MMWR 1998;47:4)
- Bacteriology: Oral flora of donor and or skin flora of recipient (S. aureus)
- Oral flora DOGS: P. multocida, C. canimorsus, anaerobes; CATS - P. multocida, anaerobes, HUMANS: Strep, Eikenella, anaerobes
- Rabies prophylaxis: worry about BATS, raccoons & skunks; dogs in developing countries; only 2 animal bites associated rabies cases in U.S. 1990-2003
- Most wounds are left open with approximation of edges using adhesive strips; suture only clean wounds & face wounds (cosmetic issue)

SELECTED READINGS

Correira K. Managing dog, cats and human bite wounds. JAAPA 2003;16:28-32

DIAGNOSIS

Andreg SM, Barra LA, Costa LJ, et al. HIV type 1 transmission by human bite. AIDS Res Hum Retroviruses 2004;20:349-50

Warrell MJ, Warrell DA. Rabies and other lyssavirus disease. Lancet 2004;363:959-69

Broder J, Jerrard D, Olshaker J, Witting M. Low risk of infection in selected human bites treated without antibiotics. An J. Emerg Med 2004;22:10-13

Talan DA, Abrahamian FM, Moran GJ, et al. Clinical presentation and bacteriologic analysis of infected human bites in patients presenting to emergency departments. Clin Infect Dis 2003;37:1481-9

Stieman KL, Lloyd KM, DeLuca-Pytell DM et al. Treatment and outcome of human bites in the head and neck. Otolaryngal Head Neck Surg 2003;128:795-801

CDC. First human death associated with raccoon rabies-Virginia 2003. MMWR 2003;52:1102

Goldstein EJC, Citron DM, Finegold SM. Dog bite wounds and infection: A prospective clinical study. Ann Emerg Med 1980;9:508-512

Talan DA, Citron DM, Abrahamian FM, et al. Bacteriologic analysis of infected dog and cat bites. Emergency Medicine Animal Bite Infection Study Group. N Engl J Med 1999;340-85-92.

Goldstein EJC, Citron DM, Wield B, et al. Bacteriology of human and animal bite wounds. J Clin Microbiol 1978;8:667-672.

BLEPHARITIS

Spyridon Marinopoulos, M.D.

DIAGNOSTIC CRITERIA

- Eyelid inflammation - assoc w/ acne rosacea, atopy, seborrhea. Anterior (outer lid) usually bacterial (Staph) or seborrheic. Posterior (inner lid) caused by meibomian gland dysfxn
- Hx (anterior): itching, burning, mild foreign body sensation, tearing, crusting & mattering of lashes & medial canthus, lid edema & erythema. +/- associated conjunctivitis
- PE (anterior): anterior lids w/ margin redness/hyperemia +/- ulcers/irregularities +/- stye formation. Lashes w/ crusting +/- madarosis(loss/thinning), poliosis (whitening), trichiasis (misdirection)
- Hx (posterior): may present w/ minimal/very mild sxs (i.e., Rx burning alone) disproportionate to PE findings or like anterior w/ burning, irritation, crusting & redness and be difficult to distinguish
- PE (posterior): posterior lid margin hyperemia, thickening & irregularity + mattering/crusting of lids/lashes + conj injection + sicca. 1/3 pts have seborrhea, 1/3 rosacea

COMMON PATHOGENS: Staphylococcus aureus

TREATMENT REGIMENS

Topical

- Lid hygiene essential. Apply warm compresses to closed lid x 5-10 min bid-qid to loosen crusts, then wash lids w/ cotton swab soaked w/ mild (baby) soap diluted 1:1 w/ water
- If associated seborrhea, use selenium-based dandruff shampoo concurrently to treat associated scalp condition
- If associated acne rosacea, treat concurrently with blepharitis using PO abx. Rosacea diagnosis suggested by presence of telangiactasias on lid margins, cheeks, nose and chin
- Anterior Blepharitis: follow lid cleansing w/ topical anti-staph Rx. Bacitracin or erythro ophth oint first line, apply to lids bid-qid immediately post cleansing. May cause transient blurred vision
- Rule of thumb - apply abx oint initially qid x 1-2 wk, bid after improvement, and finally QHS x 1 mo once eyelids appear normal

- Note: Ophthalmic ointment preferred over solution for blepharitis, but if unable to use, anti-Staph ophthalmic soln also effective (ref conjunctivitis module for details)
- Posterior Blepharitis: lid massage after lid hygiene helps meibomian gland evacuation & reestablishes normal flow
- All Patients: monitor closely for keratoconjunctivitis sicca. Suspect in refractory cases despite adequate Rx & liberalize use of artificial tears. Refer to Ophtho for Schirmer testing
- Ophthalmic steroid use is NOT indicated for the Rx of blepharitis in the primary care setting; may lead to corneal thinning/ulceration, secondary/opportunistic infections, glaucoma & cataracts
- If recurrent/unresponsive to Rx, do eyelid cx r/o resistant bugs; think atypical infxn/ sebaceous cell CA. Refer Ophtho. Also refer if visual loss, mod/sev pain, sev/chronic redness, cornea involved

Systemic antibiotics

- If assoc acne rosacea or in refractory cases of meibomian gland dysfunction: doxycycline 100mg PO bid or tetracycline 250mg PO qid - may need Rx x wks to mos then maintenance (doxy 50 qd or tetra 250 qd)

DRUG-SPECIFIC COMMENTS

Bacitracin: Ointment only. Good Staph coverage. May transiently blur vision

Doxycycline: bid dosing. May cause fetal harm. Stains teeth in pts < 8 years old. Photosensitivity.

Tetracycline: Inconvenient qid alternative to doxy. May cause fetal harm. Stains teeth in pts < 8 years old. Photosensitivity.

IMPORTANT POINTS

- Recommendations are author's opinion. Ddx includes conjunctivitis, keratoconjunctivitis sicca, contact-lens keratoconjunctivitis, preseptal cellulitis, hordeolum/chalazion, nasolacrimal duct obstruction
- Lid hygiene key to Rx blepharitis. Topical abx adjunctive. Rx anterior & posterior dz differently. Rx assoc seborrheic dermatitis/acne rosacea. Suspect lid malignancy if recurrent, esp if unilateral
- Refer to Ophtho if eye pain, dec vision, sx >2 wk, refractory. Complications hordeolum (stye)/chalazion, dry eyes (keratoconjuctivitis sicca), corneal infxn, other forms of keratitis/corneal ulceration
- Almost all bacterial blepharitis due to Staph; rare, non-Staph microbial causes: HSV blepharitis, molluscum contagiosum, phthiriasis palpebrarum (pediculosis pubis), other parasites
- Other causes: 1) isotretinoin; 2) allergic blepharitis - contact dermatitis due to cosmetics, drugs, plants, chemicals. Sxs include itching & pain +/- blurred vision. Identify/eliminate causative agent

SELECTED READINGS

Diaz-Valle D, Benitez del Castillo JM, Fernandez Acenero MJ, et al. Bilateral lid margin ulcers as the initial manifestation of Crohn disease. Am J Ophthalmol. 2004 Aug;138(2):292-4.

Selva D, Chen CS, James CL, et al. Discoid lupus erythematosus presenting as madarosis. Am J Ophthalmol. 2003 Sep; 136(3): 545-6

McCulley JP, Shine WE. Eyelid disorders: the meibomian gland, blepharitis, and contact lenses. Eye Contact Lens. 2003 Jan; 29(1 Suppl): S93-5; discussion S115-8, S192-4

Sullivan TJ, Boulton JE, Whitehead KJ. Intraepidermal carcinoma of the eyelid. Clin Experiment Ophthalmol. 2002 Feb; 30(1): 23-7

McCulley JP; Shine WE. Changing concepts in the diagnosis and management of blepharitis. Cornea 2000; 19(5):650-8

Shields SR. Managing eye disease in primary care. Part 2. How to recognize and treat common eye problems. Postgraduate Medicine 2000;108(5):83-96

Akpek EK, Polcharoen W, Chan R, et al. Ocular surface neoplasia masquerading as chronic blepharoconjunctivitis. Cornea. 1999 May; 18(3): 282-8

Carter SR. Eyelid disorders; diagnosis and management. American Family Physician 1998;57(11):2695-2702

Key JE. A comparative study of eyelid cleaning regimens in chronic blepharitis. CLAO J. 1996 Jul; 22 (3): 209-12

Smith RE; Flowers CW. Chronic blepharitis; a review. The CLAO journal ; official publication of the Contact Lens Association of Ophthalmologists, Inc 1995;21(3):200-207

BRONCHIECTASIS   David Zaas, M.D.; Paul Auwaerter, M.D.

DIAGNOSTIC CRITERIA
- Definition: pathologic, irreversible dilation of one or more proximal, medium-sized bronchi due to destruction of the bronchial walls
- Consequence of pulmonary infections (esp. bacterial pneumonia (untreated), TB, endemic fungi) or host disorders; e.g., cystic fibrosis, other structural lung dz, immune disorder/Kartagener's
- Sx: chronic cough, purulent sputum, hemoptysis, fever, weight loss. PE: fetid breath, clubbing, basilar crackles, rhonchi.
- CXR: tram tracks, toothpaste shadows, clustered cysts (may be nl in 84% of pts w/ bronchiectasis on CT)
- High Resolution CT: gold standard, dilation of bronchi >1.5 times as wide as nearby vessel, bronchial wall thickening, lack of normal tapering, cysts

COMMON PATHOGENS: S. pneumoniae ; Haemophilus influenzae ; Moraxella catarrhalis ; Mycobacterium avium complex ; Mycobacteria (atypical) ; Aspergillus fumigatus ; P. aeruginosa

TREATMENT REGIMENS

Outpatient (empiric)
- Preferred: oral fluoroquinolone
- Levofloxacin 500-750mg PO qd
- Gatifloxacin 400mg PO qd
- Moxifloxacin 400mg PO qd
- All abx recommendations are for 7-10 days. Some may treat 3-6 weeks for recurrences

Hospitalized patient (empiric)
- IV antipseudomonal beta-lactam (consider change to oral Abx once improved). Use sputum culture sensitivities to guide therapy.
- Piperacillin 3.0-4.0g IV q 4-6 hrs
- Ticarcillin 3.0g IV q 4-6 hrs
- Cefepime 1-2g IV q 12 hrs
- Ceftazidime 1-2g IV q 8-12 hrs
- All abx recommendations are for 7-10 days. Some may treat 3-12 weeks for recurrences

Pathogen-specific
- P. aeruginosa: ciprofloxacin oral or IV, antipseudomonal penicillin IV (piperacillin, ticarcillin), 3rd or 4th gen cephalosporin IV (ceftazadime, cefepime)
- H. influenzae: amox/clav, 2nd or 3rd gen cephalosporin, TMP-SMX, fluoroquinolone

- M. catarrhalis: amox/clav, 2nd or 3rd generation cephalosporin, TMP-SMX, fluoroquinolone
- MAI: clarithromycin 500mg PO BID, ethambutol 15-25 mg/kg/d PO, rifampin 600mg PO QD (rifabutin 300mg PO QD) x 12-18mos [see separate MAI (non-HIV) monograph]
- Allergic bronchopulmonary aspergillosis: corticosteroids plus itraconazole

DRUG-SPECIFIC COMMENTS

Amoxicillin: High dose amoxicillin 1g PO TID used by some with standard bacterial bronchiectasis--unclear whether this practice from the 1960's & 70's still effective in era of increasing resistance.

Amoxicillin + Clavulanate: Good coverage of most pathogens except pseudomonas.

Cefepime: Excellent IV anti-pseudomonal cephalosporin. However, most exacerbations can be adequately treated with oral antibiotics.

Ceftazidime: Excellent IV anti-pseudomonal cephalosporin. However, most exacerbations can be adequately treated with oral antibiotics.

Cefuroxime and Cefuroxime axetil: Good coverage of most pathogens except Pseudomonas. Available in oral and IV formulations.

Ciprofloxacin: Has better in vitro activity against Pseudomonas compared to the newer fluoroquinolones, though may be waning in some reports.

Clarithromycin: Good activity against most pathogens except Pseudomonas. More expensive than bactrim, cefuroxime, and doxycycline

Gatifloxacin: Good choice for empiric oral treatment of acute exacerbations.

Levofloxacin: Good choice for empiric oral treatment of acute exacerbations due to the efficacy against Pseudomonas.

Moxifloxacin: Good choice for empiric oral treatment of acute exacerbations.

Piperacillin: Excellent anti-pseudomonal pencillin which only comes in IV formulation. However, most exacerbations can be adequately treated with oral antibiotics.

Ticarcillin: Excellent anti-pseudomonal pencillin which only comes in IV formulation. However, most exacerbations can be adequately treated with oral antibiotics.

IMPORTANT POINTS

- Guidelines are authors' opinion
- Acute exacerbations (4 of the following): change in sputum, increased dyspnea, increased cough, fever, increased wheezing, fatigue, decreased PFT's, new infiltrate, change in PE.
- Inhaled tobramycin 300mg BID alternating months appears useful in CF, but not idiopathic bronchiectasis
- Recombinant human DNAase 2.5mg bid may be beneficial in tx of pts with CF
- Mucolytic therapy never proven beneficial and not recommended

SELECTED READINGS

Tsang KW, Tipoe GL. Bronchiectasis: not an orphan disease in the East. Int J Tuberc Lung Dis. 2004 Jun;8(6):691-702

J Angrill, C Agusti, R de Celis, et al. Bacterial colonization in patients with bronchiectasis: microbial pattern and risk factors. Thorax 2002. 57: 15-19

AF Barker. Bronchiectasis. NEJM 2002. 346(18)1383-93

M Pasteur, S Helliwell, S Houghton, et al. An investigation into causative factors in patients with bronchiectasis. AJRCC 2000. 162: 1277-1284

AF Barker, L Couch, SB Fiel, et al. Tobramycin solution for inhalation reduces sputum Pseudomonas aeruginosa density in bronchiectasis. AJRCC 2000. 162: 481-485

DA Stevens, HJ Schwartz, JY Lee, et al. A randomized trial of itraconazole in allergic bronchopulmonary aspergillosis. NEJM 2000. 342: 756-62

BW Ramsey, et al., The Cystic Fibrosis Inhaled Tobramycin Study Group . Intermittent administration of inhaled tobramycin in patients with cystic fibrosis. NEJM 1999. 340: 23-30

KW Tsang, WM Chan, PL Ho, et al. A comparative study on the efficacy of levofloxacin and ceftazidime in acute exacerbation of bronchiectasis. Eur Respir J 1999. 14(5):1206-9

AE O'Donnel, AF Barker, JS Ilowite, et al. Treatment of idiopathic bronchiectasis with aerosolized recombinant human DNAse I. Chest 1998. 113(5): 1329-1334

The official statement of the American Thoracic Society. Diagnosis and treatment of disease caused by nontuberculous mycobacteria. AJRCC 1997. 156(2): S1-S25

BRONCHITIS, ACUTE EXACERBATIONS OF CHRONIC

John G. Bartlett, M.D.

DIAGNOSTIC CRITERIA

- Definition: increased in cough, sputum and sputum purulence in pt with chronic bronchitis (cough + sputum x 3yrs)
- PE: Dyspnea, cyanosis, wheezing, rhonchi +/- fever
- Chest XR to R/O pneumonia, CHF, effusion, mass, pneumothorax
- Lab: Sputum gram stain and culture: not advocated; blood gases or pulse oximetry - if pt seriously ill; spirometry - probably not useful
- Severity: pulse oximetry, blood gases, FEV-1

COMMON PATHOGENS: Haemophilus influenzae ; Moraxella catarrhalis ; S.pneumoniae

TREATMENT REGIMENS

Antibacterials

- Principles: about half of AECB are caused by bacterial infection; x-ray to r/o pneumonia, Rx - albuterol/Atrovent, steroids, O2; Abx - only for severe exacerbations - preferred agents controversial
- Abx Indications: severe exacerbations - increased cough, sputum vol & sputum purulence
- Recommendations adapted ACP/ASIM Guidelines (Ann Int Med 2001;134:595)
- Preferred (ACP): amoxicillin 500-875mg PO tid or doxycycline 100mg PO bid x 10-14d
- Alternatives: amoxicillin-clavulanate (Augmentin) 875mg PO bid x 10-14d
- Azithromycin (Zithromax) 500mg, then 250mg PO qd x4d OR clarithromycin (Biaxin) 500mg PO bid or 1g PO qd x 10-14d
- Telithroycin 800mg (Ketek) PO qd x 5d
- Cefuroxime axetil (Ceftin) 500mg PO bid x 10-14d
- Cefprozil (Cefzil) 500mg PO bid x 10-14d
- Cefpodoxime (Vantin) 200-400mg PO bid x 10-14d

Severe AECB flares

- Severe + recent abx: levofloxacin (Levaquin) 750mg IV or PO qd OR
- Gatifloxacin (Tequin) 400mg PO qd or moxifloxacin (Avelox) 400mg PO qd all x 10-14 d
- Influenza (within 48h): rimantidine 100mg bid, oseltamivir (Tamiflu) 75mg bid; both x 5 days

Supportive care (most important)

- Inhaled bronchodilator: albuterol (180mcg) up to q 30min or 2 puffs qid by metered inhaler +/- spacer when stable or ipratropium (Atrovent) 0.25-0.5mg inhaled q 6h - 8h

- Hospitalized pts: methylprednisolone 125mg IV q 6h x 3d, then PO prednisone 60mg/d x 4-7d, 40mg/d x 8-11d, 20mg/d x 12-15d
- Hospitalized pts: O2 2-4L by nasal cannula; to keep pulse ox > 91%; if need increase or pCO2 > 45 - Venturi mask. Risk is resp. failure
- Smoking cessation
- Aminophylline: potentially serious side effects; avoid or use with caution and measure levels at 8-12 h
- Inhaled steroids: not indicated
- Noninvasive pos-pressure ventilation; requires trained physician
- Not effective: chest PT, methylxanthine bronchodilators, mucolytic agents

DRUG-SPECIFIC COMMENTS

Amantadine: Old agent for treatment and prevention of flu caused by Influenza A. Must be given within 48 hrs of onset of sx. Cheap, but substantial CNS side effects. Must be careful with dose in renal failure and elderly.

Amoxicillin: Good activity against most S. pneumoniae, performed well in prior studies of AECB & cheap. Concern is resistance by 5-10% of S. pneumoniae, 30-40% of H. influenzae, & 90-95% of M. catarrhalis. Recommended as a preferred agent in ACP guidelines, but supporting trials preceeded era of resistant pathogens.

Amoxicillin + Clavulanate: Expands amoxicillin activity to cover H. influenzae & M. catarrhalis, but no better than amoxicillin alone vs. S. pneumoniae.

Cefaclor: A bad choice--poor activity against S. pneumoniae relative to other oral cephalosporins.

Cefpodoxime proxetil: Active against most strains of S. pneumoniae & all strains of H. influenzae & M. catarrhalis. Somewhat less active than amoxicillin vs. S. pneumoniae. Relatively expensive; well tolerated.

Cefprozil: Active against most strains of S. pneumoniae & all strains of H. influenzae & M. catarrhalis. Somewhat less active than amoxicillin vs. S. pneumoniae. Relatively expensive; well tolerated.

Cefuroxime and cefuroxime axetil: Active against most strains of S. pneumoniae & all strains of H. influenzae & M. catarrhalis. Somewhat less active than amoxicillin vs. S. pneumoniae. Relatively expensive; well tolerated.

Clarithromycin: As active as azithromycin & erythromycin vs. S. pneumoniae; activity vs. H. influenzae is debated due to activity ascribed to a metabolic product, which is greater than that of the parent compound. FDA has approved for H. influenzae pneumonia.

Doxycycline: Risky by in vitro activity against S. pneumoniae & H. influenzae, but good historic record for AECB, well tolerated & cheap. This is usally a good choice for patients who aren't very sick. Doxycycline is recommended by the ACP guidelines for severe exacerbations of chronic bronchitis.

Gatifloxacin: Active against nearly all treatable pathogens except influenza virus including S. pneumoniae, H. influenzae, M. catarrhalis, most S. aureus, most GNB, Chlamydia pneumoniae, & Mycoplasma pneumoniae. The drug is easy to take (once daily) & well tolerated. The major concern is abuse with the consequence of resistance.

Moxifloxacin: Active against nearly all treatable pathogens except influenza virus including S. pneumoniae, H. influenzae, M. catarrhalis, most S. aureus, most GNB, Chlamydia pneumoniae, & Mycoplasma pneumoniae. The drug is easy to take (once daily) and well tolerated. The major concern is abuse with the consequence of resistance.

Diagnosis

Oseltamivir: Newer agent for treatment and prophylaxis of flu caused by influenza virus A and B. Must be given within 48 hours of onset of sx. Expensive. Main side effect in GI intolerance.

Rimantadine: Old agent for treatment and prevention of flu caused by Influenza A. Must be given within 48 hrs of onset of sx. Inactive vs influenza B. Inexpensive. Well tolerated, but may result in resistance and no activity vs influenza B. CNS toxicity is infrequent and much less problematic than amantadine.

Telithromycin: New drug (ketolide) related to the macrolide class, but effective against both high-level penicillin and macrolide resistant S. pneumoniae. Has better H. influenza coverage than azithromycin or clarithromycin.

Zanamivir: Newer agent for treatment of flu caused by influenza A or B. Given by inhalation, may not be suitable for persons with reactive airways. Must be given within 48 hrs of onset of sx. Expensive. Main side effect is bronchospasm.

Important Points

- Guidelines are from Am College Physicians (Ann Int Med 2001;134:595) and Stoller (NEJM 2002;346:988)
- Common non-bacterial causes of AECB: viral infections, allergens, pollution
- Abx in 3 categories: cheap, old & proven(amox, doxy,TMP-SMX); better activity vs S. pneumo & H. influenzae (oral cephs, azithro, clarithro, amox-clav); drugs w/clout but concern re abuse (gati, levo, moxi)
- Must r/o pneumonia (x-ray), subclinical asthma (PFT) and resp. failure (ABG)
- Main issue: Major role of H. influenzae and role of newer drugs to reduce hospitalizations to delay next exacerbation?

Selected Readings

Sethi S. Bacteria in exacerbations of chronic obstructive pulmonary disease. Proc Amer Thorac Soc 2004;1:109

Sethi S. Strain-specific response to Haemophilus influenzae in chronic obstructive lung disease. Am J Respir Crit Care Med 2004;169:448

Saint S, Bent S, Vittinghoff E, et al. Antibiotics in chronic obstructive pulmonary disease exacerbations: a meta-analysis. JAMA 1995;273:957

Jorgensen AF, Coolidge J, Pedersen PA, et al. Amoxicillin in treatment of acute uncomplicated exacerbations of chronic bronchitis. A double-blind, placebo-controlled multicentre study in general practice. Scand J Prev Health Care 1992;10:7

Anthonisen NR, Manfreda J, Warren CPW, et al. Antibiotic therapy in exacerbations of chronic obstructive pulmonary disease. Ann Intern Med 1987;106:196

Gump DW, Phillips CA, Forsyth BR, et al. Role of infection in chronic bronchitis. Am Rev Respir Dis 1976;113:465

American Thoracic Society. Standards for the diagnosis and care of patients with chronic obstructive pulmonary disease (COPD) and asthma. Am Rev Respir Dis 1987;136:225

Snow V, et al. Evidence base for management of acute exacerbations of chronic obstructive pulmonary disease. Ann Intern Med 2001;134:595

Snow V, Lascher S, Mottur-Pilson C. Evidence base for management of acute exacerbations of chronic obstructive pulmonary disease. Ann Intern Med 2001;134:595

Pines A, Raafat H, Plucinski K, et al. Antibiotic regimens in severe and acute purulent exacerbations of chronic bronchitis. Br Med J1968;168;2:735.

BRONCHITIS, ACUTE UNCOMPLICATED

John G. Bartlett, M.D.

DIAGNOSTIC CRITERIA

- Hx: acute upper respiratory tract infection with cough
- PE: Fever is most common with influenza or parainfluenza infection. Lung exam may reveal rhonchi, but no crackles.
- Indications for X-ray: Abnormal VS (P >100, T >38, RR >20) or rales or cough >3wks
- Differential dx cough: bronchitis, subclinical asthma, postnasal drip, GERD, Ca, ACE inhibitor

COMMON PATHOGENS: Rhinovirus ; Coronavirus ; Respiratory syncytial virus ; Bordetella pertussis ; Chlamydia pneumoniae ; Influenza

TREATMENT REGIMENS

Treatment for cause

- Principles: Dx - URI + cough; R/O - asthma, GERD, Ca, postnasal drip; XR if abn VS; Rx - No abx unless pertussis
- Indications for antimicrobials: suspected pertussis or anti-influenza agents
- Cough meds containing codeine or dextromethorphan
- Common cold: dexbrompheniramine + sedating antihistamine (Actifed, Contac, Dimetapp, etc.), naproxen 500mg tid x 5d and/or Atrovent nasal spray
- Allergic rhinitis: Loratadine 10mg PO qd
- Sinusitis: Above +/- antibiotic if severe or >7 days
- AECB: (see "Bronchitis, Acute Exacerbation of Chronic")
- Albuterol by inhaler 2 inhalations q4-6h
- Influenza: (See "Influenza") consider anti-flu drug if symptoms <48hrs.

Suspected or confirmed pertussis

- Antibiotics should not be used for bronchitis except for suspected or confirmed pertussis.
- Most adults with pertussis lack typical sx due to partial immunity. Major clues - cough > 3 wks, whoop or post-tussive vomiting
- Commonly available diagnostic tests to detect B. pertussis aren't sensitive.
- Pertussis (preferred): Erythro 500mg qid x 14d
- Alternative: TMP-SMX 1 DS bid x 14d; Clarithro 500 PO bid x 14d; azithro 500mg, then 250mg qd x 4d

DRUG-SPECIFIC COMMENTS

Clarithromycin: Could be used for suspected pertussis, C. pneumoniae, or Mycoplasma-- all possible causes of persistent cough and all nearly impossible to prove. Activity is similar to erythromycin which is less expensive but less well tolerated. No clinical trials show antibiotic treatment is a benefit. Potential benefit with pertussis is prevention of transmission.

Erythromycin: Preferred agent for pertussis although azithromycin and clarithromycin are probably equally effective and better tolerated. Main reason to give abx is to reduce transmission.

Oseltamivir: (Flu only). Active vs. influenza A & B, must be given within 48 hours of onset of flu symptoms, 10-20% get GI intolerance, may mask bacterial pneumonia & relatively expensive at AWP of $55/5-day course. May be used at half dose to prevent influenza.

Rimantadine: 100mg bid--this is probably the least toxic and most cost-effective treatment of influenza A. Must treat within 48 hrs. of onset of symptoms. CNS toxicity is much less than that of amantadime.

Zanamivir: Active vs. influenza A & B, delivered by aerosol, must be given within 48 hrs. of onset of symptoms. Expensive at AWP of $45/5-day course & may cause bronchospasm, especially in asthmatics. May also be used at half dose to prevent influenza, but not FDA-approved for prevention.

Important Points

- Guidelines from ACP (Ann Intern Med 2001;134:158), CDC (AIM 2001;134:521) and Irwin RS (NEJM 2000; 343:1715)
- If abnormal vital signs (T >38, P >100, RR >20) & not obviously influenza -- get chest XR to exclude pneumonia.
- Multiple well-controlled studies show antibiotics don't help.
- Patient acceptance of non-antibiotic treatment is better if it is called "a chest cold" rather than "bronchitis."
- Abx indications: severe acute exacerbation of chronic bronchitis, some influenza, or pertussis

Selected Readings

Steinman MA, Sanaia A, Maselli JH, et al. Office evaluation and treatment of elderly patients with acute bronchitis. J Am Geriatr Soc 2004;52:875-9

Linder JA, Singer DE, Stafford RS. Association between antibiotic prescribing and visit duration in adults with upper respiratory tract infections. Clin Ther 2003;25:2419-30

Metlay JP, Kapoor WN, Fine MJ. Does this patients have community acquired pneumonia? Diagnosing pneumonia by history and physical exam. JAMA 1997;278:1440.

Wipf JE, Lipsley BA, Hirschmann JV. Diagnosing pneumonia by physical examination: relevant or relic?. Arch Intern Med 1999;159:1082.

Stott NCH, West RR. Randomised controlled trial of antibiotics in patients with a cough and purulent sputum. BMJ 1976;2:556.

Orr PH, Scherer K, MacDonald A, Moffatt MEK. Randomized placebo-controlled trials of antibiotics for acute bronchitis: a critical review of the literature. J Fam Pract 1993;36:507.

Fahey T, Stocks N, Thomas T. Quantitative systemic review of randomized controlled trials comparing antibiotic with placebo for acute cough in adults. BMJ 1998;316:906.

Bent S, Saint S, Vittinghoff E, Grady D. Antibiotics in acute bronchitis: a meta-analysis. Am J Med 1999;107:62.

Sprauer MA, Cochi SL, Zell ER. Prevention of secondary transmission of pertussis in households with early use of erythromycin. Am J Dis Child 1992;146:177.

Pasternack MS. Pertussis in the 1990s: diagnosis, treatment and prevention. Curr Clin Top Infect Dis 1997;17:24.

CANDIDIASIS, OROPHARYNGEAL (THRUSH) [AIDS]

John G. Bartlett, M.D.

Diagnostic Criteria

- Hx: sore mouth, dysphasia, altered taste perception, or asymptomatic
- Risk: HIV infection with CD4 <200, antibiotic or steroid use, malnutrition
- Pseudomembranous: white plaques on oral mucosa that can be wiped away to leave erythematous base. Erythematous: patch on palate or angular cheilitis.

- Ddx: substernal odynophagia/dysphagia suggests esophagitis, oral hairy leukoplakia (white non-removable plaques on sides of tongue)
- Lab: Gram stain: mycelia. Culture for candida spp. Usually unnecessary except w/ refractory cases to confirm Dx or perform fungal sensitivity testing

COMMON PATHOGENS: Candida albicans ; Candida species

TREATMENT REGIMENS

Preferred

- Principles: RISK = CD4 <200 +/- abx/steroids; r/o esophagitis (odynophagia); DX - clinical; Rx - usually empiric
- Preferred: clotrimazole troches 10mg 5x/day x 14d
- Nystatin pastilles (1-2 flavored pastilles) suck 4-5x/d or suspension to gargle (100,000 U/mL) 4-6mL qid x 7-14d
- Fluconazole (Diflucan) 100mg PO qd 7-14 d
- Itraconazole suspension swish/swallow on empty stomach, 100-200mg qd
- HAART

Alt (fluconazole refractory or recurrent cases)

- Recurrent cases: chronic suppressive Rx: fluconazole 100mg/d effective but risks resistance
- Alt: itraconazole liquid (Sporanox) solution 200mg qd
- Refractory: ampho B 100 mg/mL 5mL swish/gargle (solution compounded by pharmacy)
- Refractory: fluconazole 200-400mg/d po/d
- Refractory: itraconazole soln on empty stomach 200-400 mg/d
- Refractory: caspofungin 50mg IV/d (loading dose not required)
- Refractory: ampho B 0.3mg/kg/d IV
- Refractory: voriconazole 200mg PO bid ($70/d); multiple drug interactions

Reversible provocative factors

- Immune suppression: improves with HAART
- Discontinue or change antibacterials: TMP/SMX predisposes, dapsone doesn't
- D/C or lower dose of TMP/SMX if possible
- Avoid steroids
- Repair poorly fitting dentures
- Azole resistance risks: chronic or repeated azole exposure, CD4 <50, chronic abx (TMP-SMX)
- In vitro sensitivity testing Candida: possible role with refractory cases

DRUG-SPECIFIC COMMENTS

Clotrimazole: (Oral tabs 10mg 5x/d) This is a preferred treatment, but complicated by the frequency of dosing. Delays exposure to azoles, which may decrease risk of resistance. Clinical trials show efficacy comparable to that of fluconazole.

Fluconazole: (100-200mg PO qid) is highly effective but continuous use leads to azole-resistant Candida

Ketoconazole: (100-200 mg/day) Cheaper than fluconazole, but absorption less predictable. There are more drug interactions and more hepatotoxicity. May also lead to azole - resistance.

Nystatin: Topical treatment with vaginal tablets (100,000 units) TID disolved slowly or oral solution (100,000 units/mL) & pastilles (200,000 units) all given 4-5 x daily. This is a preferred treatment, but may be less effective than clotrimazole.

IMPORTANT POINTS

- Recommendations of IDSA (CID 2004;38:161) + Vazquez review (HIV Clin Trials 2000;1:47) & CDC/IDSA guidelines MMWR 2004;53 RR-15
- Recurrent: consider dapsone for PCP prophylaxis instead of Bactrim
- Recurrent: chronic fluconazole works but risks resistance
- Refractory: in vitro sens test or empiric progression in dose (fluconazole) or change to different agent (itraconazole ,voriconazole, ampho B, caspofungin)
- Thrush & dysphagia: treat empirically for esophagitis with systemic Rx - (azole)

SELECTED READINGS

Pappas PG et al. Guidelines for the treatment of candidiasis. Clin Infect Dis 2004;38:161

Vazquez JA. Therapeutic options for management of oropharyngeal and esophageal candidiasis in HIV/AIDS patients. HIV Clin Trials 2000; 1:47

Pinheiro A, et al. Dental and oral lesions in HIV infected patients: a study in Brazil. Int. Dent J. 2004;54:131-7

Oude Lashof AM, et al. An open multicentre comparative study of efficacy, safety and tolerance of fluconazole and itraconazole in the treatment of cancer patients with oropharyngeal candidiasis. Eur J. Cancer 2004;40:1314-9

Hospenthal Dr, et al. The role of antifungal susceptibility testing in the therapy of candidiasis. Diagn Microbiol Infect Dis 2004;48:153-60

Walmsley S, King S, McGeer A, et al. Oropharyngeal candidiasis in patients with human immunodeficiency virus: correlation of clinical outcome with in vitro resistance, serum azole levels and immunosuppression. CID 2001;32:1554

Vazquez JA et al. Evolution of antifungal susceptibility among Candida species isolates recovered from HIV-infected women receiving fluconazole prophylaxis. CID 2001;33:1069

Magald S, Mata S, Hartung C, et al. In vitro susceptibility of 137 Candida sp isolates from HIV positive patients to several antifungal drugs. Mycopathologia 2001;149:63

Espinel-Ingroff A, Boyle K, Sheehan DJ. In vitro antifungal activities of voriconazole and reference agents as determined by NCCLS methods: review of the literature. Mycopathologia 2001;150:101

Powderly WG, Gallant JE, Ghannoum MA, et al. Oropharyngeal candidiasis in patients with HIV: suggested guidelines for therapy. AIDS Res Human Retroviruses 1999;15:1619

CARDIOVASCULAR DEVICE INFECTIONS

Khalil G. Ghanem, M.D.

DIAGNOSTIC CRITERIA

- Devices include transvenous pacemakers (TVP), implantable cardioverter defibrillators (ICD), & left ventricular assist devices (LVAD). Infection can be early (<1 mo), late, or delayed (>12 mos).
- Device-related infection classified anatomically: (1) pocket infections, 2) electrode infections (subcutaneous tissues & venous system), & 3) endocardial infections (valvular & nonvalvular)
- Infection= warmth, erythema, swelling, pain, or discharge from the device pocket, in addition to + cx from device, device pocket, or lead (reference 1); device associated endocarditis also occurs.
- Rates of infection for TVP and ICD range from 1 to 7% (reference 1); for LVAD range from 6 to 15 infections per 1000 LVAD days (reference 2).
- Risk factors for infxn include: extended duration of use, multi-organ failure, extended ICU stay, diabetes mellitus, malnutrition, malignancy, postoperative hematoma & use of a temporary electrode.

COMMON PATHOGENS: Some studies have suggested that early infections are usually due to S. aureus, and late infections are mostly due to coagulase-negative staphylococci; infections can also be due to enterococcus.

TREATMENT REGIMENS

Overview

- There is significant debate about optimal management: should the device be removed in all cases of infection, or can antibiotics alone succeed in eradicating the infection?
- Most reports of successful eradication of infection without complete removal of the device have usually been small case series, or cases of infections limited to the pocket.
- If incomplete removal is chosen, clinicians should make sure that all infected portions of the device are removed. This can be quite challenging, hence the high rate of relapse w/ partial removal.
- Except for localized early infections, complete removal is recommended. The decision, however, is based on the clinical condition of the patient.
- Recently, the availability of laser sheath technology has reduced the rate of complications associated w/ device removal.
- The type of antimicrobial depends on culture data. Early empiric therapy should cover gram-positives: vancomycin is a reasonable first choice, with modification based on culture data.

Pacemaker/ICD/LVAD infections

- The optimal route & duration of antimicrobial therapy has not been prospectively studied.
- Duration of therapy should take into consideration: 1) pathogen virulence; 2) host immune status; 3) extent of infection; 4) whether the device was completely removed; 5) early response of host to Rx.
- Patients with endocarditis should have the device completely removed and pathogen-directed parenteral therapy for 4-6 weeks.
- Patients with bacteremia and negative TEE should have the device removed & should receive at least a portion, if not all of the therapy parenterally.
- Patients with moderate infections of the pocket are usually treated initially parenterally, then orally to complete their course. Duration depends on response (usually 2-6 wks).
- Pocket infections generally necessitate local wound care as well.
- In most cases, removal of LVAD is not feasible. Long-term suppression is usually the goal until transplantation, after which time, a course of abx to cure the infection is intiated.
- If for whatever reason the device cannot be removed, the addition of rifampin to the therapeutic regimen in select cases may offer added benefit. LFTs should be monitored.

Re-implantation

- The timing of re-implantation of a new device is controversial.
- It is generally agreed upon that if no endocardial infection is present, & bacteremia has been eradicated (usually 3-5 days of abx), it is safe to proceed.
- In cases of endocardial infection during which organisms remain viable despite negative blood cx, longer parenteral courses are recommended before re-implantation (? exact duration).
- Re-implantation should occur at new clean sites.

IMPORTANT POINTS

- Echocardiography should be performed on all patients with CV devices & bacteremia or clinical evidence of endovascular infection. TEE has much higher sensitivity than a TTE
- When trying to determine route and duration of therapy, one must consider both the type of pathogen, & the immune status and response to therapy of the host.
- Up to 40% of pts with bacteremia lack fever & systemic symptoms- clinicians should be mindful of drawing blood cultures. Up to 33% of infections have positive blood cultures.
- It is often very difficult to determine whether infection from the pocket has extended more proximally. Relapse rates when the devices are not completely removed can be quite high.
- Probably, devices should be removed entirely, unless there are significant medical reasons not to do so.

SELECTED READINGS

Chua JD, et al. Diagnosis and management of infections involving implantable electrophysiologic cardiac devices. Ann Intern Med. 2000 Oct 17;133(8):604-8.

Meier-Ewert HK, et al. Endocardial pacemaker or defibrillator leads with infected vegetations: a single-center experience and consequences of transvenous extraction. Am Heart J. 2003 Aug;146(2):339-44.

Malani PN, et al. Nosocomial infections in left ventricular assist device recipients. Clin Infect Dis. 2002 May 15;34(10):1295-300.

Chamis AL, et al. Staphylococcus aureus bacteremia in patients with permanent pacemakers or implantable cardioverter-defibrillators. Circulation. 2001 Aug 28;104(9):1029-33.

Klug D, et al. Systemic infection related to endocarditis on pacemaker (PM) leads: clinical presentation and management. Circulation. 1997 Apr 15;95(8):2098-107.

Spinler SA, et al. Clinical presentation and analysis of risk factors for infectious complications of implantable cardioverter-defibrillator implantations at a university medical center. Clin Infect Dis. 1998 May;26(5):1111-6

Da Costa A, et al. Role of the preaxillary flora in pacemaker infections: a prospective study. Circulation. 1998 May 12;97(18):1791-5.

Muers MF, et al. Prophylactic antibiotics for cardiac pacemaker implantation. A prospective trial. Br Heart J. 1981 Nov;46(5):539-44

Baddour LM. Long-term suppressive antimicrobial therapy for intravascular device-related infections. Am J Med Sci. 2001 Oct;322(4):209-12.

Gordon SM, et al. Nosocomial bloodstream infections in patients with implantable left ventricular assist devices. Ann Thorac Surg. 2001 Sep;72(3):725-30

CELLULITIS/ERYSIPELAS Ciro R. Martins, M.D.

DIAGNOSTIC CRITERIA

- Clinical: acute onset of inflammatory plaque/patch with erythema, tenderness/pain, warmth & variable edema. Fever, malaise and regional lymphadenopathy common.
- PE (erysipelas): superficial inflammatory process with sharply demarcated borders usually affecting the extremities and, less commonly, the face, scalp and genitals
- PE (cellulitis): deeper infection extending into the subcutaneous tissue with less edema and demarcation
- Lab: obtain cxs/sensitivity testing if blisters or purulent secretions present. Cxs of biopsy specimens or fine needle aspirates usually negative. Blood cultures not routinely recommended.

COMMON PATHOGENS: Staphylococcus aureus ; Streptococcus pyogenes (Group A)

TREATMENT REGIMENS

Mild cases, minor systemic symptoms

- Preferred: penicillin V 500mg PO q6h x 10d; penicillin G benzathine 1.2 mU IM x1
- Amoxicillin 250-500mg PO q8h x 10d; amoxicillin/clavulanate 875/125mg PO q12h x 10d
- Cephalexin 250-500mg PO q6h x 7-10d; cefadroxil 500mg-1g PO q12h x 7-10d; cefuroxime 250-500mg PO q12h x 7-10d; cefpodoxime 100-400mg PO q12h x 7-10d; cefprozil 250-500mg PO qd/q12h x 7-10d
- Erythromycin 250-500mg PO q6h or 333mg PO q8h x 7-10d; azithromycin 500mg PO x1 followed by 250mg PO qd x 4d; clarithromycin 250mg PO q12h x 7-10d
- Clindamycin 150-450mg PO q6h x 7-10d
- Moxifloxacin (Avelox) 400mg PO qd x 7d, gatifloxacin (Tequin) 400mg PO qd x 7d, levofloxacin (Levaquin) 250-500mg PO qd x 7d

Moderate and severe cases, significant systemic sx

- Penicillin G 2- mU IM or IV q4-6h (maximum 24mil U/day)
- Cefazolin 0.5-1.5g IM or IV q6-8h (maximum 12g/day); cefuroxime 0.75-1.5g IM or IV q6-8h; cefotaxime 1-2g IV/IM q6-12h; ceftriaxone 1-2g IV qd
- Clindamycin 300-900mg IM or IV q6-8h (max 600mg/day IM or 4.8g/day IV)
- Erythromycin 15-50 mg/Kg IV qd (divided q6h)
- Gatifloxacin (Tequin) 400mg IV qd, levofloxacin (Levaquin) 500mg IV qd or 750mg PO qd x 7d
- Consider MRSA if hospital-acquired, community-acquired MRSA risk factors or non-responding cellulitis.
- Vancomycin 1g IV q12h or linezolid 600mg IV/PO q12h x 7-10 d

General measures

- Immobilization and elevation of the affected area
- Moist heat compresses
- Debridement and drainage when bullae, abscess or necrosis present

DRUG-SPECIFIC COMMENTS

Amoxicillin: Not effective against Staph aureus, but good coverage agains Group A Strep. Group A Strep is always sensitive to penicillin and amoxicillin. Inexpensive oral medication.

Amoxicillin + Clavulanate: Good oral drug for both Group A Strep and Staph aureus (except MRSA), but an expensive choice.

Ceftriaxone: If the patient is sick enough to be admitted, this drug is a good option if MRSA not suspected.

Cephalexin: Good and inexpensive oral anti-Staph aureus drug. Also effective against Group A Strep. A good choice for mild cases that do not require parenteral therapy and when Staph aureus is a possibility.

Dicloxacillin: Also a good choice for covering both Group A Strep and methicillin-sensitive Staph aureus in patients with mild disease that can be treated with oral antibiotics. Expensive drug.

Gatifloxacin: Very convenient qd dosing and short duration of Rx (7d), very effective against S. aureus and S. pyogenes, but significant list of drug interactions and side-effects.

Linezolid: Broad gram-positive activity. Use if MRSA proven/suspect. Oral dosing makes conversion from IV vancomycin attractive.

Moxifloxacin: Very convenient qd dosing and short duration of Rx (7d), very effective against S. aureus and S. pyogenes, but significant list of drug interactions and side-effects.

IMPORTANT POINTS

- The guidelines in this module represent the opinion of the author
- Both erysipelas and cellulitis are usually unifocal and unilateral processes
- Complications: frequent recurrences and rapid spread with chronic lymphedema, thrombophlebitis in older patients, gram-negative superinfection of necrotic areas
- Predisposing factors: puncture wounds, chronic lymphatic or venous obstruction, diabetes, malnutrition, burns, immunocompromise, alcohol or drug abuse, skin diseases (stasis ulcers, eczemas, tineas)
- Ddx: contact dermatitis, angioneurotic edema, asteatotic eczema, herpes zoster, osteomyelitis, inflammatory carcinoma of the breast

SELECTED READINGS

Eady EA, Cove JH. Staphylococcal resistance revisited: community-acquired methicillin resistant Staphylococcus aureus--an emerging problem for the management of skin and soft tissue infections. Curr Opin Infect Dis. 2003 Apr;16(2):103-24

Laube S, Farrell AM. Bacterial Skin Infections in the Elderly: Diagnosis and Treatment. Drugs Aging 2002: 19(5):331-42

Perl B, Gottehrer NP, Raveh D et al. Cost Effectiveness of Blood Cultures for Adult Patients with Cellulitis. Clinical Infectious Diseases, 29:1483-8, 1999

Erksson B. Anal Colonization of Group G Beta-hemolytic Streptococci in Relapsing Erysipelas of the Lower Extremity. Clinical Infectious Diseases, 29:1319-20, 1999.

CERVICAL FASCIAL (PERIMANDIBULAR) SPACE INFECTIONS

John G. Bartlett, M.D.

DIAGNOSTIC CRITERIA

- Infection involving spaces created by fascial insertions along the mandible, usually of dental origin
- Clinical: Tender swelling along the mandible--differential dx includes parotitis, actinomycosis, peritonsillar abscess, or adenitis.
- Laboratory features: CT scan defines space infections with great clarity.
- Critical space infections: submandibular (Ludwig's angina), retropharyngeal space (behind esophagus), lateral pharyngeal space + jugular vein phlebitis (Lemierre's syn).

COMMON PATHOGENS: Prevotella; Peptostreptococcus; Streptococcus species; Fusobacterium necrophorum ; Anaerobes

TREATMENT REGIMENS

Antibiotics

- Principles: Anatomic definition - CT scan; drainage - ENT/oral surg; airway protection; abx-anaerobes and strep
- Preferred: clindamycin (Cleocin) 300mg PO qid or 600 mg IV q8h
- Ampicillin-sulbactam (Unasyn) 3g IV q6h or amox-clav (Augmentin) 875mg bid
- Metronidazole (Flagyl) 500mg PO bid-qid (+ penicillin or amoxicillin)
- Imipenem (Primaxin) 0.5-1g IV q6h
- Piperacillin-tazobactam (Zosyn) 3.375g IV q6h
- Cefoxitin (Mefoxin) 0.5-2g IM or IV q4-6h

Life-threatening space infections

- Lemierre's Syndrome: Most respond to antibiotic treatment and do not require anticoagulation, vein ligation or surgical drainage
- Ludwig's: Secure airway (intubation or trach) antibiotics +/- surgical drainage

- Retropharyngeal abscess: Secure airway (tracheotomy prn) + antibiotics; surgery if unresponsive to antibiotics

Miscellaneous

- Surgery: Decision for surgery and incision site depends on space involved and cosmetics. (See "Important points")
- Dental care: Dental infections are usually the underlying cause--a tooth that needs extraction or a complication of a dental procedure.

DRUG-SPECIFIC COMMENTS

Amoxicillin: Penicillin was once regarded as the preferred drug for anaerobic infections above the diaphragm. Resistance is now a problem. Risky for severe infections.

Ampicillin + Sulbactam: Active against all clinically significant anaerobes. This is a rational choice. Other betalactam - betalactamase inhibitors are also effective.

Ceftazidime: Not a good choice. Advantage of this drug is expanded spectrum against P. aeruginosa and other GNB--bacteria that don't cause these infections; poor activity against anaerobes which do cause most of these infections.

Clindamycin: Excellent activity against pathogens in the mouth and extensive use in orodental infections. Main concern is GI side effects.

Gatifloxacin: Reasonably good in vitro activity vs. anaerobes, but clinical experience is limited and other drugs are preferred.

Imipenem/Cilastatin: Active vs. all obligate anaerobes and most strep, GNB and other bacteria of unknown significance in mixed infections.

Meropenem: Active vs. all obligate anaerobes and most strep, GNB and other bacteria of unknown significance in mixed infections.

Metronidazole: Very active against all obligate anaerobes; no activity vs. aerobic and microaerophic strep, which often must be treated. Could combine with penicillin.

Moxifloxacin: Reasonably good in vitro activity vs. anaerobes, but clinical experience is limited and other drugs are preferred.

Piperacillin + Tazobactam: Active vs. all anaerobes--a good choice although experience is limited.

Ticarcillin + Clavulanic Acid: Active vs. all anaerobes--a good choice although experience is limited.

IMPORTANT POINTS

- Recommendations are author's opinion
- Most perimandibular space infections are complications of dental infections, esp. molar tooth infections
- Some are potentially serious: lateral pharyngeal space--sepsis; submandibular space--airway obstruction; danger space--extension to mediastinum
- Multiple contiguous spaces are often involved
- Anaerobic bacteria and oral streptococci are the usual pathogens

SELECTED READINGS

Chow A. Orofacial odontogenic infections. Ann Intern Med 1978;88:392

Chow AW. Life-threatening infections of the head and neck. Clin Infect Dis 1992;14:991

Sinave CP, Hardy GJ, Fardy PW. The Lemierre syndrome: suppurative thrombophlebitis of the internal jugular vein secondary to oropharyngeal infection. Medicine 1989;68:85

Salit IE. Diagnostic approaches to head and neck infections. Infect Dis Clin N Amer 1988;2:35

Kurien M, Mathew J, Zachariah N. Ludwig's angina. Clin Otolaryngology 1997; 22:263

Kristensen H, Prag J. Human Necrobacillosis, with Emphasis on Lemierre's Syndrome. Clin Infec Dis 2000; 31:524

Weber AL, Siciliano A. CT and MR imaging evaluation of neck infections with clinical correlations. Radiol Clin North Am 2000; 38:941

Chirinos JA, et al. The evolution of Lemierre's syndrome: report of two cases and review of the literature. Medicine 2002;81:458

Chow A. Odontenogenic infections in the elderly. Infect Dis Clin Pract 1998;6:587

Lewis MA, Parkhurst CL, Douglas CS. Prevalence of penicillin-resistant bacteria in acute suppurative oral infection. J Antimicro Chemother 1995;35:785

CERVICITIS
Noreen A. Hynes, M.D., M.P.H.

DIAGNOSTIC CRITERIA

- Cervicitis: > 10 PMNs per oil-immersion field on gram-stained slide of cervical secretions collected after the endocervix has been cleaned off.
- Mucopurulent cervicitis (MPC): yellow to green coloration of the tip of a cotton-tipped swab after insertion into the endocervix, compared in good light with a clean white swab; aka endocervicitis
- Friability, bleeding after cervical contact, and edema may also be features of MPC.
- Hypertrophic cervicitis: an intensely erythematous, raised, irregular area radiating outward from the cervical os that bleeds easily with contact (common in chlamydial cervicitis)
- Routine confirmatory laboratory tests from collected cervical specimens should be performed for GC, CT and HSV. If colpitis macularis (i.e. strawberry cervix) seen, test for trichomonas.

COMMON PATHOGENS: Chlamydia trachomatis ; Neisseria gonorrhoeae ; Herpes Simplex Virus

TREATMENT REGIMENS

MPC, first episode or high-risk profile

- MPC: await GC/CT test results. If unlikely pt will return in timely manner, Rx for chlamydia and gonorrhea (See "Neisseria gonorrheae" in Pathogens section).
- See Table 3 in Appendix I

MPC, recurrent

- Wait for laboratory test results unless has high risk profile
- Treat according to lab results
- If high risk profile, treat for GC and CT at time of presentation and prior to return of laboratory results. (See "Neisseria gonorrheae" in Pathogens section for recommended Rx).
- Test for gonorrhea, chlamydia, HSV, trichomonas, collect pap smear (if none in the past year). Await results unless in high-risk group for an STD.

Gram stain c/w gonococcal infection

- Antigonococcal regimen PLUS antichlamydial regimen is the standard of care (See "Neisseria gonorrheae" in Pathogens section for recommended Rx).
- IMPORTANT! Avoid fluoroquinolone (FQ) use if gonorrhea (GC) acquired in HI, CA, MA, NYC, or Pacific Basin due to high rates of FQ-resistant GC

Friable cervix, negative gram stain

- Antichlamydial regimen
- Antigonococcal regimen if GC risk high for pt

DRUG-SPECIFIC COMMENTS

Acyclovir: Greatest experience in HSV Rx with this agent and only one with IV form. Data supports continuous suppression up to 6 years without adverse effects or resistance.

Amoxicillin: Doxycycline and ofloxacin are contraindicated in pregnant women and the safety and efficacy of azithromycin in pregnant and lactating women has not been established. Because amoxicillin may not be efficacious for all pregnant women with chlamydia, a test of cure 3 weeks after completing Rx is recommnended.

Cefixime: NEW CEFIXIME SOURCE! Lupin Pharmaceuticals (410-576-2000); only form now is 100mg/5mL suspension. Can use 20 mL to treat suspect gonococcal cervicitis. Cefixime does not attain adequate penetration of the Waldeyer's ring and should not be used to treat gonorrhea in anyone with orogenital exposure. Probenicid increases concentration.

Ceftriaxone: Single injection of 125mg provides sustained, high bactericidal levels. Treats uncomplicated gonorrhea at ALL sites, curing 99.1%. MUST concomitantly treat for chlamydia!

Ciprofloxacin: Increasing GC resistance to this agent worldwide, including in the U.S. Do NOT use drug in CA, HI, MA, New York City, or Pacific Basin unless fluorquinolone-resistant gonorrhea has been ruled out.

Doxycycline: Doxycycline and azithromycin have been shown to be equally efficacious in clinical trials. Doxycycline costs much less than azithromycin and it has been used extensively. Instruct pt to abstain from sexual intercourse until completion of the 7-day regimen. Sex partners in the last 60 days should be treated.

Famciclovir: Has high oral bioavailability but is much more expensive than acyclovir in Rx of HSV. Most acyclovir-resistant strains are also resistant to this agent. Foscarnet, 40 mg/kg body weight IV every 8 hours until clinical resolution is attained may be effective in acyclovir-resistant genital herpes. Topical cidofovir gel 1% applied to lesions once daily for 5 consecutive days may also be effective. Safety in pregnancy not established

Spectinomycin: Used in the treatment of gonorrhea, particularly in penicllin-allergic pregnant women. Expensive, must be injected. Effective in curing 98.2% of uncomplicated urogenital and anorectal gonococcal infections. Test of cure required if used to treat patient with orogenital exposure. Use in patients with gonorrhea who cannot tolerate quinolones or cephalosporins

IMPORTANT POINTS

- Recommendations based on CDC's 2002 STD Rx Guidelines; MMWR 2002; 51(RR-6)
- Approximately 40% of women with MPC have no identified pathogen. Approximately 50% of women with GC cervicitis will have a neg gram stain; Cervisitis a risk factor for HIV acquisition/transmission.
- Females <20 yrs should be strongly encouraged to return for rescreening in 3-6 mo after a CT or GC dx.
- Absence of sxs or physical or lab findings does not rule out infxn with GC or CT as most infections are asymptomatic. Lab-based DX is key! Rx most recent sex partner even if >60 days since contact.
- Nabothian cysts, benign pearly white/yellow, nonfriable entities w/clear mucus within may be seen in the transition zone of cervix and do not require Rx
- Risk Profile: Treatment decisions must consider prevalence of pathogens in the community and the risk profile of the patient examined including age, number of sexual partners, previous history of an STD, recent history of an STD or STD syndrome in any sexual partner, number of sex partners of patient's sex partners

- Additional optional laboratory tests:
- a. A cervical Pap smear or other diagnostic test for identifying cervical pathology should be collected when recurrent MPC is identified and no pathogen is identified
  b. Necrotic appearing MPC should include a Pap smear and a serologic test for syphilis or darkfield microscopic examination for evidence of Treponema pallidum

SELECTED READINGS

Centers for Disease Control and Prevention. Sexually transmitted disease treatment guidelines 2002. MMWR 2002; Vol 51(No. RR-6).

Gift TL et al. A cost-effectiveness evaluation of testing and treatment of Chlamydia trachomatis infection among asymptomatic women infected with Neisseria gonorrheae. Sex Transm Dis 2002; 29 (9):542-551

Lau C-Y and Qureshi AK. Azithromycin versus doxycycline for genital chlamydial infections: a meta-analysis of randomized clinical trials. Sex Transm Dis 2002; 29(9): 497-502

McClelland RS et al. Treatment of cervicitis is associated with decreased cervical shedding of HIV-1. AIDS 2001;15:105-10.

Prakash M et al. Macrophages are increased in cervical epithelium of women with cervicitis. Sex Transm Inf 2001;77:366-369.

Wright TC Jr et al. Human immunodeficiency virus 1 expression in the female genital tract in association with cervical inflammation and ulceration. Am J Obstet Gynecol 2001; 184:279-85.

van Valkengoed IGM et al. Cost effectiveness analysis of a population based screening programme for asymptomatic Chlamydia trachomatis infections in women by means for home obtained urine specimens. Sex Transm Inf 2001;77:276-282.

Dean D, et al. Evidence of long-term cervical persistence of Chlamydia trachomatis by omp1 genotyping. J Infect Dis 2000; 182:909-16.

Ryan CA et al. Risk assessment, symptoms, and signs as predictors of vulvovaginal and cervical infections in an urban STD clinic: implications for use of STD algorithms. Sex Transm Infect 74(Supp 1):S59-S76. 1998.

Mosure DJ et al. A re-evaluation of selective screening criteria for women attending family planning clinics in the U.S. Chlamydial Infections, Stephens RS et al (eds). San Francisco, International Chlamydia Symposium, pp 333-6. 1998.

CHOLANGITIS
Pamela A. Lipsett, M.D.; Chris Carpenter, M.D.

DIAGNOSTIC CRITERIA

- Hx: gallstones, strictures, biliary or pancreatic malignancy, sclerosing cholangitis
- Charcot's triad of intermittent chills/fever, jaundice, RUQ pain. RUQ pain less likely in patients w/ biliary stent or endoprothesis, though fever and jaundice remain common.
- Lab: leukocytosis, hyperbilirubinemia (90%), elevated alkaline phosphatase/GGT, AST, ALT
- Evaluate source of jaundice. US if gallstones suspected, CT scan if malignancy suspected
- Cholangiography needed to define etiology; treat underlying cause WHEN STABLE. Pts w/ fever, RUQ pain, jaundice, confusion, and hypotension require rapid evaluation and treatment.

COMMON PATHOGENS: Enterobacteriaceae ; E. coli ; Klebsiella species ; Enterobacter species ; Enterococcus ; Anaerobes ; Polymicrobial likely

TREATMENT REGIMENS

Treatment of acute cholangitis

- Recommendations based on authors opinion
- Piperacillin 2-3g IV q4h or piperacillin-tazobactam 3.375g IV q6h or 4.5g IV q8h

- Third or fourth-generation cephalosporins (cefotaxime, ceftriaxone, cefepime)
- Ticarcillin 4g IV q6h or ticarcillin-clavulanate 3.1g IV q6h
- Ampicillin 2g IV q6h plus gentamicin 1.7mg/kg IV q8h
- Imipenem 0.5g IV q6h
- Meropenem 1.0g IV q8h
- Pts unresponsive to abx, may require drainage (T-tube), or surgery (gallstones)

Mild-moderate disease
- Ampicillin-sulbactam 3.0g IV q6h
- Fluoroquinolones (ciprofloxacin, levofloxacin, gatifloxacin, or moxifloxacin)
- Ertapenem 1g IV qd
- Cefotetan 1-2g IV q12h
- Cefoxitin 1-2g IV q6h

DRUG-SPECIFIC COMMENTS

Ampicillin + Sulbactam: Good coverage of gram-positive, gram-negative, and anaerobic pathogens - lacks Pseudomonas aeruginosa coverage but good Enterococcus species coverage.

Cefepime: Excellent gram-negative with some gram-positive coverage

Cefotetan: Good single agent coverage of gram-positives, gram-negatives, and anaerobes, drug currently not available in the U.S.

Ertapenem: New carbapenem with excellent coverage for abdominal sepsis; does not cover resistant gram-negatives (e.g., Pseudomonas aeruginosa).

Gatifloxacin: Excellent broad spectrum coverage but clinical data limited on anaerobe coverage; does not cover resistant gram-negative rods (e.g., Pseudomonas aeruginosa).

Imipenem/Cilastatin: Good anaerobic, gram-negative and gram-positive coverage.

Meropenem: Excellent broad spectrum (gram-positive, gram-negative, and anaerobe) coverage.

Moxifloxacin: Excellent broad-spectrum coverage including some anaerobes; does not cover resistant gram-negative rods (e.g., Psuedomonas aeruginosa).

Piperacillin: Good single agent coverage of gram-positives (including some enterococcus species coverage) and gram-negatives including Pseudomonas aeruginosa; has some anaerobic coverage but not Bacteroides fragilis.

Piperacillin + Tazobactam: Improved gram-positive (including Staphylococcus aureus and coagulase negative staphylococcus species) coverage, improved gram-negative coverage (B-lactamase producing pathogens) and improved anaerobic coverage (including Bacteroides fragilis) compared to piperacillin alone.

Ticarcillin: Good single agent coverage of gram-positives (including some enterococcus species coverage) and gram-negatives including Pseudomonas aeruginosa; has some anaerobic coverage but not Bacteroides fragilis.

Ticarcillin + Clavulanic Acid: Improved gram-positive (including Staphylococcus aureus and coagulase negative staphylococcus species) coverage, improved gram-negative coverage (B-lactamase producing pathogens) and improved anaerobic coverage (including Bacteroides fragilis) compared to ticarcillin alone.

IMPORTANT POINTS
- Antibiotics are indicated in all patients with acute cholangitis. Bactibilia alone is not cholangitis.
- Patients who present seriously ill and who are not responding to antimicrobial and supportive therapy will require emergent drainage.

DIAGNOSIS

- Gallstones account for more than 50% of cases. Can occur post-cholecystectomy
- Occlusion of the bile duct from stricture (benign or malignant), bile stents, or parasites account for most non-gallstone causes
- If severe, treat for 7-10 days; modify antibiotic choice for local pathogens and resistance patterns

SELECTED READINGS

National Surgery Infection Prevention Project. Antimicrobial prophylaxis for surgery: an advisory statement from the National Surgical Infection Prevention Project. Clin Infect Dis. 2004 Jun 15;38(12): 1706-15.

The Medical Letter - Treatment Guidelines. Antimicrobial prophylaxis in surgery. Treatment Guidelines 2004 April;19:13-26.

Solomkin et al. Guidelines for the Selection of Anti-infective Agents for Complicated Intra-abdominal Infections. Clin Infect Disease 2003 October 15;37:997-1005

Mazuski J, Robert G, Sawyer RG, et al. The Surgical Infection Society Guidelines on Antimicrobial Therapy for Intra-Abdominal Infections: An Executuve Summary . Surgical Infections 2002, Vol 3

Galandi D, Schwarzer G, Bassler D, et al. Ursodeoxycholic acid and/or antibiotics for prevention of biliary stent occlusion. Cochrane Library, Issue 4, 2002

Berma D, Rauns EA, Keulemans YC, et al. Wait-and-see policy on laparoscopic cholecystectomy after endoscopic sphincterotomy for bile duct stones - a randomized trial . Lancet 2002: 360-761-5

Lee DW, Chan AC, Lam YH, et al. Biliary decompression by nasobiliary catheter or biliary stent in acute suppurative cholangitis: a prospective randomized trial. Gastrointest Endosc 2002; 56: 361-5

Khuroo MS . Hepatobiliary and pancreatic ascariasis . Ind J Gastroenterol 2001 Mar; 20 Suppl 1:C28-32

Lillemoe KD. Surgical treatment of biliary tract infections. Am Surg 2000 Feb;66(2):138-44

Westphal JF and Brogard JM. Biliary Tract Infections: a guide to treatment. Drugs. 1999 Jan;57(1):81-91

CHOLECYSTITIS   Pamela A. Lipsett, M.D.; Chris Carpenter, M.D.

DIAGNOSTIC CRITERIA

- Hx: nausea/vomiting and RUQ pain (often following fatty meal) with fever. Predisposition: female sex, multiparity, obesity, recent pregnancy, sickle cell.
- Lab: elevated WBC, variable elevation of alkaline phosphatase, bilirubin, and transaminases
- US for gallstones, edema/pericholic fluid, RUQ tenderness; color-flow doppler shows hyperemia. Tech-HIDA > expensive, slightly more sensitive. CT w/ little role except to exclude other dx.
- Hyperbilirubinemia may suggest CBD stones or Mirrizzi's syndrome (obstruction by a stone impacted in Hartman's pouch)
- Majority of patients have gallbladder-associated symptoms prior to the development of acute cholecystitis.
- Diaphragmatic irritation may lead to right shoulder pain.
- Rebound and guarding are less commonly found and indicate peritonitis.
- Murphy's sign (inspiratory arrest during deep palpation over the gallbladder) not highly sensitive but quite specific.
- Jaundice, hypoactive bowel sounds, and a palpable mass may also be present.
- Acute cholecystitis: US sensitivity greater than 92%-95%, HIDA greater than 97%. Technetium-HIDA is less specific in acalculus cholecystitis and ultrasonography plays a larger role in diagnosis as does percutaneous cholecystostomy.

COMMON PATHOGENS: Often inflammatory and noninfectious; if infectious, frequently polymicrobial: ; Enterobacteriaceae ; E. coli ; Klebsiella species ; Enterobacter species ; Enterococcus

TREATMENT REGIMENS

Antibiotic treatment of acute cholecystitis
- Authors' opinion and IDSA Guidelines Clin Infect Disease 2003 October 15;37:997.
- Acute cholecystitis often only an inflammatory process w/o infection; most patients covered with antibiotics. If infected, most are polymicrobial.
- Uncomplicated cholecystitis - treat with operation and antibiotics for 24-48 hrs, if operation delayed treat for 3-5 days. Persistent fever or illness indicates complication.
- Ampicillin 2g IV q6h plus gentamicin 1.7mg/kg IV q8h or ampicillin-sulbactam 3.0g IV q6h
- Piperacillin 4g IV q6h or piperacillin-tazobactam 3.375g IV q6h or 4.5g IV q8h
- Ticarcillin 4g IV q6h or ticarcillin-clavulanate 3.1g IV q6h
- Ertapenem 1g IV qd, meropenem 1.0g IV q8h or imipenem 0.5g IV q6h
- Third- or fourth-generation cephalosporin (cefotaxime, ceftriaxone, or cefepime)
- Fluoroquinolone (ciprofloxacin, levofloxacin, gatifloxacin, or moxifloxacin)
- Cefoxitin 1-2g IV q6h or cefotetan 1-2g IV q12h

Surgical treatment
- Laparoscopic cholecystectomy preferred if possible; early cholecystectomy can be performed in the majority of cases; some surgeons advocate delayed surgery.
- Open cholecystectomy if technically needed
- Percutaneous drainage or cholecystostomy if unable to tolerate above
- Unlike calculus cholecystitis, early/emergent intervention indicated in acalculus cholecystitis due to risk of gangrene and/or perforation: either percutaneous drainage via cholecystostomy, or CCY.

Prophylaxis for cholecystectomy
- Indicated for all cholecystectomy operations in patients with acute cholecystitis.
- Prophylaxis also indicated in high risk patients (age > 70, nonfunctioning gallbladder, obstructive jaundice, or common duct stones)
- Also advocated by many clinicians for endoscopic retrograde cholangiopancreatography
- Cefazolin 1-2g IV within 60 minutes prior to surgical incision
- Antibiotics not needed beyond the operating room time

DRUG-SPECIFIC COMMENTS

Ampicillin + Sulbactam: Good coverage of gram-positive, gram-negative, and anaerobic pathogens - lacks Pseudomonas aeruginosa coverage but good Enterococcus species coverage.

Cefepime: Excellent gram-negative coverage with some gram-positive.

Cefotetan: Good single agent coverage of gram-positives, gram-negatives, and anaerobes, drug currently not available in the U.S.

Ciprofloxacin: Good gram-negative coverage, gram-positive coverage is suboptimal for most purposes

Ertapenem: Gram-positive (except enterococcus), gram-negative (except resistant GNR, P. aeruginosa), and anaerobic coverage - good monotherapy

Gatifloxacin: Excellent broad spectrum coverage but clinical data limited on anaerobe coverage.

DIAGNOSIS

Imipenem/Cilastatin: Excellent broad spectrum (gram-positive, gram-negative, and anaerobe) coverage; would reserve for seriously ill patients.

Levofloxacin: Good gram-positive and gram-negative coverage

Meropenem: Excellent broad spectrum (gram-positive, gram-negative, and anaerobe) coverage; would reserve for seriously ill patients.

Moxifloxacin: Excellent gram-positive, gram-negative, and reasonable anaerobic coverage.

Piperacillin: Good single agent coverage of gram-positives (including some enterococcus species coverage) and gram-negatives including Pseudomonas aeruginosa; has some anaerobic coverage but not Bacteroides fragilis.

Piperacillin + Tazobactam: Improved gram-positive (including Staphylococcus aureus and coagulase negative staphylococcus species) coverage, improved gram-negative coverage (B-lactamase producing pathogens) and improved anaerobic coverage (including Bacteroides fragilis) compared to piperacillin alone.

Ticarcillin: Good single agent coverage of gram-positives (including some enterococcus species coverage) and gram-negatives including Pseudomonas aeruginosa; has some anaerobic coverage but not Bacteroides fragilis.

Ticarcillin + Clavulanic Acid: Improved gram-positive (including Staphylococcus aureus and coagulase negative staphylococcus species) coverage, improved gram-negative coverage (B-lactamase producing pathogens) and improved anaerobic coverage (including Bacteroides fragilis) compared to ticarcillin alone.

IMPORTANT POINTS

- Patients with acute cholecystitis require hospitalization, and the definitive treatment is cholecystectomy (may be required emergently, e.g., emphysematous cholecystitis, etc.)
- Early symptoms related to inflammation. Late signs, symptoms and complications likely infectious
- Over 90% of patients have calculus cholecystitis. Acalculus cholecystitis has different epidemiology (less predominant in females and often associated with other acute events, e.g., trauma).
- Chronic cholecystitis is not an indication for antibiotic treatment. Should elective cholecystectomy be performed, preoperative prophylaxis should be considered in high risk patients.

SELECTED READINGS

National Surgery Infection Prevention Project. Antimicrobial prophylaxis for surgery: an advisory statement from the National Surgical Infection Prevention Project. Clin Infect Disease 2004 Jun 15;38 (12):1706-15

The Medical Letter - Treatment Guidelines. Antimicrobial prophylaxis in surgery. Treatment Guidelines 2004 April;19:13-26.

Solomkin et al. Guidelines for the Selection of Anti-infective Agents for Complicated Intra-abdominal Infections. Clin Infect Disease 2003 October 15;37:997-1005

Mazuski JE, Sawyer RG, Nathans AB et al. The Surgical Infection Society Guidelines on Antimicrobial Therapy for Intra-Abdominal Infections: An Executuve Summary . Surgical Infections 2002, Vol 3 (3)

Indar AA, Beckingham IJ: . Acute cholecystitis . BMJ 2002; 325:639-643

Lillemoe KD. Surgical treatment of biliary tract infections. Am Surg 2000 Feb;66(2):138-44

Westphal JF and Brogard JM. Biliary Tract Infections: a guide to treatment. Drugs 1999 Jan;57(1):81-91

CHRONIC FATIGUE SYNDROME

Khalil G. Ghanem, M.D.

DIAGNOSTIC CRITERIA

- Profound disabling fatigue X 6mos + 4 of the following: impaired memory, sore throat, tender glands, stiff/aching muscles, joint pain, new headaches, unrefreshing sleep, & post-exertional fatigue.
- Chronic fatigue syndrome (CFS) is a clinical (symptom-based) dx NOT a dx made by exam or laboratory findings (except to r/o other causes). Note: 10-15% of US population c/o fatigue and muscle aches.
- Concomitant disorders that occur with CFS: fibromyalgia (35-70%), multiple chemical sensitivities, irritable bowel syndrome, Gulf War Syndrome, & TMJ disorders.
- Prevalence: 0.007% to 2.8% in general population; most commonly affects young white successful women who are 30-40 years old; children and adolescents less affected.
- Psychiatric, infectious, endocrine & sleep disorders argued; but no causality established. Post-infectious fatigue syndrome favored as term when infection (EBV, Lyme, etc.) precedes prolonged fatigue.

TREATMENT REGIMENS

Non-pharmacological

- Graded low-impact exercise programs
- Cognitive behavioral therapy
- Patient advocacy groups to educate and counsel patients have been shown to be most helpful

Pharmacological

- None of the following pharmacological regimens have shown substantial benefit in treating patients with CFS:
- Antidepressants: monoamine oxidase inhibitors (MAOI) modestly effective; serotonin-specific uptake inhibitors not as effective.
- Antidepressants: venlafaxine (titrated to 450mg qd) or pramipexole (0.125-0.5 qhs) for poor sleep may be helpful, although, no good published data.
- Immunological: IVIG (1 placebo-controlled trial); specifically configured RNA drug: poly(I):poly(C12U) (1 placebo controlled trial); corticosteroid and interferon data inconclusive.
- Antivirals: acyclovir was used in one study without clear benefit.
- Antifungals: no benefit.
- Unproven benefit: chelation therapy, anabolic steroids, megadose vitamins, chronic antibiotics or antivirals, & immune boosters.
- Some early studies of neurally mediated hypotension favored vigorous hydration, supplemental salt, & florinef, but this has fallen out of favor.

IMPORTANT POINTS

- Strict CDC definition is for research purposes only; many patients may suffer from CFS without meeting all criteria.
- Ddx of fatigue: depression, somatization, hypothyroidism, hypogonadism, adrenal insuff, hemochromatosis, orthostatic hypotension & sleep disorders. Baseline labs (CBC, chemistries, ESR) assumed nl.
- No infectious etiologies have been causally linked to CFS.
- Non-pharmacological strategies such as exercise and cognitive behavioral therapy have had modest success in treating patients with CFS.

- Pharmacological therapy, save for MAOI drugs, have had minimal documented impact on patient symptoms.

SELECTED READINGS

Blacker CV, Greenwood DT, Wesnes KA, et al. Effect of galantamine hydrobromide in chronic fatigue syndrome: a randomized controlled trial. JAMA. 2004 Sep 8;292(10):1195-204

Afari N, Buchwald D. Chronic fatigue syndrome: a review. Am J Psychiatry. 2003 Feb;160(2):221-36

Wessely S, Chalder T, Hirsch S, et al. Postinfectious fatigue: prospective cohort study in primary care. Lancet. 1995 May 27;345(8961):1333-8

Koelle DM, Barcy S, Huang ML, et al. Markers of viral infection in monozygotic twins discordant for chronic fatigue syndrome. Clin Infect Dis. 2002 Sep 1;35(5):518-25.

Straus SE, Dale JK, Tobi M, et al. Acyclovir treatment of the chronic fatigue syndrome. Lack of efficacy in a placebo-controlled trial. N Engl J Med. 1988 Dec 29;319(26):1692-8.

Reeves WC, Stamey FR, Black JB, et al. Human herpesviruses 6 and 7 in chronic fatigue syndrome: a case-control study. Clin Infect Dis. 2000 Jul;31(1):48-52. Epub 2000 Jul 24.

Rowe PC, Calkins H, DeBusk K, et al. Fludrocortisone acetate to treat neurally mediated hypotension in chronic fatigue syndrome: a randomized controlled trial. JAMA. 2001 Jan 3;285(1):52-9.

White PD, Thomas JM, Kangro HO, et al. Predictions and associations of fatigue syndromes and mood disorders that occur after infectious mononucleosis. Lancet. 2001 Dec 8;358(9297):1946-54

Swanink CM, van der Meer JW, Vercoulen JH, et al. Epstein-Barr virus (EBV) and the chronic fatigue syndrome: normal virus load in blood and normal immunologic reactivity in the EBV regression assay. Clin Infect Dis. 1995 May;20(5):1390-2.

Kerr JR, Cunniffe VS, Kelleher P, et al. Successful intravenous immunoglobulin therapy in 3 cases of parvovirus B19-associated chronic fatigue syndrome. Clin Infect Dis. 2003 May 1;36(9):e100-6.

CONJUNCTIVITIS, ACUTE   Spyridon Marinopoulos, M.D.

DIAGNOSTIC CRITERIA

- Epidemic keratoconjunctivitis (EKC): highly contagious fulminant type viral conjunctivitis. Presents w/ severe foreign-body sensation & decreased visual acuity.
- Allergic: IgE response to environment allergens. Hx: B/L redness, watery d/c, itching (hallmark), worse with rubbing. PE: diffuse injection, watery/mucoserous discharge, indistinguishable from viral
- Bacterial: Hx/PE: uni/bilateral redness. Thick, globular, purulent white, yellow or green d/c lid margin/eye corners. Eye stuck shut in AM. If tender preauricular LN, think GC/chlamydia
- Rapidly progressive redness, hyperpurulence, tenderness, lid edema & tender preauricular LN suggest gonococcal hyperacute bacterial conjuctivitis. Lab: pus w/ gram neg diplococci
- Viral: Hx: thin, watery/mucoserous rather than purulent discharge. +/- viral URI. Burning, sandy or gritty feeling common. PE: diffuse conjunctival injection & profuse tearing +/- preauricular LN

COMMON PATHOGENS: S. aureus; S. pneumoniae; Haemophilus influenzae ; Neisseria gonorrhoeae ; Chlamydia trachomatis ; Adenovirus 6, 11, and 19

TREATMENT REGIMENS

Topical antibiotics

- Comment: use for bacterial conjunctivitis. All doses while awake. Ointments may blur vision x 20 min post administration. Must use systemic abx for gonorrheal/chlamydial disease
- Trimethoprim-Polymyxin B (Polytrim) sol 1gtt q3h x 7-10d

- Bacitracin-Polymyxin B (Polysporin) ophthalmic 1gtt q3-4h x 7-10d
- Sulfacetamide (Bleph-10) 10% sol 1-2gtt q2-3h x 7-10d, taper to BID with improvement. Some staph strains may be resistant
- Erythromycin ophthalmic oint 1/2-in qid inside lower lid x 5-7d. Some staph strains may be resistant
- Fluoroquinolones: use for more serious cases, esp if suspected Pseudomonas (contact lens wearers) or corneal ulcers
- Levofloxacin (Quixin) 0.5% sol 1-2gtt q2h x 2d then 1-2gtt qid x5d or ofloxacin (Ocuflox) 0.3% sol 1-2 gtt q2-4h x 2d then 1-2gtt qid x 5d or Cipro (Ciloxan) 0.3% sol 1-2gtt q2h x 2d then 1-2gtt q4h x 5d
- Bacitracin-Neomycin-Polymyxin B (Neosporin Ophthalmic) sol 1-2gtt q4h x 7-10d. Up to 10% pts allergic to neomycin.
- Tobramycin (Tobrex) 0.3% sol 1-2gtt q4h x 7d or gentamicin (Garamycin, Genoptic) 0.3% sol 1-2gtt q4h x 7d
- AVOID: chloramphenicol (Chloroptic) 0.5% sol 1-2gtt 4-6x/d x 3d, use only if no other options avail. Bone marrow aplasia with prolonged/frequent use has resulted in death

Systemic antibiotics

- Comment: in patients with gonococcal disease, treat sexual partners & consider/treat chlamydial co-infection. Vice versa for patients w/ chlamydial conjunctivitis. Also consider/screen for other STDs
- Hyperacute bacterial conjunctivitis (Neisseria gonorrhoeae): ceftriaxone 1g IM x 1 dose
- Alternative for pen/ceph allergic patients: spectinomycin 2g IM x 1 dose (currently unavail in US)
- Only if ceph allergy & spect unavail: norfloxacin 1200mg PO x 1 dose effective in one case series BUT Asia/Pacific Basin/Hawaii/some US (esp CA) strains FQ resistant - DO NOT USE if areas of origin
- Cipro/levo/oflox used to Rx non-conj GC infxn (ref Neisseria gonorrhoeae module) but no studies re Rx of GC conjunctivitis. One case report used Cipro 500mg PO bid + Cipro drops qid x 2 wk w/ success
- Adult inclusion conjuctivitis (Chlamydia trachomatis): azithromycin 1g PO x 1 dose or doxy 100mg PO q12h or tetracycline 250mg PO q6h or erythromycin 250mg PO q6h x 14d

Miscellaneous

- Comment: there is no role for the use of steroid eye drops or antibiotic/steroid drop combinations to Rx conjunctivitis in the primary care setting. Refer to ophthalmology if contemplating use.
- All patients with red eye: discontinue contact lenses and resume only when eye is white and without discharge after Rx completed. Discard lens case and disinfect or replace lens.
- Allergic: pheniramine-naphazoline (Naphcon-A) 1-2gtt qid PRN. May try lopatadine (Patanol) 0.1% sol 1gtt bid or ketorolac tromethamine (Acular) 0.5% sol 1gtt qid if above not effective.
- Hyperacute bacterial conjunctivitis: saline lavage to clear mucopurulent debris and dilute effects of released toxins on ocular tissues. Monitor closely for possible keratitis and perforation.
- Viral conjuctivitis: instruct patient to avoid sharing personal items (towels, sheets, pillows, etc.), use meticulous hand washing & avoid close personal contact for approximately 2 weeks.
- Patients with adenoviral conjunctivitis need to dispose of unclean contact lenses as adenovirus survives chemical and hydrogen peroxide disinfection.

- Epidemic keratoconjunctivitis (EKC): refer to ophthalmology. Highly contagious disease requiring implementation of isolation and infection control procedures.

Drug-Specific Comments

Chloramphenicol: More commonly used in Europe. Avoid. Cases of bone marrow aplasia and death have been reported with prolonged/frequent use.

Ciprofloxacin: Eye drops: Big gun. Expensive. Would not use as first line unless Pseudomonas suspected, as in contact lens wearers. Approximately 20% risk of crystalline precipitate in cornea, resolves w/ discontinuation of rx. Oral: Not approved for the treatment of gonococcal conjunctivitis. Single dose effective for the treatment of gonorrhea but some strains resistant.

Doxycycline: BID dosing. Preferred for chlamydial conjunctivitis over erythro. May cause fetal harm. Stains teeth in pts < 8 years old. Photosensitivity.

Gentamicin: Treats wide range of bacterial eye infections, but may damage corneal epthelium with prolonged use. Use in treating specific gram negatives and Staph aureus.

Levofloxacin: Eye drops: Big gun. Expensive. Alternative to Cipro. Would not use as first line unless Pseudomonas suspected, as in contact lens wearers. May achieve superior microbial eradication rates vs. ofloxacin. No crystalline precipitate.

Norfloxacin: Not as well absorbed as other fluoroquinolones. Risk of crystalluria. Patients receiving norfloxacin should be well hydrated and should be instructed to drink fluids liberally. Otherwise similar to other quinolones.

Tetracycline: Inconvenient qid alternative to doxy. May cause fetal harm. Stains teeth in pts < 8 years old. Photosensitivity.

Tobramycin: May damage corneal epithelium. Alternative to gent. Use in treating specific gram negatives and Staph aureus.

Important Points

- Recommendations are author's opinion.
- Ddx subconjunctival hemorrhage, blepharitis, eyelid disorders, scleritis, episcleritis, keratitis, pterygium, acute anterior uveitis, acute angle closure glaucoma.
- Cultures not necessary for dx & Rx unless recurrent, severe sx or suspected hyperacute conjunctivitis. Consider GC/Chlamydia in sexually active pts. Refer immediately.
- Advise immediate contact lens discontinuation in any patient with red eye. Refer to ophthalmology urgently if keratitis, iritis/uveitis, scleritis or angle closure glaucoma suspected by hx or PE.
- Think of secondary conjunctivitis or pseudomonal, ulcerative keratitis & have low threshhold for referral in contact lens wearers. Foreign body sensation & corneal opacity on penlight exam.
- Red flags pain/photophobia/decreased acuity. Refer ASAP if any of above present, worse after 1-2d of Rx or no better after 7d. Exception: viral conj sx may worsen first 3-5d, reassure if no red flags.

Selected Readings

Centers for Disease Control and Prevention (CDC). Acute hemorrhagic conjunctivitis outbreak caused by Coxsackievirus A24--Puerto Rico, 2003. MMWR Morb Mortal Wkly Rep. 2004 Jul 23;53(28):632-4.

Schwab IR, Friedlaender M, McCulley J, et al. A phase III clinical trial of 0.5% levofloxacin ophthalmic solution versus 0.3% ofloxacin ophthalmic solution for the treatment of bacterial conjunctivitis. Ophthalmology 2003 Mar;110(3):457-65

Sheikh A, Hurwitz B, Cave J. Antibiotics versus placebo for acute bacterial conjunctivitis (Cochrane Review). The Cochrane Library, 2002;Issue 4

Graves A, Henry M, O'Brien TP, et al. In vitro susceptibilities of bacterial ocular isolates to fluoroquinolones. Cornea 2001 Apr;20(3):301-5

Kowalski RP, Sundar-Raj CV, Romanowski EG, et al. The disinfection of contact lenses contaminated with adenovirus. Am J Ophthalmol 2001;132:777-779

Price LM, O'Mahony C. Gonococcal ophthalmia treated with ciprofloxacin. Int J STD AIDS 2001 Dec;12 (12):829-30

Leibowitz HM. The Red Eye. NEJM 2000;343(5):345-51

Tabbara, KF, El-Sheikh, HF, Aabed, B. Extended wear contact lens related bacterial keratitis. Br J Ophthalmol 2000; 84:327-328

Raizman, MB, Rothman, IS, Maroun, F, et al. Effect of eye rubbing on signs and symptoms of allergic conjunctivitis in cat-sensitive individuals. Ophthalmology 2000; 107:2158-2161

Cheng, KH, Leung, SL, Hoekman, HW, et al. Incidence of contact-lens-associated microbial keratitis and its related morbidity. Lancet 1999; 354:179-183

CRYPTOSPORIDIOSIS [AIDS]   John G. Bartlett, M.D.

DIAGNOSTIC CRITERIA

- C. parvum and C. hominis are most common cause of severe diarrhea w/low CD4. Contaminated water is usual source, also person-person, food.
- Hx: watery diarrhea; sx are more severe & persistent with CD4 count <100
- Sx: Diarrhea +/- nausea, vomiting, fever in 1/3
- Large volume, secretory diarrhea without blood or pus. Cause of HIV cholangiopathy in AIDS. Infection otherwise self-limiting usually in the immune competent.
- Lab: cryptosporidia not seen by standard O&P exam. Must request modified AFB (they stain red), trichrome or DFA stain of stool

COMMON PATHOGENS: Cryptosporidium parvum ; C. hominis

TREATMENT REGIMENS

Antimicrobials

- RX: only proven Rx is HAART with immune reconstitution
- Preferred (IDSA Guidelines - CID 2001;32:331): paromomycin 500mg PO tid (w/food) x 14-28d + HAART
- Alt: paromomycin 1g PO bid (w/food) x 2-4 wks then 0.5-1.0g PO bid

Antiperistaltic agents

- Loperamide 4mg PO, then 2mg PO with each loose stool up to 16 mg/day max
- Lomotil 2.5mg PO qid
- Codeine 15-60mg (usually 30mg) PO q3-6h prn
- Deodorized tincture of opium (DTO) 0.3-1mL (usually 0.6mL) PO 3-4x/d prn

Non-specific treatment

- Diet: frequent small feedings, diet: low-fat, lactose- & caffeine-free, high fiber, bland foods
- Fluid support - losses up to 10 L/d
- Oral feedings to replace NaHCO3, K, Mg, P04, glucose
- Non-specific agents: NSAIDs, bismuth subsalicylate (PeptoBismol)
- Food supplements--Vivonex, TEN, etc.
- Parenteral hyperalimentation--severe refractory cases only
- Octreotide- not effective
- Prevention: boil water x 1 min, 1 um filter or bottled water; filters - call 800-673-8010 (NSF International)

DRUG-SPECIFIC COMMENTS

Atovaquone: Sometime tried in desperation. Utility unproven and cost is high. Dose: 750mg bid w/meals.

Clarithromycin: (Biaxin) Role in treating cryptosporidiosis is unclear. When combined with rifabutin for MAC prophylaxis there is a reduced rate of cryptosporidiosis, but some would question the wisdom of combining RBT & clari due to drug interaction.

Nitazoxanide: Therapeutic trial (ACTG 192) showed marginal response, but it was inadequate to convince the FDA for approval.

Paromomycin: May help control cryptosporidiosis, but not curative. Must be taken with food.

IMPORTANT POINTS

- Guidelines from NYS AIDS Institute (09/04).
- Healthy host may have self-limited disease lasting 2-3 wk; compromised hosts (CD4 <100) may have severe chronic diarrhea
- No good therapy: paromomycin, azithromycin, atovaquone and nitazoxanide tried and failed in HIV. Adequate volume replacement essential; hyperalimentation may be required.
- Best therapy is HAART with immune reconstitution; even slight increase in CD4 reduces disease
- Paromomycin must be taken with meals and rarely helps

SELECTED READINGS

Hunter, PR et al. Health sequelae of human cryptosporidiosis in immunocompetent patients. CID 2004;39:504-10

Xiao L, Ryan UM. Cryptosporidiosis: an update in molecular epidemiology. Curr Opin Infect Dis 2004;17:483

USPHS/IDSA. Guidelines for the Prevention of Opportunistic Infections in Persons with HIV. MMWR 2001 2002;51RR-1

Leav BA, et al. Cryptosporidium species: New insights and old challenges. CID 2003;36:903

Carr A, Marriott D, Field A. Treatment of HIV-1-associated microsporidiosis and cryptosporidiosis with combination antiretroviral therapy. Lancet 1998;351:256

Smith NJ, Cron S, Valdez LM, et al. Combination drug therapy for cryptosporidiosis in AIDS. J Infect Dis 1998;178:900

Dunne WM, Williams DJ, Young LS. Azithromycin and the treatment of opportunistic infections. Rev Contemp Pharmacother 1994;5:373

Vakil NB, Schwartz FN, Buggy BP,et al. Biliary cryptosporidiosis in HIV-infected people after the water-borne outbreak of cryptosporidiosis in Milwaukee. N Engl J Med 1996;334:19

Clark DP. Cryptosporidiosis. Clin Microbiol Rev 1999;12:554

Miao YM et al. Eradication of cryptosporidia and microsporidia following successful antiretroviral therapy. JAIDS 2000; 25:124

CYSTITIS, ACUTE UNCOMPLICATED BACTERIAL
Noreen A. Hynes, M.D., M.P.H.

DIAGNOSTIC CRITERIA

- Clinical: urgency, frequency, suprapubic discomfort; NO urinary sx in past 4 wk; no fever; no flank pain

- Lab: Dipstick positive leukocyte esterase test or positive nitrite (75% sensitive, 82% specific); >100 CFU/mL on midstream clean-catch urine culture; >9 WBCs/HPF of spun urine
- Uncomplicated UTI does not require culture unless apparent Rx failure noted with empiric therapy
- In sexually, active women, dysuria can be due to an STD rather than a UTI-->dysuria without pyuria suggests an STD rather than UTI. Rule out vaginitis, chlamydia, gonorrhea, HSV in sexually active

COMMON PATHOGENS: Escherichia coli ; Staphylococcus saprophyticus

TREATMENT REGIMENS

Short-course therapy

- Trimethoprim-Sulfamethoxazole 1 DS tab PO bid x 3d (Preferred for empiric Rx if prevalence of E. coli resistance to TMP-SMX <20%; if >20% use fluoroquinolone)
- Trimethoprim 300mg PO qd x 3d
- Norfloxacin 400mg PO bid x 3d
- Ciprofloxacin 250mg PO bid x 3d
- Ofloxacin 200mg PO bid x 3d
- Amoxicillin/clavulanate 500/125mg PO bid x 3d (Higher percentage of organisms resistant to amoxicillin alone).

Longer duration therapy

- Trimethoprim-Sulfamethoxazole 1 DS tab PO bid x 5-7d (Preferred for empiric Rx if prevalence of E. coli resistance to TMP-SMX <20%; if >20% use fluoroquinolone)
- Trimethoprim 100mg PO bid x 7d
- Norfloxacin 400mg PO bid x 7d
- Ciprofloxacin 250mg PO bid x 7d
- Amoxicillin/clavulanate 500/125mg PO bid x 7d (higher percentage of organisms resistant to amoxicillin alone).
- Amoxicillin 250mg PO tid x 7d
- Cephalexin 250mg PO tid x 7d

Treatment in women with diabetes and older women

- Do NOT use short-course (3-day) Rx in diabetics
- Treat for 7-10 d with any agent listed under "Longer Duration Therapy" outlined above

DRUG-SPECIFIC COMMENTS

Amoxicillin: 1. A second line therapy for the empiric Rx of uncomplicated UTI in women; 3-day Rx should be avoided. 30%-40% of E. coli isolates may be resistant to this agent. 2. First line therapy if the etiology known to be due to a gram-positive organism, e.g., S. saprophyticus 3. 25%-40% of E. coli are resistant to this agent in some U.S. locations. 4. Amoxicillin-clavulanate may be a more reasonable agent than amoxicillin in that E.coli resistance to agent is less but cost much higher.

Amoxicillin + Clavulanate: 1. A second line therapy for the empiric Rx of uncomplicated UTI in women 2. First line therapy if the etiology known to be due to a gram-positive organism, e.g., S. saprophyticus 3. 25%-40% of E. coli are resistant to this agent in some U. S. locations; resistance is higher for amoxicillin alone.

Cephalexin: 1. The cephalosporins, in general, perform much worse than TMP-SMX, FQs, amoxicillin, amox-clavulanate in the treatment of uncomplicated UTIs. 2. They are never a first-line agent. 3. They should not be used in a 3-day dosing regimen due to high recurrence rates.

DIAGNOSIS

Trimethoprim: 1. TMP alone is equivalent to TMP-SMX, at least in 7 day Rx and has a lower side effect profile. 2. A first-line therapy for the empiric treatment of uncomplicated UTI in women. 3. In some parts of the world TMP-resistant E. coli may be as high as 50%.

IMPORTANT POINTS

- Recommendations from IDSA Guidelines (CID 1999;29:745).
- The MOST common bacterial infection in women. The incidence of acute, uncomplicated UTIs in young women is 0.5-0.7 episode/yr with approximately 6 associated disability-days/episode.
- 25%-30% of women who have an initial bout of acute, uncomplicated bacterial cystitis will have recurrent infections.
- If S. saprophyticus is the suspected or known cause of the UTI, then the longer therapy (7 days) should be used due to increased efficacy.
- Older women with acute bacterial cystitis should be managed using a longer regimen
- In premenopausal women, the key risk factors for acute, uncomplicated UTI include: a) coitus, b) prior HX of UTI, c) spermicide exposure, d) recent antibiotic use.
- In premenopausal women with recurrent, uncomplicated UTI same risk factors apply as above AND a) maternal HX of UTI or b) HX of childhood UTI (both are consistent with an inherited predisposition to UTI such as nonsecretor status).
- In postmenopausal women with uncomplicated recurrent UTI the major risk factors are anatomical or functional defects including a) incontinence, b) post-void residual urine, and c) cystocele. Additional factor is the relative lack of estrogen effect. This results in loss of dominance of lactobacilli among vaginal flora with subsequent increase in vaginal pH, increased colonization of the introitus with E. coli. This provides a setting for increased number of UTIs. Studies have shown that the use of topical estrogens reverses these changes and greatly reduces the incidence of recurrent UTI in such women NOT using HRT.

SELECTED READINGS

Wilson ML and Gaido L. Laboratory diagnosis of urinary tract infections in adult patients. Clin Infect Dis 2004; 38:1150-1138.

Fihn SD. Acute uncomplicated urinary tract infection in women. N Engl J Med 2003; 349:259-66.

McIssac WJ et al. The impact of empirical management of acute cystitis on unnecessary antibiotic use. Arch Intern Med 2002; 162(5):600-5.

Gupta K et al. Antimicrobial resistance among uropathogens that cause community-acquired urinary tract infections in women: a nationwide analysis. Clin Infect Dis 2001;33:89-94.

Huovinen P. Resistance to trimethoprim-sulfamethoxazole. Clin Infect Dis 2001;32:1608-14.

Le TP and Miller LG. Empirical therapy for uncomplicated urinary tract infection in an era of increasing antimicrobial resistance: a decision and cost analysis. Clin Infect Dis 2001:33:615-621.

Stamm WE and Norrby SR. Urinary tract infections: disease panorama and challenges. J Infect Dis 2001; 183(Suppl 1):S1-4.

Hooton TM, et al. A prospective study of asymptomatic bacteriuria in sexually active young women. New Engl J Med 2000; 343:992

Echols RM, et al. Demographic, clinical, and treatment parameters influencing the outcome of acute cystitis. Clin Infect Dis 1999; 29(1):113-9

Gupta K, et al. The prevalence of antimicrobial resistance among uropathogens causing acute uncomplicated cystitis in young women. Int J Antimicrob Agents 1999; 11:305-8.

DENTAL INFECTIONS
Spyridon Marinopoulos, M.D.

DIAGNOSTIC CRITERIA
- Dental caries: no sx. Chalky white lesion turns golden-brown then dark/black with central cavitation. Pain suggests progression to pulp infection (pulpitis).
- Pulpitis: sharp-to-dull throbbing pain, tooth specific or generalized, may refer to ear/temple/neck/opposite jaw (rare). May be early/reversible or progress to late/irreversible stage with necrosis.
- Early: sensitive to temperature change, sweet stimuli, worse w/ reclining, spontaneously better in secs. Late: pain severe, persistent, often poorly localized, worse with any stimulus including air
- PE: grossly decayed tooth. If not obvious, localize by percussing with or asking pt to bite on tongue blade. Exquisite pain suggests progression to periapical abscess
- Periapical abscess Hx/PE: exquisite tooth pain w/ touch/chewing. Loss of temp sensitivity. Fever, LN, tooth mobility (tooth feels higher/longer) +/- soft tissue edema

COMMON PATHOGENS: Streptococcus mutans ; pigmented Bacteroides (Porphyromonas & Prevotella) ; Streptococcus milleri ; Actinomyces viscosus ; Peptostreptococcus

TREATMENT REGIMENS

Miscellaneous
- Warm saline rinses
- NSAIDs +/- weak opioid analgesics for pain control
- Early/reversible pulpitis: removing carious lesion and filling of cavities with inert material may be sufficient to arrest disease
- Late/irreversible pulpitis requires endodontic therapy (root canal treatment) or extraction of involved tooth
- Note: persistent root canal infxn is associated w/ Candida albicans. Eradicate w/ calcium hydroxide/camphorated paramonochlorophenol/glycerin or 0.12% chlorhexidine digluconate/zinc oxide
- Periapical abscess requires I&D + endodontic therapy (root canal treatment) or extraction of diseased tooth. Abx are adjunctive only
- Prevention is essential and involves meticulous dental care and frequent dental visits to eliminate dental caries

Antibiotics
- Comment: abx commonly used for the Rx of periapical abscess, but generally not needed in healthy pts w/ pulpitis alone. Use if systemic sxs/signs of infxn. Rx 3d, then reassess, may need 7d.
- Penicillin VK 500mg PO q6h x 7d. Switch/broaden coverage if no better after 48 hrs
- Cephalexin 500mg PO q6h x 7d. Switch/broaden coverage if no better after 48 hrs
- Clindamycin 300mg PO q6h x 7d in pen-allergic pts or if pen/ceph ineffective. First-line in more severe cases, if anaerobes predominant (after day 3) or beta-lactamase resistance a concern
- Penicillin VK 500mg PO q6h + metronidazole (Flagyl) 500mg PO q6h x 7d excellent for broader gram pos & anaerobic coverage when pen alone ineffective
- Augmentin 500mg PO q8h x 7d if pen/ceph ineffective. First-line in more severe cases, if anaerobes predominant (after day 3) or beta-lactamase resistance a concern
- Limited use: erythromycin 500mg PO q6h x 7d alternative to penicillin but less active against anaerobes & certain mouth flora and there is emerging resistance. Clinda preferred

- Azithromycin 500mg PO x1 then 250mg PO qd x4d (ZPAK) OR clarithromycin (Biaxin) 500mg PO q12h x 7d more expensive alternatives to erythro w/ similar concerns re: resistance
- Non-preferred: doxycycline 200mg PO x 1 then 100mg PO qd x 7d OR tetracycline 250mg PO q6h x 7d in pen-allergic patients. Very limited use as some strep & anaerobes resistant. Clinda preferred

DRUG-SPECIFIC COMMENTS

Amoxicillin: Easier dosing than penicillin VK, broader coverage, slightly more expensive

Amoxicillin + Clavulanate: Much costlier than penicillin or amox. Broader coverage anaerobically as well as gram negative. 500 TID regimen preferred over 875 BID regimen.

Cephalexin: Effective alternative to penicillin. Inconvenient qid dosing.

Ciprofloxacin: Use to manage severe infections in combination with clindamycin or metronidazole. Not commonly prescribed.

Doxycycline: BID dosing. Non-preferred alternative to penicillin as some strep resistant and lacks optimal anaerobic activity. Photosensitivity.

Metronidazole: Only covers anaerobes and does not fully cover oral microaerophilic spp., therefore, never used as sole agent. Watch for P450 drug-drug interactions.

Penicillin: Inexpensive, well absorbed and effective. Dosing nconvenience main drawback. 10% allergy risk.

Tetracycline: Inconvenient qid dosing. Non-preferred alternative to penicillin as some strep resistant and lacks optimal anaerobic activity. Photosensitivity.

IMPORTANT POINTS

- Recommendations represent the author's opinion. The etiology of dental infections is dental caries which can be prevented by meticulous dental hygiene and frequent dental visits
- Treatment of infection must always involve treatment of the offending tooth +/- abscess drainage if necessary. Abx may be used for periapical abscess but not needed in healthy pts with pulpitis alone
- Potential complications include sinusitis, cavernous sinus thrombosis, Ludwig's angina, retro/parapharyngeal abscess, osteomyelitis, endocarditis, brain abscess
- Infection may spread into fascial planes & extend into face/neck soft tissues if bacteria aggressive or host compromised. Dysphagia/drooling suggest retro/parapharyngeal infection, a medical emergency
- Refer to dentist ASAP if 1) severe, acute pain unrelieved with analgesics or removal of thermal stimuli; 2) trauma; 3) new or enlarging orofacial swelling; 4) uncontrolled bleeding; 5) fever

SELECTED READINGS

Siqueira JF Jr, Sen BH. Fungi in endodontic infections. Oral Surg Oral Med Oral Pathol Oral Radiol Endod. 2004 May;97(5):632-41.

Swift J, Gulden W . Antibiotic therapy-managing odontogenic infections. Dent Clin N Am 2002;46:623-633

Wynn R, Bergman S, Meiller T, et al. Antibiotics in treating oral-facial infections of odontogenic origin: An update. Gen Dent 2001;49(3):238-40,242,244

Wayne D, Trajtenberg C, Hyman D . Tooth and Periodontal Disease: A Review for the Primary-Care Physician. South Med J 2001;94(9):925-932

Flynn T. The swollen face. Severe odontogenic infections. Emerg Med Clin North Am 2000; 18(3): 481-519

Caufield P, Griffen A. Dental caries. An Infectious and Preventable disease . Ped Clin North Am 2000;47 (5)

Johnson B. Oral Infection. Principles and Practice of Antibiotic Therapy. Infect Dis Clin North Am 1999;13(4):851-870

Moore PA. Dental therapeutic indications for the newer long-acting macrolide antibiotics. J Am Dent Assoc 1999;130(9):1341-3

Peterson LR, Thomson RB . Use of the clinical microbiology laboratory for the diagnosis and management of infectious diseases related to the oral cavity. Infect Dis Clin North Am 1999;13(4):775-95

Sandor G, Low D, Judd P, et al. Antimicrobial treatment options in the management of odontogenic infections. J Can Dent Assoc 1998;64(7):508-514

DIABETIC FOOT INFECTION   Eric Nuermberger, M.D.

DIAGNOSTIC CRITERIA

- Hx: Cellulitis or ulcer usually painless due to diabetic neuropathy
- PE: a) cellulitis; b) infxn of superficial ulcer; c) deep soft tissue infxn/abscess; d) osteomyelitis (ulcer penetrating to bone); e) gangrene (demarcated necrotic tissue-wet or dry)
- Rad: Plain film insensitive for early osteo; bone scan highly sensitive, but not specific; MRI is best study (95% sens, 99% spec), but some false positives due to neuropathic osteoarthropathy.
- Tagged white cell scans have better sensitivity/specificity than bone scans
- Ability to probe to bone at base of ulcer considered diagnostic for osteo, decreasing need for radiologic testing

COMMON PATHOGENS: Staphylococcus aureus ; Streptococcus species ; Enterobacteriaceae ; Anaerobes ; Enterococcus ; P. aeruginosa

TREATMENT REGIMENS

Cellulitis or mild superficial ulcer infection

- Cephalexin 500mg PO qid x 14d
- Amoxicillin/clavulanate 875-1000mg PO bid x 14d
- Clindamycin 300mg PO tid x 14d
- Cefazolin 1-2g IV q8h x 14d
- Ampicillin/sulbactam 3g IV q6h x 14d
- Clindamycin 600mg IV q6-8h x 14d
- Nafcillin or oxacillin 2g IV q4h x 14d
- Linezolid 600mg PO bid x 14d (MRSA)

Deep soft-tissue infection or osteomyelitis

- Urgent surgical consultation
- Consider vascular evaluation
- Ampicillin/sulbactam 3g IV q6h or ticarcillin/clavulanate 3.1g IV q6h or piperacillin/ tazobactam 3.375g IV q6h
- Alt: Clindamycin 600mg IV q6h + ciprofloxacin 750mg PO (400mg IV) q12h
- Alt: Ceftazidime 2g IV q8h or cefepime 2g IV q12h + clindamycin 600mg IV q8h
- Modify regimen according to culture results from deep wound cultures, bone biopsy
- Parenteral therapy until stable, then orals for up to 4 wks in absence of osteomyelitis
- For osteomyelitis: debridement of necrotic bone and 2 wks or more of parenteral therapy and 6 wks or more total antibiotics or no debridement and 2-6 wks of parenteral therapy and 2 months or more of oral therapy

DIAGNOSIS

- Some authors still favor 10-12 wks of parenteral therapy for bone infection

Limb-/life-threatening infection

- Urgent surgical consultation, urgent vascular evaluation. Pick abx regimen based on sensitivity data (if known), likelihood of MRSA and host issues.
- Clindamycin 900mg IV q8h + ciprofloxacin 400mg IV q12h or tobramycin 2.0 mg/kg IV x 1, then 1.7 mg/kg IV q8h
- Clindamycin 900mg IV q8h + ceftazidime 2g IV q8h or cefepime 2g IV q12h or cefotaxime 2g IV q8h or ceftriaxone 2g IV qd
- Piperacillin/tazobactam 3.375g IV q4h or ticarcillin/clavulanate 3.1g IV q4h
- Imipenem 500mg IV q6h or meropenem 1g IV q8h
- Vancomycin 1g IV q12h + aztreonam 2g IV q8h + metronidazole 500mg IV q6h
- Vancomycin 1g IV q12h + cefepime 2g IV q12h or ceftazidime 2g IV q8h + metronidazole 500mg IV q6h
- Treatment generally requires prolonged parenteral and oral therapy, duration determined by outcome and presence or absence of osteomyelitis

DRUG-SPECIFIC COMMENTS

Amoxicillin + Clavulanate: Good oral option for polymicrobial infections. New formulation allows increasing dose of amox (to 1000mg) without increasing dose of diarrhea-causing clavulanate.

Ampicillin + Sulbactam: Like other beta-lactam/lactamase inhibitor combinations, it provides broad coverage (gram-positive cocci, gram-negative bacilli, and anaerobes). A good choice for polymicrobial infections or infections with resistant nosocomial organisms. Shown in a double-blind, randomized trial to be as effective as, though less expensive than, imipenem in the treatment of the diabetic foot.

Aztreonam: Broad activity against gram-negative bacilli, but no gram-positive or anaerobic activity. Good penetration into blister fluid, infected bone, and synovial fluid. An alternative for resistant nosocomial pathogens. Must accompany with agent(s) active against gram-positive and anaerobic organisms for polymicrobial infections.

Cefepime: Fourth generation cephalosporin with further enhanced spectrum against gram-negative pathogens, including Pseudomonas aeruginosa. Use should be reserved for pathogens resistant to third generation cephalosporins. Poor activity against most gram-negative anaerobic pathogens.

Ceftazidime: Third generation cephalosporin with the greatest activity against Pseudomonas aeruginosa, though less active against Staphylococcus aureus. Therefore, a better choice when pseudomonas is suspected (diabetic foot with chronic ulcer, recent antibiotic usage).

Cephalexin: First-line oral agent for cellulitis or infected superficial ulcers. Increasingly threatened by rising incidence of MRSA infections in outpatients with health-care associated risk factors.

Ciprofloxacin: Most active fluoroquinolone against Pseudomonas and Enterobacteriaceae, though one of the least active against Staph. Therefore, best paired with a gram-positive/anaerobe agent (e.g., clindamycin) for polymicrobial infections. Use IV or high-dose oral (750mg) formulations to improve penetration.

Daptomycin: Parenteral agent remains relatively untested in osteomyelitis, but it may be useful in other soft tissue infections when MRSA is identified. There is more evidence to support the use of linezolid, however.

Gatifloxacin: Fluoroquinolone with greater potency vs. gram-positives compared to ciprofloxacin. Could be an alternative for listed regimens to treat superficial infections.

Good choice for osteomyelitis, especially oral therapy. For deep polymicrobial infections, it is best paired with metronidazole.

Imipenem/Cilastatin: Broad-spectrum, including anaerobes, make this agent an attractive alternative for polymicrobial infections or infections with resistant organisms. No better than ampicillin/sulbactam in a double-blind randomized trial. Meropenem is an alternative.

Levofloxacin: At the 750mg dose, levofloxacin has activity against Pseudomonas aeruginosa and Enterobacteriaceae similar to that of ciprofloxacin. Good choice for treatment of osteomyelitis, especially for oral therapy.

Linezolid: Only available antibiotic actually approved for diabetic foot infections. Good evidence for efficacy in cellulitis and infected ulcers. Limited data for osteomyelitis. Must be paired with other agent if gram-negative pathogens suspected or present.

Metronidazole: Highly potent agent for anaerobes. Excellent oral bioavailability and tissue distribution. Best paired with a fluoroquinolone or vancomycin+beta-lactam with little anaerobic activity.

Moxifloxacin: Fluoroquinolone with greater potency vs. gram-positives compared to ciprofloxacin. Could be an alternative for listed regimens to treat superficial infections. Good choice for osteomyelitis, especially oral therapy. For deep polymicrobial infections, it is best paired with metronidazole.

Piperacillin + Tazobactam: Like other beta-lactam/lactamase inhibitor combinations, it provides broad coverage. A good choice for polymicrobial infections or infections with resistant nosocomial organisms. More reliable anti-pseudomonal coverage than other penicillins, but should be used with four-hour dosing interval when Pseudomonas is suspected.

Ticarcillin + Clavulanic Acid: Like other beta-lactam/lactamase inhibitor combinations, it provides broad coverage, although coverage of Staph. aureus weaker than others. A good choice for polymicrobial infections or infections with resistant nosocomial organisms. Use four-hour dosing interval when treating severe infection or Pseudomonas.

IMPORTANT POINTS

- Guidelines: IDSA (CID 2004;39;104)
- Deep tissue specimens (e.g., bone biopsy, abscess fluid) give most reliable culture/susceptibility data. Superficial cultures (e.g., swabs) do not correlate reliably with deep cultures.
- Antimicrobial therapy best if combined with enforced non-weight bearing status (e.g., contact casting), glycemic control and complete debridement or resection of infected bone
- Choose IV antibiotics when systemically ill w/ severe infection, unable to take PO

SELECTED READINGS

Lipsky BA. Medical treatment of diabetic foot infections. Clin Infect Dis 2004;39(Suppl 2):104-14

Lipsky BA, Itani K, Norden C, et al. Treating foot infections in diabetic patients: a randomized, multicenter, open-label trial of linezolid versus ampicillin-sulbactam/amoxicillin-clavulanate. Clin Infect Dis 2004;38:17-24

Senneville E, Yazdanpanah Y, Cazaubiel M et al. Rifampicin-ofloxacin oral regimen for the treatment of mild to moderate diabetic foot osteomyelitis. J Antimicrob Chemother 2001;48:927-30.

Gough A, Clapperton M, Rolando N, et al. Randomized placebo-controlled trial of granulocyte-colony stimulating factor in diabetic foot infections. Lancet 1997;350:855

Tan JS, Fiedman NM, Hazelton-Miller C, et al. Can aggressive treatment of diabetic foot infections reduce the need for above-ankle amputation? . Clin Infect Dis 1996;23:286

Eckman MH, Greenfield S, Mackey WC, et al. Foot infections in diabetic patients: Decision and cost-effectiveness analyses. JAMA 1995;273:712

Grayson ML, Gibbons GW, Balogh K, et al. Probing to bone in infected pedal ulcers: A clinical sign of underlying osteomyelitis in diabetic patients. JAMA 1995;273:721

Grayson ML, Gibbons GW, Habershaw GM, et al;. Use of ampicillin/sulbactam versus imipenem/cilastatin in the treatment of limb-threatening foot infections in diabetic patients. Clin Infect Dis 1994;19:820

Seabrook GR, Edmiston CE, Schmitt DD, et al. Comparison of serum and tissue antibiotic levels in diabetes-related foot infections. Surgery 1991;110:671

Lipsky BA, Pecoraro RE, Larson SA, et al. Outpatient management of uncomplicated lower-extremity infections in diabetic patients. Arch Intern Med 1990;150:790

DIARRHEA, ANTIBIOTIC-ASSOCIATED

John G. Bartlett, M.D.

DIAGNOSTIC CRITERIA

- Clinical: Diarrhea ascribed to antibiotic use that is usually due to C. difficile or is enigmatic.
- Clinical features that suggest C. difficile are: fever, cramps, evidence of colitis, leukocytosis, hypoalbuminemia, endoscopy showing colitis or pseudomembraneous colitis (nearly diagnostic).
- Laboratory: Positive stool C. difficile toxin assay.

COMMON PATHOGENS: C. difficile ; Salmonella species ; Clostridium perfringens ; P. aeruginosa

TREATMENT REGIMENS

General

- Principles: AAD is C dif pos-20%, may be serious (colitis, toxic megacolon) & treatable w/metronidazole; C. difficile neg-80%, usually not serious, symptomatic Rx
- Clostridium difficile positive: guidelines IDSA (CID 2001;32:331): D/C implicated ABX +/- metronidazole PO 250mg qid or 500mg tid x 10d + AVOID ANTIPERISTALTIC AGENTS + infection control
- C. difficile neg: Quality of test variable - if strong suspicion treat and repeat a neg toxin assay. If test neg x 2-3x - D/C implicated abx or switch give fluid support + loparamide 4mg then 2mg q loose stool
- Deit: Oral rehydration - soups + clear fluids. Diet - lactose & caffeine free, bland, small feedings
- If abx necessary for original infection: AVOID suspected drug and clind, cephalosporins + broad spectrum penicillins (amp, pip); MORE SAFE: IV aminogly, IV vanco, metro, sulfas, doxy

C. difficile

- Outbreaks: wash hands, single rooms or cohorting, wash toilet facility with sporocidal agent. May need to control clindamycin use. D/C rectal temp.
- Surgery: Usually for ileus or toxic megacolon, indication - toxic & unresponsive to PO vanco, procedure -total colectomy
- Metro & vanco Rx: Impose 25% risk of relapse
- Refractory cases: vanco PO always works unless ileus or concurrent cause (IBD, lactose deficiency, etc)
- Ileus: vanco 500mg PO qid +/- NG tube or enema +/- metronidazole 750mg IV q 12h (in vitro resistance to metro - 6%, vanco - never reported)

- Infection control: Single room + bathroom, contact isolation, clean room w/sporicidal

C. difficile relapses

- Relapse: Retreat w/ metro or vanco, equally effective, equally likely to cause relapse
- Multiple relapses: Standard Rx metro/vanco x 10d, then 1) vanco 125mg QOD x 6 wks
- Multiple relapses: Standard Rx metro/vanco x 10d then cholestyramine 4g PO tid +/- lactinex 1g qid x 6wks
- Multiple relapses: vanco 500mg PO qid + saccharomyces boulardii (CVS pharmacies) 500mg bid day 7 to 4-8wks
- Multiple relapses: Standard Rx metro/vanco x 10d then lactobacillus GG ("Culturelle"; 888-828-4242) 1 tab/d x 4-6wks
- Multiple relapses: IVIG 300mg/kg IV q 3wks (experimental)

Drug-Specific Comments

Bacitracin: This drug is active against most strains of C. difficile and is not absorbed so it provides the desired high levels in the colon. It's not often used because the published experience is limited, metronidazole is cheaper, and most patients don't need it.

Metronidazole: This drug is generally preferred for C. difficile-associated diarrhea or colitis; efficacy is about the same as with vancomycin, but metronidazole is cheaper and avoids possible abuse of vancomycin. The rate of response and post-treatment relapses are about the same for metronidazole and vancomycin.

Vancomycin: Only FDA approved drug for C. difficile. Ideal pharmacology and activity; it is not absorbed so colon lumen levels are very high and all strains are sensitive. Concerns are: cost, difficulty getting parvules, and possible abuse of vancomycin with promotion of VRE.

Important Points

- Guidelines from IDSA: C. difficile Rx (CID 2001;32:331) & SHEA - C. difficile testing & inf control (Inf Cont Hosp Epid 1995;16:459)
- C. difficile: only common identifiable cause of nosocomial diarrhea; may cause outbreaks
- C. difficile clues: colitis, PMC, fecal WBC, cramps, ileus, toxic megacolon, WBC increase, albumin decrease, fever
- C. difficile neg: usual cause is reduced colon anaerobes - altered CHO metabolism (osmotic diarrhea) or bile acid metabolism (secretory diarrhea)
- C difficile: metro preferred abx by IDSA, CDC and SHEA
- Many reports since 2004 suggest C. difficile–associated diarrhea is more common, more serious, and more refractory to therapy. This may be strain related and variable in geographic distribution. These cases are preferentially treated with oral vancomycin.

Selected Readings

Bartlett JG. Clinical Practice: Antibiotic-associated diarrhea. N Engl J Med 2002;346:334

Pepin J, Valiquette L, Alary ME, Villemure P, Pelletier A, et al. Clostridium difficile-associated diarrhea in a region of Quebec from 1991 to 2003: a changing pattern of disease severity. CMAJ 2004; Aug 31;171 (5):466-472

Pepin J, Alary ME, Valiquette L, Raiche E, Ruel J, Fulop K et al. Increasing risk of relapse after treatment of Clostridium difficile colitis in Quebec, Canada. Clin Infect Dis 2005; Jun 1:40(11):1591-1597

Bartlett JG. Antibiotic-associated diarrhea. Clin Infect Dis 1992;15:573

Bartlett JG. Treatment of Clostridium difficile colitis. Gastroenterology 1985;89:1192

Lipsett PA, Samantaray DK, Tam ML, et al. Pseudomembraneous colitis: A surgical disease?. Surgery 1994;116:491

Fekety R, Shah AR. Diagnosis and treatment of Clostridium difficile colitis. JAMA 1993;269:71

Barbut F, et al. Epidemiology of recurrences or reinfections of Clostridium difficile-associated diarrhea. J Clin Micro 2000;38:2386

Kyne L, et al. Asymptomatic carriage of C. difficile and serum levels of IgG antibody to toxin A. N Engl J Med 2000;342:390

Pittman EF. Lomotil and antibiotic colitis. Ann Intern Med 1975;83:124

DIARRHEA, COMMUNITY-ACQUIRED, ACUTE
John G. Bartlett, M.D.

DIAGNOSTIC CRITERIA

- Hx (Epidemiology): outbreak, travel, antibiotic exposure, underlying disease
- Lab: stool cx - salmonella, shigella, C. jejuni +/- E. coli 0157, yersinia, vibrio
- Lab (if abx exposure): C. difficile - EIA for toxin A & B +/- fecal WBCs or lactoferrin.
- Lab (parasite): AFB stain/trichrome - cryptosporidia, isospora, cyclospora; EIA - giardia antigen; O & P - E. histolytica.
- Hx (symptoms): severity, blood, duration, fever, tenesmus, sx dehydration

COMMON PATHOGENS: Norovirus ; Campylobacter jejuni ; Salmonella species ; Shigella species ; Enterohemorrhagic Escherichia coli (EHEC) ; Cryptosporidia ; Giardia lamblia

TREATMENT REGIMENS

Sequential evaluation

- Reference: (NEJM 2004;350:38)
- Assessment: dehydration, duration, evidence of inflammation (fever, blood, tenesmus)
- Symptomatic Rx: hydration + loparamide - initial 4mg PO, then 2mg q each loose stool (16mg/d max).
- Management by setting: travel, outbreak, nosocomial, abx
- Stool study: Association – Travel: E. coli; outbreak: Salmonella, norovirus; Abx hx?: C. difficile; bloody: E. coli 0157
- Empiric abx if indicated: severe - cipro 500mg bid x 3d; Travel - cipro/levo 1-3d; Sx >7d - Metro 500mg tid x 7-10d
- Reportable infections: Salmonella, Shigella, E. coli 0157:H7, cyclospora, giardia, cryptosporidia

Pathogen-specific therapy

- Reference: (IDSA CID 2001;32:331)
- Shigella: ciprofloxacin 500mg PO bid x 1-3d or levofloxacin 500mg qd x 1-3d
- Salmonella: (abx treatment if severe, >50yrs, valve dis, severe atherosclerosis, CA, AIDS, uremia): cipro 500mg bid x 5-7d, TMP-SMX DS bid x 5-7d, ceftriaxone 100mg/kg/d x 5-7d
- C. jejuni: erythro 500mg PO bid x 5d
- E. coli: enterohemorrhagic (Shiga toxin - bloody diarrhea): NO antibiotic, may increase toxin release
- C. difficile: stop implicated drug + metronidazole 250mg qid x 10d
- Giardia: metronidazole 250-750mg tid PO x 7-10d; tinidazole 2g PO x 1 dose
- Cyclospora: TMP-SMX 1DS PO bid x 7-10d
- E. histolytica: metronidazole 750mg tid PO x 5-10d + paromomycin 500mg tid PO x 7d; tinidazole 2g PO qd x 3d followed by followed by paromomycin, iodoquinol, or diloxanide furoate.
- Isospora: TMP-SMX 1DS bid PO x 7-10d

- Aeromonas & Pleisomonas (severe or prolonged): cipro 500mg PO bid x 3d or TMP-SMX 1DS bid x 3d or ofloxacin 300mg PO bid x 3d

Nonspecific therapy

- Rehydration: mild diarrhea - clear juices & soups; severe - Ceralyte, Pedialyte
- Food should match stool: watery - soups, broth, yogurt, soft drinks, Jello +- saltines; some form - rice, bread, broiled fish, chicken, baked potato
- Avoid milk, milk products, caffeine, fried food, spicy food
- Antimotility agents: Avoid w/ E. coli 0157 (bloody diarrhea) & C. difficile. Loperamide (OTC) 4mg, then 2mg q loose stool (16mg/d max). Lomotil or Bismuth subsalicylate

DRUG-SPECIFIC COMMENTS

Ciprofloxacin: Appropriate for empiric treatment of nearly all treatable enteric bacterial pathogens except for C. jejuni but this is an important pathogen.

Doxycycline: Use in pathogen-specific treatment; avoid use in persons <18yrs. Drug of choice for cholera.

Erythromycin: Preferred drug for C. jejuni but little else that causes diarrhea.

Metronidazole: Main uses are for C. difficile, amebiasis and giardia.

IMPORTANT POINTS

- Recommendations based on guidelines: IDSA (CID 2001;32:331) and Guerrant (NEJM 2004;350:38)
- Highest priorities: Rehydration, antibiotic treatment of shigellosis (fluoroquinolone), avoid antibiotics with bloody diarrhea (E. coli 0157)
- Inflammatory diarrhea (fecal WBC, tenesmus, fever): think Salmonella, Shigella, C. jejuni, C. difficile, Yersinia if bloody or severe consider stool cx.
- Most common: norovirus sporadic & epidemic (hosp, nursing homes, cruise ships, events)
- Foodborne outbreaks: salmonella, E. coli 0157, norovirus, Yersinia, Vibrio (seafood), C. jejuni (poultry)
- Traveler's diarrhea (developing countries): Enterotoxigenic E. coli (dx and Rx empirically) fluoroquinolone; other - Salmonella, Shigella, Giardia, C. jejuni.
- Outbreak: Salmonella & Norovirus; notify health dept.
- Bloody stool: E. coli 0157 (avoid abx), E. histolytica, inflammatory bowel disease
- Fecal leukocytes: C. jejuni, C. difficile, Salmonella, Shigella
- Reportable: Cholera, Cryptosporidia, Salmonella, Shigella, E. coli 0157, Giardia

SELECTED READINGS

Thielman NM and Guerrant RL. Acute diarrhea. N Engl J Med 2004;350:38

Chattergee NK, et al. Molecular epidemiology of outbreaks of viral gastroenteritis in New York State, 1998-99. Clin Infect Dis 2004;38(Suppl 3): S303-10

CDC. Norovirus activity - US 2002. MMWR 2003;52:41

CDC. Preliminary FoodNet data on the incidence of infection with pathogens in food-selected sites, United States, 2003. MMWR 2004;53:338

Widdowson M-A, Cramer EH, Hadley L, et al. Outbreaks of acute gastroenteritis on cruise ships and on land: Identification of a predominant circulating strain of Norovirus - US 2002. J Infect Dis 2004;190:27-36

Gallimore CI, et al. Diversity of noroviruses circulating in the north of England from 1998 to 2001. J Clin Microbiol 2004;42:1396-401

Svenungsson B, et al. Enteropathogens in adult patients with diarrhea and healthy subjects: A 1yr prospective study in a Swedish clinic for infectious diarrhea. Clin Infect Dis 2000;30:770

Green KY, et al. A predominant role for noroviruses as agents of epidemic gastroenteritis in Maryland nursing homes for the elderly. JID 2002;185:133

Young VB, Schmidt TM. Antibiotic-associated diarrhea accompanied by large-scale alterations in Microbiota. J Clin Micro 2004;42:1203

Yarma JK, et al. An outbreak of E. coli 0157 infection following exposure to a contaminated building. JAMA 2003;290:2709

DIARRHEA, COMMUNITY-ACQUIRED, PERSISTENT/CHRONIC

Cynthia Sears, M.D.; Chris Carpenter, M.D.

Diagnostic Criteria

- Persistent diarrhea is defined as diarrheal disease lasting longer than 1-2 weeks but less than 4 weeks; diarrhea lasting longer than 4 weeks is considered chronic diarrhea.
- Most infectious causes of acute diarrhea generally resolve within 2 weeks of onset; on the other hand, most of the causes of acute diarrhea can cause persistent or chronic diarrhea.
- Definitions of diarrhea in the United States or Western Europe, where low residual diets are the norm, may include: stools weighing >200g, >3 stools/day, and decreased fecal consistency.
- Noninfectious causes of diarrhea are increasingly common as the duration of diarrhea increases.
- Irritable bowel syndrome should be considered in patients with persistent or chronic complaints and associated abdominal pain.
- IBS = abd. pain and abnormal bowel habits (constipation, diarrhea, or both) w/o source
- Organic (vs. functional) diarrhea: high output (>400 g/day in western countries), shorter duration (<3 mos), nocturnal, continual, sudden onset, wt. loss >5 kg, high ESR/CRP, anemia, low albumin
- Initial eval: fecal leukocytes, lactoferrin, occult blood, ova and parasites, AFB stain, Giardia ag., C. difficile toxin; also consider pH, wt. (g/day), 72 hr fecal fat (on 75-100g/day fat)
- 2nd tier eval: trial lactose-free diet, CBC w/ diff., ESR/CRP, metabolic panel, TSH, T4, gastrin, radiographs (AXR, Abd. CT, UGI w/ SBFT, contrast enema), sigmoid/colon endoscopy w/ biopsies
- 3rd tier eval: VIP, substance P, calcitonin, histamine (high output and hypokalemia); urine 5-HIA acids (flushing); alkalinization assays, phenolphthalein, and anthraquinone (?laxative abuse); fecal electrolytes/osmolality; urine studies w/ thin-layer chromatography for bisacodyl; enteroclysis, bile acid or other breath tests for bacterial overgrowth.

COMMON PATHOGENS: Giardia lamblia ; Entamoeba histolytica ; Clostridium difficile ; Campylobacter jejuni ; Salmonella species ; Shigella species ; Enterohemorrhagic Escherichia coli (EHEC)

Treatment Regimens

Empiric therapy

- In cases where an initial evaluation has been unrevealing and further studies are more invasive and place the patient at risk, consideration of an empiric trial is reasonable.
- Use metronidazole for suspected protozoal diarrhea or a fluoroquinolone for suspected bacterial diarrhea as empiric therapy with the potential risks and benefits explained to the patient.

- Ciprofloxacin 500mg PO bid for 3-5 days, norfloxacin. 400mg PO bid for 3-5 days, or ofloxacin 300mg PO bid for 3-5 days are reasonable empiric choices.
- Metronidazole 250-500mg PO tid for 10 days.
- Trimethoprim-sulfamethoxazole may be considered for empiric treatment of patients at risk for Cyclospora infections.

Pathogen-specific therapy

- Specific therapy for the three most common causes of infectious persistent or chronic diarrhea (Giardia, Amebiasis, and C. difficile) is generally indicated.
- First-line therapy for all three includes metronidazole; amebiasis requires the addition of an agent active against cysts (paromomycin or iodoquinol or diloxanide furoate).
- Specific treatment is indicated for bacterial enteritis caused by Shigella sp. and possibly C. jejuni; isolated Salmonella sp. intestinal disease should not be treated with antibiotics.
- EHEC treatment is controversial and we recommend holding treatment due to concern that certain antibiotics have been demonstrated to induce toxin synthesis and release.
- Furthermore, both trimethoprim-sulfamethoxazole and fluoroquinolones may promote hemolytic uremic syndrome.
- Fluoroquinolone-resistant strains of C. jejuni have been identified in many parts of the world.

Symptomatic medications and measures

- Fluid replacement is an important component of treatment, especially in patients with significant dehydration where it is often the most important component.
- Oral replacement with oral rehydration solutions (ORS); commercially available packets include Cera Lyte generic ORS, the WHO ORS, Rehydralyte, Pedialyte, Resol, and Rice-Lyte.
- IV replacement with 0.9% NS with 20 mEq KCL or with Lactated Ringers solution should be used in patients with moderate to severe diarrhea or in patients not tolerating oral replacement.
- Antimotility agents, such as loperamide 4mg po, then 2mg PO post each loose stool to a maximum of 16mg/day are of benefit; avoid with C. difficile diarrhea, enterohemorrhagic E. coli diarrhea.
- Diphenoxylate with atropine and tincture of opium offer no major advantage over loperamide; all of these agents should be avoided in patients with dysentery and/or EHEC infection (may -> HUS).
- Other recommendations: lactose-free (e.g., milk, cheese) diet, caffeine avoidance, Metamucil, bismuth subsalicylate, Kaolin-containing agents, and probiotics.
- Gatorade, fruit juices, and soft drinks are hyperosmolar and deficient in electrolytes and thus are suboptimal replacements patients with significant dehydration
- These drinks may be sufficient in otherwise healthy patients who are mildly ill; additional electrolytes from soups or saltine crackers will be supplemental.

IMPORTANT POINTS

- Chronic diarrhea is generally caused by noninfectious etiologies, whereas acute diarrhea is mostly due to self-limited infections.
- Depending on the definition used, chronic diarrhea occurs in 3-18% of Americans; irritable bowel syndrome with abdominal pain makes up a majority in the higher estimates.
- With an extensive workup including hospital evaluation when required, only approximately 10% of patients with chronic diarrhea remain undiagnosed.

- Immunocompromised patients (e.g., HIV-infected patients) with persistent/chronic diarrhea: consider CMV, Giardia, Cryptosporidium, Cyclospora, Isospora belli, Microsporidia, and M. avium complex.

SELECTED READINGS

Schiller LR. Chronic Diarrhea. Gastroenterology 2004;127:287-293

Thomas et al. Guidelines for the investigation of chronic diarrhoea, 2nd edition. Gut 2003;52(Supp V): v1-v15

Guerrant et al. Practice guidelines for the Management of Infectious Diarrhea. Clin Infect Disease February 2001;32:331-50

Fine KD, Schiller LR. American Gastroenterological Association Medical Position Statement: Guidelines for the Evaluation and Management of Chronic Diarrhea. 1999; 116:1461-3.

Fine KD, Schiller LR. AGA Technical Review on the Evaluation and Management of Chronic Diarrhea. 1999; 116:1464-86.

Donowitz M, Kokke FT, Saidi R. Evaluation of Patients with Chronic Diarrhea. New England Journal of Medicine, 1995 Vol. 332(11):725-9

DIARRHEA, TRAVELER'S   Lisa Spacek, M.D., Ph.D.

DIAGNOSTIC CRITERIA

- Definition: 3 or more unformed stools in 24 hrs with 1 or more symptoms of enteric disease: nausea, vomiting, abdominal cramps, fever, fecal urgency, tenesmus, or bloody, mucoid stools (10-20%)
- Hx: onset 5-15d after arrival at destination, illness often benign and self-limited; duration 1-5d, severity based on stool frequency and presence of fever or bloody stools
- PE: fever, anorexia, malaise and abd tenderness +/- nausea and vomiting
- Lab: usually none needed; if diagnostics pursued for those with severe/bloody diarrhea or high fever, consider obtaining fecal leukocytes, stool cx (E. coli, Shigella, Salmonella, Campylobacter, Aeromonas), Shiga toxin assay, Giardia antigen, stool for ova and parasites.
- Epi: host factors increasing risk: immunosuppression, hypochlorhydria, inflammatory bowel disease, diabetes mellitus, AIDS
- Epi: bacterial enteric pathogens most commonly isolated, viral outbreaks sporadic, parasitic pathogens rare

COMMON PATHOGENS: Enterotoxigenic Escherichia coli ; Salmonella species ; Shigella species ; Campylobacter jejuni ; Aeromonas species ; Rotavirus ; Norovirus; other viruses ; Giardia lamblia ; Cyclospora ; Cryptosporidium parvum

TREATMENT REGIMENS

Nonspecific therapy

- Rx based on symptoms (Intl J Antimicrob Agents 2003;21:116)
- Mild illness, 1-2 stools/24h, min symptoms - loperamide 4mg loading dose, then 2mg after each loose stool max 16mg/24h or bismuth subsalicylate two 262mg tabs chewed qid or 30mL q1h max 8 doses/24h
- Moderate illness, >2 stools/24h, watery diarrhea - fluoroquinolone, single dose of once-daily fluoroquinolone may be adequate plus loperamide, if ongoing dysentery, complete 3d course of abx
- Severe illness/dysentery, >6 stools/24 h, fever, bloody stools - fluoroquinolone therapy to complete 3d course
- Avoid bismuth subsalicylate with fluoroquinolone, combination will chelate fluoroquinolone

- Bismuth preparations contain salicylate, two tabs qid comparable to 3-4 adult aspirins, avoid combination and do not use bismuth with oral anticoagulants
- Attapulgite (Kaopectate), a hydrated aluminum silicate clay preparation, 30mL after each loose stool up to 7 doses/d, is not absorbed and causes more formed stool, for use in mild illness
- Prevention: handwashing, water purification, avoid raw fruits and vegetables unless peeled, choose steaming hot foods
- Rifaximin, a nonabsorbed antibiotic for noninvasive E. coli, is NOT recommended for systemic infections, diarrhea complicated by fever or bloody stool or persistent symptoms > 24-48 hrs

Pathogen-specific therapy

- Enterotoxigenic E. coli: TMP-SMX 1DS bid x 3d, worldwide resistance limits effectiveness, fluoroquinolone more effective, ciprofloxacin 500mg bid x 3d or 750mg single dose, rifamixin 200mg tid x 3d
- Salmonella, non-typhi: Rx severe illness, pt >50yrs, prostheses, valvular heart disease, severe atherosclerosis, ca, uremia; TMP-SMX 1DS bid x5-7d or ciprofloxacin 500mg bid x5-7d
- Shigella: TMP-SMX 1DS bid x 3d or ciprofloxacin 500mg bid x 3d
- C. jejuni: erythromycin 500mg bid x 5d, fluoroquinolones x 5d, increased resistance to fluoroquinolones in SE Asia
- Enterohemorrhagic E. coli: AVOID antibiotics and antimotility agents, reserve antibiotics for severe illness
- Giardia - metronidazole 250-750mg tid x7-10d or tinidazole 2mg PO x 1 dose
- Cyclospora: TMP-SMX 1DS bid x 7d
- Cryptosporidium: if severe, paromomycin 500mg tid x7d (uncertain effectiveness)
- E. histolytica: metronidazole 750mg tid 5-10d followed by luminal agent, paromomycin 500mg tid x 7d (NEJM 2003;348:1565); tinidazole 2g p.o daily with food x 3d
- Vibrio cholerae - doxycycline 300mg x1 dose or tetracycline 500mg qid x3d or TMP-SMX 1DS bid x3d or ciprofloxacin 500mg x1 dose

IMPORTANT POINTS

- IDSA treatment guidelines in CID 2001;32;331.
- Prevent and treat dehydration, reduce symptoms and duration of illness with empirical self-therapy (CID 2000;31:1079)
- Dysentery or inflammatory diarrhea likely bacterial, culture stool and treat with antibiotics. AVOID antibiotics in proven or suspected Enterohemorrhagic E. coli (STEC)
- Persistent diarrhea >2wks likely parasitic infection. Check giardia ELISA, serial stool exams for ova and parasites, C. difficile toxin assay (if Abx taken)
- Worldwide resistance to TMP/SMX limits effectiveness as empiric therapy, increased resistance of Campylobacter to fluoroquinolones documented in SE Asia

SELECTED READINGS

DuPont HL et al. A randomized, double-blind, placebo-controlled trial of rifaximin to prevent travelers' diarrhea. Ann Intern Med 2005; May 17;142(10):805-812

Haque R, et al. Amebiasis. N Engl J Med 2003; 348: 1565-1573

Vila J, et al. Aeromonas spp and traveler's diarrhea; clinical features and antimicrobial resistance. Emerg Infect Dis 2003; 9:552-555

Ericsson CD. Travellers' diarrhoea. International J Antimicrobial Agents 2003; 21: 116-124

Ryan ET, et al. Illness after international travel. N Engl J Med 2002; 347: 505-516

Rendi-Wagner P and Kollaritsch H. Drug prophylaxis for travelers' diarrhea. CID 2002; 34: 628-33

Guerrant RL, et al. Practice guidelines for the management of infectious diarrhea. CID 2001; 32: 331-351

DuPont HL, et al. Rifamixin versus ciprofloxacin for the treatment of traveler's diarrhea: a randomized, double-blind clinical trial. CID 2001; 33: 1807-15

Adachi JA, et al. Empirical antimicrobial therapy for traveler's diarrhea. CID 2000; 31: 1079-1083

von Sonnenburg F, et al. Risk and etiology of diarrhea at various tourist destinations. Lancet 2000; 356: 133-134

DIVERTICULITIS Pamela A. Lipsett, M.D.; Chris Carpenter, M.D.

Diagnostic Criteria

- Diverticulosis increases with age: 50% of people > 60 yrs old have diverticulosis, and 10-25% of those with diverticulosis develop diverticulitis.
- Symptoms include LLQ pain that can be intermittent or constant, fever, and altered bowel habits (either diarrhea or constipation)
- PE: fever, LLQ tenderness - may localize +/- rebound and guarding; mass may be palpable
- Lab: leukocytosis w/ left shift frequent
- Dx: often clinical (like appendicitis); CT used in pts with atypical presentations or severe/complicated illness (unresponsive to abx or concern of abscess/rupture)

Common Pathogens: Enterobacteriaceae; Enterococcus; Streptococcus species; Anaerobes

Treatment Regimens

Inpatient treatment: 7 to 10 days

- Recommendations based upon authors' opinion
- Cefoxitin 1-2g IV q6h
- Ampicillin-sulbactam 3.0g IV q6h or ticarcillin-clavulanate 3.1g IV q6h or piperacillin-tazobactam 3.375g IV q6h or 4.5g IV q8h
- Imipenem 0.5g IV q6h or meropenem 1g IV q8h or ertapenem 1g IV qd
- 3rd or 4th generation cephalosporin or fluoroquinolone or aztreonam, plus metronidazole
- Ampicillin 2g IV q6h plus gentamicin 1.7g IV q8h plus metronidazole 1.0g IV loading dose then 0.5g IV q6h or clindamycin 450-900mg IV q6h

Outpatient treatment: 5 to 10 days

- Amoxicillin-clavulanic acid 500mg PO tid or 875mg PO bid
- Ciprofloxacin 500mg bid or levofloxacin 500mg qd plus metronidazole 500mg PO q6h; or gatifloxacin 400mg qd or moxifloxacin 400 +/- metronidazole 500mg PO q6h.
- Trimethoprim-sulfamethoxazole DS bid PO plus metronidazole 500mg PO q6h

Surgical treatment

- If abscess present, percutaneous drainage may offer temporizing intervention for localized perforation w/o generalized peritonitis or severe illness; resection performed later.
- Resection +/- diversion may be required for perforation with generalized peritonitis and/or pneumoperitoneum
- Recurrence after 1st attack 20-30%; after 2nd >50%; resection is thus recommended after 2nd/3rd attack
- Perforation rates in immunosuppressed and post-operative patients higher

DRUG-SPECIFIC COMMENTS

Ampicillin + Sulbactam: Good coverage of gram-positive, gram-negative, and anaerobic pathogens; lacks Pseudomonas aeruginosa coverage but good Enterococcus species coverage (significance in diverticulitis uncertain).

Aztreonam: Excellent gram-negative coverage; use in combination with anaerobic agent; would reserve for seriously ill patients with B-lactam allergies and no other reasonable alternatives.

Cefepime: Excellent coverage of gram-negative pathogens; use in combination with anaerobic agent.

Cefotetan: Good single agent coverage of gram-positives, gram-negatives, and anaerobes. Would not use with serious intra-abdominal infection due to B. fragilis resistance 30-40%.

Ertapenem: Newer carbapenem with excellent gram-positive, gram-negative, and anaerobic coverage; doesn't cover Enterococcus or some resistant gram-negative rods, e.g., pseudomonas.

Gatifloxacin: Excellent broad spectrum coverage but clinical data limited on anaerobe coverage

Imipenem/Cilastatin: Excellent broad spectrum (gram-positive, gram-negative, and anaerobe) coverage; would reserve for seriously ill patients.

Meropenem: Excellent broad spectrum (gram-positive, gram-negative, and anaerobe) coverage; would reserve for seriously ill patients.

Metronidazole: Excellent anaerobic coverage

Moxifloxacin: Advanced generation fluoroquinolone available IV/PO. Sufficient gram-positive, gram-negative coverage with reasonable anaerobic spectrum

Piperacillin + Tazobactam: Excellent broad spectrum coverage including gram-positive coverage, gram-negative coverage (including Pseudomonas aeruginosa and B-lactamase producing pathogens) and anaerobic coverage.

Ticarcillin + Clavulanic Acid: Broad spectrum coverage including gram-positive coverage, gram-negative coverage (including Pseudomonas aeruginosa and B-lactamase producing pathogens) and anaerobic coverage.

IMPORTANT POINTS

- High fiber diets (fruits, vegetables, etc.) may reduce the risk of developing diverticular disease.
- Diverticulosis alone without signs or symptoms of diverticulitis does not warrant the use of antibiotics
- Consider pts acceptable for outpatient management: mild illness, tolerating oral intake, supportive social situation, and no significant comorbidity or other risk factors for complications.
- Patients w/ severe disease, who cannot tolerate oral intake, or have risk factors for complicated course (immunosuppression, elderly, significant comorbid illness) should be hospitalized.
- Patients with recurrent attacks, fistula or abscess development, younger age, or immunocompromise may require surgical intervention.

SELECTED READINGS

Solompkin et al. Guidelines for the Selection of Anti-infective Agents for Complicated Intra-abdominal infections. Clin Infect Disease 2003 October 15;37:997-1005

Mazuski, JE Sawyer RG. Nathens AB et al, . The Surgical Infection Society Guidelines on Antimicrobial Therapy for Intra-Abdominal Infections: an Executive Summary. Surgical Infections 2002, Vol 3

Richardo RJ, Hammitt JK. Timing of prophylactic surgery in prevention of diverticulitis recurrence cost-effectiveness analysis. Dig Dis Sci 2002 Sep; 47(():1903-8

Tursi A, Brandimarte G, Daffina R . Long-term treatment with mesalazine and rifaximin versus rifaximin for patients with recurrent attacks of acute diverticulitis of colon. Dig Liver Dis 2002:34:510-5

Ambrosetti P, Becker C, Terrier F : . Colonic diverticulitis : impact of imaging on surgical management- a prospective study of 542 patients. Eur Radiol 2002; 12:1145-9

Schilling MK, Maurer CA, Kollmar O, et al: . Primary vs, secondary anastamosis after sigmoid colon resection for perforated diverticulitis (Hinchey Stage III and IV): a prospective outcome and cost analysis. Dis Colon Rectum 2001;44 699-703, 703-5

Stollman NH and Raskin JB. Diagnosis and Management of Diverticular Disease of the Colon in Adults. The American Journal of Gastroenterology, Vol. 94, No 11, 1999

The Standards Task Force of the American Society of Colon and Rectal Surgeons. Practice parameters for sigmoid diverticulitis - supporting documentation. Diseases of the Colon and Rectum 1995;38:126-32

The Medical Letter, Inc. Choice of Antibacterial Drugs. Treatment Guidelines from The Medical Letter, March 2004;vol. 2 (Issue 19)

EMPYEMA

John G. Bartlett, M.D.

Diagnostic Criteria

- Clinical: symptoms of pneumonia + pleurisy; PE shows signs of effusion
- Laboratory: Chest XR shows effusion, but dx requires pleural fluid analysis showing pus, + GS or cult for likely pathogen or effusion pH <7.0
- Thoracentesis if fluid >10mm lat decubitus x-ray
- Tests of pleural fluid: GS, cult, pH, WBC, LDH, AFB stain/cult, glucose, cytology

Common Pathogens: S. pneumoniae ; S. aureus; Anaerobes ; Streptococcus milleri ; Mycobacterium tuberculosis

Treatment Regimens

Antibiotics: anaerobes +/- aerobes

- Principles: Dx: pleural fluid shows pus, pH <7 or pos cult/GS. Rx: drainage + Abx. Recovery: slow
- Empiric: (covers most anaerobes, MSSA, GMB & GNB): imipenem 0.5-1g IV q 6h or pip-tazo 3.375g q 6h IV
- Abx - anaerobes (putrid, mixed bact GS): clind 600mg IV q8h, then clind 300mg PO tid
- Anaerobes Alt: amp/sulbactam (Unasyn) 1.5-3g IV q 6h (or Zosyn or Timentin) then Augmentin 875 PO bid
- S. pneumoniae/S. milleri: cefotaxime 1g IV q8h/ceftriaxone 1g IV QD then amox 500-750mg PO qid
- S. pneumoniae: alternative choice or pen-resistant: gatiflox 400mg PO IV/d, moxiflox 400mg PO IV/d or levoflox 750mg IV or PO/d
- S. aureus: ox/naf 2g IV q 4-6h IV, then cephalexin (Keflex) 500mg qid
- S. aureus - MRSA or pen allergy: vanco 1g q12h
- MRSA: vanco, linezolid; if sensitive - clind, TMP-SMX, FQ
- GNB: cefotaxime/ceftriaxone/fluoroquinolone (see S. pneumoniae for doses)

Pleural drainage

- Guidelines from R Light (Chest 1991;100:892)
- CT evidence of pleural peel - usually requires decortication
- Fibrinolytics (not generally recommended): streptokinase, (250,000 IU/d) urokinase (100 IU/d) or streptokinase plus streptodornase (Varidase)
- Loculated effusions: tube + thrombolytics - drainage incomplete: thoracotomy

- pH 7.0-7.2 or LDH >1000: consider chest tube if loculated or large effusion
- pH <7.0 or glucose <40 or pus: chest tube
- pH >7.2, glucose >40, LDH <1000: (repeat) thoracentesis

DRUG-SPECIFIC COMMENTS

Amoxicillin + Clavulanate: (Augmentin) A good oral agent for anaerobic lung infection, although experience is greater with clindamycin.

Aztreonam: Good choice +/- aminoglycoside for nosocomial empyemas that yield P. aeruginosa or Enterobacteriaceae or shows typical GNB on gram stain.

Ceftazidime: Good choice +/- aminoglycoside for nosocomial empyemas that yield P. aeruginosa or Enterobacteriaceae or shows typical GNB on gram stain.

Gatifloxacin: (Tequin) Has good in vitro activity vs. anaerobes, good against coliforms, and variable against S. aureus. Use if justified by bacteriology and sensitivity test results of aerobes.

Imipenem/Cilastatin: (Primaxin) Good choice +/- aminoglycoside for nosocomial empyemas that yield P. aeruginosa or Enterobacteriaceae or shows typical GNB on gram stain.

Moxifloxacin: (Avelox) Has good in vitro activity vs. anaerobes, good against coliforms, and variable against S. aureus. Use if justified by bacteriology and sensitivity test results of aerobes.

Piperacillin: Good choice +/- aminoglycoside for nosocomial empyemas that yield P. aeruginosa or Enterobacteriaceae or shows typical GNB on gram stain.

Piperacillin + Tazobactam: (Zosyn) Good choice +/- aminoglycoside for nosocomial empyemas that yield P. aeruginosa or Enterobacteriaceae or shows typical GNB on gram stain.

Ticarcillin + Clavulanic Acid: (Timentin) Good choice +/- aminoglycoside for nosocomial empyemas that yield P. aeruginosa or Enterobacteriaceae or shows typical GNB on gram stain.

IMPORTANT POINTS

- Recommendations: IDSA for abx selection (CID 2003;37:1405) & R. Light (Chest 1991;100:892) for drainage.
- THE critical facet is adequate drainage with thoracentesis +/- tube placement, thoracotomy tube (open or closed) or decortication. Delay in surgical drainage is major cause of long LOS.
- Empyemas are rare--pleural effusions in 30-40% of pneumonias; empyemas in 0.5-2%.
- Major empyema cause in CAP is anaerobic bacteria, the major cause in nosocomial empyema (usually after chest surgery) is S. aureus.
- Gram stain - important clues for bacteriology & abx selection on day 1. Polymicrobial flora often indicates anaerobes; "putrid" empyema always means anaerobes.

SELECTED READINGS

Chapman SJ and Davies RJ. Recent advances in parapneumonic effusion and empyema. Curr Opin Pul Med 2004;10:299-304

Anstadt MP, et al. Surgical versus nonsurgical treatment of empyema thoracis: an outcome analysis. Am J Med Sci 2003;326:9

Petrakis IE, et al. Video-assisted thorascopic surgery for thoracic empyema: primarily or after fibrinolytic therapy failure. Am J Surg 2004;1187:471-4

Melloni G, et al. Decortication for chronic parapneumonic empyema: results of a prospective study. World J Surg 2004;28:488-93

DIAGNOSIS

Wei CJ, et al. Computed tomography features of acute pulmonary tuberculosis. Am J Emerg Med 2004;22:171

Diacon AH, et al. Intrapleural streptokinase for empyema and uncomplicated parapneumonic effusions. Am J Respir Crit Care 2004;170:49-53

Porcel JM and Vives M. Etiology and pleural fluid characteristics of large and massive effusions. Chest 2003;124:978-83

Fartoukh M, Azoulay E, Galliot R, et al. Clinically documented pleural effusion in medical ICU patients: how useful is routine thoracentesis. Chest 2002;121:178

Tuncozgur B, et al. Intrapleural urokinase in the management of parapneumonic empyema: a randomized, controlled trial. Int J Clin Prat 2001;55:658-60

Ko SC, Chen KY, Hsueh PR, et al. Fungal empyema thoracis: an emerging entity. Chest 2000;117:1672.

ENCEPHALITIS   Paul Auwaerter, M.D.

DIAGNOSTIC CRITERIA

- Clinical: fever, cognitive deficits, focal neurologic signs (often rapidly progressive), and/or seizures preceded by non-specific/flu-like prodrome. Review travel, sexual contact, tick/insect hx.
- PE: Meningeal signs (meningoencephalitis); abnormal mental status with ataxia, hemiparesis, aphasia, cranial nerve involvement and psychosis possible.
- Lab: CSF usually w/ mononuclear cells & increased protein; CSF PCR, CSF culture, or serology (HSV, West Nile virus etc); typical viral pathogen by brain biopsy.
- Ddx: Among most common--arboviruses (summer-fall), HSV (most common sporadic cause), enterovirus (summer-fall), toxic/metabolic explanations, CNS SLE. See pathogens for more comprehensive list.
- MRI normal in many cases early on. May show temporal lobe changes (HSV) or more diffuse involvement. EEG abnl in many cases HSV encephalitis with characteristic temporal lobe spikes.

COMMON PATHOGENS: Herpes Simplex Virus ; Arboviruses ; West Nile Virus ; Enteroviruses ; Rabies ; HIV ; Bartonella species ; Listeria monocytogenes ; Toxoplasma gondii ; Common arboviruses causing encephalitis in the US are: St. Louis, Eastern Equine encephalitis virus, Western Equine, La Crosse, Colorado tick fever, and now, West Nile virus.; Other less common viral etiologies include: mumps, measles, rubella, influenza, rabies, human herpesvirus-6, EBV. CMV, VZV possible esp. in immune suppressed. B virus (post-monkey bite). Acute HIV infection may occasionally present with encephalitis.; Amoebic encephalitis is most commonly caused by Naegleria fowleri or Acanthamoeba species.

TREATMENT REGIMENS

Viral encephalitis: treatable causes

- HSV or VZV: acyclovir 10mg/kg IV q8h x 14-21d
- Herpes B virus: ganciclovir 5mg/kg IV bid or acyclovir 15mg/kg IV q8h x > 10d, then acyclovir 800mg PO 5 times daily or valacyclovir 1 g PO tid indefinitely
- CMV, HHV6 (preferred): ganciclovir 5mg/kg IV q12h x 10-14 days; then 5mg/kg IV qd for maintenance
- CMV, HHV6 (alternative): foscarnet 40-60mg/kg IV q8h x 10-14 days; then 90-120mg/kg IV qd for maintenance

Nonviral encephalitis

- Listeria: Ampicillin 2mg IV q4h + gentamicin 5mg/kg/d IV divided q8h x 3-6 weeks.
- Listeria (alternative): TMP/SMX 15mg/kg/d IV divided q6h x 6 weeks
- Naegleria fowlerii: Amphotericin B 1.0-1.5mg/kg/d IV + intrathecal therapy

- Toxoplasmosis (preferred): Pyrimethamine 100-200mg PO once (loading dose), then 50-100mg PO qd + sulfadiazine 1-2g PO qid + folinic acid 10mg PO qd x minimum 6 weeks
- Toxoplasmosis (alternative): Pyrimethamine 100-200mg PO once (loading dose), then 50-100mg PO qd + clindamycin 900mg IV q6h + folinic acid 10mg PO qd x minimum 6 weeks

DRUG-SPECIFIC COMMENTS

Acyclovir: Always initiate in suspected encephalitis cases until HSV comfortably ruled-out by PCR studies other clinical information.

Meropenem: Meropenem and imipenem have been shown to be bactericidal for listeria and may be considered as alternatives when ampicillin, penicillin, and trimethoprim/sulfamethoxazole are not tolerated. These drugs are virtually untested clinically, however. Meropenem appears to have less potential to lower the seizure threshold and is thus the favored carbapenem for treating CNS infections.

IMPORTANT POINTS

- HSV is critical to treat rapidly; clues-fever, sz, MS/personality change, focal neuro deficits, temporal lobe involvement on MRI. ALWAYS start empiric acyclovir while awaiting test results.
- More HSV clues: CSF showing RBCs and elevated protein; no HSV skin lesions
- Suspected or proven HSV: acyclovir IV; if dx studies neg - may need brain bx
- Treatable causes: HSV, VZV, B virus, HHV6, CMV, (AIDS), Naeglaria, Listeria, Lyme. Arboviral, enteroviral causes: supportive care.
- Guidelines are author's opinion

SELECTED READINGS

Solomon T. Flavivirus encephalitis. N Engl J Med. 2004 Jul 22;351(4):370-8

Petersen LR, Marfin AA, Gubler DJ. West Nile virus . JAMA. 2003 Jul 23;290(4):524-8

Anonymous. Update: West Nile virus encephalitis--New York, 1999. MMWR Morb Mortal Wkly Rep 1999;48:944

Rotbart HA, O'Connell JF, McKinlay MA. Treatment of human enterovirus infections. Antiviral Res 1998;38:11

Domingues RB, Tsanaclis AC, Pannuti CS, et al. Evaluation of the range of clinical presentations of herpes simplex encephalitis by using polymerase chain reaction assay of cerebrospinal fluid samples. Clin Infect Dis 1997;25:86

Johnson RT. Acute encephalitis. Clin Infect Dis 1996;23:219

Whitley FJ, Lakeman F. Herpes simplex virus infections of the central nervous system: Therapeutic and diagnostic considerations. Clin Infect Dis 1995;20:414.

Lakeman FD, Whitley RJ. Diagnosis of herpes simplex virus encephalitis: Application of polymerase chain reaction to cerebrospinal fluid from brain-biopsied patients and correlation with disease. J Infect Dis 1995;171:857.

Poscher ME. Successful treatment of varicella-zoster virus in meningoencephalitis in patients with AIDS: Report of 4 cases and review. AIDS 1994;8:1115.

Armstrong RW, Fung PC. Brainstem encephalitis (rhombencephalitis) due to Listeria monocytogenes: Case report and review. Clin Infect Dis 1993;16:689

ENDOCARDITIS IN INJECTION DRUG USERS

John G. Bartlett, M.D.

DIAGNOSTIC CRITERIA

- Sx: fever, malaise, chest/back pain, cough, dyspnea, arthralgia, myalgia, neurologic sx, wt loss, night sweats
- PE & Lab: Duke criteria = [2 Major] or [1 Major + 3 Minor] or [5 minor]; and below (see Tables 1a-1b in Appendix I)
- Major (microbiologic): 1) typical orgs x 2 blood cx (S. viridans, S. bovis, HACEK, S. aureus, Enterococcus w/o other primary source); OR 2) persistent bacteremia 12h or more); OR 3) 3/3 or 3/4 pos. bld cx
- Major (Valve): 1. Pos. echo; OR 2. new valve regurgitation
- Minor: 1) Predisposing heart cond. or IDU; 2) Fever 38C (100.4F) or higher; 3) Vascular phenomenon; 4) Immune phenomenon; 5) Pos. bld cx not meeting above criteria; 6) Echo abnl but not diagnostic

COMMON PATHOGENS: Staphylococcus aureus ; Enterococcus ; Streptococcus species ; Candida

TREATMENT REGIMENS

Antibiotics: empiric

- Preferred (empiric Rx). oxacillin/nafcillin 2g IV q4h + gentamicin 1mg/kg IV q8h
- Alternative: vancomycin 1g IV q12h + gentamicin 1mg/kg IV q8h

Pathogen-specific

- S. aureus (preferred): oxacillin/nafcillin 2g IV q4h x 4wks, gentamicin 1mg/kg IV q8h x 3-5d
- S. aureus (2wk course for tricuspid valve): nafcillin/oxacillin 2g IV q4h x 2wks + gentamicin 1mg/kg IV q8h x 2wks
- S. aureus (alternative--MRSA suspected/confirmed or pen hypersensitivity): vancomycin 1g IV q 12h x 4-6 wks + gent 1mg/kg IV q8h x 3d +/or rifampin 300mg IV or PO bid.
- Strep viridans (pen sens, MIC <0.1): Aq pen G 12-18mU IV/d x 4wks; OR ceftriaxone 2g/d IV x 4wks; OR Aq pen 12-18mU IV/d + gent 1mg/kg q8h x 2wks; OR vanco 2g/d IV x 4wks
- Strep viridans (pen MIC >0.5 or Enterococcus, amp + gent x 4 wks): Aq pen G 18-30mU/d IV + gent 1mg/kg q8h x 4wks OR Vanco 2g/d IV + gent (enterococcus only) 1mg/kg q8h x 4wks
- Candida (preferred): amphotericin B 0.8-1mg/kg/d IV + flucytosine 100-150mg/kg/d + surgery; Alt: fluconazole 400mg IV/d + surgery
- P. aeruginosa: (use in vitro data) preferred: tobramycin 2.5mg/kg IV q8h IV (high dose, peak 15-20mcg/mL) + piperacillin, 4g IV q4h OR ceftazidime 2g IV q8h x 4-6wks
- P. aeruginosa (alternatives) aztreonam, ciprofloxacin , or imipenem, each + tobra/gent

Surgery

- Indications: severe heart failure, uncontrolled infection, persistent bacteremia despite abx, fungal endocarditis, unstable prosthetic valve, periannular extension
- Procedure: tricuspid valve - valvectomy or vegetectomy + valvuloplasty; aortic/mitral-valve replacement
- Issues: Some heart surgeons are reluctant to operate on addicts for IE, some require assurance there will be drug rehab

IMPORTANT POINTS

- Treatment guidelines from AMA Council on IE (JAMA 1995;274:1706) and Mayo Clin guidelines (Mayo Clin Proc 1997;72:532)
- Suspect endocarditis in any IDU with FUO. Usual presentation: fever, chest x ray - embolic lesions, blood cult - S. aureus, echo - tricuspid valve vegetations
- Pathogens: S. aureus - 60%, Strep - 20%, P. aeruginosa - 10%, Candida - 5%, S. epi - 2%; Valves - tricuspid - 60%
- Surgery: Prognosis for prosthetic valve without drug rehab is poor. For tricuspid valve - valvectomy is option
- Concurrent HIV infection increases mortality rate with CD4 counts <200

SELECTED READINGS

Moreillon P and Que Y-A. Infective endocarditis. Lancet 2004;363:139

Bassetti S, Battegay M. Staphylococcus aureus infections in injection drug users: risk factors and prevention strategies. Infections 2004;32:163-9

Durack DT, Lukes AS, Bright DK. New criteria for diagnosis of infective endocarditis of specific endocardiographic findings. Am J Med 1994;96:200-9

Miro JM, delRio A, Mestres CA. Infective endocarditis and cardiac surgery in intravenous drug abusers and HIV-1 infected patients. Cardiol Clin 2003;21:167-84.

Heldman AW, Hartert TV, Ray S et al. Oral antibiotic treatment of right sided staphylococcal endocarditis in injection drug users. Am J Med 1996;101:68

Korzeniowski OM, Sande MA. The National Collaborative Endocarditis Study Group. Combination antimicrobial therapy for S. aureus endocarditis in patients addicted to parenteral drugs and in nonaddicts. A prospective study. Ann Intern Med 1982;97:496

Reisberg BE. Infective endocarditis in the narcotic addict. Prog Cardiovasc Dis 1979;22:193

Graves MK, Soto L. Left sided endocarditis in parenteral drug abusers: Recent experience in a large community hospital. S Med J 1992;85:387

Chambers HF, Korzeniowski OM, Sande MA, et al. Staphylococcus aureus endocarditis: Clinical manifestations in addicts and non-addicts. Medicine 1983;62:170

Straumann E, Stulz P, Jenzer HR. Tricuspid valve endocarditis in the drug addict: A reconstructive approach ("vegetectomy"). Thorac Cardiovasc Surg 1990;38:291

ENDOCARDITIS, NATIVE VALVE (NOT IDU)

John G. Bartlett, M.D.

DIAGNOSTIC CRITERIA

- Sx: fever, malaise, chest/back pain, cough, dyspnea, arthralgias, myalgias, neurologic sx, wt loss, night sweats
- PE & lab: Duke criteria = [2 Major] or [1 Major + 3 Minor] or [5 Minor]; (see Table 1a-1b in Appendix I)
- Major (microbiologic) 1) typical organisms x 2 blood cx (S. viridans, S. bovis, HACEK, S. aureus, Enterococcus, no other id'd source OR 2) persistent bacteremia (12h or more); OR 3) 3/3 or 3/4 (+) blood cx
- Major (valve): 1) echo w/ valvular vegetation; OR 2) new valve regurgitation
- Minor: 1) predisposing heart cond. or IDU; 2) fever 38C (100.4F) or more; 3) vascular phenomenon; 4) immune phenomenon; 5) (+) blood cx not meeting above criteria; 6) ECHO abnl but not diagnostic

COMMON PATHOGENS: S.aureus ; S. viridans ; S. bovis ; S. epidermidis ; HACEK ; Enterococcus

TREATMENT REGIMENS

Antibiotic therapy (empiric)

- Empiric Rx acute: [nafcillin or oxacillin 2g IV q4h + gentamicin or tobramycin 1mg/kg IV q8h] OR [vancomycin 1g IV q12h + gentamicin 1mg/kg IV q8h]
- Empiric Rx subacute: [ampicillin/sulbactam 3g IV q 4-6h + gentamicin or tobramycin 1mg/kg IV q8h] OR [vancomycin 1g q12h + ceftriaxone 2g IV q12h] OR [cefotaxime 2g IV q6h + gent/tobra 1 mg/kg IV q8h]
- Culture and sensitivity results when available will define treatment

Cardiac valve replacement

- Indications for surgery: CHF, hemodynamic compromise, fungal etiology, unresolving bacteremia, continuing embolization, progressive heart block, valvular ring abscess, relapse.
- Prognosis for IDU with artificial valve depends on rehabilitative potential from IV drug abuse
- Post-surgical antibiotic therapy: 2 wks or more postop. Consider full 4-6 wk abx course if micro culture of valve or blood cx is positive at time of surgery.
- Streptococcus viridans or Enterococci: same as for native valve endocarditis. Therapy is guided by resistance profile (quantitative or qualitative).
- Pseudomonas aeruginosa: tobramycin or amikacin plus piperacillin-tazobactam or ticarcillin-clavulanic acid or ceftazidime or cefoperazone.
- Candida or Aspergillus species: amphotericin B with fluconazole or itraconazole. Valvular surgery necessary.

DRUG-SPECIFIC COMMENTS

Cefotaxime: Good activity against penicillin sensitive staph and strep, synergistic with aminoglycosides extensive and favorable experience with endocarditis

Ceftazidime: Anti-Pseudomonal. Combine with Tobramycin or Gentamicin.

Daptomycin: Can be used for Vancomycin-resistant enterococci.

Linezolid: Disadvantages are the lack of experience and static rather than cidal activity

Nafcillin: Common empirical choice for Staph (MSSA) and Strep coverage while awaiting culture results.

Oxacillin: Common empirical choice for Staph (MSSA) and Strep coverage while awaiting culture results.

Tobramycin: Recommended as synergistic treatment with beta-lactams as anti-Pseudomonal therapy.

Vancomycin: Increasing empirically choosen in populations at higher risk for MRSA, e.g., IDU, nosocomially-related endocarditis.

IMPORTANT POINTS

- Predisposing conditions: IDU, rheumatic heart disease, valvular insufficiency, indwelling catheters, pacemakers, prosthetic heart valves, congenital heart disease, prior endocarditis
- Mycotic aneurysm: concern if focal headaches & neurologic changes, especially if also w/ meningitis. 75% in middle cerebral artery, 20% multiple locations.
- Special cx requirements: HACEK, Legionella, Mycoplasma, nutritionally variant strep (Abiotrophia), Bartonella, Coxiella, Brucella, Gonococci, Listeria, Nocardia, Corynebacteria, TB
- Penicillin allergic pts: skin test for allergy. Consider cephalosporins. Vancomycin common if documented anaphylaxis. Consider PCN desensitization.

- See "Endocarditis in Injection Drug Users" and "Prosthetic Valve Endocarditis"
- Mycotic Aneurysm: CT scan and lumbar puncture to determine aneurysmal rupture. Consider angiography for those with suspected hemorrhage or those with persistent focal headache and CSF pleocytosis. If possible, delay valve replacement surgery and resultant anticoagulation if documented aneurysm to allow healing of aneurysm. Highest risk for intracranial infectious aneurysms are those with S. aureus infection, especially those with S. aureus meningitis.
- Dominant pathogen now is S. aureus and most common source is "healthcare associated" due to IV lines and dialysis.

SELECTED READINGS

Fowler VG Jr, Miro JM, Hoen B, Cabell CH, Abrutyn F, et al. Staphylococcus aureus endocarditis: a consequence of medical progress. JAMA 2005; Jun 22;293(24):3021-3021

Durack DT, Lukes AS, Bright DK. New Criteria for Diagnosis of Infective Endocarditis: Utilization of Specific Echocardiographic Findings. Am J Med, 1994;96:200-9

Moreillan P, Que Y-A. Infective endocarditis. Lancet 2004;363:139-49

Vikram HR, Buenconsejo J, Hasbun R, Quagliarello VJ. Impact of valve surgery on 6 month mortality in adults with complicated left sided native valve endocarditis: A propensity analysis. JAMA 2003;290:3207-14

Le T, Bayer AS. Combination antibiotic therapy for infective endocarditis. Clin Infect Dis 2003;36:615-21

Bayer AS, Bolger AF, Taubert KA, et al. Diagnosis and management of infective endocarditis and its complications. Circulation 1998;98:2936

Wilson WR, Karchmer A, Dajani AS, Taubert KA, Bayer A, Kaye D, Bisno AL, Ferrieri P, Shulman ST, Dur. Antibiotic Treatment of Adults with Infective Endocarditis Due to Streptococci, Enterococci, Staphylococci, and HACEK Organisms . JAMA 1995;274:1706-13

Dajani AS, Taubert KA, Wilson W, et. al. Prevention of Bacterial Endocarditis: Recommendations by the American Heart Association. JAMA Vol277 1997;277:1794-01

Hasburn R, Vikram HR, Barakat LA, et al. Complicated left-sided native valve endocarditis in adults: Risk classification for mortality. JAMA 2003;289:1933-40

Pruitt AA. Neurologic complications of infective endocarditis: a review of an evolving disease and its management issues in the 1990s. The Neurologist 1995;1:20-34.

ENDOCARDITIS, PROPHYLAXIS John G. Bartlett, M.D.

DIAGNOSTIC CRITERIA

- Indications: existing prosthetic valve or
- Prior hx of endocarditis or
- Congenital cardiac malformations or
- Rheumatic & other acquired valve dysfunction or
- Mitral valve prolapse + murmur

TREATMENT REGIMENS

Procedure Indications

- Principles: guidelines from AHA/IDSA based on valve lesion, procedure (dental, resp vs GI/GU), and anticpated pathogen (S. viridans: above diaphragm ; enterococcus : below diaph)
- Guidelines from Amer. Heart Assoc./IDSA (JAMA 1997;277:1794)
- Dental extractions: periodontal surgery, scaling, root planing, implant, root canal, orthodontic bands, tooth cleaning with bleeding, abx strip placement, local anaesthesia-intraligamentory
- Surgery: T&A, incision of intestine or respiratory mucosa, gall bladder surgery

- Endoscopy: bronchpscopy with rigid scope, cystoscopy
- Misc: esophageal dilatation, urethral dilatation, sclerotherapy esophageal varices, ERCP with biliary obstruction

Abx for oral, dental & respiratory procedures

- Amoxicillin 2g PO 1h pre-procedure
- Alternative: penicillin V 2g 1h pre-procedure & 1g 6h later PO
- Pen allergy: clindamycin 600mg PO 1h pre-procedure or cephalexin/cefadroxil 2g PO 1h pre-procedure or azithromycin/clarithro 500mg PO 1h pre-procedure
- Intolerant oral meds: ampicillin 2g IM or IV 30min pre-procedure

Abx for GI & GU procedures or high-risk patient

- High risk (prosthetic valve, prior endocarditis, surgical shunt): ampicillin 2g IM/IV + gent 1.5mg/kg IV/IM 30min pre-procedure
- High risk + pen allergy: vancomycin 1g IV over 1-2h complete 30min pre-procedure + gent 1.5mg/kg IV 30min pre-procedure
- Moderate risk: amoxicillin 2g PO 1hr pre-procedure
- Moderate risk + pen allergy: vancomycin 1g IV over 1-2h complete 30 min pre-procedure

DRUG-SPECIFIC COMMENTS

Amoxicillin: This drug is used because it is well absorbed and it is active against the major anticipated bacterial pathogen - Viridans streptococci. Need a single high dose (2g) 1hr pre-procedure.

IMPORTANT POINTS

- Source: Am Heart Assoc & IDSA (JAMA 1997;277:1794 & Med Letter 2001;43:98)
- Target of prophylaxis for oral/respiratory procedures - alpha strep; GI & GU procedures - enterococcus
- Principle of prophylaxis: high dose abx 30-60 minutes pre-procedure +/- 1 additional dose (if high risk or long procedure beyond half life of agent used)
- Controversy with mitral valve prolapse due to frequency, offer prophylaxis with valvular thickening or redundancy or presence of murmur.
- Highest risks: prosthetic valve, prior endocarditis, surgical shunt

SELECTED READINGS

Mylonakis E, Calderwood. Infective endocarditis in adults. N Engl J Med 2001;345:1318-30

Durack D. Prophylaxis of infective endocarditis. Principles & Practice of Infect Dis, Chp 67, Mandell G, Bennett J, Dolin R (Editors), 5th Ed, Churchill Livingstone, Phil 2000, pg 917

Simmons NA. Recommendations for endocarditis. J Antimicrob Chemother 1993;31:437

Strom BL, Abrutyn E, Berlin JA, et al. Dental and cardiac risk factors fear infective endocarditis. A population-based case control study. Ann Intern Med 1998;129:761

Marks AR, Choong CY, Sanfilippo AJ, et al. Identification of the risk of bacterial endocarditis in persons with mitral-valve prolapse. NEJM 1982;307:776

Clemens JD, Ransohoff DF. A quantitative assessment of pre-dental antibiotic prophylaxis for patients with mitral valve prolapse. J Chron Dis 1984;37:531

Durack DT, Kaplan EL, Bisno AL. Apparent failures of endocarditis prophylaxis: analysis of 52 cases admitted to a national registry. JAMA 1983;250:2318

Lockhart PB, et al. Decision-making on the use of antimicrobial prophylaxis for dental procedures. CID 2002;34:1621

Guntheroth WG. How important are dental procedures as a cause of endocarditis. Am J Cardiol 1984;54:797

Medical Letter. Prevention of bacterial endocarditis. Medical Letter 2001;43:98

ENDOCARDITIS, PROSTHETIC VALVE

Richard Nettles, M.D.

DIAGNOSTIC CRITERIA

- Sx: fever, malaise, chest/back pain, cough, dyspnea, arthralgia, neurologic sx, wt loss, night sweats; in early infection (<2 months after surgery) CHF or shock may predominate over subtle symptoms
- PE & Lab: Duke criteria = [2 Major] or [1 Major + 3 Minor] or [5 minor]; per below (see Tables 1a-1b in Appendix I)
- Major (microbiologic): 1. typical orgs x 2 blood cx; OR 2. persistent bacteremia (>=12h); OR 3. 3/3 or 3/4 pos. bld cx OR 4. blood cx + or IgG Ab titer >1:800 for Coxiella burnetii
- Major (Valve): 1. vegetation seen on echocardiography; OR 2. new valve regurgitation
- Minor: 1. Predisposing heart cond. or IDU; 2. Fever >38C (100.4F); 3. Vascular phenomenon 4. Immune phenomenon 5. Pos. bld cx not meeting above criteria

COMMON PATHOGENS: Coagulase-negative Staphylococcus ; Staphylococcus aureus; Streptococcus species ; Enterococcus

TREATMENT REGIMENS

Antibiotic therapy

- Methicillin Sensitive Staphylococcus: nafcillin or oxacillin 2g IV q4h x 6 wks plus rifampin 300mg PO q8h x 6 wks plus gentamicin 1.0mg/kg IV or IM q8h x 2 wks.
- Methicillin Resistant Staphylococcus: vancomycin 15mg/kg IV q12h x 6 wks plus rifampin 300mg PO q8h x 6 wks plus gentamicin 1.0mg/kg IV or IM q8h x 2 wks.
- Penicillin Sensitive Streptococcus (MIC< 0.1mcg/mL): penicillin G 18-24 mU IV/24h (continuously or divided q4h) x 6 wks + gentamicin 1mg/kg IV/IM q8h x 2 wks.
- Penicillin Resistant Streptococcus (MIC > 0.1mcg/mL): penicillin G 24-30 mU/24h (continuously or divided q4h) x 6 wks + gentamicin 1mg/kg IV/IM q8h x 4 wks.
- Enterococci: ampicillin 2g IV q4h + gentamicin 1mg/kg IV/IM q8h x 6 wks or if resistant to pen, vancomycin 15 mg/kg IV q12h + gentamicin 1mg/kg IV/IM q8h x 6 wks
- HACEK organisms: ceftriaxone 2g IV/IM q24h x 6 wks
- Culture-negative: vancomycin 15mg/kg IV q12h + gentamicin 1mg/kg IV or IM q8h x 6wks +/- ceftriaxone 2 g IV/IM q24h x 6 wks

Surgical intervention

- Indications for surgery: moderate to severe CHF, unstable prosthesis, paravalvular extension, persistent bacteremia despite optimal ABX, certain organisms (fungi, P. aeruginosa, S. aureus), relapse
- Relative surgical indications: vegetations >10mm, culture negative PVE with unexplained fever >10d
- Timing of surgery depends on optimization of hemodynamic status prior to surgery, not sterilization of blood cultures or duration of ABX. Risk low of infecting new valve, some prefer bioprostheses.
- In the setting of neurologic complications, the risk of hemorrhagic transformation is decreased by delaying surgery if cardiac hemodynamics permit

Special considerations

- Infection <2 months following cardiac surgery are often nosocomially linked, the micro of these episodes is distinct from episodes acquired later, which is more similar to native valve endocarditis.

DIAGNOSIS

- Legionella pneumophila and Legionella dumoffii PVE is linked to tap water exposure of postoperative (sternal) wounds or chest tubes
- Mycobacterium chelonae PVE is linked to contamination of the bioprosthesis during manufacturing
- Anticoagulation is controversial, but probably indicated with PVE involving valves that require anticoagulation when not infected (mechanical valves)
- Bioprosthetic valves that typically do not require anticoagulation do not warrant anticoagulation when infected.
- Anticoagulation must be very carefully controlled for fear of hemorrhagic infarcts

IMPORTANT POINTS

- Vancomycin is considered inferior to oxacillin or nafcillin for methicillin-sensitive strains of S. aureus
- TEE (transesophageal echocardiography) is diagnostically superior in PVE and preferred over TTE (transthoracic echocardiography)
- Length of ABX after surgery is determined by operative findings; if there is evidence of ongoing infection then treat with a full course of standard antibiotics postoperatively.
- If there is no sign of ongoing infection at surgery, the sum of the pre and post operative antibiotic course should equal the recommended duration of therapy for the specific causative organism
- Recommendations based upon JAMA, 1995;274(21):1706.

SELECTED READINGS

Chirouze C, Cabell CH, Fowler VG, et al. Prognostic Factors in 61 cases of Staphylococcal aureus prosthetic valve infective endocarditis from the international collaboration on endocarditis merged database. Clin Infect Dis. Vol 38, 2004, pp1323-7.

Chien JW, Kucia ML, Salata RA. Use of linezolid, an oxazolidinone, in the treatment of multi-drug resistant gram positive bacterial infections. Clin Infect Dis. Vol 31(1), 2000, pp.208-9

Li JS, Sexton DJ, Mick N, et al. Proposed Modifications to the Duke Criteria for the Diagnosis of Infective Endocarditis. Clin Infect Dis. Vol 30, 2000, pp. 633-8

Tornos P, Almirante B, Mirabet S, et al. Infective endocarditis due to Staphylococcus aureus: Deleterious effect of anticoagulation therapy. Arch Intern Med. Vol 159, 1999 pp.473-75

John MD, Hibberd PL, Karchmer AW, et al. Staphylococcus aureus prosthetic valve endocarditis: Optimal management and risk factors for death. Clin Infect Dis. Vol. 26. 1998, pp. 1302-9

Nettles RE, McCarty DE, Corey RG, et al. An evaluation of the Duke Criteria in 25 pathologically confirmed cases of prosthetic valve endocarditis. Clin Infect Dis. Vol. 25, 1997, pp1401-3

Wilson WR, Karchmer A, Dajani AS, et al. Antibiotic Treatment of Adults with Infective Endocarditis Due to Streptococci, Enterococci, Staphylococci, and HACEK Organisms . JAMA, vol. 274, no. 21, Dec, 1995, p.1706-13

Grover FL, Cohen DJ, Oprian C, et al. Determinants of the occurrence of and survival from prosthetic valve endocarditis. Experience of the Veterans Affairs Cooperative study on valvular heart disease. J Thorac Cardiovasc Surg. Vol. 108(2), 1994, pp 207-14

Durack DT, Lukes AS, Bright DK. New Criteria for Diagnosis of Infective Endocarditis: Utilization of Specific Echocardiographic Findings. Am J Med, vol. 96, March 1994, p. 200-209

Levine DP, Fromm Bs, Reddy BR . Slow Response to Vancomycin or Vancomycin plus Rifampin in Methicillin-sensitive S. aureus endocarditis. Ann Int Med, vol 115, no. 9, November, 1991, pp. 674-80

ENDOPHTHALMITIS
Aimee Zaas, M.D.

DIAGNOSTIC CRITERIA

- Ocular inflammation due to introduction of an infectious agent into posterior segment of eye
- Types: post-operative, post-traumatic (penetrating globe injury) and hematogenous spread ("endogenous endophthalmitis")
- Diagnosis: sampling and culture of vitreous imperative for etiology and sensitivities; 70% yield positive culture
- Presentation: depends on virulence; range from mild irritation to profound pain, exophthalmos, periorbital extension
- Diagnosis: PCR of vitreous samples can identify pathogen in nearly 100% of cases; use as adjunct to cx if available

COMMON PATHOGENS: Propionibacterium species ; Enterococcus ; Bacillus cereus ; Fusarium

TREATMENT REGIMENS

Endogenous endophthalmitis (EE)

- Bacterial: intravitreal antibiotics - ceftazidime 2.2mg in 0.1mL (gram-negative), vancomycin 1.0mg in 0.1mL (gram-positive)
- Systemic fluoroquinolones penetrate vitreous; no trials to support use
- Repeat vitreal tap at 48-72 hours and redose antibiotics if no improvement/worsening
- Candida: early vitrectomy combined with systemic antifungal therapy (amphotericin B or fluconazole) recommended
- Candida: 6-12 weeks systemic therapy with amphotericin B 0.7-1.0mg/kg or fluconazole 400mg/day IV/PO; ampho has renal toxicity
- Candida: intravitreal amphotericin B controversial; dose is 5-10ug
- Candida: caspofungin may be effective (see references), but not well studied as yet
- Aspergillus: intravitreal amphotericin B 5-10ug with dexamethasone 400ug; repeat in 2 days post vitrectomy; no studies of voriconazole or caspofungin
- Fusarium: successful case report of posaconazole (systemic and ocular); see references
- Bacillus: systemic and intra-vitreal vancomycin; vitrectomy

Post-operative endophthalmitis

- Intra-vitreal antibiotics alone generally suffice, based on large randomized trial (see references)
- Coagulase-negative staphylococci, gram-negative rods and streptococci most common
- Empiric therapy: intra-vitreal vancomycin plus ceftazidime
- Gram-positive: vancomycin 1mg/0.1mL; may repeat at 48-72 hours if not improving
- Gram-negative: amikacin 0.4mg/0.1mL may be used; has risk of retinal microvasculitis
- Gram-negative: ceftazidime 2.25mg/0.1mL is drug of choice; may repeat at 48-72 hours if not improving
- Oral fluoroquinolones penetrate vitreous; have not been studied in treatment trials
- Intravitreal corticosteroids controversial
- Despite recommendation for intra-vitreal antibiotics alone, many clinicians use systemic abx as well for severe cases

Post-traumatic endophthalmitis

- Immediate vitrectomy with bacterial/fungal cultures, remove foreign bodies and necrotic tissue
- Empiric intravitreal antibiotics: vancomycin 1mg and ceftazidime 2.25 mg; consider amphotericin B 5ug if rural/vegetable matter injury

- Systemic broad-spectrum antibiotics recommended: vancomycin and ceftazidime are a good choice

IMPORTANT POINTS

- Post-operative: late infections (years after surgery) often due to Propionobacterium acne
- P. acnes often causes a white plaque on the posterior lens capsule; can be biopsied for culture
- Post traumatic: risks are foreign body, delayed globe closure and extent of globe laceration
- EE is result of systemic infection; risks are immune compromise, intravenous lines, hyperalimentation, IDU, malignancy; 25% bilateral
- EE can be caused by S. pneumoniae, H. influenzae, N. meningitidis in otherwise healthy patients
- Endophthalmitis can present mildly as painless floaters/visual change or fulminantly with pain, chemosis, visual loss and fevers.

SELECTED READINGS

Marangon FB, Miller D, Giaconi JA, Alfonso EC. In vitro investigation of voriconazole susceptibility for keratitis and endophthalmitis fungal pathogens. Am J Ophthalmol. 2004 May;137(5):820-5

Goldblum D, Rohrer K, Frueh BE, et al. Ocular distribution of intravenously administered lipid formulations of amphotericin B in a rabbit model. Antimicrob Agents Chemother 2002;Dec 46(12)3719-3723

Sponsel WE, Graybill JR, Nevarez HL, & Dang D. Ocular and systemic posaconazole (SCH-56592) treatment of invasive Fusarium solani keratitis and endophthalmitis. British Journal of Ophthalmology 2002; Jul 86(7):829-30

Durand ML. The post-endophthalmitis vitrectomy study era. Archives of Ophthalmology 2002;120:233-4

Scott IU, Flynn HW Jr, MIller D, et al. Exogenous endophthalmitis caused by amphotericin-b-resistant Paecilomyces lilacinus: treatment options and visual outcomes. Arch Ophthalmol 2001;Jun 119(6):916-919

Sternberg P & Martin DF. Management of endophthalmitis in the post-endophthalmitis vitrectomy study era. Archives of Ophthalmology 2001;119:754-5

Gonzalez CA, Scott IU, Chaudhry NA, et al. Endogenous endophthalmitis caused by Histoplasma capsulatum var. capsulatum: case report and literature review. Ophthalomology 2000 Apr;107(4):725-9

Majji AB, Jalali S, Gopinathan U. Role of intravitreal dexamethasone in exogenous fungal endophthalmitis. Eye 1999 Oct 13 (pt 5):660-5

Martinez-Vazquez C, Fernandez-Ulloa J, Bordon J, et al. Candida albicans endophthalmitis in brown heroin addicts: response to early vitrectomy proceeded and followed by antifungal therapy. Clinical Infectious Diseases 1998;Nov 27(5):1130-3

Boldt HC, Pulido JS, Blodi CF, et al. Rural Endophthalmitis. Ophthalmology 1989;96:1722-26

EPIDIDYMITIS

Noreen A. Hynes, M.D., M.P.H.

DIAGNOSTIC CRITERIA

- Clinical sx: Severe scrotal pain, usually unilateral, with or without inguinal pain.
- Clinical hx: 1/3 will report sudden onset; 2/3 gradual onset; may have history of urethral discharge and/or dysuria.
- PE findings: Testicle usually in normal position in scrotum; swollen, tender epididymis on palpation; scrotum of affected side may be erythematous and edematous.

- Lab eval: gram stain for dx of urethritis; CX of intraurethral exudate or nucleic acid amplification test for GC/CT; exam of unspun FVU for WBC if gram stain neg; syphilis serology; HIV test
- RULE OUT TESTICULAR TORSION IN ALL CASES. This is a surgical emergency. In severe epididymitis cases with acute swelling of spermatic cord, flank pain if obstruction of ureter as it crosses cord.

COMMON PATHOGENS: Chlamydia trachomatis ; Neisseria gonorrhoeae ; Enteric pathogens

TREATMENT REGIMENS

Gonorrhea or chlamydia most likely (age <35 yrs)
- Ceftriaxone 250mg IM once PLUS doxycycline 100mg PO bid x 10d
- Ofloxacin 300mg PO bid x 10d
- Allergy to cephalosporins or doxycycline: Levofloxacin 500mg PO qd x 10d

Enteric organism most likely (Age >34 yrs)
- Levofloxacin 500mg PO qd x 10d
- Ofloxacin 300mg PO bid x 10d

Adjunctive therapy for all
- Bed rest
- Scrotal elevation
- Analgesics until fever and local inflammation subside
- Reexamine EVERY patient within 72h to assess original dx and Rx.

DRUG-SPECIFIC COMMENTS

Ceftriaxone: Single injection of 250mg provides sustained, high bactericidal levels. Must be coupled with doxycycline to provide coverage for Chlamydia trachomatis.

Doxycycline: The antichlamydial agent in this epididymitis treatment regimen. No studies have yet been reported comparing doxycycline with azithromycin in the treatment regimen for epididymitis.

Levofloxacin: Use in epididymitis where enteric gram negative rods are suspected in the etiology. This is the L-isomer of ofloxain. Fluroquinolones should not be used to Rx suspect GC epididymitis if acquired in the MA, New York City, HI, CA, or the Pacific Basin due to fluoroquinolone resistant GC in these areas.

IMPORTANT POINTS
- Recommendations based on CDC's 2002 STD Rx Guidelines (MMWR 2002; 51 (RR-6) and revised recommendations for gonorrhea treatment (MMWR 2004 53:335-338).
- Ddx: testicular torsion (a surgical emergency!), abscess, hydrocele, spermatocele, hernia, trauma, testicular cancer, drugs, esp. amiodarone.
- MEN <35 YRS: usual etiology is C. trachomatis and N. gonorrhoeae. In men who engage in insertive rectal intercourse, coliforms are also likely; more unusual organisms--P. aeruginosa, M. tuberculosis.
- MEN >34 YRS: the most common pathogens--coliforms and P. aeruginosa but CT and GC must always be considered; underlying structural pathology or chronic bacterial prostatitis must be considered.
- Persistent swelling and tenderness after completion of RX requires evaluation. Differential diagnosis includes tumor, abscess, testicular cancer, infarction, TB or fungal epididymitis.
- Some, rare organisms can be spread hematogenously: S. pneumoniae, Brucella spp, N. meningitidis, T. pallidum, Nocardia spp, H. influenzae type B, histoplasmosis, Coccidioides, blastomycosis, cryptococcosis, candidiasis, CMV.

- Unless patient exam is early in course of evolving acute process, physical exam may not be able to tell epididymitis from torsion.
- Examination of urine helps differentiate epididymitis from torsion; former usually shows bacteriuria or WBCs in urine.
- Sex partners of patients should be referred if their contact with the index patient was within 60 days preceding the onset of symptoms in the patient.
- Fungi and mycobacterial causes more HIV-infected men than HIV-uninfected men.
- Epididymo-orchitis has been described in 12% to 19% of men with Behcet's disease. This is non infective and thought to be part of the disease process.

SELECTED READINGS

Chen F et al. Tuberculous epididymo-orchitis presenting within the setting of a sexually transmitted disease clinic. Sex Transm Dis 2004 31:163-165.

Donzella JG et al. Epididymitis after transrectal ultrasound-guided needle biopsy of prostate gland. Urology 2004 62:306-308.

Centers for Disease Control and Prevention. Sexually transmitted diseases treatment guidelines. MMWR 2002; 51(RR-6).

Clinical Effectiveness Group (AGM/MSSVD). 2001 National guideline for the management of epididymo-orchitis. http://www.mssvd.org.uk/PDF/CEG2001/epididymoorchitis%200601.PDF

Kaklamani VG et al. Recurrent epididymo-orchitis in patients with Behcet's disease. J Urol 2000; 163:487-9.

Berger RE et al. Etiology, manifestations and therapy of acute epididymitis: prospective study of 50 cases. J Urol 1996; 121:750-754.

Sadek I et al. Amiodarone-induced epididymitis: report of a new case and literature review of 12 cases. Can J Cardiol 1993; 9(9):833-6.

Bowie WR. Approach to men with urethritis and urologic complications of sexually transmitted diseases. Med Clin North Amer 1990; 74(6):1543-57.

Berger RE et al. Etiology and manifestations of epididymitis in young men: correlations with sexual orientation. J Infect Dis 1987; 155:1341-43.

Berger RE et al. Chlamydia trachomatis as a cause of acute "idiopathic" epididymitis. N Engl J Med 1978; 298:301-4.

EPIGLOTTITIS
John G. Bartlett, M.D.

DIAGNOSTIC CRITERIA

- Hx: sore throat with odynophagia & fever,+/- drooling, stridor, dyspnea, hoarseness
- PE: Direct visualization shows cherry red epiglottis with tongue blade exam, or by direct or indirect laryngoscopy (caution: don't attempt this exam unless there's setup for airway control)
- Lab: XR of lateral neck shows enlarged epiglottis, but not sensitive or specific
- Leukocytosis with shift--prognostic; chest XR--accompanying pneumonia in up to 25%
- Has become a rare condition in children since the mandatory introduction of H. influenza type b vaccination.

COMMON PATHOGENS: Haemophilus influenzae ; Respiratory tract viruses ; Influenza

TREATMENT REGIMENS

Antibiotic

- Principles: maintain airway + empiric abx targeting H. influenzae
- Preferred abx: cefotaxime 2-3g IV q6-8h x 7-10d or ceftriaxone 1-2g IV qd x 7-10d
- Cefuroxime 0.75-1.5g IV q6-8h x 7-10d

- Ampicillin-sulbactam (Unasyn) 1.5-3g IV q6h x 7-10d
- Ticarcillin-clavulanate (Timentin) 3.1g IV q4-6h x 7-10d
- Piperacillin-tazobactam (Zosyn) 3.375g IV q 4-6h x 7-10d
- Levofloxacin (Levaquin) 500mg IV qd x 7-10d
- Gatifloxacin (Tequin) 400mg IV qd x 7-10d

Maintain airway
- Manage in ICU, maintaining airway is most critical
- Indications for intubation or tracheostomy: dyspnea, stridor and/or drooling

Anti-inflammatory and miscellaneous agents
- Prednisone (or other steroid) is often given although utility is not known and dose is arbitrary
- Hydration, oxygen, analgesics

DRUG-SPECIFIC COMMENTS

Ampicillin + Sulbactam: A good choice for anticipated pathogens--primarily H. influenzae. Also covers most less common alternative pathogens.

Chloramphenicol: Cephalosporins or betalactam-betalactamase inhibitors usually preferred. Severity of this infection justifies chloramphenicol when there is contraindication to betalactams.

Gatifloxacin: A good choice for anticipated pathogens--primarily H. influenzae. Also covers most less common alternative pathogens. Experience in serious H. influenzae infections is limited.

Piperacillin + Tazobactam: A good choice for anticipated pathogens--primarily H. influenzae. Also covers most less common alternative pathogens.

Ticarcillin + Clavulanic Acid: A good choice for anticipated pathogens--primarily H. influenzae. Also covers most less common alternative pathogens.

IMPORTANT POINTS

- Guidelines are the author's opinion and MayoSmith (Chest 1995; 108:1640)
- Major decision is managing airway - trach or intubate or observation in ICU - adults usually observed
- H. influenzae is the major identifiable treatable pathogen; many cases in adults are culture negative & are thought to be viral
- Diagnosis requires visualization of epiglottis with tongue blade, laryngoscope or lateral neck XR--don't manipulate airway or send for XR without being prepared for emergent intubation

SELECTED READINGS

MayoSmith MF , Spinale JW, Donskey CJ et al. Acute epiglottitis. Chest 1995; 108:1640

Sengor A, et al. Isolated necrotizing epiglottitis. Ann Otol Rhinol Laryngol 2004;113:225-8

MayoSmith MF, et al. Acute epiglottis in adults. An eight year experience in the state of Rhode Island. N Engl J Med 1986;314:1133-9

Carey MJ. Epiglottitis in adults. Am J Emerg Med 1996:14:421.

Ozanne A, et al. Acute epiglottitis: MRI. Neuroradiol 2004;46:153-5

Sack JL, Brock CD. Identifying acute epiglottitis in adults. Post Grad Med 2002;112:81-86

Smith MM, et al. CT in adult epiglottis. Am J Neurorad 1996;17:1355-8

Frantz TD, Rasgon BM, Quesenberry CP. Acute epiglottitis in adults: analysis of 129 cases. JAMA 1994;272:1358.

Rothrock SG, Pignatiello GA, Howard RM. Radiographic diagnosis of epiglottitis: objective criteria for all ages. Ann Emg Med 1990;19:978

Pedersen BK, Pedersen C. Epiglottitis as a manifestation of acute HIV infection. J Acquir Immunodef Synd 1994;7:1210.

ESOPHAGITIS [AIDS]

John G. Bartlett, M.D.

DIAGNOSTIC CRITERIA

- Hx: substernal dysphagia or odynophagia
- Causes: candida, CMV & aphthous esophagitis are most common; herpes esophagitis less common.
- Clues: candida--thrush, diffuse odynophagia/dysphagia & CD4 <100; CMV--fevers, focal pain & CD4 <50; aphthous--focal odynophagia, no fever & variable CD4.
- CD4 >200: GERD, NSAIDS, pill ulcers (ddC, tetracycline, doxycycline, potassium, iron, TB, cancer, lymphoma)
- Lab findings: endoscopy showing plaque-like lesions (candida) or ulcers (CMV, aphthous or HSV); if ulcer, need bx.

COMMON PATHOGENS: Candida ; Cytomegalovirus ; Herpes Simplex Virus

TREATMENT REGIMENS

Candidiasis

- Principles: thrush + odynophagia - treat empirically with azole; endoscopy if no response after 7-10d or atypical features.
- Preferred: fluconazole 200-400mg/d PO/IV x 2-3 wks
- Alternative: itraconazole 200mg/d or voriconazole 200mg PO bid
- Refractory: caspofungin 70mg IV x 1, then 50mg qd x 7 d
- Refractory: Ampho B 0.3-0.7 mg/kg/d IV
- Maintenance: For recurring disease, fluconazole 100-200mg/d

Ulcerative disease

- Preferred for CMV: valganciclovir 900mg PO bid with food or ganciclovir 5 mg/kg IV q12h x 2-3 weeks
- Alternative for CMV: foscarnet 90 mg/kg/d IV q12h x 2-3 wks
- Maintenance: indication- recurrent CMV esophagitis, valganciclovir 900 mg/d PO w/ food until immune recovery
- HSV: acyclovir 5 mg/kg IV tid or PO valacyclovir 1g po tid or famciclovir 500mg PO tid
- Aphthous (preferred): prednisone 40 mg/d PO, tapering 10 mg/wk, x 1 mo.
- Aphthous (refractory): thalidomide 200 mg/d PO. 100-200 mg PO/d, titrate up to 400-600/d (but poorly tolerated) x 7-28d +/- 50 mg/d maintenance. For thalidomide call 888-423-5436.

DRUG-SPECIFIC COMMENTS

Clotrimazole: Clotrimazole troches are not a good choice for Candida esophagitis since a systemic treatment is required. This drug is used for topical treatment of oral candidiasis (thrush).

Fluconazole: Advantages of fluconazole are that absorption is more predictable, experience is greater and there are fewer drug interactions than ketoconazole. Both IV and PO formulations are now available generically. NOTE: Maintenance fluconazole not generally used due to resistance -- use for severe recurrence only.

Itraconazole: Advantage is activity vs some fluconazole-resistant Candida species; disadvantage is less reliable absorption

Ketoconazole: Sometimes advocated as first-line therapy for Candida esophagitis due to reduced cost; however, advantages of fluconazole are that absorption is more predictable, experience is greater and there are fewer drug interactions.

IMPORTANT POINTS

- Guidelines from NYS AIDS Institute (9/04).
- Most common: candida - CD4 <100 + thrush + odynophagia = treat empirically w/ fluconazole.
- Endoscope pts with atypical odynophagia or fluconazole failure.
- Refractory candidiasis: high dose fluconazole (400-800mg/d), IV Amphotericin B, IV caspofungin, voriconazole or itraconazole. Most important: HAART.
- If able to swallow, oral Rx with azole (candida) valganciclovir (CMV), valacyclovir (HSV) or prednisone

SELECTED READINGS

Pappas PG, et al. Guidelines for the treatment of candidaisis. Clin Infect Dis 2004;38:161

Wilcox CM, et al. Prospective comparison for brush cytology, viral culture and histology for the diagnosis of ulcerative esophagitis in AIDS. Clin Gastroenterol Hepal 2004;564-7

Hospenthal DR, et al. The role of antifungal susceptibility testing in the therapy of candidiasis. Diagn Microbiol Infect Dis 2004;48:153-650

Kartsonis N, et al. Efficacy of caspofungin in the treatment of esophageal candidiasis resistant to fluconazole. JAMA 2002;31:183

Arathoon EG, et al. Randomized, double-blind multicenter study of caspofungin versus amphotericin B for treatment of oropharyngeal and esophageal candidiasis. Antimic Ag Chemother 2002;46:451

Bini EJ, Micate PL,. Weinshel EH. Natural history of HIV-associated esophageal disease in the era of protease inhibitor therapy. Dig Dis Sci 2000;45:1301

Monkemuller KE, Wilcox CM. Esophageal ulcer caused by cytomegalovirus: resolution during combination antiretroviral therapy for acquired immunodeficiency syndrome. South Med J 2000;93:818

Martinez C, Tobal GF, Ruiz-Irastorza G. Risk factors for esophageal candidiasis. Eur J Clin Microbial Infect Dis 2000;19:96.

Barbaro G, Barbarini G, Calderon W, et al. Fluconazole versus itraconazole for candida esophagitis in AIDS. Gastroenterology 1996;111:1169.

Wilcox CM, Straub RF, Alexander LN. Etiology of esophageal disease in HIV infected patients who fail antifungal therapy. Am J Med 1996;101:599.

FEVER AND NEUTROPENIA   Khalil G. Ghanem, M.D.

DIAGNOSTIC CRITERIA

- Fever: single oral temp 38.3C (101F) or higher or temp 38C (100.4F) or higher for 1h or more AND
- Neutropenia: Absolute neutrophil count (ANC)<500 cells/mm^3 OR <1000 cells/mm3 with predicted decline to <500 cells/mm^3.
- History: correlate date fever onset to date of cytotoxic Rx to predict duration of neutropenia (nadir count usually 10-14 d after chemo).
- PE: exam esp. periodontium, pharynx, lungs, perineum/anus, skin, eyes, vascular access sites, BM bx sites.
- Labs: 2 sets bacterial & fungal blood cx. Central line, cx lumen & peripheral vein; gram stain exudates; UA w/micro; CBC w/diff; LFTs; electrolytes. CXR; scans (CT, US, MRI) as per signs/symptoms

COMMON PATHOGENS: Gram-negative bacillis; Staphylococcus aureus; Enterococcus

Treatment Regimens

Oral therapy
- Adults who are low risk pts (see "Important Points" below) may use: ciprofloxacin + amox/clav. Make sure pts observed carefully & have access to appropriate medical care 24/7.
- Oral therapy: ciprofloxacin 500mg PO BID and amox/clav 500mg PO q8h.

Monotherapy & combination therapy
- No difference between combination or monotherapy for empirical Rx of uncomplicated febrile neutropenia.
- Choice of empiric therapy should be based on local patterns of infection and antibiotic susceptibilities.
- Monotherapy: cefepime, ceftazidime or carbapenem (imipenem/ meropenem) approved; carbapenems are preferred if ESBL rate is high (AVOID cephalosporins).
- Combination: aminoglycoside + [antipseudomonal PCN or cefepime or ceftazidime or carbapenem]
- Potential advantages of combination Rx: synergistic effects against GNRs & decrease in the emergence of drug-resistance. Balance with the potential for nephro- and ototoxicity.
- Vancomycin considered if: clinically suspected serious cath-related infxn, known MRSA colonization, + BC results w/GPC prior final id, or hypotension. O/W follow initial cx data & add vanco as needed.
- Quinolones are NOT recommended as routine initial monotherapy agents due to lack of prospective data, & use of quinolones as routine prophylaxis in many centers.
- Intravenous therapy: ceftazidime 2g IV q8H OR cefepime 2g IV q12h OR imipenem 1g IV q6h (caution in patients with renal insufficiency in view of seizure potential).
- Addition of aminoglycoside for combination therapy: gentamicin 2mg/kg q8h or 5mg/kg q 24h (once daily preferred: less toxicity) OR amikacin 15mg/kg/day or divided q8-12h.
- Other drugs used: vanco 1g q12h; fluconazole 400mg IV q24h; amphotericin B 0.5-1mg/kg/day OR abelcet 5mg/kg/day or ambisome 3mg/kg/day.

Approach to Rx
- 1) Hx, PE, labs (cx) 2) assess risk of patient & determine if PO or IV Rx; begin Abx (mono or combo) & continue at least 3-5d before any changes if no new cx data or clinical deterioration.
- 3) decide if vancomycin warranted; 4) if pt afebrile in 3-5d, continue abx at least 7d or IDEALLY until ANC>500 or suspected source treated. If pt LOW RISK, can switch to PO cipro + amox/clav.
- 5) persistent fever: Clinical reassessment incl cx & scans;decide if continue abx (pt stable) OR change/add abx (dz progress, or vanc criteria met) OR add antifungal (febrile and ANC>500 NOT imminent)
- 6) Antifungal Rx= ampho B (or lipid formulations); fluconazole if resistance pattern permits; new data on voriconazole very encouraging. Prior to antifungal therapy, work-up for fungal infxn should be complete: bx of skin lesions, CT of chest, abdomen, sinuses, nasal endoscopy (if indicated), & cx.
- 7) persistent fever: can D/C abx 4-5 days after ANC>500; continue X14d if ANC<500 & febrile (continually reassess). At 14d, if stable and cx neg, can stop Abx and follow carefully.
- The single most important determinant of sucessful D/C OF ABX is neutophil count.

- Routine granulocyte transfusions not recommended; routine antivirals not indicated unless herpes/VZV lesions (acyclovir); CMV rare except in BMT pts (use ganciclovir).
- Colony-Stimulating Factors (G-CSF): can shorten duration of neutropenia but NOT duration of fever or decrease infection mortality;routine use NOT recommended.
- Consider use of G-CSF in severely neutropenic patients w/documented infections that do not respond to appropriate rx, or when prolonged delay in marrow recovery is anticipated.

IMPORTANT POINTS

- Signs and symptoms (induration, erythema, pustulation, CXR infiltrates, CSF pleocytosis) may be absent in patients with neutropenia.
- Low risk pts:ANC>100; monocytes>100; nl CXR; nl LFTs and Cr; no IV site infxn; temp<39C; no abd pain; evidence of BM recovery; no comorbidities; neutropenia to last <10d.
- Median time to defervescence in adequately treated pts is 5d (range 2-7 days). DO NOT modify initial abx choice unless clinical deterioration or new cx data dictate it.
- Sinusitis should be aggressively diagnosed and treated as neutropenia is a risk factor for aspergillus infections.
- 50% of febrile neutropenics will have an established or occult infection and 1/5 with ANC<100 cells/mm^3 will have bacteremia.

SELECTED READINGS

Hughes WT. 2002 guidelines for the use of antimicrobial agents in neutropenic patients with cancer. Clin Infect Dis 2002 Mar 15;34(6):730-51

Bodey GP, et al. Quantitative relationships between circulating leukocytes and infection in patients with acute leukemia. Ann Intern Med 1966 Feb;64(2):328-40

Cordonnier C, et al. Epidemiology and risk factors for gram-positive coccal infections in neutropenia: toward a more targeted antibiotic strategy. Clin Infect Dis 2003 Jan 15;36(2):149-58

Rolston KV et al. Pseudomonas aeruginosa--still a frequent pathogen in patients with cancer: 11-year experience at a comprehensive cancer center. Clin Infect Dis 1999 Aug;29(2):463-4

Santolaya ME, et al. Discontinuation of antimicrobial therapy for febrile, neutropenic children with cancer: a prospective study. Clin Infect Dis 1997 Jul;25(1):92-7

Maher DW, et al. Filgrastim in patients with chemotherapy-induced febrile neutropenia. A double-blind, placebo-controlled trial. Ann Intern Med 1994 Oct 1;121(7):492-501

Ozer H, et al. 2000 update of recommendations for the use of hematopoietic colony-stimulating factors: evidence-based, clinical practice guidelines. American Society of Clinical Oncology. J Clin Oncol 2000 Oct 15;18(20):3558-85

Lucas KG, et al. The identification of febrile, neutropenic children with neoplastic disease at low risk for bacteremia and complications of sepsis. Cancer 1996 Feb 15;77(4):791-8

Peacock JE, et al. Ciprofloxacin plus piperacillin compared with tobramycin plus piperacillin as empirical therapy in febrile neutropenic patients. A randomized, double-blind trial. Ann Intern Med 2002 Jul 16;137(2):77-87

Engels EA, et al. Efficacy of quinolone prophylaxis in neutropenic cancer patients: a meta-analysis. J Clin Oncol 1998 Mar;16(3):1179-87

FEVER OF UNKNOWN ORIGIN (FUO)

John G. Bartlett, M.D.

DIAGNOSTIC CRITERIA

- FUO definition: Temp >38.3C + >3 wks duration + no dx w/2 outpt visits or 3 hosp days

Diagnosis

- PE: verify fever, exam - mouth, temporal arteries (esp age >50), abd, spleen, liver, skin, nodes
- Lab - initial: CBC, CRP, ESR, chem panel, chest x-ray, U/A, ANA, Blood cult x 3, HIV
- Scans: CT abd (other: WBC scan? Gallium scan?, ultrasound biliary tract?)
- Next tests: Abn LFT - liver bx; Abn CBC - marrow bx + cxs, temp art bx if > 50yrs
- See Tables 2a-2d in Appendix I

Treatment Regimens

Treatment: based on dx: infectious dis

- Abd abscess: CT scan. Rx Abx + drainage
- TB & MOTT - dx: PPD, chest x-ray, LP, liver bx, marrow bx - granulomas; Rx: 4 drugs
- Cult neg endocarditis - consider HACEK, nutritionally variant strep (cx); Bartonella, Q fever, Legionella, Brucella (serology), fungi. Dx: Echo (TEE), Abx - empiric [see "Endocarditis"]
- Mononucleosis syndromes: 80% EBV (atypical lymphs + Mono spot), CMV, toxo, acute HIV

Treatment: granulomas & collagen vascular disease

- Temporal arteritis - sx: age >50, ESR >50, wt. loss, PMR sx, vision sx; dx - artery bx - Rx pred 60mg/d ASAP to avoid blindness
- Polymyalgia rheumatica - dx: age >50, ESR >50, pain (neck, shoulder, pelvis); clinical diagnosis; Rx: Pred 10-20mg/d
- Still's dis - dx: arthralgia, faint fleeting rash, nodes, WBC increased, anemia, ANA neg, remittent fever; high ESR/CRP, ferritin; ASA or steroid responsive; Rx: NSAID or steroids
- Sarcoid - dx: chest x-ray, bx of tissue - granuloma. R/O TB
- Crohn's dis: dx: endoscopy + bx; Rx: steroids, etc.
- Granulomatous hepatitis - sx: ESR >50, increased alk phos, wt loss, dx: liver bx - Rx steroids

Treatment: tumors/miscellaneous

- "Omas" - lymphoma, myeloma, hypernephroma, dx: CT scan, serum immunoglobulins, SPEP/UPEP
- Hodgkins/Lymphoma - sx: intermittent fever, nodes, liver/spleen enlarged, naproxen response, dx: node, liver or marrow bx
- Solid tissue tumors: CT scan abd, & LFTs for liver mets; DX: Bx
- Drug fever: looks well for temp, low pulse. Occurs typically 1-3wks post start of drug (phenytoin, sulfa, betalactam, barbiturate, clind, dapsone, ampho). D/C = response within 48hrs.
- Factitious: fraudulent - polymicrobial bacteremia, young adult; appears healthy
- Factitious: deceit - healthy young adult, neg labs, ESR nl., no diurnal change, urine temp nl. Rx: confrontation
- Embolism: increased RR or dyspnea, edema, atelectasis or effusion. Dx vent-perfusion scan or angiography (chronic PE not well dx by CT). Rx anticoagulation.
- Familial Med Fever: Jews, Armenians, Turks. Attacks of fever & pain w/no alternative cause +/- serositis, amyloidosis. Rx: colchicine

Important Points

- Guidelines from author
- Classic description: >38 degree C (101F) temp x 3 wks x neg w/u in 3 day hosp or 2 clinic visits
- No diagnosis in 20-40%; prognosis for them is good

- Special categories: nosocomial, immunosuppressed, HIV, travelers
- Most common: ID- TB, endocarditis. CVD- Stills dis, GCA/PMR, granulomatous hepatitis. Tumor- lymphoma. Other-drug, PE, FMF, factitious

SELECTED READINGS

Petersdorf RG, Beeson PB. Fever of unexplained origin: Report on 100 cases . Medicine. 1961;40:1-30

Larson EB, Featherstone HJ, Petersdorf RG. Fever of undetermined origin: Diagnosis and follow-up of 105 cases, 1970-1980. Medicine. 1982;61:269-292

Mackowiak PA, and Durack DT. Fever of unknown origin. In Mandell, Douglas , Dolin eds. Principles and Practice of Infectious Diseases. Churchill Livingstone, pp.622-633.

Aduan RP, Fauci AC, Dale DC, et al. Factitious fever and self-induced infection, a report of 32 cases and review of the literature. Ann Intern Med 1979;90:230

Mackowiak PA, LeMaistre CF. Drug fever: A critical appraisal of conventional concepts. Ann Intern Med 1987;106:728

Chang JC, Hawley BH. Neutropenic fever of undetermined origin (N-FUO): Why not use the naproxen test?. Cancer Invest 1995;13:448

Tsukahara M, Tsuneoka H, Iino H, et al. Bartonella henselae infection as a cause of fever of unknown origin. J Clin Micro 2000;38:1990

McDermott MF, Frenkel J. Hereditary periodic fever syndromes. Neth J Med 2001;59:118

Gonzaolez-Gay MA, Garcia-Porrua C, Salvarani Z, et al. The spectrum of conditions mimicking polymyalgia rheumatica in Northern Spaces. J Rheumatol 2000;27:2179

Klemda E, von Essen R, Heule G, et al. Infectious mononucleosis - like disease with negative heterophile agglutination test. J Infect Dis 1970;121:608

FOLLICULITIS   Ciro R. Martins, M.D.

DIAGNOSTIC CRITERIA

- PE: erythematous papules and/or pustules centered by hair follicles mainly on the back, buttocks, chest, neck and thighs
- Superficial folliculitis: superficial, fragile pustules are predominant (fewer inflammatory lesions)
- Deep folliculitis: inflammatory papules and/or nodules are predominant
- Usually localized and mildly symptomatic process. Can be generalized and significantly pruritic in immunocompromised states.
- Studies: gram stain, cultures, KOH prep and saline examination recommended only when usual treatment fails, especially in immunocompromised individuals.

COMMON PATHOGENS: Staphylococcus aureus

TREATMENT REGIMENS

Topical therapy

- Topical route preferred treatment
- Erythromycin 2% (solution, lotion, gel) bid
- Clindamycin (solution, lotion, gel) bid
- Mupirocin 2% cream bid
- Benzoyl peroxide 2.5, 4.0, 5.0, or 10% (cream, lotion, gel, wash) qd-bid
- Sodium sulfacetamide 10% lotion bid
- Antiseptic/antibacterial soaps can be used in conjunction with above meds qd/bid

• Continue treatment until complete clinical cure

Systemic therapy

• Recommended in generalized, persistent or recurrent cases or when topical therapy fails
• Minocycline or doxycycline 50-100mg PO bid x 2-4 wk
• Cephalexin 500mg PO qid x 7-10d
• Dicloxacillin 500mg PO qid x 7-10d
• Azithromycin 500mg, then 250mg qd x 4d
• Clarithromycin XL 1g PO qd or 500mg PO bid x 7-10d
• Clindamycin 300mg PO tid x 7-10d
• Amoxicillin-clavulanate 875/125mg PO bid x 7-10d
• Trimethoprim/sulfamethoxazole (TMP/SMX) 1 DS PO bid x 7-10d

HIV-infected patients

• Pityrosporum: ketoconazole topical qd-bid (shampoo, cream) or itraconazole 100-400mg PO qd x 2 wk
• Demodex: permethrin topical cream qHS X 7 d or metronidazole 0.75 - 1% topical (lotion, cream, gel) qHS x 4-8 wks
• Eosinophilic folliculitis: cetirizine 20-40mg PO qd, hydroxizine 25-50mg PO qHS, metronidazole 250mg PO tid X 3-4 wk and mid-potency (class III-IV) topical corticosteroids for inflammatory lesions.
• Recurrent Staph folliculitis: Staph-carrying areas of the body (nares) should be treated with mupirocin cream bid x 1w repeated q3 months
• Phototherapy (PUVA or UVB) is effective in cases unresponsive to other treatments

DRUG-SPECIFIC COMMENTS

Amoxicillin + Clavulanate: Very good choice for treating cases due to S. aureus or GNB, but expensive.

Cephalexin: Good oral anti-S. aureus drug and relatively inexpensive

Clarithromycin: Reasonable choice in penicillin-allergic patients; better tolerated than erythromycin but also more expensive

Dicloxacillin: Reasonable oral anti-S. aureus drug, but expensive. No MRSA activity.

Doxycycline: Variable activity against S. aureus (80-85% are susceptible). Very effective and can be used for a long period of time in cases of acne. Potentially photosensitizing drug.

Metronidazole: Relapse rates are high when using this drug orally to treat HIV-associated folliculitis. It seems to work better topically for these patients.

IMPORTANT POINTS

• These guidelines represent the author's opinion
• Both superficial and deep folliculitis usually respond to topical therapy alone
• Predisposing factors: frequent shaving, occlusion (tight clothes, prosthesis), prolonged decubitus, diabetes, immunosuppression and chronic exposure to topical corticosteroids, ointments and greases
• Differential diagnosis: insect bites, papular urticaria, drug reactions, scabies, varicella, disseminated zoster, molluscum contagiosum
• Folliculitis in HIV-infected individuals can cause intense pruritus. It usually requires a combination of multiple topical and systemic meds and recurs frequently
• Recurrent folliculitis: in immunocompetent individuals suggests chronic S. aureus carriage.

- Gram (-) folliculitis: develops abruptly in individuals with acne vulgaris undergoing chronic systemic antibiotic therapy with development of very inflammatory lesions affecting the "T-zone" of the face.
- Pseudomonas folliculitis: develops 6 h to 3 d after swimming in inadequately chlorinated hot tubs, whirlpools and heated swimming pools.
- Eosinophilic folliculitis: histologic diagnosis where the hair follicle is permeated by multiple eosinophils. It is seen mainly in HIV-infected individuals as a very pruritic papular eruption. Its cause remains unknown and controversial. It is not the most common type of folliculitis seen in these patients.
- Drug-induced folliculitis: monomorphic lesions on head, upper trunk and proximal upper extremities. Drugs commonly associated: corticosteroids, androgens, ACTH, lithium, isoniazid (INH), phenytoin, B-complex vitamins

SELECTED READINGS

Sadick, NS. Current Aspects of Bacterial Infections of the Skin. Derm Clinics, 15(2):341-9, April 1997

Carroll, JA. Common Bacterial Pyodermas: Taking aim against the most likely pathogens. Postgrad Med, 100(3):311-22, September 1996

Johnson, RA. Infectious Folliculitis. Fitzpatrick's Journal of Clinical Dermatology, 3(3):38-42, May/June 1995.

Fearfield LA, Rowe A, Francis N. et al. Itchy Folliculitis and Immunodeficiency Virus Infection: Clinicopathological and immunological Features, Pathogenesis and Treatment. Brit J Derm 1999; 141:3-11

FURUNCLE/CARBUNCLE

Ciro R. Martins, M.D.

DIAGNOSTIC CRITERIA

- Furuncle: deep seated, firm, tender nodule that enlarges, becomes erythematous, painful and fluctuant after several days
- Carbuncle: deeper and wider lesions with interconnecting subcutaneous abscesses and multiple draining sinuses which may develop into ulcers that heal with scarring
- Surrounding cellulitis and systemic sx of fever and malaise may be present (more often seen with carbuncles)
- PE: most commonly affected areas are the neck, axillae, groin, buttocks and thighs
- Lab: cx and sensitivity testing are usually not necessary. Perform in toxic patient, HIV, recurrences: consider community-acquired MRSA infection

COMMON PATHOGENS: Staphylococcus aureus

TREATMENT REGIMENS

General management/topical care

- Moist heat (compresses) or hot packs tid-qid until drainage or resolution
- Surgical incision and drainage when fluctuation is palpable
- After drainage, wash area w/ antiseptic/antibacterial soap followed by application of Mupirocin 2% ointment bid
- Keep the area covered with gauze until wound closes.
- Topical care usually curative for single lesions not associated with cellulitis or systemic symptoms
- "Community-acquired MRSA" - Epidemic strain (USA 300). New clone that causes severe furunculosis and less frequently necrotizing fasciitis. Usually needs surgical drainage.

Diagnosis

- Most strains are sensitive to TMP-SMX, rifampin, clindamycin and doxycycline.

Systemic therapy

- Indicated only in cases with associated systemic symptoms or extensive cellulitis
- Mild systemic sxs/mild cellulitis: cephalexin 250-500mg PO qid, dicloxacillin 500mg PO qid, cefuroxime axetil 250-500mg PO bid, TMP-SMX 1 DS PO bid or clindamycin 300mg PO tid; all x 7-10d
- Extensive cellulitis or sepsis: cefazolin 1g IV q8h, cefuroxime 750-1500mg IV q8h, nafcillin 2g IV q4-6h, oxacillin 2g IV q4-6h, clindamycin 600mg IV q8h or vancomycin 1g IV q12h; all x 7-10d

Recurrent furunculosis

- Treatment goal: eradicate chronic S. aureus carriage
- Use nasal swab to assess for S. aureus carriage, presence of MRSA and guide abx selection
- General measures: antiseptic soaps such as chlorhexidine or hexachlorophene; loose-fitting clothes; frequent changes of underwear and linens; avoidance of trauma/irritation of skin
- Topical: intranasal application of Mupirocin 2% cream bid x 5d q 2-3 mo.
- Systemic (if above measures fail): TMP-SMX 1 DS PO qd x 3 mos OR clindamycin 150-300mg PO qd x 3 mos OR rifampin 600mg PO qd AND dicloxacillin 500mg PO qid x 10d

Drug-Specific Comments

Cefadroxil: A good choice for oral therapy of methicillin-sensitive S. aureus. Twice day regimen is a plus.

Cefixime: Poor choice for this type of infection. Drug is relatively inactive against S. aureus as compared to alterantive medications such as cephalexin.

Cephalexin: Very good choice for treating methicillin-sensitive S. aureus. The drug is inexpensive and very well tolerated though qid dosing.

Clarithromycin: Reasonable choice as a second line agent in penicillin-allergic patients. More expensive than erythromycin, but fewer GI symptoms.

Dicloxacillin: This is the standard oral drug for treating S. aureus and should be effective against most community-acquired strains, but be wary of community-acquired MRSA risk factors: IVU, children, local outbreaks.

Doxycycline: Reasonable anti-staphylococcal activity including many community-acquired MRSA strains.

Linezolid: Recommended only in severe systemic infection by a methicillin-resistant strain of S. aureus that is vancomycin-resistant (rare). Also a choice in cases of methicillin-resistance where there are contraindications or intolerance to vancomycin.

Trimethoprim + Sulfamethoxazole: Reasonable Staph activity, and usually active in community-acquired MRSA strains.

Important Points

- These guidelines represent the author's opinion
- Local predisposing factors (recurrent furunculosis): hyperhydrosis, poor hygiene, constant friction and pressure, ingrown hairs
- Systemic predisposing factors (recurrent furunculosis): obesity, blood dyscrasias, malnutrition, immunodeficiency, diabetes, chronic dialysis, IV drug abuse
- Recurrent furunculosis NOT due to more virulent strain of S aureus or host immune deficiency (w/u unnecessary in 95% of cases) , but develops as a consequence of local skin factors instead.

- Ddx: erythema nodosum, other forms of panniculitis, arthropod bite hypersensitivity reaction, vasculitis, mycobacterial infections, cutaneous B-cell lymphomas
- The USA 300 strain of S. aureus is a clonal epidemic strain in the US. This strain has genes for the Pantine Valentine Leukociden toxin thought to account for unique virulence. It is methicillin-resistant but usually sensitive to TMP-SMX, doxycycline, aminoglycosides and clindamycin. Over 12,000 cases of soft-tissue infections were reported in 2004, most were furunculosis. They usually respond to drainage; if abx are given, most recommend TMP-SMX or doxycycline, but not a beta-lactam. Hygiene is important in control-cover wounds and hand hygiene especially.

SELECTED READINGS

Turnidge J, Grayson L. Optimum Treatment of Staphylococcal Infections. Drugs, 45(3):353-66, 1993

Feingold DS. Staphylococcal and Streptococcal Pyodermas. Seminars in Dermatology, 12(4):331-5, December 1993

Reagan DR, Doebbeling BN, Pfaller AW. Elimination of coincident S. aureus nasal and hand carriage with intranasal application of mupirocin calcium ointment. Annals of Internal Medicine, 114:101, 1991

Daroulche R, Wright C, Hammill R. Eradication of colonization by methicillin-resistant S. aureus using oral minocycline-rifampin and topical mupirocin. Antimicrobial Agents and Chemotherapy, 35:1612, 1991

Klempnor MS, Styrt B. Prevention of recurrent Staphylococcal skin infections with low-dose oral clindamycin therapy. JAMA 260:2682, 1988

GAS GANGRENE
John G. Bartlett, M.D.

DIAGNOSTIC CRITERIA

- Clinical: severe pain then rapid progression w/fever, shock, hemolysis, renal failure; wound shows tense edema that changes color: white to bronze to dark with blebs.
- Lab: cx of blood, muscle or bullae yield Clostridia, usually C. perfringens. Aspirates of bullae or muscle show "box-car" GPB on gram stain.
- Other: hemolytic anemia, leukocytosis and renal failure. CT scan will show myonecrosis; x ray shows gas in tissue; clinical course rapid.
- Ddx: Streptococcal myonecrosis, necrotizing fasciitis, Vibrio vulnificus, Aeromonas sp.
- Less than 1% of blood cxs and cx of infected tissue yielding Clostridia represent gas gangrene; most are contaminants & some are mixed infections. Must correlate cx with clinical scenario.

COMMON PATHOGENS: Clostridium perfringens ; Clostridium novyi ; Clostridium septicum ; Clostridium bifermentans ; Clostridium histolyticum ; Clostridium fallax

TREATMENT REGIMENS

Antibiotics
- Principles: rare but critical to dx early. Dx based on injury/surgery + SEVERE PAIN + soft tissue changes + CT/MRI. Need surgeon + Abx ASAP.
- Preferred: clindamycin 600mg IV q6h + penicillin 2-4 million units IV q4h x 10-28 days (covers clostridia + strep)
- Alt: clindamycin 600mg IV q6h + cefotaxime 2-4g IV q8h or imipenem 0.5-1g IV q8h x 10-28 days (covers clostridia, strep, potential mixed infection w/ GNB)
- PCN allergy: clindamycin or chloramphenicol 1g IV q6h
- Most active in vitro: pen G, ampicillin, piperacillin, chloramphenicol, cefotaxime, imipenem; clindamycin is best to reduce toxin production.

- Clostridia antitoxin: no longer available

Surgery

- Mutilating surgery or amputations often required; may need re-op daily to debride necrotic tissue.
- Uterine gas gangrene: total hysterectomy
- Typhlitis (cecal inflammation): C. tertium - usually medical management; C. septicum - may require laparotomy with resection.

Hyperbaric oxygen

- Role of hyperbaric O2 debated.
- Advantages: often demarcates viable tissue to facilitate surgery; surgeons at O2 chambers often have extensive experience.
- Disadvantages: pt transportation may delay critical surgery; unconvincing clinical response data.

Drug-Specific Comments

Ampicillin + sulbactam: Active against virtually all anaerobes including Clostridia. Experience with gas gangrene is nil compared to penicillin, chloramphenicol and clindamycin. Main justification is concern of another etiologic agent(s), e.g., gram-negatives.

Ceftazidime: Cephalosporins are not good drugs for Clostridial infections, and this drug may be the worst of the class for gas gangrene.

Chloramphenicol: Excellent choice, especially for a patient with penicillin allergy. Don't worry about aplastic anemia (1/40,000) when using chloroamphenicol for a life-threatening infection.

Imipenem/cilastatin: Active against virtually all anaerobes including Clostridia. Experience with gas gangrene is nil compared to penicillin, chloramphenicol and clindamycin. Main justification is concern of another etiologic agent(s), e.g., gram-negatives.

Piperacillin + tazobactam: Active against virtually all anaerobes including Clostridia. Experience with gas gangrene is nil compared to penicillin, chloramphenicol and clindamycin. Main justification is concern of another etiologic agent(s), e.g., gram-negatives.

Ticarcillin + clavulanic Acid: Active against virtually all anaerobes including Clostridia. Experience with gas gangrene is nil compared to penicillin, chloramphenicol and clindamycin. Main justification is concern of another etiologic agent(s), e.g., gram-negatives.

Important Points

- Guidelines are author's opinion.
- Skin lesions with bullae ddx: necrotizing fasciitis, Aeromonas infections, necrotizing synergistic cellulitis, Vibrio vulnificus
- Need surgical consultation immediately.
- Other serious soft tissue infxns: necrotizing fasciitis (mixed coliforms + anaerobes or strep), myonecrosis (strep or clost), Aeromonas (fresh/brackish water exposure) Vibrio sp (sea/oyster exp).

Selected Readings

Stevens DL, Bryant AE. The role of clostridial toxins in the pathogenesis of gas gangrene. Clin Infect Dis 2002;35Suppl1:S93

Kimura AC, et al. Outbreak of necrotizing fasciitis due to Clostridium sordelli among black for heroin users. Clin Infect Dis 2004;38:87-91

Caplan ES, Kluge RM. Gas gangrene: review of 34 cases. Arch Intern Med 1976;136:788

Stevens DL, Bryant AE, Adams K. Evaluation of therapy with hyperbaric oxygen for experimental infection with Clostridium perfringens. Clin Infect Dis 1993;17:231

Riseman JA, Zamboni WA, Curtis A, et al. Hyperbaric oxygen therapy for necrotizing fasciitis reduces the mortality and needs for debridement. Surgery 1990;108:847.

Rudge FW. The role of hyperbaric oxygenization in the treatment of clostridial myonecrosis. Military Med 1993;158:80.

MacLennan JD. The histotoxic clostridial infections of man. Bacterol Rev 1962;26:177.

Kindwall EP. Uses of hyperbaric oxygen therapy in the 1990's. Cleveland Clin J Med 1992;59:517.

Altemier WA, Fullen WD. Prevention and treatment of gas gangrene. JAMA 1971;217:806.

Bangsberg DR, et al. Clostridial myonecrosis cluster among injection drug users. Arch Intern Med 2002;162:517

GENITAL ULCER ADENOPATHY SYNDROME

Noreen A. Hynes, M.D., M.P.H.

DIAGNOSTIC CRITERIA

- Lab Dx is a must: Considerable overlap in ulcer characteristics mandate lab-based DX
- Genital herpes: Cx or antigen detection by ELISA or DFA of ulcer fluid; ulcer usually painful; tender regional adenopathy w/ 1st episode
- Primary syphilis: Positive darkfield microscopy, direct IF staining, RPR/VDRL variably positive at this stage; ulcer usually painless; firm, nontender, bilateral lymphadenopathy
- Chancroid: Experimental PCR available, cx of selective media about 70% sensitive; ulcers (usually >1 ulcer) has undermined, ragged edges; nodes may suppurate
- Uncommon: LGV--CF test is useful, PCR/LCR available; ulcer often precedes adenopathy. Donovaniasis: Giemsa or Wright stain of secretions or cx; non-painful ulcer w/red ulcer, bleeds easily

COMMON PATHOGENS: Herpes Simplex Virus ; Treponema pallidum (syphilis) ; Haemophilus ducreyi (Chancroid)

TREATMENT REGIMENS

Herpes simplex virus infection

- 1st clin episode: acyclovir 400mg PO tid x 7-10d OR acyclovir 200 PO 5id x 7-10d OR famciclovir 250mg PO tid x 7-10d OR Valacyclovir 1g PO bid x 7-10d
- Episodic Rx of recurrent HSV: Use 5d (5-10d in HIV +)--acyclovir 200mg PO 5 x d; acyclovir 800mg PO bid; famciclovir 125mg PO bid; valacyclovir 1g PO bid; OR valacyclovir 500mg PO bid x 3-5d
- Suppressive daily therapy for recurrent disease (without HIV): acyclovir 400mg PO bid; famciclovir 250 PO bid; valacyclovir 500mg PO qd; valacyclovir 1.0 g PO
- Suppressive daily therapy for recurrent disease (HIV infected): acyclovir 400-800mg PO tid-bid; famciclovir 500 PO bid; valacyclovir 500mg PO qd (DO NOT USE 1G BID DOSING)
- Acyclovir resistant HSV (other oral Rx don't work): Foscarnet 40 mg/kg IV q8h until clinical resolution; Cidofovir gel 1% to lesions qd x 5d may work (requires pharmacy compounding)

- Severe disease or complications requiring hospitalization: Acyclovir 5-10 mg/kg IV q8h x 2-7d or until clinical improvement. Change to PO to complete 10d.

Primary syphilis

- Benzathine penicillin G (BPG) 2.4mU IM x 1
- Penicillin Allergy: doxycycline 100mg PO bid x 14d; OR ceftriaxone 1g IV or IM qd x 8-10d;OR azithromycin 2g PO once
- HIV-infected: Benzathine penicillin G 2.4mU IM x 1 (some recommend q wk x 3. Use PCN only in pen allergic if at all possible by desensitizing. Otherwise try Rx outlined for non-HIV.
- Pregnant woman: Must ALWAYS be treated with penicillin; desensitize if penicillin-allergic.

Chancroid Regimens

- Azithromycin 1g orally x 1
- Ceftriaxone 250mg IM x 1
- Ciprofloxacin 500mg PO bid x 3d
- Erythromycin base 500mg PO qid x 7d

DRUG-SPECIFIC COMMENTS

Acyclovir: Greatest experience in HSV Rx with this agent and only IV acyclovir available for parenteral routine use. Data supports continuous suppression up to 6 years without adverse effects. Disadvantage is multiple daily dosing with oral form.

Ceftriaxone: Can be used to treat chancroid (250 mg) or as a possible alternative to treat early syphilis in penicillin-allergic, non-cephalosporin allergic patients (1g IM or IV qd x 8-10 d). For this latter use, there have only been limited studies. However biologic and pharmacologic considerations suggest that it should be effective in early syphilis.

Ciprofloxacin: Has been shown to be effective in the treatment of chancroid in HIV-infected and HIV-uninfected persons. Ceftriaxone and azithromycin have the advantage in being single dose regimens. Also, worldwide, some isolates have demonstrated intermediate resistance to ciprofloxacin.

Doxycycline: Doxycycline is considered a second-line drug for the treatment of syphilis and should only be used in penicillin allergic persons with early syphilis. It is not as efficacious as parenteral penicillin. This agent should NEVER be used in pregnant women with syphilis --- only penicillin is indicated. HIV-infected persons should also receive penicillin rather than this agent.

Famciclovir: Has high oral bioavailability but is much more expensive than acyclovir. Most acyclovir-resistant strains are also resistant to this agent. Foscarnet, 40 mg/kg body weight IV q8h until clinical resolution is attained may be effective in acyclovir-resistant genital herpes. Topical cidofovir gel 1% applied to lesions qd x 5d may also be effective. Safety in pregnancy not established.

Penicillin: Parenteral penicillin G has been used effectively for >50 yrs to acheive clinical resolution of primary syphilis and to prevent sequelae. However, NO adequately conducted comparative trials have been performed to guide selection of an optimal penicillin regimen, re: dose, duration, or preparation. Even fewer data are available for nonpenicillin regimens.

IMPORTANT POINTS

- Recommendations based on CDC's 2002 STD Rx Guidelines (MMWR 2002; 51(RR-6).
- No single agent affords reliable therapy for all causes of genital ulcer adenopathy syndrome
- All genital ulcer diseases facilitate the acquisition and transmission of HIV infection.

- HSV is the most common cause of GUD in U.S. Recurrent painful ulcers preceded by vesicles is usually HSV.
- In an area with a high incidence or increasing incidence of syphilis, all patients presenting with genital ulcers with or without adenopathy should be treated for syphilis at the time of presentation.
- The inner 2/3 of the vagina and the cervix drain to the sacral and perirectal lymph nodes. Therefore ulcers at these locations will not be associated with palpable lymphadenopathy
- The lymphadenopathy seen in syphilis is usually non-tender, bilateral, firm; the ulcer is classically painless with undermined, clean edges.
- Genital HSV is usually associated with painful lymphadenopathy
- The "groove sign" seen when there is involvement of both the inguinal and femoral lymph nodes separated by a valley is often seen with LGV but may, at times be seen with chancroid. The associated adenopathy is painful with both LGV and chancroid.
- Donovoniasis is not associated with true lymphadenopathy. Rather there is subcutaneous spread of granulomata (hence the other name granuloma inguinale) which leads to pseudobubo formation.

SELECTED READINGS

Steen R and Dallabetta G. Genital ulcer disease control and HIV prevention. J Clin Virol 2004 29:143-151.

Usatine RP. Painful genital ulcers. J Fam Pract 2003 52:951-4.

Centers for Disease Control and Prevention. Sexually Transmitted Diseases Treatment Guidelines 2002. MMWR 2002; 51 (No. RR-6).

O'Farrell N. Donovanosis: an update. Int J STD AIDS 2001:12:423-7.

Spotswood SL et al. Application of a topical immune response modifier, resiquimod gel, to modify the recurrence rate of recurrent genital herpes: a pilot study. J Infect Dis 2001;184:196-200.

Ballard RC. Genital ulcer adenopathy syndrome. In Holmes KK et al (eds) Sexually Transmitted Diseases, 3rd ed. McGraw-Hill, New York. pp 887-892. 1999.

Carter JS, et al. Phylogenetic evidence for reclassification of Calymmatobacterium granulomatis as Klebsiella granulomatis comb.nov. Int J Syst Bacteriol 1999; 49 Pt 4(4):1695-1700.

Trees DL and Morse SA. Chancroid and Haemophilus ducreyi: an update . Clin Microbiol Rev 8:375-80. 1995

Dangor Y et al. Accuracy of clinical diagnosis of genital ulcer disease. Sex Transm Dis 17:184-88. 1990.

GINGIVITIS/PERIODONTITIS

Spyridon Marinopoulos, M.D.

DIAGNOSTIC CRITERIA

- GINGIVITIS: gums bleed with minor injury/spontaneously +/- edema/erythema. HIV gingivitis (linear gingival erythema): brightly inflamed band of marginal gingiva +/- bleeding/pain/rapid destruction
- Acute necrotizing ulcerative gingivitis (NUG) or trench mouth:fetid breath, blunting of interdental papillae & ulcerative necrotic gingival sloughing +/- fever/regional LN. Noma precursor
- PERIODONTITIS: inflamed gingiva w/ loss of supportive connective tissues. No sx. PE: bone craters w/ increased gingival pocket (probing) depth & tooth mobility. XR may show bone loss
- Necrotizing ulcerative periodontitis (NUP): rapidly progressive painful gingival tissue & alveolar bone destruction w/ eventual necrosis, progresses from NUG. Impaired host. If HIV, CD4 usually <200

- PERIODONTAL ABSCESS: acute, tender, purulent inflammation in gingival wall of periodontal pocket + fluctuance +/- sinus tract +/- regional LN +/- tender/sensitive adjacent teeth + fever if severe

COMMON PATHOGENS: Prevotella gingivalis and intermedia ; Actinobacillus actinomycetemcomitans ; Treponema denticola ; Bacteroides forsythus ; Capnocytophaga sp. ; Peptostreptococcus micros ; Spirochetes ; Gram negative anaerobes

TREATMENT REGIMENS

Miscellaneous/topical antibacterial

- Gingivitis/Periodonitis: plaque removal w/ scaling & root planing (SRP) q3-6mo can Rx most pts w/ no need for abx. Prevention involves meticulous hygiene w/ brushing, flossing & regular dental visit
- Initiate Rx w/ scaling and root planing (SRP)+ home hygiene. Consider antibacterial mouthwash (see below) if pts unwilling/unable to comply w/ home hygiene measures. Assess for response 1-3mo post rx
- Exceptions: 1) fulminant types 2) disease caused by A. Actinomycetemcomitans (Aa) - inc juvenile & some adult - not responsive to SRP alone & requires post-SRP adjunctive systemic abx
- Chlorhexidine (PerioGard) 0.12% oral rinse 15cc bid between dental visits reduces bacterial flora/prevents plaque advancement. May cause tooth staining & promote bacterial resistance w/ prolonged use
- Refactory +/- Recurrent Periodontitis: cx prior to initiation of Rx. If sites of disease few, Rx SRP+local-delivery abx. If extensive disease, Rx SRP+systemic abx (see separate section)
- Local delivery adjunct to SRP (applied once): minocycline 1mg microsphere (Arestin)/ tetracycline 12.7mg fiber (Actisite)/doxycycline 10% gel (Atridox)/chlorhexidine 2.5mg chip (PerioChip)
- Other Rx: (Submicrobial dose) doxycycline hyclate (Periostat) 20mg PO q12h x 90d (up to 9mo) reduces periodontitis by inhibiting collagenase. Effect small but significant. Useful as adjunct to SRP
- Periodontal Abscess: NSAIDs +/- weak narcotic opioids for pain control. I&D is primary treatment w/ abx supportive if systemic sx (fever, LN etc). Refer to dentist within 24h

Systemic antibiotics

- Comment: although scaling & root planing (SRP) alone is effective in most pts w/ periodontal disease, strong evidence exists for use of abx as adjunct to SRP in severe/ refractory/aggressive cases
- Juvenile Periodontitis: tetracycline 250mg PO q6h or doxy/minocycline 200mg PO x 1 then 100mg PO qd x 14d. If no success/aggressive disease: amox 375mg + metronidazole 250mg PO q8 x 7d
- Refractory+/- Recurrent Periodonitis: Cx prior to initiation of rx. If sites of disease few, Rx SRP+local-delivery abx (see separate section). If extensive disease, Rx SRP +systemic abx (below)
- If c+s unavail & no prior abx hx: tetracycline 250mg PO q6h OR doxy/minocycline 200mg PO x 1 then 100mg PO qd x 14d. Alt: amox/clav 250-500mg PO q8h x 10d. PCN ALLERGY: clinda 150-300mg PO q6h x 7-10d
- More aggressive disease: amox 375mg+metronidazole 250mg PO q8h x 7d. PCN ALLERGY: clinda 150-300mg PO q6h x 10d very effective. Alternative: metronidazole 500mg+Cipro 500mg PO q12h x 7d

- ANUG (Trench Mouth) /NUP/HIV-NUG/HIV-NUP: metronidazole 250mg + amox/clav 250mg PO q8h x 7d (+nystatin rinses 5mL qid or flucon 200mg PO qd x 7-14d if HIV+ esp given candida overgrowth w/ abx use)
- Pen allergy: metronidazole 500mg PO+ciprofloxacin 500mg PO q12h x 7d (+Nystatin rinses 5mL qid or Diflucan 200mg PO qd x 7-14d if HIV+ esp given Candida overgrowth w/ abx use)
- Periodontal Abscess. Abx controversial. Use if severe/systemic Sx always in conjunction w/ I&D. Cover anaerobes. Tradition Rx 7d, but also acceptable Rx 3d then reassess if further Rx req
- Augmentin 500mg PO q8h or (PCN allergy) metronidazole 500mg PO q8h. Rx failure: when possible, obtain c+s and tailor abx accordingly. Rx failure empiric rx: clindamycin 300mg PO q6h

DRUG-SPECIFIC COMMENTS

Amoxicillin + Clavulanate: Good for the Rx of aggresive periodontitis when beta lactamase resistance a concern. Good alternative to clinda. Used in combination with metronidazole to treat necrotizing ulcerative periodontitis in HIV; tid better than bid dosing.

Ciprofloxacin: Used in combination with metronidazole in penicillin allergic patients to treat refractory and/or aggressive disease. Excellent coverage of enteric gram-negatives.

Doxycycline: Alternative to tetracycline with better absorption and more convenient dosing.

Metronidazole: Great choice for mouth anaerobes. May arrest disease progression in refractory periodontitis patients with Porphyromonas gingivalis and/or Prevotella intermedia. Used in combination with amox, Augmentin or Cipro to Rx aggressive or necrotizing forms of periodontal disease. Avoid alcohol (Antabuse potential). P450 metabolism.

Nystatin: Use in combination with PO abx in HIV patients to suppress/treat Candida.

Penicillin: Although preferred for tooth infections, not the agent of choice for periodontal disease as it does not cover mouth anaerobes and there is significant resistance.

Tetracycline: Excellent accumulation into crevicular fluid, better than any other abx class. Good agent for periodontal disease caused by A. Actinomycetemcomitans, but there is emerging resistance. GI side effects. May stain teeth. Photosensitivity. Food restrictions and qid dosing inconvenient.

IMPORTANT POINTS

- Recommendations are the author's opinion. Gingivitis & periodontitis are preventable; meticulous oral hygiene & regular dental visits are key. Rx consists of scaling & root planing +/- adjunctive abx
- Use abx adjunctively in fulminant/aggressive/recurrent disease. Prefer topical if few teeth involved, but systemic justified in more diffuse/severe disease. C+s may aid appropriate abx selection
- Gingivitis/periodontitis may represent initial presentation of systemic illness: DM, HIV, leukemia, other immune. Also consider meds causing gingival hyperplasia: dilantin, nifedipine, cyclosporin etc
- HIV positive patients present with fulminant disease. Unique bacterial flora includes gram negative anaerobes, enterics and fungi. Must cover Candida. Refer urgently
- Potential complications include tooth loss, sinusitis, cavernous sinus thrombosis, Ludwig's angina, retro/parapharyngeal abscess, osteomyelitis, endocarditis, brain abscess. CVA risk assoc reported

Diagnosis

Selected Readings

Grau AJ, Becher H, Ziegler CM, et al. Periodontal disease as a risk factor for ischemic stroke. Stroke. 2004 Feb;35(2):496-501. Epub 2004 Jan 05.

Loesche W, Giordano J, Soehren S, et al. The nonsurgical treatment of patients with periodontal disease. Results after five years. JADA 2002;(133):311-320

Dahlen G. Microbiology and treatment of dental abscesses and periodontal-endodontic lesions. Periodontology 2000 2002;28:206-239

Walker C, Karpinia K. Rationale for Use of Antibiotics in Periodontics. J Periodontol 2002;73(10):1188-1196

Wynn R, Bergman S, Meiller T, et al. Antibiotics in treating oral-facial infections of odontogenic origin: An update. Gen Dent 2001;49(3):238-40,242,244

Loesche W, Grossman N. Periodontal Disease as a Specific, albeit Chronic, Infection: Diagnosis and Treatment. Clinical Microbiology Reviews 2001;14(4):727-752

Purucker P, Mertes H, Goodson J, et al. Local Versus Systemic Adjunctive Antibiotic Therapy in 28 Patients With Generalized Aggressive Periodontitis. J Periodontol 2001;72(9):1241-1245

Research, Science and Therapy Committee of the American Academy of Periodontology. Treatment of plaque-induced gingivitis, chronic periodontitis, and other clinical conditions. J Periodontol 2001 Dec;72(12):1790-800

Lamster I. Current concepts and future trends for periodontal disease and periodontal therapy, part 2: classification, diagnosis, and nonsurgical and surgical therapy. Dent Today 2001;20(3):86-91

Wayne D, Trajtenberg C, Hyman D . Tooth and Periodontal Disease: A Review for the Primary-Care Physician. South Med J 2001;94(9):925-932

HEMORRHAGIC FEVER VIRUSES John G. Bartlett, M.D.

Diagnostic Criteria

- Main agents: Ebola, Marburg, Lassa, Rift Valley, Yellow fever, Omsk HF, Kyasanur Forest
- Person-toperson TX: Ebola/Marburg - contact; Lassa - aerosol; Rift Valley/Omsk/Kyasanur - none
- Clinical Dx: Fever, severely ill, hemorrhage, decreased platelets, no other cause
- Culture-Need BSL4 (4 in U.S. Lab - increase WBC, decreased platelets, D/C)
- Differential - Flu, dengue, malaria, salmonella, plague, toxic shock, hantavirus

Treatment Regimens

Infection Control

- Person-person tx: Ebola, Marburg Lassa, NO person-person tx, rift valley, yellow fever, Omsk, Kyasanur Forest
- Never acquired in U.S.; acquired within 21 days of travel or bioterrorism. Report immediately
- Enhanced barrier & airborne precautions until Marburg & Ebola ruled out
- Barrier: Double glove, impermeable gowns, face shield, goggles, leg & shoe cover
- Airborne: N-95 mask or air-purifying respirators (PAPR)
- If available: Neg pressure room w/6-12 air exchanges/hr
- Surveillance of those exposed for febrile disease for 21 days post contact
- Lab: Aerosol risk - essential tests only, prefer point-of-care analyzers, no pneumatic tube. Lab techs use airborne & contact precautions, blood spec- pretreat w/Triton X-100
- Cadavers: trained personnel, airborne & contact precautions, prompt burial or cremation, no embalming

• Environment: surfaces - household bleach 1:100; cloth - double bag & wash hot cycle w/bleach; autoclave or incinerate

Patient Care

• Support: IV, mech. vent, dialysis, pressor, anti-seizure meds
• AVOID: ASA, NSAIDS
• Ribavirin: Lassa, Rift Valley Fever (only) IV 2g x 1, then 1 gm/d x 6d then 500mg/d (Need Treatment IND for IV form)
• Ribavirin PO: >75kg 600mg bid; <75kg 1000 mg/d in 2 doses
• Ebola, Marburg, Yellow fever, Omsk, Kyasanur - no antiviral

Contact of Patients

• Monitor temps bid x 21 days post contact
• Temp >101: Ribavirin (above doses) unless known to be Ebola/Marburg/Yellow fever/ Omsk/Kyasanur
• Vaccines - Yellow fever only; not effective post exposure

DRUG-SPECIFIC COMMENTS

Ribavirin: Active in vitro & in vivo vs. Lassa fever, Rift Valley Fever & Argentine HF Viruses; no activity vs. Ebola, Marburg, Yellow Fever, Omsk or Kyasanur viruses. Available in PO form in U.S. (for hepatitis C). IV form available from ICN, but need treatment IND. Contraindicated in pregnancy. May cause hemolytic anemia. Results with early treatment of Lassa fever are good.

IMPORTANT POINTS

• Source: Hopkins Center for Biodefense, JAMA 2002;287:2391
• Epidemiology: These viruses are not in U.S.; must be imported or bioterrorism
• Clinical sx: Flu-like illness, then bleeding (hemoptysis, petecchiae, melena, hematuria) + DIC
• Tx: Ebola/Marburg - very contagious w/contact w/pt & body fluids: need enhanced barrier cautions, PAPR or M95 mask, Lab cautions
• Risk for natural disease: Travel Asia or Africa plus animal carcass contact, tick/mosquito bite
• Mortality: Ebola 50-90%, Marburg 30-60^, Lassa 15-20%, Yellow fever 20%, Omsk 2%, Kyasanur 3-10%.

SELECTED READINGS

Borio L, et al. The agents of viral hemorrhagic fever as biological weapons: medical & public health management. JAMA 2002;287:2391

Shou S, Hansen AK. Marburg & Ebola virus infections in laboratory non-human primates: a literature review. Comp Med 2000;50:108

Roels TH, et al. Ebola hemorrhagic fever, Kikwit, Democratic Republic of Congo 1995; risk factors for pts without a reported exposure. JID 1999; Suppl 1: S92

Gear JS, et al. Outbreak of Marburg virus disease in Johannesburg. Brit Med J 1975;4:489

Centers for Disease Control. Outbreak of Ebola hemorrhagic fever Uganda Aug 2000 - Jan 2001. MMWR 2001;50:73

Rowe AK, et al. Clinical, virologic and immunologic follow-up of convalescent Ebola hemorrhagic fever patients and their household contacts. JID 1999;179:Suppl 1:S28

White HA. Lassa fever. A study of 23 hospital cases. Trans R Soc Trop Med Hyg 1972:66:390

Zweighaft RM, et al. Lassa fever: response to an imported case. NEJM 1977;297:803

Woods CW, et al. An outbreak of Rift Valley fever in northeast Kenya 1997-98. Emerg Infect Dis 2002;8:138

Chen JP, Cosgriff TM. Hemorrhagic fever virus induced changes in hemostasis and vascular biology. Blood Coagul Fibr 2000;11:461

HEPATITIS A
Mark Sulkowski, M.D.; Lucy Wilson, M.D.

Diagnostic Criteria

- Virus from exposure to high risk source: contaminated food/water, travel-endemic areas, undercooked shellfish, institutionalized patients, daycare, homosexual men, floods/water disasters, IDU
- Clinical signs: 15-49d incubation period; acute hepatitis: dark urine, jaundice, fever, malaise, nausea, vomiting, abdominal pain, arthralgia, acolic stools; usually self-limited, ~3 weeks.
- Clinical sxs: asymptomatic vs. hepatomegaly, splenomegaly, bradycardia, elevated ALT/AST, elevated bilirubins, lymphocytosis, atypical mononuclear cells. ALT returns to normal in about 7 wks.
- Antibody testing: during jaundice phase, HAV IgM antibody elevation by radioimmunoassay. IgM anti-HAV remains elevated for 3-12 months. HAV IgG (+) in 20-80% of asymptomatic U.S. adults.
- Complications: cholestasis, relapsing disease, fulminant hepatitis, chronic active autoimmune hepatitis, autoimmune extrahepatic disease, depression.

Treatment Regimens

Acute infection

- Supportive care: bed rest, fluids.
- Approximately 10-15% of symptomatic cases of HAV infection require hospitalization.
- Acute HAV may be severe in persons with underlying liver disease (hepatitis C)

Post-exposure prophylaxis

- Passive immunization: pooled human immunoglobulin.
- Immunoglobulin should be administered within 2 wks of exposure. IG: 0.02mL/kg IM into gluteus muscle.
- Immunoglobulin prophylaxis: point source outbreaks, close contacts of index cases, daycare center contacts, institutional contacts.
- Can be given as pre-exposure prophylaxis with HAV vaccine if exposure is expected in less than 2 weeks: 0.02mL/kg IM.
- Can be given to children <2 yrs or in those with contraindications to vaccination: 0.02mL/kg - 0.06 mL/kg (lower dose offers about 3 months protection, higher dose up to 6 months).

Pre-exposure prophylaxis

- Active immunization: inactivated hepatitis A vaccine.
- Hepatitis A vaccine must be administered 2 weeks before expected exposure: 1mL IM into deltoid muscle, with 1mL IM booster within 6-12 months (for 10 yr duration of prophylaxis).
- Immunosuppressed patients may be unable to develop antibodies or may require additional boosters.
- Recommended: at-risk international travelers, high-risk geographic populations, male homosexuals, frequent blood/plasma recipients, chronic liver disease (incl. Hep B and C), high risk employment
- Hepatitis A and B combination vaccine (Twinrix) available; three doses: given on a 0-, 1-, and 6-month schedule (same as hep B vaccine).

IMPORTANT POINTS

- HAV neither causes carrier state nor chronic infection. Immunity is believed to be lifelong.
- Death in approximately 2/1,000 symptomatic (icteric) cases. Risk may be increased in patients with underlying liver disease.
- Fecal-orally spread virus; shed in feces for up to 21d before onset of jaundice and 8d after onset of jaundice.
- HAV causes viremia, detectable in one study for prolonged period of time > 1 yr

SELECTED READINGS

Fiore AE. Hepatitis A transmitted by food. Clin Infect Dis. 2004 Mar 1;38(5):705-15. Epub 2004 Feb 11

Feinstone SM, Gust IA. Chapter 161: Hepatitis A Virus. 5th Edition, Principles and Practice of Infectious Diseases, eds: Mandell, Bennett, Dolin, Churchhill Livingstone, 1999, pp. 1920-1940

Advisory Committee on Immunization Practices (ACIP). Prevention of Hepatitis A through Active or Passive Immunization: Recommendations of the Advisory Committee on Immunization Practices (ACIP). MMWR, 48 (RR-12), October 1, 1999, pp. 1-37

HEPATITIS B

Mark Sulkowski, M.D.; Lucy Wilson, M.D.

DIAGNOSTIC CRITERIA

- Symptoms of Acute Hepatitis B Viral Infection: 60-110 d after acute infection, 2-10 d of erythematous maculopapular rash, urticaria, arthralgia, fever, symmetric distal joint arthritis can occur, followed by headache, malaise, anorexia, nausea, vomiting, fever. Next, jaundice and right upper quadrant pain, with acolic stools, dark urine, and pruritis can occur. Laboratory abnormalities include ALT>AST, elevated direct and total bilirubin, moderate elevation in alkaline phosphatase. Less common lab abnormalities include: reduced hematocrit, mild hemolysis, granulocytopenia, lymphocytosis, proteinuria, urobilinogenuria, biliruinuria, steatorrhea, hypergammaglobulinemia, hypoalbuminemia.
- Fulminant course is often fatal, especially if accompanied by HDV infection.
- Acute Hepatitis B: HBsAg positive, Anti-HBs negative, Anti-HBc IgG positive, Anti-HBc IgM positive, HBeAg positive, Anti-HBe negative.
- Late Incubation Period of Hepatitis B: HBsAg positive, Anti-HBs negative, Anti-HBc IgG negative, Anti-HBc IgM negative, HBeAg positive or negative, Anti-HBe negative.
- Healthy HBsAg carrier: HBsAg positive, Anti-HBs negative, Anti-HBc IgG highly positive, Anti-HBc IgM positive or negative, HBeAg negative, Anti-HBe positive.
- Chronic Hepatitis B: HBsAg positive, Anti-HBs negative, Anti-HBc IgG highly positive, Anti-HBc IgM positive or negative, HBeAg positive, Anti-HBe negative.
- Recent HBV Vaccination: HBsAg negative, Anti-HBs positive, Anti-HBc IgG negative, Anti-HBc IgM negative, HBeAg negative, Anti-HBe negative.
- Continuation of Serologic Diagnosis Markers, (adapted from Table 135-2 in Mandell et. al., eds, Principles and Practice of Infectious Diseases, 5th Edition)
- Recent HBV Infection: HBsAg negative, Anti-HBs high positive, Anti-HBc IgG high positive, Anti-HBc IgM positve or negative, HBeAg negative, Anti-HBe positive.
- Distant HBV Infection: HBsAg negative, Anti-HBs positive or negative, Anti-HBc IgG positive or negative, Anti-HBc IgM negative, HBeAg negative, Anti-HBe negative.

TREATMENT REGIMENS

For chronic hepatitis B: Interferon (standard): alpha-2b/Pegylated: alfa

- Goal of Interferon therapy: sustained suppression of HBeAg and HBV DNA (markers of active viral replication). Suppression of these markers signifies clinical, biochemical & histologic remission.
- Eligibility: evidence of active viral replication > 6 months (positive HbeAg and HBV DNA), persistently elevated aminotransferases, and signs of chronic active hepatitis on liver biopsy.
- Dose: 5 mU SC qd or 10 mU SC thrice weekly x 16 weeks. Peginterferon alfa-2a 180mcg SC weekly is more effective than standard IFN
- Serial monitoring: HBV DNA, HBeAG, anti-HBe, ALT, CBC, thyroid (q3 months).
- Sustained Response: sustained negative HBV DNA, loss of HBeAg, development of Anti-HBe. Response Rate: sustained loss of HBeAg and HBV DNA occurs in approximately 30-40% of treated patients.
- Histologic improvement is seen even in those with partial response, but more often in those with sustained response.
- Side effects: fever, myalgia, bone marrow suppression, depression, thyroid abnormalities. Thrombocytopenia, granulocytopenia, fatigue and depression may respond to dose adjustment.
- Successful Response: predicted by HBV DNA < 200 pg/mL pretreatment, AST & ALT >100U/L, liver biopsy with active necrosis and active inflammation.
- Not eligible for Interferon therapy: HIV positive, normal aminotransferase levels, decompensated cirrhosis, those infected perinatally, those infected with HBeAg-negative pre-core mutations.
- Not affected by YMDD resistance (see Lamivudine Therapy).

Lamivudine

- Goal of LAM therapy: sustained suppression of HBeAg and HBV DNA (markers of active viral replication). Suppression of these markers signifies clinical, biochemical & histologic remission.
- Eligibility: evidence of active viral replication > 6 months (positive HbeAg and HBV DNA), persistently elevated aminotransferases, and signs of chronic active hepatitis on liver biopsy.
- Dose: 100mg PO qd until HBeAg conversion to Anti-HBe occurs, or lifelong treatment.
- Response: seroconversion of HBeAg occurs in about 17% in first year and total of 27% in second year. 70-90% of these responders maintain seroconversion status.
- Sustained Response: sustained negative HBV DNA, loss of HBeAg, development of Anti-HBe.
- Histologic improvement occurs regardless of HBeAg treatment response, thus prolonged treatment despite no immune response recommended. Shown to be beneficial in decompensated cirrhosis.
- Can treat those with precore mutant strains of HBV who are ineligible for IFN. Also can treat those with immunosuppression, perinatal acquisition, normal ALT and decompensated cirrhosis.
- HBV DNA usually suppressed within first 2 weeks, but often become detectable after 2 years of treatment, indicating development of YMDD resistance mutation.
- Despite YMDD resistance, partial suppression of HBV DNA attainable. Reversion to wild-type virus occurs with discontinuation. Thus, continued therapy recommended despite development of resistance.

- Side effects are few. ALT elevation can occur after withdrawal of therapy.

Adefovir

- Adefovir: adenine nucleotide analogue. FDA-approved for the treatment of HBeAg+ and - disease. ADV 10mg PO daily
- HBeAg+: ADV 10mg PO daily x 48 wks- HBV DNA decrease median 3.52 log c/mL; HBeAg loss 24%: HBeAb seroconversion, 12%
- HBeAg neg: HBV DNA decrease 3.91 log10 c/mL; histologic improvement, 64% with ADV > 33% with placebo
- ADV resistance mutation - uncommon ~ 3.9% at 3 yrs; novel mutation rtN236T in the D domain of HBV RT confers resistance to adefovir in vitro and in vivo. LAM remains active
- ADV is active versus LAM resistant HBV - YMDD.

DRUG-SPECIFIC COMMENTS

Famciclovir: Nucleoside analog with weaker anti-HBV action than lamivudine. Less frequent HBeAg seroconversion. Famciclovir resistance overlaps with lamivudine resistance.

Interferon alpha: Good first line treatment for HBV infection in those who are immunocompetent, non-cirrhotic, with high aminotransferases, non-perinatally acquired, with HBeAg positive wild type virus, and with YMDD mutations to lamivudine, with HBV DNA < 200pg/mL. Side effects may limit its use.

IMPORTANT POINTS

- Recent studies suggest entecavir or tenofovir may be preferred drugs, but durability of responses of any treatment with cessation of therapy does not appear good.
- Immunization: HBV vaccine for those with increased risk (hemodialysis, exposed household members, group home residents, health care workers, risky sex behaviors, injection drug users)
- Hepatocellular carcinoma associated w/ chronic HBV, especially in endemic Southeast Asia, Japan, sub-Saharan Africa, Greece, Italy & Oceania. Found especially in perinatally acquired infection.
- Vaccination has been shown to decrease the incidence of hepatocellular carcinoma in Taiwan.
- Extrahepatic manifestations of HBV: serum sickness-like syndrome, polyarteritis nodosa, membranous glomerulonephritis, aplastic anemia.
- Postexposure Prophylaxis: Specific for type of exposure, host characteristics and source characteristics. Follow CDC guidelines for HBIG and HBV vaccination (see Vaccines and Prophylaxis section).

SELECTED READINGS

Kanwal F, Grainek IM, Martin P, Dulai GS, Farid M, Speigel BM. Treatment alternatives for chronic hepatitis B virus infection: a cost-effective analysis. Ann Intern Med 2005; May 17;142(10):821-831

Peters MG, Hann Hw H, Martin P, Heathcote EJ, Buggisch P, Rubin R, Bourliere M, Kowdley K, Trepo C, . Adefovir dipivoxil alone or in combination with lamivudine in patients with lamivudine-resistant chronic hepatitis B. Gastroenterology. 2004 Jan;126(1):91-101.

Marcellin P, Chang TT, Lim SG, Tong MJ, Sievert W, Shiffman ML, Jeffers L, Goodman Z, Wulfsohn MS, X. Adefovir dipivoxil for the treatment of hepatitis B e antigen-positive chronic hepatitis B. N Engl J Med. 2003 Feb 27;348(9):808-16.

Hadziyannis SJ, Tassopoulos NC, Heathcote EJ, Chang TT, Kitis G, Rizzetto M, Marcellin P, Lim SG, Go. Adefovir dipivoxil for the treatment of hepatitis B e antigen-negative chronic hepatitis B. N Engl J Med. 2003 Feb 27;348(9):800-7

Malik AH and Lee AM. Chronic Hepatitis B Virus Infection: Treatment Strategies for the Next Millennium. Ann Int Med, 132 (9), May, 2000, 723

Hunt CM, McGill JM, Allen MI, Condreay LD. "Clinical Relevance of Hepatitis B Viral Mutations". Hepatology, 31 (5), May, 2000, 1037

Schalm SW, Heathcote J, Cianciara J, et.al., . "Lamivudine and alpha interferon combination treatment of patients with chronic hepatitis B infection: a randomised trial". Gut, 46, 2000, 562

Villeneuve J, Condreay LD, Willems, et.al.,. "Lamivudine Treatment for Decompensated Cirrhosis Resulting from Chronic Hepatitis B". Hepatology, 31 (1), Jan, 2000, 207

Dienstag JL, Schiff ER, Wright TL, et.al.,. "Lamivudine as Initial Treatment for Chronic Hepatitis B in the United States". NEJM, 341(17), October, 1999, 1256

Robinson, WS. Chapter 135: Hepatitis B Virus and Hepatitis D Virus. Principles and Practice of Infectious Diseases, 5th Edition, eds. Mandell, Bennett, Dolin, Churchhill Livingstone, 1999, 1652

HEPATITIS C
Mark Sulkowski, M.D.

DIAGNOSTIC CRITERIA

- Screen: exposure to blood/organs before July, 1992; Hx IDU at any time; elevated ALT; hemodialysis; other exposure
- Diagnostic tests: 1) screen with HCV antibody; > 99% sensitivity; (False neg if <70 days since exposure, dialysis, HIV pos); 2) confirm with HCV RNA (need repeated negative to exclude infection)
- Clinical: acute - 20% jaundice; chronic - most asymptomatic until liver failure; extrahepatic findings - cyroglobulinemia +/- vasculitis and glomerulonephritis; porphyria cutanea tarda
- Evaluation: ALT/AST, Alb, PT, TBili, platelet ct; HCV genotype and viral load - predict treatment response; liver biopsy - best indicator of disease stage
- Supplemental tests: exclude other liver diseases: iron, autoimmune, HBV, alpha-1 AT def, Wilson's. Consider TSH, alpha-feto protein if cirrhotic.

TREATMENT REGIMENS

HCV treatment

- Standard of care (2004): pegylated IFN alfa-2b 1.5mcg/kg (wt-adjusted) or PEG alfa-2a 180mcg (fixed) SC injection wkly + ribavirin (RBV) PO.
- Indications: + HCV RNA and necroinflammation and fibrosis on biopsy. Biopsy: indicated - genotype 1; controversial -genotypes 2/3. Normal ALT and HIV + are candidates for Rx based on biopsy findings
- Contraindications (some relative): severe psych. disease, decompensated liver disease, poor adherence, severe cytopenia (wbc, plt, Hgb), pregnancy possible, severe comorbid disease
- HIV is not contraindicated
- Pre-tx work-up: hx (comorbidity); PE (decompensation); CBC w/plt, ALT/AST, PT, PTT, TBr, TSH, HCV viral load, HCV genotype; liver biopsy - for many patients; consider no biopsy with genotypes 2/3.
- Tx objectives: 1) HCV eradication (cure); 2) slow fibrosis progression - prevent end-stage liver disease, hepatocellular CA, etc
- Outcomes: sustained viral response (SVR) - neg HCV RNA at end of tx (EOT) and 6 mo post; Relapse - neg HCV RNA EOT but + HCV RNA after d/c; Non-response - HCV RNA not neg during tx
- Response indicators: SVR rare (< 2%) if by wk 12 - HCV RNA still + and < 2 log drop or by wk 24 - HCV RNA still +. Consider d/c Rx if viral failure at wk 12.

- Cure rate: PEG alfa-2a/alfa-2b + RIBA, overall 54-56%; genotype 1 - 42/46% for 48 week tx; genotype 2/3 - 76/82% for 24 week tx.
- FDA-approved regimens - IFN monotherapy: IFN alfa 2a, 2b, alfacon-1 (consensus), PEG-IFN alfa-2b, PEG-IFN alfa-2a; Combination therapy: IFN alfa-2b + RBV, PEG-IFN alfa-2b + RBV

Pegylated +/- ribavirin

- Pegylated interferon: long half life, once weekly injection. Two types PEG alfa-2b - 12 kd, linear PEG, wt-based dosing; PEG alfa-2a - 40 kd, branched PEG, fixed dosing. Both FDA approved +/- RIBA
- PEG-IFN alfa-2b dosing (weight-based): monotherapy use 1.0 mcg/kg/wk; PEG alfa-2b + RIBA combination use 1.5 mcg/kg/wk; PEG alfa-2a (fixed dose) 180 mcg/wk for both mono and combo with RIBA
- Both PEG IFN alfa-2a and 2b monotherapy - approx. 2-fold higher sustained response rate (SVR) compared to standard IFN alone; similar side effects
- PEG IFN monotherapy indicated for "maintenance" therapy in viral non-responders (experimental use) and pts with contraindication to RBV (heart, lung, hemoglobinopathy).
- Combo PEG alfa-2b or PEG alfa-2a + RBV is the most effective therapy; standard of care for HCV 2004. Strader DB. Hepatology 2004
- Standard regimen: PEG alfa-2b (1.5mcg/kg/week) or PEG alfa-2a (180mcg/wk) + RIBA 1000 mg/d (< 75kg) or 1200 mg/d (> 75kg) for geno 1 (48 wks Rx)and RBV 800 mg/d all pts with geno 2/3 (24 wks Rx)
- Wt < 40 kg (88 lbs): PEG2b = vial size 100mcg - use 0.5 mL/wk; RBV 800 mg/day
- Wt=40-50 kg (88-110 lbs): PEG2b = vial size 160mcg - use 0.4 mL/wk; RBV 800 mg/d; Wt=51-64 kg (112-141 lbs): PEG2b = vial size 160 use 0.5 mL/wk; RBV 800mg/d
- Wt=65-75 kg (142-166 lbs): PEG2b = vial size 240mcg - use 0.4mL/wk; RBV 1000mg/d; Wt=76-85 kg (167-187 lbs): PEG2b = vial size 240 use 0.5mL/wk; RBV 1000mg/d
- Wt=86-105 kg (188-231 lbs): PEG2b = vial size 300mcg - use 0.5mL/wk; RBV 1200mg/d; Wt > 105 kg (>231 lbs): PEG2b = vial size 300 use 0. mL/wk; RBV 1400mg/d

Experimental and future HCV treatment options

- Viramidine - RBV "pro-drug;" concentrated in the liver; less in RBCs - less anemia. 2004 - phase 3 studies with PEG-2a and PEG-2b. Expected to be next "new" hep C drug
- HCV protease - phase 1 data presented oral PI; BILN 2061 - 2 day oral dosing > 2 log10 decrease HCV RNA pts with genotype 1. Terminated - toxicity in primates. Other PIs: Vertex VX-950, phase 1 2004
- HCV polymerase inhibitors - several drugs in phase 1/2 development. Idenix NM283 orally available; achieve 1-2 log10 reduction in HCV RNA in genotype 1 pts - IFN naive and failures.
- Amantadine - influenza drug; no rationale for use and no in vitro effect; clinical studies mixed results.
- Thymosin-alpha-1: non-specific immune modulator; limited data on effectiveness
- Iron reduction: not effective; phlebotomy indicated only with iron overload (hemochromatosis or HCV-related porphyria)

DRUG-SPECIFIC COMMENTS

Interferon alpha: Side effects: flu-like symptoms, fatigue, depression, cognitive changes, hair thinning, bone marrow suppression with anemia, thrombocytopenia and neutropenia. Approximately 1% manifest thyroid disease, diabetes, psychosis, autoimmune disease, seizures, cardiovascular disease. Approximately 0.1% develop liver failure, sepsis with neutropenia or suicide. Antidotes include: dose adjustment for bone marrow suppression, epogen for anemia, anti-depressant medications for depression.

Peginterferon alfa: FDA approved dose of 1.0mcg/kg/wk not generally recommended.

Ribavirin: Major side effect: hemolytic anemia. Follow CBC. Dose adjustment may be necessary: if hemoglobin < 10g/dL (or Hct<30%) decrease ribavirin dose by 200mg each time and if hemoglobin < 8.5g/dL (or Hct < 26%) stop Ribavirin treatment. Teratogenic: patient must agree and adhere to effective birth control. rHu-EPO 40,000 IU SC Wkly - 2 studies assoc. w/ 2.5g - 3g increase Hb after 4 wks. Also, inc riba dose

IMPORTANT POINTS

- PEG-IFN side effects: "flu-like" - respond to NSAIDS, tylenol; fatigue; depression and irritability - respond to SSRIs; insomnia - responds to trazodone (avoid benzos); thyroid (hypo-5%/hyper-1%)
- PEG-IFN - neutropenia (< 500 cells in 1%) - respond to decrease dose PEG; consider G-CSF (filgrastim) 300 mcg SC injection 2-3x per wk
- Ribavirin side effects: dyspepsia - responds to antacids; dry cough; gout; anemia - dose-related, reversible hemolytic anemia - develops 2-4 wks; avg drop 2.5 - 3g Hb
- Anemia due to PEG (bone marrow) + Riba (hemolytic) - respond rHu-EPO 40,000 IU SC weekly; avg increase 2.8 g over 4 wks; maintain RBV dose

SELECTED READINGS

Muir AJ, Bornstein JD, Killenberg PG; et al. Peginterferon alfa-2b and ribavirin for the treatment of chronic hepatitis C in blacks and non-Hispanic whites. N Engl J Med. 2004 Sep 16;351(12):1268

Hadziyannis SJ, Sette H Jr, Morgan TR, et al. Peginterferon-alpha2a and ribavirin combination therapy in chronic hepatitis C: a randomized study of treatment duration and ribavirin dose. Ann Intern Med. 2004 Mar 2;140(5):346-55

Fried MW, Shiffman ML, Reddy KR, et al. Peginterferon alfa-2a plus ribavirin for chronic hepatitis C virus infection. N Engl J Med 2002 Sep 26;347(13):975-82

Consensus Panel. NIH Consensus Development Conference Statement Management of Hepatitis C: 2002 June 10-12, 2002 . http://consensus.nih.gov/cons/116/091202116cdc_statement.htm

Manns MP, McHutchison JG, Gordon SC, et al. Peginterferon alfa-2b plus ribavirin compared with interferon alfa-2b plus ribavirin for initial treatment of chronic hepatitis C: a randomised trial. Lancet 2001 Sep 22;358(9286):958-65

Trepo C, Lindsay K, Neiderau C, et.al., . "Pegylated Interferon Alfa-2b (PEG-Intron) Monotherapy is Superior to Interferon Alfa-2b (Intron A) for the Treatment of Chronic Hepatitis C, . Abstract number GS2/07, EASL, 2000.

Zeuzem S, Feinman SV, Rasenack J, et.al., . "Evaluation of the Safety and Efficacy of Once-Weekly PEG/ Interferon Alfa-2a (PEGASYS, TM) for Chronic Hepatitis C. A Multinational, Randomized Study". Abstract number GS2/08, EASL, 2000.

Nelson DR, Lauwers GY, Lau JY, et al. "Interleukin 10 Treatment Reduces Fibrosis in Patients with Chronic Hepatitis C: A Pilot Trial of Interferon Nonresponders". Gastroenterology, 118 (4), April, 2000, pp. 655-60.

Shiratori Y, Imazeki F, Moriyam M, . "Histologic Improvement of Fibrosis in Patients with Hepatitis C who have Sustained Response to Interferon Therapy". Ann Intern Med, 132 (7), Apr, 2000, pp. 517-24.

Thomas DL, Lemon SM,. Chapter 143: Hepatitis C, in: 5th Edition, Principles and Practice of Infectious Diseases, eds.,. Mandell, Bennett, Dolin, Churchill Livingstone, 1999, pp. 1736-1760.

HEPATITIS D

Mark Sulkowski, M.D.; Christopher Carpenter, M.D.

DIAGNOSTIC CRITERIA

- A defective RNA virus, HDV requires hepatitis B for replication; infection occurs either as coinfection (acute hepatitis B) or superinfection (upon chronic hepatitis B), both with increased morbidity.
- Evaluation for hepatitis virus D (HDV) should be undertaken in patients with severe acute hepatitis B or during an exacerbation of chronic hepatitis B who have traveled to a HDV endemic region.
- HDV should also be considered during hepatitis B surface antigen negative but IgM antibody to hepatitis B core antigen positive hepatitis.
- The only FDA-approved assay is for total antibody to HDV; it does not distinguish between acute, chronic, or resolved infection unless seroconversion is documented (indicating acute infection).
- Research assays are available to detect HDV RNA or antigen in the serum or liver or IgM anti-HDV; the latter usually persists in chronic infection and thus is not specific for acute infection.

COMMON PATHOGENS: Hepatitis B virus ; Hepatitis D virus

TREATMENT REGIMENS

Treatment of acute HDV infection (coinfection)

- No evidence of benefit giving interferon alpha for acute HDV coinfection or superinfection.
- Orthotopic liver transplantation should be considered in patients with fulminant acute hepatitis D.

Treatment of chronic HDV infection

- May be from superinfection (more likely) or coinfection.
- Interferon alpha has shown benefit in chronic HDV infection.
- Early treatment of chronic disease appears to result in improved response
- High dose (4-5mU/day, or 9-10mU three times/week) improves serum transaminases, liver histopathologic changes, and/or serum HDV RNA levels in nearly one-half of patients.
- One third have sustained reduction of their transaminase levels.
- Other forms of treatment - immunosuppressives (corticosteroids, azathioprim), immunomodulatory drugs (levamisole), ribavirin, and lamivudine (3-thiacytidine) have not proven effective.
- Lamivudine does have proven benefit for treating chronic hepatitis B.
- Orthotopic liver transplantation should be considered in patients with end-stage chronic disease.

Prevention

- HDV coinfection is effectively prevented by HBV vaccination as well as other HBV preventive measures.
- There is no HDV vaccine to protect HBV carriers from superinfection.

DRUG-SPECIFIC COMMENTS

Interferon alpha: Currently the only available treatment for hepatitis D infection, and only in patients with chronic hepatitis D; significant side effects, especially with high dose regimen, which diminish over time.

DIAGNOSIS

IMPORTANT POINTS

- Fulminant hepatitis occurs at higher incidence during coinfection than during acute hepatitis B, though fewer (< 5%) develop chronic infection.
- Most patients with superinfection, however, develop chronic HDV hepatitis (up to 95%).
- Patients with elevated transaminases, histopathologic evidence of chronic hepatitis, and HDV antigen in the liver should be considered for treatment with interferon alpha.
- If after three months a decline of 50% in transaminases is not achieved (within 1.5 times the upper limit of normal) consideration should be given to discontinuing interferon alpha.
- Otherwise, treatment should be continued for one year as tolerated. Yearly treatment interruptions should be scheduled to assess for relapse.

SELECTED READINGS

Dodson SF, Issa S, Bonham A. Liver transplantation for chronic viral hepatitis. Surg Clin North Am 1999; 79(1):131-145

Karayiannis P. Hepatitis D virus. Rev Med Virol 1998; 8(1):13-24

Koff RS, editors Gorbach SL, Bartlett JG, Blacklow NR. Hepatitis B and Hepatitis D. Infectious Diseases. Philadelphia: W.B. Saunders Company, 1998: 850-863

Hoofnagle JH. Therapy of acute and chronic viral hepatitis. Adv Intern Med 1994; 39:241-275

HEPATITIS E
Mark Sulkowski, M.D.; Christopher Carpenter, M.D.

DIAGNOSTIC CRITERIA

- RNA virus transmitted predominantly via enteric routes similar to hepatitis A. Highest incidences noted in Asia, Africa, Middle East and Central America.
- Evaluation for hepatitis E virus (HEV) infection should be undertaken in patients with acute hepatitis and a negative workup for hepatitis A, B, or C who have traveled to a HEV endemic region.
- IgM or IgG anti-HEV testing is available at the Hepatitis Branch of the Centers for Disease Control and Prevention [http://www.cdc.gov/ncidod/diseases/hepatitis/; 800-311-3435].
- IgM is detectable during acute and early convalescent phases, IgG is usually detectable when the patient has acute hepatitis and may persist but often decreases over time.
- HEV RNA may be detected in the serum or feces of patients during the early acute phase of hepatitis but replication usually diminishes by the time symptoms of hepatitis develop.

COMMON PATHOGENS: Hepatitis E virus

TREATMENT REGIMENS

General principles

- Most patients develop a benign or mild and self-limited infection. There is no specific therapy. Care is supportive.
- Preganant women appear to be more likely to develop fulminant Hepatitis E.
- Aggressive supportive management is indicated in severe cases.
- Orthotopic liver transplantation should be considered in patients who develop fulminant hepatitis E.

Prevention

- No vaccine is currently available; efforts are underway

- Given the enteral rout of transmission, routine hand washing, consuming water and ice only from safe sources, and avoiding uncooked shellfish, fruits, and vegetables likely aid in prevention.
- Pregnant women should avoid any contact with potential sources of hepatitis E, including patients or their specimens and laboratory exposure.

Important Points

- Typical illness is subclinical or mild to moderate in nature.
- Generally self-limited although pregnant women appear to be at much higher risk than men and non-pregnant women for developing fulminant hepatitis E.
- During pregnancy, the mortality rate is approximately 20% and peaks during the third trimester.
- HEV hepatitis may have a cholestatic component.
- Control of hepatitis E outbreaks is likely aided by public health measures such as chlorination of water supplies.

Selected Readings

Wang L, Zhuang H. Hepatitis E: an overview and recent advances in vaccine research. World J Gastroenterol. 2004 Aug 1;10(15):2157-62.

Harrison TJ. Hepatitis E virus - an update. Liver 1999; 19(3):171-176

Mast EE, Krawczynski K. Hepatitis E: an overview. Annu Rev Med 1996; 47:257-266

Balayan MS. Epidemiology of hepatitis E virus infection. J Viral Hepat 1997; 4(3):155-165

Kwo PY, Schlauder GG, Carpenter HA, Murphy PJ, Rosenblatt JE, Dawson GJ et al. Acute hepatitis E by a new isolate acquired in the United States. Mayo Clin Proc 1997; 72(12):1133-1136

HIV, OCCUPATIONAL EXPOSURE

John G. Bartlett, M.D.

Diagnostic Criteria

- Healthcare workers with exposure to bloodborne pathogen: candidate for post-exposure prophylaxis (PEP)
- Source: HIV positive or HIV unknown, hepatitis B or hepatitis C
- Injury: percutaneous ("sharps") or mucous membrane/non-intact skin
- Fluid: blood, bloody body fluid or viral cultures (all cases to date)

Treatment Regimens

Evaluation

- Guidelines: CDC (MMWR 2001; 50RR-11, Hotline: 888-448-4911)
- Principles: Cleanse injury fast then assess source for HIV (rapid HIV serology) HCV (anti-HCV) and HBV (HBsAg)
- Risk review: Exposure (blood) or bloody body fluid + sharps injury or exposure of mucous membrane or non-intact skin
- PEP: for HIV if 1) blood exposure, 2) source HIV positive or unknown serostatus and 3) <36 hours
- High HIV risk: 1) sharps - deep, hollow bare needle, visible blood; 2) source - AIDS, sx, high viral load

- Fluids @ risk: Blood, bloody fluids, HIV cultures (these account for all cases so far); others - semen, vaginal, CSF, joint pericard, peritoneal, amniotic fluids (risk is unknown but PEP recommended)

Treatment: HIV PEP indications

- Percutaneous, low risk injury (solid needle/superficial) source HIV or high risk: 2 drug PEP
- Percutaneous, high risk injury (deep, visible blood, large bore) source HIV + high risk source: 3 drug PEP
- Percutaneous, low risk injury, source HIV + high risk source (AIDS, high VL, sx): 3 drug PEP
- Percutaneous, high risk injury, source HIV + low risk source: 3 drug PEP
- Percutaneous, high/low risk, source ?: usually none or consider 2 drug PEP
- Mucous/non-intact skin + small volume, HIV + source: 2 drug PEP if source high risk
- Mucous/non-intact skin, large volume HIV + source: 2 or 3 drug depending on source
- Source - high risk if AIDS, high viral load, acute HIV, symptomatic HIV
- NY State AIDS Institute Guidelines: 3 drugs for all HCW exposures that qualify

Treatment: atiretrovirals/monitoring

- 2 drug PEP: AZT/3TC, d4T/3TC or TDF/FTC
- 3 drug PEP: 2 NRTIs (above) + IDV/r, LPV/r, ATV/r or FPV/r, NFV
- Start ASAP; Modify - based on tolerance and source assessment - resistance; stop - 4wks
- Follow-up: HIV serology 0, 3 & 6 mo w/PEP - CBC & chem profile 0 & 2 wks
- Counseling: Risk 0.3% with percutaneous AZT efficacy 80%, drug toxicity, safe/no sex x 6-12wks
- Avoid: ddC & nevirapine; pregnancy - ddI + d4T and efavirenz
- Avoid NVP (hepatic necrosis) & ABC (hypersensitivity); use EFV w/caution (CNS) and consider T20

DRUG-SPECIFIC COMMENTS

Abacavir (ABC): This NRTI is included in the list of options for the 3rd drug for PEP. The main concern is the hypersensitivity reaction which is characterized by red eyes, rash, abd pain, nausea, vomiting and most importantly, hypotension. This usually occurs in the first 6 wks of therapy and may occur with the 1st dose.

Didanosine (ddI): Good HIV drug - preferably the Videx EC 400mg qd formulation which is better tolerated & has fewer drug interactions. Major complications are peripheral neuropathy and pancreatitis - neither are likely with the 1-wk course.

Efavirenz (EFV): This is a theoretically attractive inclusion in the 3 drug PEP when the source has established or suspected resistance to PIs. The problem is that 50% have CNS toxicity which is usually self-limited, but it occurs immediately with the first dose usually lasts 2-3 wks in a regimen that is given only 4 wks. It is not clear if HCWs can easily take this drug and do their jobs.

Fosamprenavir (FPV): PI with potency and often attractive for patients who have resistance or intolerance to other PIs. Main problems are high rates of reactions - GI intol, rash & paresthesias.

Indinavir (IDV): This is 1 of 2 CDC-recommended PIs for post-exposure prophylaxis based on the philosophy that 3 drugs ("triple therapy") are much more potent than 2 nucleosides in HIV-infected patients. Problems are: 1) risk of nephrolithiasis of about 3% in a 1-month course; warn healthcare worker & advise to take 1.5 liters or more fluids daily. 2) Must take IDV on an empty stomach or with low-fat meal. 3) Must take IDV q8h.

Lamivudine (3TC): Combined with AZT in the "basic prophylactic regimen" since this combination is known to be more potent in HIV-infected patients than AZT alone and 3TC is well tolerated. A concern is resistance if the source has received 3TC and has a high viral load or is known to have the 184 codon mutation. Support for AZT + 3TC vs AZT alone is with data from a perinatal transmission study in which AZT + 3TC was superior to AZT alone.

Lopinavir (LPV): (Kaletra) This drug makes a lot of sense for PEP, especially when the source has had exposures to multiple regimens. Kaletra is well tolerated except for mild diarrhea that can usually be controlled by Imodium. It is also potent and has a great pharmacologic profile.

Nelfinavir (NFV): An alternative PI to indinavir in the CDC recommendations for the 3-drug regimen. This drug is usually well-tolerated, but causes diarrhea that can often be controlled with imodium.

Nevirapine (NVP): (Viramine) This drug was associated with fulminant hepatic failure in 2 health care workers including one who required a liver transplant. It is not clear that the drug was given properly with the phase in dose scheme. Nevertheless, the CDC has taken a strong stand in discouraging NVP for post-exposure prophylaxis.

Ritonavir (RTV): Not in the CDC guidelines, but often combined with indinavir to improve the pharmacokinetic profile and reduce administrations from q8h to bid. Dose regimen could be 800 IDV/100-200 RTV bid (may risk increased nephrolithiases due to high IDV peaks) or 400 IDV/400 RTV bid (poor GI tolerance to this much RTV).

Stavudine (d4T): Often used in place of AZT when intolerance of AZT precludes use. d4T has no established track record for prophylaxis, but many feel it should work as well as AZT. It cannot be used in combination with AZT due to pharmacologic antagonism.

Zidovudine (AZT): This is the only drug with verified benefit in reducing HIV transmission in the workplace. The retrospective analysis by CDC showed 80% efficacy when adjusted for other risk factors. These data are supported by the 076 trial showing 70% efficacy of AZT in preventing perinatal transmission, including activity when the maternal HIV strain was resistant to AZT and there was no reduction in viral load. Main problem is toxicity - nausea, headache and asthenia. GI toxicity may be improved by multiple administrations/day or taking with meals. Some will require switch to d4T.

Important Points

- Source: CDC (MMWR 2001;50; RR-11) - updated by author for drugs
- Risk: w/needlestick infected source: HIV - 0.3%, HCV 1.8%, HBV (eAg pos + unvaccinated HCW) 50%
- Higher risk: deep injury, visible blood on device, needle from artery/vein, source high VL
- HIV prophylaxis: AZT decreased HIV transmission 80%
- HIV experience: 57 known cases - all exposures to blood or HIV cultures including 6 HCWs given PEP within 2 hours
- Other bloodborne pathogens to consider: HCV and HBV
- PEPline: 1-888-HIV-4911

Selected Readings

Centers for Disease Control. Updated US Public Health Service Guidelines for the management of occupational exposure to HBV, HCV and HIV and recommendations for post-exposure prophylaxis. MMWR 2001;50: RR-11

Gerberding JL. Clinical Practice. Occupational exposure to HIV in health care settings. N Engl J Med 2003;348:826

Moyle G, Boffito M. Unexpected drug interactions and adverse events with antiretroviral drugs. Lancet 2004;364:8

Panlilio AL. Estimate of the annual number of percutaneous injuries among hospital-based healthcare workers in the U.S., 1997-1998. Infect Control Hosp Epidemiol 2004;25:556

Busch MP, Satten GA. Time course of viremia and antibody seroconversion following human immunodeficiency virus exposure. Am J Med 1997;102(suppl 5B):117

Ridzon R, Gallagher K, Ciesielski C, et al. Simultaneous transmission of HIV and hepatitis C virus from a needlestick injury. N Engl J Med 1997;336:919

Jochimsen EM. Failures of zidovudine postexposure prophylaxis. Am J Med 1997;102(Suppl 5B):52

Wang SA, Paulilio AL, Doi PA. Experience of healthcare workers taking post-exposure prophylaxis after occupational HIV exposures: findings of the HIV post-exposure prophylaxis registry . Infect Control Hosp Epidemiol 2000;21:780

Beltrami EM, et al. Antiretroviral drug resistance in human immunodeficiency virus - infected source patients for occupational exposures to healthcare workers. Infect Control Hosp Epidemiol 2003;24:724

Puro V. Post-exposure prophylaxis of HIV infection in healthcare workers: recommendations for the European setting. Euro J Epidemiol 2004;19:577

HORDEOLUM (STYE)/CHALAZION

Spyridon Marinopoulos, M.D.

DIAGNOSTIC CRITERIA

- Hordeolum (stye): infection of Zeiss/Moll tear glands in eyelid margin (external) or meibomian gland in tarsal plate (internal hordeolum). Acute inflammation of eyelid with abscess formation.
- Clinical: tender swelling of eyelid & erythema. Abscess points internally or externally. Self-limited, spontaneously drains in 5-7d, but may progress to cellulitis or chalazion esp if internal
- Ddx eyelid tumor, blepharitis, conjunctivitis, periorbital cellulitis. Predisposing factors: hordeolum - staph blepharitis; chalazion - seborrheic blepharitis and rosacea
- Chalazion: granuloma develops as foreign body reaction to lipid produced by meibomian gland. May arise from internal hordeolum or with sebum plugging tear gland opening and causing obstruction
- Clinical: painless, rubbery, palpable nodule at margin of lid or higher. If large, may cause visual disturbance by pressing on and deforming the cornea

COMMON PATHOGENS: Hordeolum: S. aureus ; Chalazion: Non-ID causes

TREATMENT REGIMENS

General measures

- Hordeolum (stye): most will drain spontaneously within 3-4 days following pointing, especially if external. Internal may persist and progress to chalazion
- Warm compresses 4-5 x / day x 10-15 min per session essential to help open pore and promote drainage. Scrubbing eye with neutral soap (Dove, Ivory or baby shampoo) may hasten recovery
- If external, relief of pain and resolution are hastened if pointing lesion is pricked with fine sterile needle. Apply antibiotic ointment post procedure. Do not attempt for internal hordeolum
- Refer to Ophtho for I&D if no improvement by day 3 of conservative therapy +/- antibiotics

- Chalazion: may resolve spontaneously if duct of gland opens. Warm compresses 4-5 x / day x 10-15 min per session x 1 month will help soften plug. ~50% will resolve. If no resolution, refer to Ophtho
- Ophthalmologists may Rx by incision and curettage, intralesional steroid injection or both
- Intralesional steroid injection with 0.05-0.3 mL of 5mg/dL triamcinolone effective, but may depigment overlying skin in darkly pigmented individuals. Expect resolution in 1-2 wks
- Steroid inj good for children, pts allergic to local anesthesia & lesions close to lacrimal drainage system. Also no eye patching required, less in-office time/cost & can Rx mult lesions in same visit
- Outpt incision and curettage preferred for hard lesions of >6 months duration, for possibly infected chalazia, when skin depigmentation is a concern & is the only recourse if steroid inj ineffective
- Combined incision, curettage and intralesional corticosteroid injection may be more effective for patients with large, recurrent and multiple chalazia

Antibiotics

- Hordeolum (stye): generally systemic abx unnecessary unless there is associated periorbital cellulitis (rare). However, oral abx may be indicated in moderate to severe cases of internal hordeola
- Hordeolum (external): erythromycin ophthalmic oint (E-mycin, Eryc) 0.5-inch into conjunctival sac bid-qid x 7d or sulfacetamide 10% ophthalmic oint 0.5-in ribbon bid-qid x 7d
- Hordeolum (internal, mild cases): erythromycin ophthalmic oint (E-mycin, Eryc) 0.5-inch into conjunctival sac bid-qid x 7d or sulfacetamide 10% ophthalmic oint 0.5-in ribbon bid-qid x 7d
- Hordeolum (internal, moderate or severe cases): dicloxacillin 500mg PO q6h x 7d or cephalexin 500mg PO q6h x 7d
- Alternatives (pen or ceph allergy): clindamycin 300mg PO q6h x 7d or clarithromycin 500mg PO q12h x 7d or azithromycin 500mg PO once then 250mg PO qd x 5d (Z-PAK)
- Chalazion: not an infectious disease as lesion generally is sterile. However, chronic PO tetracycline or doxy may treat recurrent chalazia ? via effect on fatty acid production by tear glands

DRUG-SPECIFIC COMMENTS

Cephalexin: First generation cephalosporin with excellent methicillin-sensitive staph coverage. Do not use in patients with severe penicillin allergy

Clarithromycin: Better methicillin-sensitive staph coverage than erythromycin, easier dosing regimen, more expensive

Dicloxacillin: Synthetic penicillin with excellent methicillin-sensitive staph coverage, first-line agent

IMPORTANT POINTS

- Recommendations represent the author's opinion
- Hordeolum (stye): Warm compresses primary Rx with topical abx secondary and PO abx only in moderate to severe cases if hordeolum internal. Refer if no improvement by day 3 of Rx
- Preauricular lymph node involvement and fever are not consistent with diagnosis and may suggest a more serious infection (e.g., periorbital cellulitis) requiring aggressive systemic therapy

Diagnosis

- **Chalazion:** Refer for incision and curettage or intralesional steroids if compresses not effective. R/O sebaceous cell, basal cell or meibomian gland CA if persistent or recurrent

Selected Readings

Crama N, Toolens AM, van der Meer JW, et al. Giant chalazia in the hyperimmunoglobulinemia E (hyper-IgE) syndrome. Eur J Ophthalmol. 2004 May-Jun;14(3):258-60.

Ozdal PC, Codere F, Callejo S, et al. Accuracy of the clinical diagnosis of chalazion. Eye. 2004 Feb;18 (2):135-8.

Cunniffe G, Chang BY, Kennedy S, et al. Beware the empty curette!. Orbit 2002 Jun;21(2):177-80

Jackson T, Beun L. A prospective study of cost, patient satisfaction and outcome of treatment of chalazion by medical and nursing staff. Br J Ophthalmol 2000;84(7):782-5.

Lederman C, Miller M. Hordeola and Chalazia . C - Pediatr Rev - 01-Aug-1999; 20(8): 283-4

Olson M. The Common Stye. Journal of School Health 1991;61(2):95-97

Epstein GA, Putterman AM. Combined excision and drainage with intralesional corticosteroid injection in the treatment of chronic chalazia. Arch Ophthalmol 1988 Apr;106(4):514-6

Diegel JT. Eyelid problems. Blepharitis, hordeola, and chalazia. Postgrad Med 1986 Aug; 80(2): 271-2

Pavan-Langston D. Diagnosis and therapy of common eye infections: bacterial, viral, fungal. Compr Ther 1983 May; 9(5): 33-42

Perry H, Serniuk R. Conservative Treatment of Chalazia. Ophthalmology 1980; 87:218-221.

IMPETIGO

Ciro R. Martins, M.D.

Diagnostic Criteria

- PE (non-bullous impetigo): single or multiple, isolated or coalescent, small, superficial pustules progressing to erosions covered by stuck-on, honey-colored crusts, surrounded by erythematous halo
- PE (bullous impetigo): bullae with minimal or no inflammation. Denuded areas after the blisters rupture are covered by thin, varnish-like light brown crusts
- Clinical: frequent regional lymphadenopathy usually NOT associated with systemic symptoms
- Lab: gram stain of pus or base of the lesions reveal GPC. Cx and sensitivity testing indicated, especially if treatment failure, or if gram negative organisms seen on Gram stain.
- Most common agent non-bullous impetigo = S. pyogenes, followed by an association of S. pyogenes + S. aureus. Bullous impetigo = S. aureus.

Common Pathogens: Streptococcus pyogenes (Group A) ; Staphylococcus aureus

Treatment Regimens

Topical therapy
- Usually effective in treating mild and localized disease
- Mupirocin 2% (Bactroban) ointment or cream tid-qid until clear

Systemic therapy
- Indicated in cases of bullous impetigo or extensive disease +/- regional lymphadenopathy
- Non-bullous impetigo (preferred): penicillin VK 250-500mg PO q6-8h x 7d, Penicillin G- benzathine 1.2 million U IM x1, amoxicillin 250-500mg PO q8h or 500-875mg PO q12h x 7d, ampicillin 250mg PO q6h x 7d
- Bullous impetigo or cx-proven Staphylococcal impetigo: cephalexin 250-500mg PO q6h, cefadroxil 500mg-1g PO q12h, or dicloxacillin 500mg PO q6h--all x 7d. Consider community-acquired MRSA in toxic pt.

- Alt: amoxicillin/clavulanate 875/125mg PO q12h x 7d
- Alt: erythromycin 250-500mg PO q6h or 333mg PO q8h x 7d; azithromycin 500mg PO x1 followed by 250mg PO qd x 4d; clarithromycin PO 250mg PO q12h x 7d

General management

- Soften crusts with vaseline or antibiotic ointment several times /day
- Wash individual lesions with antibacterial soap or antiseptic solution and water trying to gently remove crusts twice a day
- Instruct the patient not to touch lesions and to wash hands frequently
- Clip fingernails short to decrease risks of excoriation, self-inoculation and contagion spread
- Keep out of school until crusted lesions have healed
- Cleanliness and prompt care of minor skin wounds such as minor cuts, abrasions and insect bites prevents the disease.

DRUG-SPECIFIC COMMENTS

Amoxicillin: May have slight advantage over penicillin VK due to better absorption, but also has higher risk of diarrhea.

Amoxicillin + Clavulanate: This drug offers good coverage for both S. aureus and Strep spp. but it is an expensive choice.

Cefadroxil: Good choice for both Strep and Staph impetigo. Twice a day regimen is convenient.

Cephalexin: Rational choice for either Strep or Staph impetigo but qid dosing.

Clarithromycin: Good choice for penicillin-allergic individuals, but the experience in Strep skin infections is limited. Less GI intolerance than erythromycin.

Dicloxacillin: Rational choice for for S. aureus but not dependable for Strep impetigo.

Mupirocin: The best choice for topical treatment alone, but not an inexpensive drug. Ointment vehicle helps removing the crusts and should be used in combination with systemic therapy.

IMPORTANT POINTS

- These guidelines represent the author's opinion
- Most common skin infection in children; highly contagious, especially w/ poor hygiene and crowding (schools, day-care centers, orphanages); more common in hot and humid weather.
- Ecthyma is a form of impetigo characterized by deeper ulcer that heals with scarring
- Ddx: varicella, herpes simplex infection, atopic dermatitis, contact dermatitis, scabies, candidiasis, guttate psoriasis

SELECTED READINGS

Veien NK. The clinician's choice of antibiotics in the treatment of bacterial skin infections. Bri J Derm, 139:30-6, 1998.

Sadick NS. Current Aspects of Bacterial Skin Infections. Derm Clinics, 15(2):341-9, 1997

Raz R, Miron D, Colodner R et al. A 1 year trial of nasal mupirocin in the prevention of recurrent staphylococcal nasal colonization and skin infection. Arch Int Med 156:1109-12, 1996

Wortman PD. Bacterial Infections of the Skin. Curr Prob in Derm 5:193-228, 1993

INFLUENZA

John G. Bartlett, M.D.

DIAGNOSTIC CRITERIA

- Respiratory virus. Types: A (major disease, mortality); B (milder) and C (mildest)

DIAGNOSIS

- Hx: epidemic of flu + fever + cough = 70% probability of flu
- Common complications: bacterial sinusitis, otitis, exacerbations of chronic bronchitis, pneumonia, asthma, deterioration of cardiovascular disease, diabetes or other chronic disease
- Laboratory confirmation: positive nasopharyngeal cx for influenza virus, positive DFA stain, positive rapid diagnostic test or seroconversion
- Physician dx flu (epidemic, fever, typical sx) as good as rapid flu test: ~70% sensitivity. Fever especially important sign in clinical dx.

COMMON PATHOGENS: Influenza

TREATMENT REGIMENS

Anti-flu agent--must be given <48 hrs of onset
- Principles: vaccine best to prevent; antiflu agents must be within 48hrs sx onset
- Influenza A: amantadine 100mg PO bid x 5d; >65 yrs, 100mg PO qd x 5
- Influenza A: rimantadine 100mg PO bid x 5d; >65 yrs., renal failure, hepatic failure-- 100mg PO qd x 3-5d
- Anti Flu A&B (preferred): oseltamivir (Tamiflu) 75mg PO bid x 5d
- Anti Flu A&B (alt): zanamivir (Relenza) 10mg bid inhaled x 5d
- Relative merits - see Important Points and Table 4 in Appendix I
- Amantadine-CNS toxicity, Flu A only, APW $6/5d; rimantadine-Flu A, AWP $22/5d; oseltamivir-GI initial, Flu A & B - $70/5d.

Flu prophylaxis
- Preferred (by everybody): vaccination, esp persons >50, chronic diseases and healthcare workers; 2 weeks for response
- Immunization: inactivated vaccine given yearly, reformulated annually; live-attenuated given intranasally (only age 4-49yrs). See "Influenza Immunization and Prophylaxis" in the Vaccines section.
- 2004-05 priority (short vaccine supply): persons >65 yrs or <23 mo, chronic illness, pregnancy or health care workers
- Immediate protection: antiviral (70-90% effective) + vaccine as 2 weeks required until antibody response
- Preferred antiviral (R Couch NEJM 2000; 343:1778): Influenza A - rimantadine (Flumadine)100mg PO bid; >65 yrs, renal failure, hepatic failure, 100mg PO qd
- Alternative amantadine 100mg PO bid; >65 yrs, 100mg PO qd
- Preferred for flu A & B: oseltamivir (Tamiflu) 75mg PO qd, Influenza A & B, FDA approved for prophylaxis, expensive
- Alternate for A & B: zanamivir (Relenza) 10mg inhaled qd, Influenza A & B, not FDA approved for prophylaxis (but works)
- Oseltamivir/Zanamivir effective in half-daily dose for protecting family members of an index case.

Symptomatic treatment
- Naprosyn 500mg tid, ASA etc
- Cough - meds with codeine or dextromethorphan
- Sedating antihistamine - Actifed, Contact, Dimetapp, etc
- Atrovent nasal spray
- Albuterol nasal spray 2 whiffs q4-6h prn

DRUG-SPECIFIC COMMENTS

Amantadine: FDA-approved for treatment of influenza in 1966. Least expensive, but has significant CNS toxicity with confusion, reduced ability to concentrate, etc. Some feel that the drug is acceptable with dose adjustment so that persons >65 yrs. get 100 mg/d.

Oseltamivir: FDA approved in 1999 as the first available neuraminidase inhibitor for influenza which, like zanamivir, is active vs. both influenza A & B. Main side effect is GI intolerance. Approved for treatment and prophylaxis (age > 13yrs).

Rimantadine: FDA-approved for treatment of influenza in 1993. Much less expensive than Zanamivir & oseltamivir (AWP $16 vs. $50-55 for 5-day course), has some CNS toxicity as does amantadine, but less frequent & severe. FDA approved for treatment and prophylaxis

Zanamivir: FDA approved in 1999. Must be inhaled with a tricky gadget. Major side effect is bronchospasm, primarily in asthmatics. FDA approved only for treatment, but it works for prophylaxis

IMPORTANT POINTS

- Guidelines from CDC (MMWR 2000;52:RR-8) and R. Couch (NEJM 2000;343:1778)
- Main current concern is Avian flu A (H5N1) in Asia--highly lethal and no vaccine
- Influenza is major cause of serious dx in persons >65 yrs, nursing home residents, and persons w/chronic dx - lung, heart, liver/renal failure, diabetes, etc.
- All 4 anti-flu drugs reduce duration of sx by 1-2 days if started <48 hours of onset of sx; benefit is greater if started early & if sx severe.
- Remember that bacterial pneumonia may complicate influenza esp, S. pneumoniae & S. aureus.
- CDC weekly updates: phone: 888-232-3228, fax: 888-232-3299 (doc. #361100), or www.cdc.gov/ncidod/diseases/flu/weekly.htm

SELECTED READINGS

CDC. Prevention and Control of Influenza . MMWR 2003;52RR8:1-36

CDC. When to use antiviral drug for the flu. www.cdc.gov/flu/protect/antiviral/index/htm;accessed 9/13/04

CDC: . Avian Influenza. www.cdc.gov/flu/about/avainflu.htm accessed 9/10/04

CDC. Avian influenza infection in humans. www.cdc.gov/flu/avian/gen-info/avian-flu-humans.htm; accessed 9/13/04

CDC. Avian influenza viruses. cdc.gov/flu/avian/gen-info/avian-influenza.htm; accessed 9/14/04

Ault, A. Shifting tactics in the battle against influenza. Science 2004;303:1280

CDC. Update: Influenza Activity-US and Worldwide 2003-04 season and composition of the 2004-05 vaccine. MMWR 2004;53:547

Armstrong BG, et al. Effect of influenza vaccination on excess deaths occurring during periods of high circulation of influenza: cohort study in elderly people. BMJ 2004; (pre-print on web)

Cooper NJ, et al. Effectiveness of neuraminidase inhibitors in treatment and prevention of influenza A & B: systematic review and meta-analysis of randomized controlled trials. BMJ 2003;326:1235

Koopmans M, et al. Transmission of H/7 N/7 avian influenza A virus to human beings during a large outbreak in commercial poultry farms in the Netherlands. Lancet 2004;363-587

LARYNGITIS

John G. Bartlett, M.D.

DIAGNOSTIC CRITERIA

- Hoarseness or harsh voice with deep pitch +/- episodic aphonia
- Usually accompanied by symptoms of an URI
- Laryngoscopy-demonstrated hyperemic vocal cords (for enigmatic cases)

DIAGNOSIS

- Most common non-ID cause: GERD

COMMON PATHOGENS: Rhinovirus ; Coronavirus ; Parainfluenza virus ; Influenza ; Adenovirus

TREATMENT REGIMENS

Other treatments

- Principles: Rx - voice rest. Common cause - viral URI & GERD; r/o TB, malignancy in persistent cases.
- Humidity may improve speech and throat pain
- Antibiotics are not useful. Exceptions: HSV, TB, Candida, M. catarrhalis
- Prednisone: 60-80mg/d with rapid taper (may be tried for opera singers and others who need their voice)
- Rx common cold if appropriate - see below
- Non-ID causes: GERD (trial antiacid Rx), allergy, tumors

Treatment for viral URI

- Nasal decongestant - pseudoephedrine 120mg bid. Also - Actifed, Cardec or sprays - Afrin, Dristan, Neo-Synephrine
- Antihistamine - 1st gen. benedryl, Atarax, etc.
- Ipratropium (Atrovent) 2 sprays each nostril 3-4 x/d
- Allergic rhinitis - loratadine (Claritin) 10mg/d and nasal steroids
- NSAIDs - naproxen (Aleve) not ibuprofen

IMPORTANT POINTS

- Guidelines based on CDC recommendations (Ann Intern Med 2001;134:487)
- Antibiotic trials have not shown benefit despite possible role for treatable pathogens.
- Symptomatic treatment is voice rest and humidification. Patients who need their voice-- prednisone 60-80 mg/d w/rapid taper
- Most common non-ID cause: GERD - Rx w/antacids. Rare cause is tuberculosis-- laryngeal TB is the most contagious form of TB.
- Prolonged laryngitis requires referral to ENT to see if vocal cord structural abnormality exists.

SELECTED READINGS

Williams RB, et al. Predictors of outcome in an open label, therapeutic trial of high-dose omeprazole in laryngitis. Am J Gastroenterol 2004;99:777-85

Heikkimen T and Jarvinen A. The common cold. Lancet 2003;361:51

Greenberg SB. Respiratory consequences of rhinovirus infection. Arch Intern Med 2003;163:278

Hayden FG, et al. Efficacy and safety of oral pleconaril for treatment of colds due to picornaviruses in adults. Clin Infect Dis 2003;36:1523

Snow V, Mottur-Pilson C, Gonzales R. Principles of appropriate antibiotic use for treatment of non-specific upper respiratory tract infections in adults. Ann Intern Med 2001;134:487

Neuenschwander MC, Cooney A, Spiegel JR, et al. Laryngeal candidiasis. Ear Nose Throat 2001;80:138

Ulualp SO, Toohill RJ, Shaker R. Outcomes of acid suppressive therapy in patients with posterior laryngitis. Otolaryngol Head Neck Surg 2001;124:16

Spiegel JR, Hawkshaw M, Markiewiez A, Sataloff RT. Acute Laryngitis. Ear Nose Throat J 2000; 79:488

Mishra S, Rosen CA, Murry T. 24 hours prior to curtain. J Voice 2000; 114:92

Vrabec JT, Molina CP, West B. Herpes simplex viral laryngitis. Ann Otol Rhinol Laryngol 2000; 109:611

LEGIONNAIRES' DISEASE
John G. Bartlett, M.D.

DIAGNOSTIC CRITERIA

- Clinical suspicion: severe or life-threatening pneumonia, especially in patients with risk factors. Compared to pneumococcal pneumonia > extrapulmonary signs i.e., headache, diarrhea, renal failure.
- Risk factors: age >50 years, smoking, compromised cell-mediated immunity (chronic corticosteroids, organ or marrow transplant, cancer chemo Rx) or exposure to epidemic source
- Lab: special cx media (buffered charcoal yeast extract) required, difficult and requires >3 days for growth.
- Lab: urine antigen for L. pneumophila serogroup 1 detects 70% of cases; easy for lab and fast.
- Lab: sputum or NP swab PCR for L. pneumophila; new and fast.
- See Table 11 in Appendix I

COMMON PATHOGENS: Legionella pneumophila serogroup 1-70% of cases ; Legionella pneumophila serogroup 2-6 ; Legionella micdadei

TREATMENT REGIMENS

Antibiotics

- Preferred: respiratory fluoroquinolone or azithromycin
- Levofloxacin (Levaquin) 750mg IV qd then 750mg PO qd x 10d total
- Gatifloxacin (Tequin) 400mg IV qd, then 400mg PO qd x 10d total
- Moxifloxacin (Avelox) 400mg IV qd, then 400mg PO qd x 10d total
- Azithromycin (Zithromax) 500mg IV, then 500mg PO x 7-10d total
- Rifampin 300mg IV or PO bid plus any of the above, used mainly w/ severe illness

Nosocomial cases

- No patient isolation (because there is no patient-patient transmission), but nosocomial cases need evaluation for a common source--notify infection control.
- Usual source: water-surveillance cultures are sometimes advocated but not by CDC except with cases
- Methods to clear water: heat to 70 degrees, hyperchlorination, chlorine dioxide, electrodes, or ultraviolet light.

DRUG-SPECIFIC COMMENTS

Azithromycin: A preferred drug

Clarithromycin: (Biaxin) Good in vitro activity for Legionnaires' disease, but available only in oral form.

Doxycycline: A better drug for Legionella than commonly thought. Good activity in vitro, good activity in the animal model, available in oral & parenteral forms. Clinical experience is limited.

Gatifloxacin: Many authorities consider the fluoroquinolones to be the drugs of choice for Legionnaires' disease. Advantage here is availability of oral and parenteral forms & FDA approval for this indication.

Levofloxacin: Comparable to moxifloxacin and gatifloxacin

Moxifloxacin: Good in vitro activity, many authorities consider the fluoroquinolones to be the drugs of choice for Legionnaires' disease. Advantage includes availability of oral and parenteral forms.

Rifampin: Often added to fluoroquinolone or azithromycin although efficacy of combination is not proven.

IMPORTANT POINTS

- Guidelines of IDSA (CID 2003;37;405)
- Empiric Rx of critically ill adult with pneumonia - cover S. pneumoniae & Legionella
- Recognition is important for epidemiologic implications, requires specific abx (fluoroquinolones or azithromycin) & is potentially lethal.
- Lab tests (cx, DFA stain, urine Ag) can rule in, but neg tests don't rule out. Best dx tests are urinary antigen and cx (takes >3d and insensitive). Both have great specificity but poor sensitivity.
- Nosocomial Legionella: alert hospital Infection Control to investigate for an environmental source.

SELECTED READINGS

Sopena N, et al. Comparative study of community acquired pneumonia caused by streptococcus pneumoniae. Legionella pneumophila or chlamydia pneumoniae. Scand J.Infect.Dis.2004;36-330

Joseph CA, et al. Legionnaires' disease in Europe 2000-02. Epidemiol Infect 2004;132-417

Mandell LA. Update of practice guidelines for the management of community-acquired pneumonia in immunocompetent adults. CID 2003;37:1405-33

Murdock DR. Diagnosis of Legionella Infections. Clin Infect Dis 2003;36-64

Lettinga KD, et al. Legionnaires' disease at a Dutch flower show. Emerg Infect Dis 2002;8:1448

Helbig JH, et al. Clinical utility of urinary antigen detection for diagnosis of community-acquired, travel associated and nosocomial Legionnaires' disease. J Clin Micro 2003;41:838

Marston BJ, Lipman HB, Breiman RF, et al. Surveillance for Legionnaires' disease. Arch Intern Med 1994;154:2117

Yu V. Legionellosis. N Engl J Med 1997;337:682

Yu VL. Legionnaires' disease: seek and ye shall find. Cleve Clin J Med 2001;68:318

Fernandez-Sabe N, et al. Clinical diagnosis of Legionella pneumonia revisited. CID 2003;37:483

LYME DISEASE

John G. Bartlett, M.D.

DIAGNOSTIC CRITERIA

- Early (3-30 days after tick bite): erythema migrans with red lesion at tick bite site--no serology necessary
- Late complications: positive serology (EIA + Western blot) plus arthritis, neuropathy, encephalopathy or carditis
- Arthritis: joint swelling esp knee - joint swelling & pain, recurrent. Carditis: A-V block.
- Neuropathy: encephalopathy, cranial nerve palsy including Bell's palsy, lymphocytic meningitis or radiculopathy w/pain, paresis or paresthesias
- Vector=Ixodes scapularis (deer tick), highly endemic regions include river/costal regions of NE, MidAtlantic and Wisc/Minn. Less common in West, transmitted by black-legged tick, I. pacificus.

COMMON PATHOGENS: Borrelia burgdorferi

TREATMENT REGIMENS

Treatment: early localized or early disseminated

- Principles: dx - EM rash or pos serology + objective Lyme complications; NOT chronic fatigue

- Tick exposure: Prompt tick removal, no antibiotics. Single dose doxycycline 200mg if: <72hr in epidemic area (NEJM 2001;345:79)
- Erythema migrans: Preferred - doxycycline 100mg PO bid x 10-14d
- EM: Alternatives - Amoxicillin 500mg PO tid x 21d or cefuroxime axetil (Ceftin) 500mg PO bid x 21d
- Late Lyme - arthritis, CNS, heart block: see late complications

Early disseminated or late complications

- Bells palsy: Doxycycline 100mg PO bid x 21-28d or amoxicillin 500mg PO tid x 21-28d
- CNS (other): Ceftriaxone 2g IV q12h x 14-28d or cefotaxime 2g IV q6h x 14-28d or PCN G 4 mU IV q4h x 14-28d
- Cor, 1st degree block: doxycycline 100mg PO bid x 21-28d or amoxicillin 500mg PO tid x 21-28d
- Cor, 2/3 degree block: Ceftriaxone 2g IV qd x 14-28d or pen G 3-4 mU IV q 4h x 14-21d
- Arthritis, oral: Doxycycline 100mg PO bid x 28d or amoxicillin 500mg PO tid x 28d
- Arthritis, IV: Cefotaxime 2g IV q8h x 14-28d or pen G 18-24 mU IV qd x 14-28d
- Chronic fatigue: Don't test or treat (NEJM 2001;345:85)

Prevention

- Tick checks daily - removal within 36hrs is most effective prevention
- Prophylactic doxycycline 200mg x 1 within 72 hrs post tick bite - 87% effective, best only in highly endemic region
- Tick control: acaricide starting in early May
- DEET repellants, esp Edtiar (Ultrathon) for skin
- Permethrin (Nix) as spray for skin or applied to clothes, tents, etc
- Lyme vaccine - no longer available

DRUG-SPECIFIC COMMENTS

Amoxicillin: One of the 2 preferred agents for oral therapy of early Lyme disease and Lyme arthritis (doxycycline is the other)

Ceftriaxone: Parenteral drug of choice (along with penicillin) for lyme disease with late complications.

Clarithromycin: No macrolide is considered 1st-line for any form of Lyme disease, but they can be used for patients who cannot take doxycycline or amoxicillin

Doxycycline: One of the 2 preferred agents for oral therapy of early Lyme disease and Lyme arthritis. This drug could also be given IV in patients who merit parenteral therapy but can't take beta-lactams.

IMPORTANT POINTS

- Guidelines from Medical Letter (2005;47:41) & IDSA (CID 2000;31:S1) for tests CDC (JAMA 1999;282:62) for tick bite (NEJM 2003;348:2424)
- Dx based on epidemiology (endemic area +/- tick bite), pos. serology (except w/ erythema migrans or acute neurologic disease--early) & typical symptoms
- Patients with chronic fatigue, joint stiffness &/or muscle aches should not have Lyme disease serology & should not receive Lyme disease treatment
- Serology: EIA or IFA and western blot - takes 4-6 wks for seroconversion (reliable test)
- Tick bite: coinfection risk ~1-3%; Lyme, ehrlichiosis, babesiosis, RMSF; proph doxy 200mg x 1 for Lyme risk
- LYMErix vaccine discontinued by manufacturer March 2002 due to poor sales.

SELECTED READINGS

CDC. Lyme disease - US 2001-02. MMWR 2004;53:365

Wormser GP, et al. Duration of antibiotic therapy for early Lyme diseases. Ann Intern Med 2003;138:697

Hayes EB, Plesman J. How can we prevent Lyme disease? . N Engl J Med 2003;348;2424

Anonymous. Recommendations for treatment of Lyme disease. Medical Letter 2000;42:34

American College of Physicians. Guidelines for laboratory evaluation in the diagnosis of Lyme disease. Ann Intern Med 1997;127:1106

Smith RP, et al. Clinical characteristics and treatment outcome of early Lyme disease in patients with microbiologically confirmed erythema migrans. Ann Intern Med 2002;136:421

Steere A. Lyme Disease. NEJM 2001;345:115

Klempner MS, Hu LT, Evans J, et al. Two controlled trials of antibiotic treatment in patients with persistent symptoms and a history of Lyme disease. NEJM 2001;345:85

Seltzer EG et al. Long-term Outcomes of Persons With Lyme Disease . JAMA 2000; 283:609

Wormser GP, Nadelman RB, Dattwyler RJ, et al. IDSA practice guidelines for the treatment of Lyme disease. Clin Infect Dis 2000 31; Suppl 1:1

LYMPHADENOPATHY
Jeremy Gradon, M.D.

DIAGNOSTIC CRITERIA
- Palpable lymph nodes (> 1cm abnormal). Must distinguish generalized vs. localized; chronic vs. acute
- Painful = inflammation, suppuration or bleed into necrotic area; rubbery = lymphoma; stony hard = cancer or actinomycosis; LN may be single or "matted" (several nodes moveable as a group)
- PE - temperature, inspect mucus membranes, organomegaly & genitalia
- Lab: CBC, HIV, RPR, CMV, EBV and other tests as indicated by hx:
- Syphilis: RPR/FTA
- Group A streptococcus: culture, rapid antigen testing
- EBV: Monospot, anti-VCA IgM antibodies
- CMV: serology (IgM)
- HIV: serology, PCR (in acute seroconversion illness)
- Cat scratch disease: node biopsy, culture, serology (anti-Bartonella henselae Abs), PCR
- Brucella: serology, culture
- TB: culture, histology
- Whipple's: bx, PCR
- Tularemia: serology, PCR (experimental), culture is dangerous in routine labs!
- LN bx if unexplained nodes persist >4wks or have malignant characteristics or rapidly enlarging, +PPD, FUO-associated. Fine needle aspiration ok but less dx tissue.

COMMON PATHOGENS: ACUTE GENERALIZED: HIV, syphilis, EBV, CMV, Toxo, brucella, cat scratch; Sarcoid, lymphoma, Stills, IBD, Whipple's, hypersensitivity rxn; HAART-associated immune reconstitution syndrome in HIV+; ACUTE LOCALIZED: CERVICAL: group A strep, EBV, TB, cat scratch, Lymphoma, Temporal arteritis; PRE-AURICULAR: adenovirus conjunctivitis, tularemia, cat scratch (Parinaud's syndrome) ; EPITROCHLEAR: hand infection (medial 3 fingers) - staph/strep; Inguinal: syphilis, herpes, LGV, chancroid, HIV, lymphoma, tularemia, plague; CHRONIC GENERALIZED: Syphilis, TB, histoplasma, cryptococcosis, CGD; Lymphoma, HIV, sarcoid, hyperthyroidism, chronic fatigue syndrome, posttransplant lymphoproliferative disorder; CHRONIC LOCALIZED: TB, cryptococcus, histoplasma, cat scratch, lymphoma, metastatic cancer, Kikuchi-Fujimoto disease, Rosai-Dorman disease

IMPORTANT POINTS
- Lymphadenopathy due to infection - treat infection and nodes should resolve
- Watch for secondary malignancies and unusual OI's in HIV+ not on HAART

- Immune-Reconstitution Syndrome is a hard dx to prove
- Keep low threshold for diagnostic biopsy-supraclav., cervical or axillary LN if possible, largest node, remove entire node (incl. capsule) discuss with pathologist/microbiologist in advance.
- Follow pt with chronic lymphadenopathy and negative node bx closely, re-biopsy if nodes persist

Selected Readings

Leung AK, Robson WL. Childhood cervical lymphadenopathy. J Pediatr Health Care 2004; 18: 3-7

Veerapand P, Chotimanvijit N, Muennooch W. Percutaneous ultrasound-guided fine needle aspiration of abdominal lymphadenopathy in AIDS patients. J Med Assoc Thai 2004; 87: 400-404

Zwischenberger JB, Savage C, Alpard SK et al. Mediastinal transthoracic needle and core lymph node biopsy: Should it replace mediastinoscopy? . Chest 2002; 121: 1165-1170

Ngom A, Dumont P, Diot P, et al. Benign mediastinal lymphadenopathy in congestive heart failure. Chest 2001; 119: 653-656

Vassilakopoulos TP, Pangalis PA. Application of a prediction rule to select which patients presenting with lymphadenopathy should undergo a lymph node biopsy. Medicine 2000: 79: 338-347

Jasmer RM, Edinburgh KJ, Gotway MB et al. Clinical and radiographic predictors of the etiology of pulmonary nodules in HIV-infected patients. Chest 2000; 117: 1023-1030

de kleijn EMHA, van Lier HJJ, van der meer JWM. Fever of unknown origin (FUO)II: Diagnostic procedures in a prospective multicenter study of 167 patients. Medicine 1997; 76: 401-414

Nikanne E, Ruoppi P, Vornanen M. Kikuchi's disease: Report of three cases and an overview. Laryngoscope 1997; 107: 273-276

LYMPHANGITIS
Ciro R. Martins, M.D.

Diagnostic Criteria

- Hx: frequently hx of trauma or skin lesion distal to the affected area followed by acute onset of symptoms.
- Clinical: painful/tender erythematous linear streak on the skin progressing towards draining regional lymph nodes. Tender lymphadenopathy commonly with fever, chills and malaise
- Lab: Gram stain and cx of pus if infected wound or suppurative lymph node present. Leukocytosis with marked increase in PMN's.
- Lymphangitis of hands and arms associated with higher morbidity since infection can bypass elbow nodes progressing directly to subpectoral nodes.

COMMON PATHOGENS: Streptococcus pyogenes (Group A) ; Group A Strep is by far the most common. Other streptococcal species and S. aureus may also occur.; Pasturella multocida or anaerobes possible if lymphangitis due to animal bite.; Uncommon causes (usually more indolent): Sporothrix. Nocardia, atypical Mycobacteria

Treatment Regimens

Systemic

- Penicillin G benzathine 1.2 mU IM x1 or penicillin G 1-2 mU IV q4-6h followed by amoxicillin 500mg PO q6h to complete 10-14d
- Cefazolin 1g IV q6-8h followed by amoxicillin or cefuroxime 500mg PO bid to complete 10-14d
- Clindamycin 600mg IV q8h followed by 300mg PO qid to complete 10-14d
- Amoxicillin 500mg PO q6h x 10-14d

General care

- Immobilization

- Elevation of the affected area
- Hot packs or hot compresses q4h

DRUG-SPECIFIC COMMENTS

Amoxicillin: Good choice in mild, non-progressing cases not associated with systemic symptoms. Can also be used after the initial parenteral therapy to complete a treatment course.

IMPORTANT POINTS

- These guidelines represent the author's opinion
- Lymphangitis is a potentially serious disease with frequent development of bacteremia, sepsis and metastatic infection
- Therapy has to be instituted promptly and parenterally when systemic symptoms are present. Evaluate for deeper tissue process.
- Animal bites are a common cause of lymphangitis and, in this setting, Pasteurella multocida, S. aureus and anaerobic bacteria can also be involved
- Ddx: thrombophlebitis, contact dermatitis, linear bruises, other infections with lymphangitic spread such as sporotrichosis and atypical mycobacterial infections

SELECTED READINGS

Sadick NS. Current aspects of bacterial infections of the skin. Dermatology Clinics, 15(2):341-9, 1997

Heller HM, Swartz MN. Nodular lymphangitis: clinical features, differential diagnosis and management. Current Topics in Infectious Diseases, 14:142-58, 1994

MASTITIS

Paul Auwaerter, M.D.

DIAGNOSTIC CRITERIA

- Breast infection ranging from erythematous nodule to abscess formation. Bacterial mastitis usually with unilateral wedge-shaped induration, erythema, warmth, elicitable pain and fever.
- Common affliction (2-33%) of nursing mothers, usually 1st 3 mos., peak = 2-3 wks postpartum.
- Lactation mastitis may or may not be infectious as acute inflammation of breast tissue. Sx may include malaise, fever, unilateral redness & tenderness of breast tissue.
- Ddx: breast engorgement/milk stasis that is often bilateral and lacking fever/erythema. Breast CA must be considered in unilateral findings esp. nonlacting women. TB mastitis--consider in endemic area.
- Mastitis usually clinical diagnosis, but breast milk cx may discriminate infectious vs. noninfectious--but normal milk may have >1000colonies/cc organisms skin flora.

COMMON PATHOGENS: Staphylococcus aureus; Peptostreptococcus ; Prevotella species ; Group A beta hemolytic strep ; Noninfectious

TREATMENT REGIMENS

Nursing mothers

- Supportive: analgesics (ibuprofen preferred as not transferred to milk) & hot compresses. Also change breastfeeding patterns, ensure drainage of breast milk by regular emptying.
- To facilitate let down, initiate nursing w/uninfected breast first.
- No consensus on where nursing should be discontinued during active infection, most favor continued nursing as it may aid response.

- If bacterial usually staphylococcal use beta-lactamase stable penicillin (since breastfeeding). Dicloxacillin 500mg PO qid or cephalexin 500mg PO qid 10-14 days.
- If abscess formation occurs, I&D, stop nursing, consider IV abx: nafcillin or oxacillin 2.0g IV q4h or cefazolin 1.0g q8h IV. Clindamycin 600mg q8 or vancomycin 1g q12h IV altern. if PCN allergic
- With abscess, use breastpump to empty q2h or when engorged. May resume feeding when abscess, erythema resolved.
- Full antibiotic course should be taken even if symptoms resolve within 24-48h.
- True fungal mastitis rare but can occur. Yeast often cultured from sore/cracked nipples but of unclear significance.

Recurrent mastitis

- Cause may be inadequate Rx or breast abscess. Assess for breast abscess by USG before assuming due to resistant bacteria and changing abx.
- USG may be unhelpful as features of breast abscess nonspecific, and focal tenderness alone may be indicative of need for drainage.

Nonpuerperal mastitis or abscess

- Often bilateral black/green nipple discharge. Duct ectasia, aging breast w/ varicoeles may be cause. Bxp may show plasma cell mastitis w/necrosis and inflammation, may also r/o CA.
- May be self-limited. Some authorities believe antibiotics unhelpful, and frequent I&D offers only temporary relief. Definitive treatment with complete excision of involved duct system.
- Subaureolar location may include anaerobes, otherwise likely staphylococcal.
- Frank abscess require drainage.
- If abx employed, clindamycin 600mg IVq8 or 300mg PO q6h, or amox/clav 500mg PO tid.

DRUG-SPECIFIC COMMENTS

Cephalexin: Inexpensive, favored antibiotic for breastfeeding women with good coverage of strep and staph. Will not treat MRSA, but would not suspect unless patient with frequent hospitalization or IVDA.

Dicloxacillin: Inexpensive, favored antibiotic for breastfeeding women with good coverage of strep and staph. Will not treat MRSA, but would not suspect unless patient with frequent hospitalization or IVDA.

Doxycycline: Although doxycycline produces measurable milk levels, it is not contraindicated during the nursing period. No harmful effects have been reported in breastfeeding infants (Anon, 1994). The manufacturer contradicts this statement. Tetracyclines are excreted in human milk. Due to the POTENTIAL for serious adverse reactions in nursing infants from doxycycline, the risks and benefits of therapy must be assessed. Would not routinely use.

Gatifloxacin: Though little formal data, fluoroquinolones probably excreted into breastmilk and therefore not suggested for use.

IMPORTANT POINTS

- Recommendations based upon author opinion.
- For primary care practitioner, safest to assume all mastitis in nonlactating patient is inflammatory carcinoma until proven otherwise.
- Decreased lactation mastitis seen over past few years often ascribed to increased breastfeeding rather than infant formula practices.

Diagnosis

- Milk stasis major risk factor for mastitis: e.g., changing or skipped feedings, poor positioning, switching breasts prior to complete drainage, maternal or infant illness, abundant milk supply.
- Antibiotics may control bacterial infection if present, but w/lactation mastitis does not correct underlying cause. MUST promote milk drainage.

Selected Readings

Heer R, Shrimankar J, Griffith CD. Granulomatous mastitis can mimic breast cancer on clinical, radiological or cytological examination: a cautionary tale. Breast. 2003 Aug;12(4):283-6

Barbosa-Cesnik C, Schwartz K, Foxman B. Lactation mastitis. JAMA. 2003 Apr 2;289(13):1609-12

Foxman B, D'Arcy H, Gillespie B, Bobo JK, Schwartz K. Lactation mastitis: occurrence and medical management among 946 breastfeeding women in the United States. Am J Epidemiol. 2002 Jan 15;155 (2):103-14

Osterman KL, Rahm VA. Lactation mastitis: bacterial cultivation of breast milk, symptoms, treatment, and outcome. J Hum Lact. 2000 Nov;16(4):297-302

Marchant DJ. Inflammation of the Breast. Ob Gyn Clinics. 2002 Mar; 29(1):1-14.

6. Karstrup S, Solvig J, Nolsoe CP, Nilsson P, Khattar S, Loren I, Nilsson A, Court-Payen M. Acute puerperal breast abscesses: US-guided drainage. Radiology. 1993 Sep;188(3):807-9

Thomsen AC, Espersen T, Maigaard S. Course and treatment of milk stasis, noninfectious inflammation of the breast, and infectious mastitis in nursing women. Am J Obstet Gynecol. 1984 Jul 1;149(5):492-5

MASTOIDITIS
Daniel J. Lee, M.D.

Diagnostic Criteria

- Clinical: mastoid tenderness with erythema, fluctuance, increased projection of outer ear accompanied by otalgia with aural fullness/decreased hearing, middle ear pus/fluid/bubbles
- Main indications for abxs: pain, erythema, fever. Abx-steroid ear drops not indicated unless tympanic membrane (TM) perforation present with otorrhea-otherwise, TM erythema/middle ear fluid not treated with drops
- Culture not routine (and not obtainable) until spontaneous TM rupture, myringotomy, or mastoidectomy performed - cultures may be helpful in chronic infection, or failure to multiple therapies.
- Imaging: fine-cut temporal bone CT (1mm cuts, axial and true coronals) indicated in most cases-to r/o coalescent mastoiditis / abscess
- Complications: spontaneous TM perforation, coalescent mastoiditis (mastoid abscess dx'ed by CT), labyrinthitis, neck abscess, meningitis, facial nerve palsy, sigmoid sinus thrombosis, epidural abscess
- Myringotomy in clinic setting for adult patients will aid in obtaining cx, guiding abx therapy, and improve pain. Topical antibiotic drops can then be used with oral/IV abxs.
- Brain MR often reveals incidental "mastoid" inflammation; unless patient is symptomatic, this is not mastoiditis as MR imaging is sensitive to minimal mucosal imaging, often seen in the mastoids or sinuses. MR + contrast is helpful to rule out intracranial involvement of mastoiditis, when indicated.

Common Pathogens: S. pneumoniae ; Haemophilus influenzae

TREATMENT REGIMENS

Uncomplicated acute infection

- PO abx, close followup indicated for healthy patient with otitis media and mild mastoid tenderness, erythema. Obtain t-bone CT to r/o abscess (if so requires IV abx's/ tympanostomy/drainage).
- Presence of opacified mastoid air cells common in otitis media, and not clinically significant unless associated symptoms of mastoiditis seen.
- Amoxicillin-clavulanate 875mg PO bid x 14d
- Cefuroxime axetil 500mg PO bid x 14d
- Clindamycin 300mg PO tid x 14d

Recurrent or complicated infection

- IV abx's, temporal bone CT, otology consultation for tympanostomy +/- mastoidectomy indicated for severe pain, recurrent infection, proptotic ear, complications (meningitis or immunocompromised)
- Duration of IV abx based on clinical improvement, and timing of tympanostomy/ mastoidectomy
- Following surgery, PO abx's given for 3-4 weeks and selection guided by surgical cultures
- Clindamycin 600mg IV q8h + cefuroxime 0.75-1.5g IV q6-8h
- Vancomycin 1g IV q12h + ceftriaxone 1-2g IV q24h
- Gatifloxacin 400mg IV/PO qd
- Ampicillin/sulbactam 1.5-3g IV q6h

IMPORTANT POINTS

- Guidelines based on author's opinion and Current Therapy in Otolaryngology-Head and Neck Surgery (6th Edition, 1998, Gates, G., Editor)
- Acute mastoiditis almost always accompanied by acute/chronic otitis media.
- Fluid in mastoid air cells on CT not acute mastoiditis unless mastoid erythema/ tenderness/fluctuance seen. Otitis media often has fluid in mastoid (middle ear is continuous with mastoid air cells).
- Fluid in mastoid air cells with mild erythema/tenderness may be managed with oral abx and close followup - low threshold for IV abx/tympanostomy for increasing pain/ fever/swelling.
- Prompt referral to otologist/otolaryngologist important for tympanostomy +/- mastoidectomy; complications are common in undertreated cases.

SELECTED READINGS

Roche M, Humphreys H, Smyth E, et al. aetiology. Clin Microbiol Infect. 2003 Aug;9(8):803-9.

Kvestad, E., Kvaerner, K. J. and Mair, I. W. Otologic facial palsy: etiology, onset, and symptom duration. Ann Otol Rhinol Laryngol 2002 Jul 111(7 Pt 1): 598-602

Luntz, M., Brodsky, A., Nusem, S., et al. Acute mastoiditis--the antibiotic era: a multicenter study. Int J Pediatr Otorhinolaryngol 2001 Jan 57(1): 1-9

Rocha, J. L., Kondo, W., Gracia, C. M., et al. Central venous sinus thrombosis following mastoiditis: report of 4 cases and literature review. Braz J Infect Dis 2000 Dec 4(6): 307-12

Lee, E. S., Chae, S. W., Lim, H. H., et al. Clinical experiences with acute mastoiditis--1988 through 1998. ." Ear Nose Throat J 2000 Nov 79(11): 884-8, 890-2

Dhooge, I. J., Vandenbussche, T. and Lemmerling, M. Value of computed tomography of the temporal bone in acute otomastoiditis. Rev Laryngol Otol Rhinol (Bord) 119(2): 91-4

MENINGITIS, ACUTE COMMUNITY-ACQUIRED BACTERIAL

Paul Auwaerter, M.D.

DIAGNOSTIC CRITERIA

- Clinical sx: neck stiffness, headache and altered mental status usually present, fever common but may be absent especially in elderly.
- Signs: Kernig's/Brudzinski's sign (present in 5% or more), nuchal rigidity (30%), jolt accentuation of headache, cranial nerve palsies or other focal neurologic findings, rash, headache, seizures + myalgia.
- LP: Perform promptly in all pts; consider CT first if focal neuro findings, papilledema, or severely depressed sensorium.
- CSF: typical results OP >30cm (nl <17cm), WBC >500/mL with >80% neutrophils, glucose <40mg/dL (or < 2/3 plasma), and protein >200mg/dL.
- Gram stain and sensitivities of blood and CSF direct later decisions.
- Other adjunctive laboratory studies: blood and CSF cultures, antigen detection (rarely helpful for adults except partially-treated meningitis), CSF PCR (viral)
- Kernig's sign - patient's leg flexed at knee and hip, straighten knee; discomfort behind the knee with full extension is a pos Kernig's sign.
- Brudzinski's sign - patient supine, flex the neck; flexion of the hips and knees is pos Brudzinski's sign.
- CSF Normal values

  OP = 5 - 15 mm Hg or 65 - 195 mm H_2O

  WBC = < 5-10 monos, no polys

  protein = 15 - 45mg/dL, may be higher in elderly

  glucose = 40 - 80 mg/dL; CSF/blood ratio > 0.6 (with abruptly high serum glucose, usual ratio is 0.3)
- See also Meningitis: Aseptic, Cryptococcal, and TB

COMMON PATHOGENS: S. pneumoniae ; N. meningitidis ; Listeria monocytogenes ; Haemophilus influenzae ; Enterococcus ; Streptococcus agalactiae (Group B) ; OVERALL INFECTION RATES by species (from 1995 U.S. data from CDC): Streptococcus pneumoniae 47%, Neisseria meningitidis 25%, Group B streptococcus 12%, Listeria monocytogenes 8%, and Haemophilus influenzae 7%, with an overall incidence of 2.4 cases per 100,000 population. (Inclusive of neonates, children and adults); Note the incidence of Haemophilus influenzae type b meningitis in children has been dramatically reduced with the introduction of the vaccine in 1986; most cases of H. influenzae meningitis are secondary to non serotype b organisms or serotype b infections in non-vaccinated children and adults.; Community-acquired INFECTION RATES with specific pathogens strongly influenced BY AGE; CHILDREN and YOUNG ADULTS 2-29 yrs: N. meningitidis 60%, S. pneumoniae 27%, group B streptococcus 5%, H. influenzae 5%, L. monocytogenes 2%. ; ADULTS 30-59 yrs: S. pneumoniae 61%, N. meningitidis 18%, H. influenzae 12%, L. monocytogenes 2%.; ADULTS >60: S. pneumoniae 61%, N. meningitidis 18%, H. influenzae 12%, L. monocytogenes 6%, Group B streptococcus 3%.

TREATMENT REGIMENS

Empiric treatment, children 3 mos. to 18 years:

- Sequencing: No focal defect & no papilledema - LP then Rx; Focal defect or papilledema - Rx then CT then LP
- Most likely are N. meningitidis, S. pneumoniae: vancomycin 15mg/kg IV q6h (up to 2g/d) plus either cefotaxime 50mg/kg IV q4-6h (max 2g IV q4h) or ceftriaxone 50-100mg/kg IV q12h (max 2g IV q12h)
- Pen/ceph allergy: chloramphenicol 1g IV q6h + vancomycin

- Other considerations: 1) dexamethasone 0.4mg/kg q12h x 2d given 30 min prior to abx; 2) rifampin

Empiric treatment, adults 18-50 and >50 years:

- Age 18-50 yrs likely etiologies = S. pneumoniae and N. meningitidis: vancomycin 1g IV q12h plus either ceftriaxone 2g IV q12h or cefotaxime 2g IV 4-6h.
- Age >50 likely etiologies = S. pneumoniae, L. monocytogenes, & GNB: amp 2g IV q4h + vanco 1g IV q12h plus either cefotaxime 2g IV q4-6h or ceftriaxone 2g IV q 24 or q12h (4g/d max)
- Pen/ceph allergy: chloramphenicol 1g IV q6h + vanco +/- rifampin 300mg PO or IV bid
- Dexamethasone (10mg IV q6h x 4d) recommended 15-20 min. prior/along side first abx infusion for suspected pneumococcal meningitis. Some would give to all cases of bacterial meningitis (controversial)
- Pen/ceph allergy: chloramphenicol 1g IV q6h + vancomycin +/- rifampin

Pathogen-specific treatment

- S. pneumoniae (pcn sens - MIC < 0.1 mcg/mL): pcn G, cefotaxime, ceftriaxone, chloramphenicol. Rx > 10 days.
- S. pneumoniae (pcn MIC > 0.1mcg/mL): vancomycin +/- rifampin
- N. meningitidis: penicillin, cefotaxime, ceftriaxone; Rx 7 days min.
- H. influenzae: cefotaxime, ceftriaxone, chloramphenicol; Rx 10 days min.
- Listeria: ampicillin +/- gentamicin, (2nd line alt. TMP-SMX). Rx 14-21 days.
- Enterobacteriaceae (E. coli, etc.): cefotaxime, ceftriaxone, meropenem, aztreonam, any +/- aminoglycoside, Rx at least 21d.
- P. aeruginosa: ceftazidime, cefepime, piperacillin, aztreonam, meropenem + aminoglycoside IV (consider intrathecal only in refractory cases).

DRUG-SPECIFIC COMMENTS

Cefotaxime: Acceptable 3rd generation cephalosporin for bacterial meningitis. Must be dosed more frequently then ceftriaxone.

Ceftriaxone: Despite being highly-protein bound, this parenteral drug is a cornerstone for the treatment of community-acquired meningitis in combination with vancomycin (to cover drug-resistant pneumococci) +/- ampicillin). Dosing ought to be 2g IV q 12h.

Meropenem: Used more commonly in pediatrics, this carbapenem has good CNS penetration and perhaps less seizure risk than imipenem. May not cover high-level PCN resistance with S. pneumoniae, so still use vancomycin. Drug probably offers more broad-spectrum than commonly needed for community-acquired meningitis; however, good choice for those with gram-negative bacilli seen on CSF gram-stain, or for those with noscomially-acquired meningitis.

Vancomycin: Standard empiric choice, despite poor CNS penetration, to cover the possibility of high-level penicillin resistant S. pneumoniae.

IMPORTANT POINTS

- Empiric choices may be narrowed by gram stain and culture and sensitivity results. Recommendations based in part on Medical Letter (1999;41:95) and author's opinion.
- Must give Abx rapidly - Main issue is sequence of CT, LP and Abx. Most cases: LP > Abx; If papilledema, non-cranial focal neurologic or severe CNS suppression: Abx > CT > LP
- CSF: Predictors of pyogenic meningitis: WBC > 2000 or PMNs > 1200; glucose < 34, protein > 220 (JAMA 1989; 262:2700)
- N. meningitidis: prophylaxis for household, daycare & intimate contacts & HCW with secretion contact (intubation etc): cipro 500mg PO x 1or rifampin 600mg q12h x 4 doses

- ONLY CLOSE CONTACTS (individuals who frequently sleep and eat in the same dwelling with an index case, e.g., family, day care contacts, boyfriend/girlfriend) of patients with H. influenzae type b or N. meningitidis should be considered for prophylaxis.
- H. influenzae prophylaxis (rifampin 20mg/kg - up to max of 600mg/d - qdx4) - considered in unvaccinated household contacts < 4years old; unvaccinated day care contacts < 2years old, multiple cases should prompt prophylaxis for all children and personnel.
- N. meningitidis prophylaxis (cipro 500mg x 1; rifampin 600mg q12h x 4 or ceftriaxone 250mg IM x 1) considered in household and daycare contacts and in others with intimate contact e.g., via kissing, mouth-to-mouth resuscitation, intubation, or nasopharyngeal aspiration.
- H. influenzae vaccine recommended in all children (0.5mL at 2, 4, 6, and 12-15 months)
- N. meningitidis vaccine (most commonly used vaccine covers serotypes A,C,Y, W-135, not B) considered if traveling to areas with epidemic meningococcal meningitis (e.g., sub-Saharan Africa, Northern India, Nepal); and with high risk: complement deficiency, asplenia, outbreaks of type C. Consider for all collegiate students in residences.
- Since dexamethasone now considered standard for pneumococcal meningitis, most patients will receive at least one dose of dexamethasone if antibiotics expeditiously administered before return of any diagnostic studies (gram stain, CSF antigen studies). Some authorities suggest not using dexamethasone when vancomycin is administered (because of concerns about impairing drug flow into CSF)

SELECTED READINGS

van de Beek D, de Gans J, McIntyre P et al. Steroids in adults with acute bacterial meningitis: a systematic review. Lancet Infect Dis. 2004 Mar;4(3):139-43

Thomas KE, Hasbun R, Jekel J, et al. The diagnostic accuracy of Kernig's sign, Brudzinski's sign, and nuchal rigidity in adults with suspected meningitis. Clin Infect Dis 2002 Jul 1;35(1):46-52

de Gans J and van de Beek D. Dexamethasone in adults with bacterial meningitis. N Eng J Med, 2002, 347 (20): 1549-1556

Hasbun R, Abrahams J, Jekel J, et al. Computed tomobgraphy of the head before lumbar puncture in adults with suspected meningitis. N Engl J Med, 2001; 345: 1727-1733

The Medical Letter, inc. The Choice of Antibacterial Drugs. The Medical Letter, 1999, Vol. 41 (Issue 1064);95-104.

Attia J, Hatala R, Cook DJ, et al. Does this patient have Acute Meningitis?. JAMA, 1999, Vol 282(2):175-81

Durand ML, Claderwood SB, Weber DJ, et al. Acute bacterial meningitis in adults: a review of 493 episodes. N Engl J Med 1993; 328: 21-8

MENINGITIS, ASEPTIC   Paul Auwaerter, M.D.

DIAGNOSTIC CRITERIA

- Annually 36,000 hospitalizations. Most commonly viral w/ enteroviruses leading cause (55-70%), mostly summer & fall
- Clinical: Fever, headache, photophobia, meningeal signs and lethargy without obtundation
- Hx Travel and exposure: rodents (LCMV, lepto); ticks (Lyme); TB; sexual activity (HSV, HIV, syphilis); epidemic (West Nile virus); IDU (HIV, endocarditis).
- Other etiologies: drug-induced meningitis (NSAIDs, co-trimoxazole), parameningeal foci (epidural abscess, epidermoid cyst), and malignancy (lymphoma, carcinoma).

- Lab: CSF - 10-<1,000 WBC typical, mostly monos (but PMNs may be seen early in course), elevated protein, glucose nl., neg culture and gram stain. Enterovirus PCR superior to cx. Consider WNV studies.

COMMON PATHOGENS: VIRUSES (enteroviruses, herpes simplex virus, West Nile virus; Other viruses (HSV is primarily Type 2, arboviruses, LCMV, mumps, influenza, paraflu, measles, EBV, CMV, HHV-6); MISC. BACTERIA (Lyme, rickettsia spp, leptospira, endocarditis, TB, brucella); Most common FUNGI (cryptococcus, coccidiodes, candida, histoplasma, blastomycosis); PARASITES (Toxoplasma gondii [more commonly encephalitic]); NONINFECTIOUS causes (Malignancy [primary, metastatic, lymphoma, leukemia], CNS vasculitis, CNS sarcoidosis, drug induced, Bechet's syndrome, benign lymphocytic); RECURRENT (Mollarets [most cases likely HSV, check HSV-PCR])

TREATMENT REGIMENS

Viral meningitides

- Supportive care for most (hydration). Observe for SIADH. Seizures rare. Progressive downhill course argues against most viral meningitis.
- Enteroviral meningitis: Pleconaril (not FDA approved and no longer available for compassionate use).
- Agammaglobulinemic pts with chronic enteroviral meningitis: IVIG-administer 350->400 mg/kg IV q3weeks to maintain serum IgG >500-800 mg/dL +/- initial intrathecal therapy.
- HSV-2 meningitis: Rx for neurologic sx, such as urinary retention or weakness: acyclovir 10 mg/kg IV q8h x 10-14d, can likely switch to valacyclovir 1g PO tid w/improvement (experience limited)
- Recurrent HSV-2 meningitis (Mollaret): prevent with acyclovir 400mg bid/tid PO, famciclovir 250mg PO bid, or valacyclovir 500mg PO qd.
- VZV meningitis: Rx compromised hosts & severe infx: acyclovir 10 mg/kg IV q8h x 10-14d.
- Acute HIV infection: HAART (See Acute Retroviral Syndrome)

Bacterial/fungal/mycobacterial meningitis

- Refer to specific pathogen or diagnosis module

IMPORTANT POINTS

- Guidelines are authors opinion
- Suspect w/ CSF WBC <500/mL, monos, protein <80. Enteroviral PCR helpful, can shorten abx administration, speed hospital discharge.
- Confusion may arise with partially treated meningitis: may Rx empirically for bacterial meningitis or preferably repeat LP in 12h off therapy.
- Dx studies should include: CSF - WBC, protein, glucose, VDRL, crypt Ag, cult +/- PCR Enterovirus, HSV, VZV; Serum Lyme, RPR as min. usual studies. Other tests per suspicions.
- Craniocervical and sinus imaging (MRI or CT) should also be performed to rule out parameningeal focus.
- Blood: VDRL and HIV RNA
- Fungi: Histo Ag blood and urine, cocci serology blood and CSF

SELECTED READINGS

Worthington MG, Ross JJ. Aseptic meningitis and acute HIV syndrome after interruption of antiretroviral therapy: implications for structured treatment interruptions. AIDS. 2003 Sep 26;17(14): 2145

Sejvar JJ, Haddad MB, Tierney BC et al. Neurologic manifestations and outcome of West Nile virus infection. JAMA. 2003 Jul 23;290(4):511-5

Ramers C, Billman G, Hartin H et al. Impact of a Diagnostic Cerebrospinal Fluid Enterovirus Polymerase Chain Reaction Test on Patient Management. JAMA. 2000;283:2680-2685

Bergstrom T, Alestig K. Treatment of primary and recurrent herpes simples virus type 2 induced meningitis with acyclovir. Scand J Infect Dis 1990;22:239

Rotbart HA, O'Connell JF, McKinlay MA. Treatment of human enterovirus infections. Antiviral Res 1998;38:1

Rotbart HA. Viral meningitis and the aseptic meningitis syndrome. In: Infections of the central nervous system (2nd ed), Scheld M, Whitley R, Durack D (Eds), Raven, New York, 1997, p23

MENINGITIS, TB
Paul Auwaerter, M.D.

DIAGNOSTIC CRITERIA

- Risk factors: age, alcoholism, HIV infection, malnutrition, drug abuse, homelessness, travel to/ residence in a country with high TB prevalence, exposure to person with pulmonary TB
- Clinical: unrelenting headache (28%), fever (13%), stiff neck (2%), lethargy, confusion, seizures (due to hydrocephalus, hyponatremia, tuberculoma, cerebral edema); cranial nerve palsies (25%)
- In children, TB meningitis often presents with personality change, irritability, signs and symptoms of increased intracranial pressure, and seizures
- CSF: high opening pressure, lymphocytic pleiocytosis (10-500 cells/mm3), high protein (100-500 mg/dL), low glucose (35-45mg/dL), AFB smear (+) in 10-40%; culture (+) in 30-88%; > 1 LP sample raises yield.
- Studies: labs-hyponatremia from SIADH; CXR-pulmonary TB in 25-55% adults (50-90% children); PPD unreactive in >25% , CT/MRI Brain may show meningeal enhancement, hydrocephalus, tuberculoma, infarct

COMMON PATHOGENS: Mycobacterium tuberculosis

TREATMENT REGIMENS

Adult antitubercular therapy

- Four-drug daily therapy: isoniazid 300mg qd (+ pyridoxine 50mg qd), rifampin 600mg qd, pyrazinamide 15-30mg/kg/d or 2.0g qd max, and ethambutol 15-25mg/kg/day.
- Streptomycin 15mg/kg/day (max 1g) can be used in place of ethambutol
- ETB may be discontinued, if INH and RIF susceptible, due to poor CSF penetration. Ethionamide may be substituted for ETB.
- The optimum length of tx unknown, though 9-12mos Rx common. Some suggest in uncomplicated TBM, rifampin and isoniazid for 12 mos after initial 8-wk four-drug therapy if organism pan-sensitive.
- With HIV co-infection, always treat active TB immediately. If on HAART, add TB drugs and modify HAART for drug interactions with rifampin. If HIV untreated + CD4 greater than 200, delay HAART 2 wks – 2 months RIF can be given with EFV but not NVP or any PI.

Pediatric antitubercular therapy

- Initiate with: 1) isoniazid 10-15mg/kg/day (max 300mg qd); 2) rifampin 10-20mg/kg/day (max 600mg qd); 3) pyrazinamide 30mg/kg/day (max 2g qd); 4) streptomycin 20-40mg/kg/day (max 1g qd); 5) pyridoxine 50mg q
- Streptomycin can be stopped if CSF antimicrobial susceptibility testing reveals that the isolate is susceptible to isoniazid, rifampin and pyrazinamide
- Pyrazinamide usually discontinued after 2 months of therapy.

- American Academy of Pediatrics recommends a 12-month regimen

Other nonantimicrobial therapy

- The use adjunctive corticosteroids remains somewhat controversial due to small study sizes. See 2003 MMWR statement in reference section.
- Corticosteroids recommended especially with decreased level of consciousness
- Recommended: dexamethasone 8 mg/day for children (< 25 kg) and 12 mg/day (if >25 kg or more and for adults x 3 wks, then taper over 3wks (6wk total).

IMPORTANT POINTS

- Diagnosis is dependent upon CSF smear and culture. The yield can be increased by doing multiple, large volume (>10mL) LPs for mycobacterial culture
- As smear and culture of CSF may be negative and delay in treatment can result in death or substantial morbidity, empirical therapy should be initiated if there is a high index of clinical suspicion.
- The purpose of oral pyridoxine is to prevent the neuropathy associated with isoniazid
- Please refer to the general TB module for information on adverse effects of TB drugs and for advice on the management of multidrug-resistant TB.
- Hydrocephalus is a common complication that if left untreated may lead to permanent neurological damage. Close monitoring by repeated cranial imaging (to evaluate change in ventricular size) and LPs (with OP measurement) is advocated. Early drainage by ventriculoatrial or ventriculoperitoneal shunt has been advised.

SELECTED READINGS

Thwaites GE, Bang ND, Dung NH et al. Dexamethasone for the treatment of tuberculous meningitis in adolescents and adults. NEJM 2004;351: 1741-51

Pai M, Flores LL, Pai N et al. Diagnostic accuracy of nucleic acid amplification tests for tuberculous meningitis: a systematic review and meta-analysis. Lancet Infect Dis. 2003 Oct;3(10):633-43

American Thoracic Society, CDC and Infectious Disease Society of America. Treatment of Tuberculosis. MMWR June 20, 2003 / 52(RR11);1-77

Roos KL. Mycobacterium tuberculosis meningitis and other etiologies of the aseptic meningitis syndrome. Seminars in Neurology 2000;20(3):329-335

Thwaites G, Chau TTH, Mai NTH, et al. Tuberculous meningitis. J Neurol Neurosurg Psychiatry 2000;68:289-299

Prasad K, Volmink J, Menon GR. Steroids for treating tuberculous meningitis. Cochrane Database Syst Rev 2000;(3):CD002244

Starke JR. Tuberculosis of the central nervous system in children. Semin Pediatr Neurol 1999;6:318-331

Joint Tuberculosis Committee of the British Thoracic Society. Chemotherapy and management of tuberculoiss in the United Kingdom: recommendations 1998. Thorax 1998;53:536-548

Schoeman JF, Van Zyl LE, Laubscher JA, et al. Effect of corticosteroids on intracranial pressure, computed tomographic findings and clinical outcome in young children with tuberculous meningitis. Paediatrics 1997;99:226-31

Dooley DP, Carpenter JL, Radenader S. Adjunctive corticosteroid therapy for tuberculosis: a critical reappraisal of the literature. Clin Infect Dis 1997;25(4):872-887

MYCOBACTERIUM AVIUM BACTEREMIA [HIV]

John G. Bartlett, M.D.

DIAGNOSTIC CRITERIA

- Clinical: CD4 <50/mm^3, fever, night sweats, weight loss +/- diarrhea, abdominal pain, marrow suppression, hepatitis &/or adenopathy. Pancytopenia common.

- Avg CD4 is 10-20/mm^3; nearly always <50/mm^3
- Lab: positive cultures from blood or other normally sterile site, e.g., marrow, lymph node, or liver; cx AFB request.
- Blood cx usually requires 5d-3wks to grow MAC; biopsy of normally sterile tissue may establish dx earlier, e.g., marrow, LN, liver, etc.
- Sputum & stool are unreliable cx sources; growth of MAC from these sites not dx of either local or disseminated disease due to high colonization rates.

Treatment Regimens

Antimicrobial agents

- Principles: suspect if FUO + CD4 <50 + fever & wt loss. Dx: (+) blood cx, but takes 1-2wks. Rx until CD4 >100 x 6mos, or Rx >12 mos & asymptomatic.
- Preferred: Clarithromycin 500mg PO bid + ethambutol 15mg/kg/d + rifabutin 300mg/d indefinitely
- Alternative: Azithromycin 500mg/d + ethambutol 15mg/kg/d +/- rifabutin (above doses) indefinitely
- Refractory/recurrent: clarithromycin/azithromycin + ethambutol + either rifabutin + ciprofloxacin 500-750mg PO bid or levofloxacin 500mg/d PO or amikacin 10-15mg/kg/d IV.
- Drug interactions: w/clari & rifabutin see below

Antiretroviral agents + clarithro or rifabutin

- Clarithromycin: EFV decreases clari levels 40% (clinical sig. unk.); standard dose other PIs. Clari + rifabutin: decrease clari 50%; consider azithro: no interactions with HAART or rifabutin (RBT)
- RBT: Efavirenz (standard) + rifabutin 450-600mg/d
- RBT: Ritonavir + any PI - standard PI dose + RBT 150mg qod
- RBT: Atazanavir (standard) + ribavirin 150mg qod or 3x/wk
- RBT: Nevirapine (standard) + rifabutin (300mg/d)
- RBT: Indinavir 1000mg q8h + rifabutin 150mg qd
- RBT: Nelfinavir 1000mg tid or 1250mg bid + rifabutin 150mg qd
- RBT: Fosamprenavir (standard) + rifabutin 150mg qd
- RBT: Kaletra (standard) + rifabutin 150mg qod

Miscellaneous issues

- Systemic complaints (fever, myalgias, headache, etc)--ibuprofen, Tylenol, ASA, etc.
- Diarrhea--loperamide or lomotil
- Immune reconstitution syndrome: continue HAART and MAC therapy + NSAIDS; prednisone 20-40mg/day if necessary
- Stop rules: CD4 >100 x >6mo + MAC Rx >12 mo + asymptomatic
- Restart: CD4 <100

Drug-Specific Comments

Amikacin: Active in vitro vs. MAC. Main problems are parenteral administration, marginal data to document in vivo efficacy, toxicity and cost. Main use is when other options have failed.

Azithromycin: Favored for MAC prophylaxis but clarithromycin is generally preferred for treatment - it is a close call.

Clarithromycin: The most important agent for therapy of MAC, but must be combined with ethambutol to prevent resistance. Clarithromycin-resistant MAC may complicate therapy or prophylaxis with this drug. Usually not combined with rifabutin due to drug interaction with reduced clari levels by 50%. Nevertheless the CDC guidelines endorse clari + eth + rifabutin as a rational combination. IDV, SQV, RTV increase clari levels 45-73%, but no dose adjustment recommended. No problems with azithro.

Rifabutin: Sometimes used in combination with azithromycin + ethambutol or clarithro + ethambutol. Mortality benefit in one trial. May protect against macrolide resistance. Note dose adjustments when used with PIs or NNRTIs.

IMPORTANT POINTS

- Guidelines from NYS AIDS Institute and CDC/MMWR 2004;RR15:1-112.
- MAC common in immunocompetent pts w/lung only; AIDS pts get bacteremia & involvement of lymph nodes, liver, spleen, marrow & small bowel, usually not lung
- MAC occurs in >50% of patients with late stage HIV w/o proph
- Susceptibility tests: not helpful except with clarithromycin
- Rifabutin: adjust dose with PI & NNRTI (see Treatment Regimens)
- No isolation required.
- Treatment is with multiple agents: 2-3 directed against MAC and 3-4 antiretroviral agents.

SELECTED READINGS

Benson C, et al. US Public Health Service - Infectious Diseases Society of America (IDSA) guidelines for the treatment of opportunistic infections in adults and adolescents infected with HIV. Clin Infect Dis 2004 (in press)

Karakousis PC, et al. Mycobacterium avium complex in patients with HIV infection in the era of HAART. Lancet Infect Dis 2004;4:557-65

Green H, et al. A prospective multicenter study of discontinuing prophylaxis for opportunistic infections after effective anti-retroviral therapy. HIV Med 2004;5:278-83

Ward TT, Rimland D, Kauffman C, et al. Randomized open-label trial of azithromycin plus ethambutol vs. clarithromycin plus ethambutol as therapy for MAC bacteremia in patients with AIDS. Clin Infect Dis 1998;27:1278

Chaisson RE, Benson CA, Dube MP et al. Clarithromycin therapy for bacteremic Mycobacterium avium complex disease. Ann Intern Med 1994;121:905

Cohn DL. A prospective randomized trial of four three-drug regimens in the treatment of disseminated MAC disease in AIDS patients. Clin Infect Dis 1999;29:125

Benson CA, Williams PL, Cohn DL, et al. Clarithromycin or rifabutin alone or in combination for primary prophylaxis of MAC disease in patients with AIDS. J Infect Dis 2000;181:1289

Currier JS et al. Discontinuation of Mycobacterium avium complex prophylaxis in patients with antiretroviral therapy-induced increases in CD4 cell count: A randomized, double-blind, placebo-controlled trial. Ann Intern Med 2000; 133:493

Liao CH, et al. Discontinuation of secondary prophylaxis in AIDS patients with disseminated non-tuberculous mycobacteria infection. J Microbiol Immunol Infect 2004;51:50-6

Aberg JA, Yajko, DM, Jacobson MP. Eradication of AIDS-related disseminated Mycobacterium avium complex infection after 12 months of antimycobacterial therapy combined with highly active antiretroviral therapy. J Infect Dis 1998;178:1446

MYELITIS
Paul Auwaerter, M.D.

DIAGNOSTIC CRITERIA

- Inflammation of spinal cord, often immune-mediated; many cases are idiopathic. Often called transverse myelitis (TM).
- May be related to infection, idiopathic or associated with existing inflammatory dz, e.g., SLE, MS, Sjogren's, sarcoid.

Diagnosis

- Sx: leg weakness, sphincter dysfunction, abnl DTR's [acutely may be absent, but hyperreflexia the rule]. Sensory level helps distinguish from polio/Guillain-Barre (GB).
- May be confused w/ acute inflammatory demyelinating polyradiculoneuropathy (AIDP) or GB. R/o compressive or vascular explanation, tropical spastic paraparesis (HTLV-I) or vacuolar myelopathy (HIV).
- Dx: MRI, LP incl VDRL, AFB & fungal cx, PCR (HSV, VZV, CMV, EBV, enteroviral); Lyme serology; ?Schisto serology or O&P if exposure hx

Common Pathogens: Varicella-zoster virus ; Herpes Simplex Virus ; Cytomegalovirus ; Epstein-Barr Virus ; Enteroviruses ; Mycobacterium tuberculosis ; Treponema pallidum (syphilis) ; Borrelia burgdorferi ; Mycoplasma pneumoniae ; Schistosoma species

Treatment Regimens

General principles

- Consult w/ neurology. Usual ID consult question is to r/o infectious etiology. Note that post-infectious TM described with measles, mumps, rubella and post-URI viral illness.
- Cases may be parainfectious, but many idiopathic
- Idiopathic/inflammatory TM may be treated with steroids, plasma exchange, cyclophosphamide.
- If infection diagnosed, consider therapy for specific agent (see Specific Pathogens). Corticosteroids often considered helping quell inflammation.

Infectious-related myelitis

- See pathogen-specific module for detailed therapy
- Common infectious etiologies listed in common pathogen section.

Important Points

- Polio may be similar to TM w/ flaccid paralysis, but lack sensory findings.
- Most cases idiopathic or inflammatory; however, need to rule-out infectious etiology, HIV or HTLV1 associated process.
- CSF examination and PCR for viruses helpful. Occasionally, serologies helpful (EBV, Schisto, CMV, HTLV1). Obtain HIV EIA.
- CMV-related myelitis (or radiculopathy) in HIV often associated w/ impressive neutrophilic CSF pleiocytosis. Strong consideration should be made to initiating HAART in all HIV CMV myelitis cases.
- Treatment recommendations from Front Biosci. 2004 May 01;9:1483-99 (see refs).

Selected Readings

Krishnan C, Kaplin AI, Deshpande DM, et al. Transverse Myelitis: pathogenesis, diagnosis and treatment. Front Biosci. 2004 May 01;9:1483-99

Gilden D. Varicella zoster virus and central nervous system syndromes. Herpes. 2004 Jun;11 Suppl 2:89A-94A

Di Rocco A. Diseases of the spinal cord in human immunodeficiency virus infection. Semin Neurol. 1999;19(2):151-5

Jeffery DR, Mandler RN, Davis LE. Transverse myelitis. Retrospective analysis of 33 cases, with differentiation of cases associated with multiple sclerosis and parainfectious events. Arch Neurol. 1993 May;50(5):532-5

Haribhai HC, Bhigjee AI, Bill PL., et al. Spinal cord schistosomiasis. A clinical, laboratory and radiological study, with a note on therapeutic aspects. Brain. 1991 Apr;114 (Pt 2):709-26

MYOCARDITIS

Richard Nettles, M.D.

DIAGNOSTIC CRITERIA

- Clinical symptoms: Asymptomatic vs. fever, malaise, arthralgia, dyspnea, palpitations, precordial discomfort, upper respiratory symptoms.
- Clinical signs: prolonged elevation of CK-MB and Troponin T levels, fever, cardiomegaly, mitral/tricuspid murmurs, ECG abnormalities (ST/T wave change, heart block, dysrhythmias), shock, heart failure
- Radiographic data: chest XR-cardiomegaly; echocardiogram-change over time in movement and function; MRI-edema; Indium 111-labelled antimyosin antibody imaging-abnormal.
- Endomyocardial biopsy: early biopsies may be more sensitive, serial biopsies can help diagnosis, Dallas criteria includes myocyte necrosis and lymphocytic infiltration.
- Isolation of organism: viral isolation can be difficult, viral serum antibody titers can aid diagnosis, as can molecular techniques. Lyme serologies useful in endemic areas.

COMMON PATHOGENS: Infectious Causes of Myocarditis (from Mandell Principles & Practice of Infectious Diseases); VIRAL: coxsackie A or B, echoviruses, HIV, polio, mumps, rubeola, influenza A or B, rabies, rubella, dengue, lymphocytic choriomeningitis, adenovirus, varicella zoster, CMV, EBV, vaccinia, hepatitis B or C, RSV, parvovirus B19, yellow fever.; BACTERIAL/rickettsial: C. diphtheriae, C. perfringens, S pyogenes, N. meningitidis, Salmonella, Brucella, S. aureus, Listeria, Legionella, Mycoplasma, Chlamydia, Rickettsia, Ehrlichia, Vibrio cholerae, Borrelia burgdorferi; FUNGI: Aspergillus, Candida, Cryptococcus; PARASITES: T. cruzi, T. gambiense, T. rhodesiense, T. spiralis, T. gondii

TREATMENT REGIMENS

Viral myocarditis

- Supportive therapy: bed rest, intravascular volume control, arrhythmia management, heart failure management
- Corticosteroids: very controversial role in treatment of viral myocarditis. Some recommend in later course of illness if progressive left ventricular dysfunction exists.
- Cytomegalovirus Myocarditis: Ganciclovir can be used for severe CMV myocarditis
- Cardiac Transplantation: may be necessary in severe cases, however, the majority of cases resolve without further sequelae.
- Experimental Therapy includes hyperimmunoglobulin and interferon therapy.
- HIV-associated myocarditis: HAART & ACE inhibitors; steroids are controversial; consider neoplastic or secondary infectious cause (T. gondii, M. tuberculosis, C. neoformans, CMV)

Lyme myocarditis

- For first-degree heart block (PR interval >0.3 seconds): Doxycycline 100mg PO bid, or amoxicillin 500 250mg PO qid x 21-28 days.
- High-degree atrio-ventricular block: Ceftriaxone 2g IV qd x 14-28d or penicillin G 20 mU IV (divided q6h) x 28d + cardiac monitoring.
- Complete Heart Block is reversible, therefore permanent pacemaker not usually recommended.
- After 24 hrs of antibiotics, if complete heart block or heart failure does not improve, some recommend corticosteroid therapy.
- Myocarditis is a rare complication of Lyme disease. Chronic complications or death are extremely rare.

IMPORTANT POINTS

- Most patients with viral myocarditis recover completely

339

- Corticosteroid use is very controversial, especially in acute phase of myocarditis (possible rapid clinical deterioration). Randomized controlled trials are needed.
- Noninfectious causes: collagen vascular disease, thyrotoxicosis, TTP, peripartum, radiation induced, drug induced, pheochromocytoma, giant cell myocarditis, sarcoid, Kawasaki disease, insect bites
- NSAIDs are not effective, and may be detrimental in myocarditis
- Vaccinia-related myocarditis: incidence after smallpox vaccination is about 1:15,000. In certain cases, steroids or vaccinia immune globulin (CDC,404-639-3670) may be useful.

SELECTED READINGS

Halsell JS, Riddle JR, Atwood JE, et al. Myopericarditis following smallpox vaccination among vaccinia-naive US military personnel. JAMA. 289 (24). June 25 2003. pp. 3283-9.

Rotbart AH, Webster AD. Treatment of Potentially Life-Threatening Enterovirus Infections with Pleconaril. Clin Infect Dis. 32, 2001, pp.228-35

MERIT-HF Study Group. Effect of metoprolol CR/XL in chronic heart failure: metoprolol CR/XL randomized intervention trial in congestive heart failure (MERIT-HF). Lancet. 353, 1999. pp. 2001-7

Steere AC. Lyme Disease. N Engl J Med. 345 (2), July, 2001, pp. 115-25

Tayal SC, Ghosh SK, and Reaich D. Asymptomatic HIV patient with Cardiomyopathy and Nephropathy: Case report and Literature Review. J Infect. 42(4), May. 2001. pp. 288-90

Wormser GP, Nadelman RB, Dattwyler RJ, et al. Practice guidelines for the treatment of Lyme disease. Clin Infect Dis. 31, 2000, pp.s1-s14

NG TTC, Morris DJ, Wilkins EGL. Successful Diagnosis and Management of Cytomegalovirus Carditis. J Infection, 34, 1997, pp. 243-247.

Mason JW, O'connell JB, Herskowitz A, et al. A Clinical Trial of Immunosuppressive Therapy for Myocarditis. N Engl J Med. 333, August, 1995, pp. 269-275

Levy WS, Varghese J, Anderson D, et al. Myocarditis diagnosed by endomyocardial biopsy in HIV infection with cardiac dysfunction. AM J Cardiol 62, 1988, pp. 658-9

The SOLVD Investigators. Effect of enalapril on survival in patients with left ventricular ejection fractions and congestive heart failure. N Engl J Med. 325, 1991, pp. 293-302

NECROTIZING FASCIITIS John G. Bartlett, M.D.

DIAGNOSTIC CRITERIA

- Infection extending along fascial plane--usually extremity, perianal area, genitals (Fournier's).
- Clinical: severe pain, severe systemic toxicity, rapid spread, fever, skin necrosis with bullae, tense edema &/or black-blue discoloration.
- Lab: CT scan or MRI showing fascial plane infection.
- 2 major bacterial patterns--group A strep or mixed anaerobes + coliforms; distinguish by GS & cx of exudate, bullae, aspirate or blood
- Pus with anaerobic infection is "dishwater gray," has a characteristic putrid smell & Gram stain/culture of pus shows mixed flora.

COMMON PATHOGENS: Mixed aerobic-anaerobic bacteria ; Clostridium perfringens ; Group A strep ; MRSA (USA 300 strains)

TREATMENT REGIMENS

Antibiotic treatment

- Principles: Dx by CT/MRI or surg incision, need surgery now, abx vs. strep (clind) or anaerobes + coliforms (intra-abd sepsis regimens)

- Preferred: Mixed infection with coliforms + anaerobes - cefotaxime 2-4g IV q 8h + either clind 600mg IV q8h or metronidazole 2g/d IV/PO
- Alternative: Ampicillin + sulbactam 1.5-3g IV q6h or pip-tazo (Zosyn) or ticar-clav (Timentin) or imipenem 1-2 g/d
- Group A strep--clindamycin 600mg IV q8h + penicillin 2-4 mU IV q4h
- See Table 8 in Appendix I

Surgery--mandatory

- Incision + debridement
- May require daily re-op

Other treatment

- Toxic-shock (strep): IVIG (>2 batches: some use 50g/dose, others 0.4g/kg q6h)
- Hyperbaric O2--merit is debated. Problem is transfer of seriously ill patient & uncertain benefit. A possible benefit is that physicians at hyperbaric facilities often know a great deal about the management of serious soft tissue infections--especially the need for extensive & repeated surgery.
- Supportive care--hydration, treatment of renal failure, wound care.
- Modify antibiotic regimen when the pathogen is defined: 1) strep--clindamycin + penicillin, 2) mixed anaerobes + coliforms--regimen for intra-abdominal sepsis
- Infection control--Some consider Gr A strep transferable to family members, household contacts & healthcare workers, but risk is small.

DRUG-SPECIFIC COMMENTS

Ampicillin + Sulbactam: Good activity against all anaerobes and many coliforms. May prefer ticarcillin-clavulanate or piperacillin-tazobactam to increase coverage vs. GNB.

Clindamycin: Preferred for strep infections characterized by toxin production because it stops protein synthesis. Penicillin acts only against replicating bacteria.

Imipenem/Cilastatin: Good activity against all anticipated pathogens.

Penicillin: Active vs all strep, but does not stop toxin production like clindamycin does.

Piperacillin + Tazobactam: Good activity against all anticipated pathogens.

Ticarcillin + Clavulanic Acid: Good activity against all anticipated pathogens.

IMPORTANT POINTS

- Recommendations are based on author's opinion.
- Immediate Rx: 1) initiate abx vs. strep (clind +/- pen) & anaerobes + coliforms (regimens for intra-abd sepsis), 2) need surgeon, 3) if time available--CT scan or MRI to define lesion.
- 2 major complications with strep--rapid extension with necrosis & toxic shock syndrome.
- Causes for alarm with soft tissue infection: 1) severe pain, 2) systemic toxicity, 3) bullae, 4) cutaneous necrosis, 5) gas in tissue, 6) tense edema.

SELECTED READINGS

Wong CH, et al. Necrotizing fasciitis: clinical presentation, microbiology and determinants of mortality. J. Bone Joint Surg Am 2003;85:1454

Stevens, DL. Streptococcal toxic shock syndrome associated with necrotizing fasciitis. Annu Rev Med 2000;51:271

Kimura AC, et al. Outbreak of necrotizing fasciitis due to Clostridium sordelli among black tar heroin users. Clin Infect Dis 2004;38:87-91

Wong CH, et al. The LRINC(Laboratory Risk Indicator for Necrotizing Fasciitis) score: a tool for distinguishing necrotizing fasciitis from other soft tissue infections. Crit. Care Med 2004;32:1618-9

DIAGNOSIS

Laupland KB, et al. Intravenous immunoglobulin for severe infection: A survey of Canadian specialists. J. Crit Care 2004;19:75-81

Schmid MR, Kossman T, Duewell S. Differentiation of necrotizing fasciitis and cellulitis using MRI imaging. Am J Roentgen 1998;170:613.

Walshaw CF, Deans H. CT findings in necrotizing fasciitis--a report of 4 cases. Clin Radiol 1996;51:429.

O'Brien K, Beall B, Barrett NL, et al. Epidemiology of invasive group A streptococcus disease in the United States, 1995-1999. Clin Infect Dis 2002;35:268

Chen JL et al. Necrotizing fasciitis associated with injection drug use. CID 2001;33:6

Rea WJ, Wyrick WJ, Jr. Necrotizing fasciitis. Ann Surg 1970;72:957

OCULAR KERATITIS
Khalil G. Ghanem, M.D.

DIAGNOSTIC CRITERIA

- Keratitis=inflammation of cornea; ~50% of cases are infectious (~80% bacterial). Epithelium of cornea and conjunctiva continuous- same agents can cause both diseases.
- Signs/Symptoms: pain, +/- decreased vision, tearing, photophobia, blepharospasm; loss of transparency, ulcerated epithelium, stromal inflammation & keratolysis (loss of substance) & corneal scar/tear
- Exam: topical anesthetic, slit lamp [inflammation +/- hypopyon (WBC in anterior chamber), hyphema, synechiae, & glaucoma]; w/ advanced disease: endophthalmitis.
- Lab: corneal scrapings (multiple samples for gram, giemsa, AFB,& GMS stains & culture) ; corneal bx (in nonsuppurative cases); if no dx, then therapeutic keratoplasty for dx & Rx.
- Gram stain: diagnostic accuracy is 75% if 1 organism & only ~35% if >1 organism.

COMMON PATHOGENS: Gram-positive cocci ; Gram-positive bacilli ; Mycobacteria ; Spirochetes ; Varicella-zoster virus ; Fusarium ; Onchocerca

TREATMENT REGIMENS

Antimicrobial agents

- Routes of administration: solutions, subconjunctival, continuous lavage, hydrophilic contact lenses.
- All the following choices are ophthalmic solutions except where specifically noted
- While awaiting cx data, & if suspect bacterial cause, start broad (cephalosporin & aminoglycoside) & narrow spectrum later.
- Gram-positives: cephalosporin (cefazolin) or topical vancomycin (if resistant) for Staph; PCN-G for S. pneumo.
- Gram-negatives: aminoglycosides [gentamicin (0.3%-1.5%), amikacin, tobramycin], ciprofloxacin 0.3%, norfloxacin 0.3% & ofloxacin 0.3%.
- Antifungals: AmphoB 1.5mg/mL; Fluconazole solution; Chlorhexidine gluconate 0.2%; natamycin (not available in US); Oral antifungals often necessary depending on infection.
- Acanthamoeba: polyhexamethylene biguanide; chlorhexadine gluconate or hexamidine + surgery; length of antibiotic Rx: 3-4 weeks. Onchocerciasis: PO Ivermectin.
- Herpes: debridement + Trifluridine or Acyclovir opth soln X 10 days+ corticosteroids for stromal keratitis; consider Acyclovir 400mg PO BID X 1yr to prevent recurrence.

• Duration of therapy depends on disease: frequent slit lamp exams necessary. Early on, frequent (q30min) applications necessary: hospitalization for mod to severe dz strongly recommended.

Other modalities

• Steroids Ophthalmic Solution: controversial in bacterial keratitis excpt in syphilis and lyme; avoid in fungal keratitis; very effective for HSV stromal keratitis.
• Keratoplasty-adjunct in severe bacterial dz; frequently necessary w/ acanthamoeba to remove cysts.

IMPORTANT POINTS

• Infectious keratitis can lead to blindness; IMMEDIATE ophtho consult is mandatory and hospitalization strongly recommended in moderate to severe cases to monitor for corneal perforation.
• Interpretation of MIC resistance patterns should take into account the VERY HIGH concentrations of drug that can be achieved using OS.
• Contact lens-associated keratitis: in addition to Pseudomonas, one must consider Acanthamoeba in this setting.

SELECTED READINGS

Martins EN, et al. Infectious keratitis: correlation between corneal and contact lens cultures. CLAO J 2002 Jul;28(3):146-8

Wilhelmus KR. Indecision about corticosteroids for bacterial keratitis: an evidence-based update. Ophthalmology 2002 May;109(5):835-42

Alexandrakis G, et al. Corneal biopsy in the management of progressive microbial keratitis. Am J Ophthalmol 2000 May;129(5):571-6

Herpetic Eye Disease Study Group. Oral acyclovir for herpes simplex virus eye disease: effect on prevention of epithelial keratitis and stromal keratitis. Herpetic Eye Disease Study Group. Arch Ophthalmol 2000 Aug;118(8):1030-6

Wilhelmus K. R, et al. Acyclovir for the Prevention of Recurrent Herpes Simplex Virus Eye Disease . N Engl J Med 1998; 339:300-306, Jul 30, 1998

Kumar R, Lloyd D. Recent advances in the treatment of Acanthamoeba keratitis. Clin Infect Dis 2002 Aug 15;35(4):434-41

Parmar P, et al. Pneumococcal keratitis: a clinical profile. Clin Experiment Ophthalmol 2003 Feb;31 (1):44-7

Freitas D, et al. An outbreak of Mycobacterium chelonae infection after LASIK. Ophthalmology 2003 Feb;110(2):276-85

Ohashi Y. Treatment of herpetic keratitis with acyclovir: benefits and problems. Ophthalmologica 1997;211 Suppl 1:29-32

Chynn EW, et al. Acanthamoeba keratitis. Contact lens and noncontact lens characteristics. Ophthalmology 1995 Sep;102(9):1369-73

ONYCHOMYCOSIS
Ciro R. Martins, M.D.

DIAGNOSTIC CRITERIA

• PE: separation of the nail plate(s) from the nail bed; thickening and/or destruction and/or discoloration of the nail plate(s); accumulation of debris and keratotic material under nail(s).
• PE: one, several or all fingernails and/or toenails affected. Toenail infections are much more common.
• PE: affected nails may be tender, especially if the periungual tissue inflamed or secondarily infected by Candida (paronychia).

DIAGNOSIS

- Dx: KOH prep subungueal keratotic debris, scales from underside of affected portion of nail or nail clippings showing septated hyphae (dermatophytes) or yeasts (candida).
- Dx: fungal cx in Sabouraud's medium of nail clippings and/or subungual scrapings is more sensitive than KOH prep

COMMON PATHOGENS: Trichophyton rubrum ; Trichophyton mentagrophytes

TREATMENT REGIMENS

Systemic therapy

- Terbinafine (Lamisil) 250mg PO qd x 6 wk (fingernails) or x 12 wk (toenails). Durable 1 yr response rate 42-60%.
- Itraconazole (Sporanox) 100mg PO bid or 200mg PO qd x 8 wk (fingernails) or x 12 wk (toenails). Pulse regimen: 200mg PO bid x 1 wk per mo, for 2 mos (fingernails) or 3 mos (toenails).
- Fluconazole (Diflucan) 150-300mg PO q wk x 6-12 mos (until complete nail growth)
- Griseofulvin microsize caps (Grifulvin v) 750-1000mg PO qd x 6-9 mos (fingernails) or x 12-18 mos (toenails)
- Griseofulvin ultramicrosize (Gris-PEG) 250mg PO tid x 4-6 mos (fingernails) or x 8-12 mos (toenails)

Topical therapy

- Topical medications are not curative
- Ciclopirox 8% (Penlac) nail lacquer topically bid x 48 wks. Response rate at 1 yr 5-20%.
- Naftifine (Naftin) gel topically bid
- Urea 40% gel applied to the nails qHS in conjunction with the above topicals

Adjuvant measures

- Clipping free and detached nail borders, filing down excessive thickness of nail plate using an emery board weekly.
- Urea 40% cream (Carmol 40) on nail under occlusion every night followed by mechanical curettage of the softened nail plate. It is important to protect the periungueal tissue with tape or vaseline.
- After systemic treatment completed, pts should be encouraged to discard old shoes, especially the ones worn without socks to prevent recurrences.
- Topical antifungal powders applied to socks and shoes daily, helps decrease recurrences after successful treatment is achieved.

DRUG-SPECIFIC COMMENTS

Griseofulvin: Not as effective as the newer oral antifungals and treatment duration is extremely long. Significant list of side effects and adverse reactions.

Ketoconazole: Poor choice. Long treatment duration and risks of potentially serious liver toxicity. Significant drug interactions.

Terbinafine: Excellent choice. Baseline and monthly liver function tests and CBC are needed. Very few drug interactions and very well tolerated. Relatively short treatment duration. Expensive.

IMPORTANT POINTS

- These guidelines are based on the guidelines of the American Academy of Dermatology
- More than 80% onychomycosis caused by dermatophytes, but other agents possible: Candida albicans and, rarely, non-dermatophyte molds such as Scopulariopsis, Acremonium, etc.
- Incidence of onychomycosis increases with old age; up to 48% of those over 70 yrs affected.

- Susceptibility to acquiring onychomycosis appears to be genetically determined. Susceptible individuals have frequent recurrences and less than optimal response to treatment.
- DDx: traumatic nail dystrophies, psoriasis, lichen planus, contact dermatitis due to nail polish, Darier's disease, Reiter's syndrome and crusted ("Norwegian") scabies.
- Systemic treatment should be weighed against potential for hepatitis.

SELECTED READINGS

Crawford F, Young P, Godfrey BA et al. Oral Treatments for Toenail Onychomycosis - A Systematic Review. Arch Derm 2002; 138:811-6

Kejda J. Itraconazole pulse therapy vs continuous terbinafine dosing for toenail onychomycosis. Postgraduate Medicine - Special Report - Update on Superficial Fungal Infections, 12-16, July 1999

Scher R.K. Onychomycosis: Therapeutic Update. Journal of the American Academy of Dermatology, 40 (6) part 2, supplement, S21-6, June 1999

Drake L.A.,Dinehart S.M. et al. Guidelines of Care for Superficial Mycotic Infections of the Skin: Onychomycosis. Guidelines of Care - Dermatology World Supplement, American Academy of Dermatology, 27-32, April 1995

OPPORTUNISTIC INFECTION PROPHYLAXIS [HIV]

John G. Bartlett, M.D.

DIAGNOSTIC CRITERIA

- Indications based on CD4 count, PPD, toxo serology & hx of OI's.
- Primary prophylaxis: (no hx of infection) PCP, toxo, TB, MAC, VZV, influenza, HBV, HAV, S. pneumo
- Secondary prophylaxis: hx of prior PCP, toxo, MAC, crypt, CMV, histo, cocci, HSV, candida
- "Stop" guidelines - may stop prophylaxis with durable immune reconstitution

COMMON PATHOGENS: Pneumocystis carinii ; Mycobacterium avium complex ; Mycobacterium tuberculosis ; Toxoplasma gondii

TREATMENT REGIMENS

Primary prophylaxis

- PCP - indications: AIDS, when CD4 <200 or thrush. STOP: CD4 when >200 x 3 mos.
- PCP - preferred: TMP-SMX 1DS/d or 1SS/d. ALT: dapsone 100mg/d; aerosolized pentamidine 300mg q mo; atovaquone 1500mg/d, or dapsone 50qd + pyrimeth 50mg/wk + folinic acid 25mg/wk (also rx's toxo)
- TOXO - indications: CD4 <100 + toxo IgG. STOP: CD4 >200 x 3mos.
- TOXO - preferred: TMP-SMX 1 DS/d; ALT: TMP-SMX 1 SS/d, dapsone + pyrimeth + folinic acid (above) or atovaquone 1500mg/d +/- pyrimeth 25mg/d + folinic acid 10mg/d.
- TB - indication: PPD >5mm induration or exposure
- TB - preferred: INH 300mg/d + pyridoxine 50mg/d x 9 mo, or INH 900mg PO + pyrid 100mg 2x/wk x 9 mo, or rifampin x 4 mo.
- TB alternate: Rifampin 600mg/d x 4mo
- MAC - indications: CD4 <50. STOP: CD4 >100 x 3 mos.
- MAC - preferred: azithro 1200mg/wk or clarithromycin 500mg bid; ALT: RBT 300mg/d or azithro + RBT

- VZV - indications: significant exposure to chicken pox or shingles in pts with no prior hx or negative VZV Ab. VZV exposure prophylaxis: VZIG, 5 vials (1.25mL each) IM within 96 hours of exposure.

Prophylactic vaccines

- Pneumovax indications: CD4 >200; give 0.5mL x 1, repeat at 5 years
- Hepatitis B indications: anti-HBsAb or anti HBcAb neg - give 3 doses at 0,1 & 6 mo; neg ab titer @ 2 mo post 3rd dose - repeat 3 doses.
- Influenza indications: annual, all pts, Oct/Nov optimal
- Hepatitis A indications: anti-HAV neg + risk (IDU, gay male, HBV/HCV hepatitis, chronic liver dis); give HAV vaccine x 2 doses, 0 & 6 mos.

Secondary prophylaxis (hx of designated OI)

- MAC: (see MAC module); STOP when CD4>100 x 6mo, Rx >12mo, & asymptomatic
- Cryptococcal meningitis: drugs - fluconazole 200mg po qd; STOP when CD4 100-200 > 6 mos, Rx >8 wks & asx.
- CMV: (see CMV module); drugs: valganciclovir +/- ocular implant; STOP when CD4 >100 x 6 mos, Rx >12 mos, & asx.
- PCP: TMP-SMX or alternatives; STOP when CD4 >200 x 3 mos
- TOXO: drugs - see toxo; STOP when CD4 >200 x 6 mos, completed initial Rx + asx

IMPORTANT POINTS

- Guidelines from CDC/IDSA (MMWR 2002;51 RR-8). Pamphlets for pts: 800-448-0400 & www.cdc.gov/hiv
- Primary prophylaxis - no hx of disease
- Secondary prophylaxis - hx of disease - w/ maintenance therapy
- "Generally recommended" vaccines: cover S. pneumo, HBV, HAV, influenza
- Safety of discontinuation with immune reconstitution is well established.
- "Standard of Care": prophylaxis for PCP, TB, toxo, MAC
- "Standard of Care": prophylaxis for PCP, TB, toxo, MAC

SELECTED READINGS

Aberg J, et al. Primary care guidelines for the management of persons infected with HIV. Clin Infect Dis 2004;39:609

Green H, et al. A prospective multicenter study of discontinuing prophylaxis for opportunistic infections after effective antiretroviral therapy. HIV Med 2004;5:278

Hirsch HH, et al. Immune reconstitution in HIV-infected patients. Clin Infect Dis 2004;38:1159

Centers for Disease Control. Guidelines for preventing opportunistic infections among HIV-infected persons - 2002. MMWR 2002;51 RR-8

Kirk O, Reiss P, Uberti-Foppa C, et al. Safe interruption of maintenance therapy against previous infection with four common HIV-associated opportunistic pathogens during potent antiretroviral therapy. Ann Intern Med 2002;137:239

Seage GR III, et al. The relationship of preventable opportunistic infections, HIV-1, RNA & CD4 cell counts to chronic morbidity. JAIDS 2002;30:421

Lopez JC, Micro JM, Pena JM, et al. A randomized trial of the discontinuation of primary and secondary prophylaxis against Pneumocystis carinii pneumonia after HAART in patients with HIV infection. NEJM 2001;344(3):159

El-Sadr W, Murphy RL, Yurik RM, et al. Atovaquone compared with dapsone for the prevention of Pneumocystis carinii pneumonia in patients with HIV infection who cannot tolerate trimethoprim, sulfonamides, or both. NEJM 1998;338:1889

Wakefield AE, et al. Limited asymptomatic carriage of Pneumocystis jiroveci in HIV-infected patients. J Infect Dis 2003;187:901

Trikalinos TA, Ioannidis JP. Meta-analysis of 14 controlled trial to determine safety of stopping PCP prophylaxis. Clin Infect Dis 2001;33:1901

ORAL CANDIDIASIS

Ciro R. Martins, M.D.

DIAGNOSTIC CRITERIA

- PE: Pseudomembranous type (thrush)-- white curd-like plaques most commonly on the buccal mucosa, oropharynx, gingiva and dorsum of the tongue. Easily scraped off, leaving a raw, reddish, tender patch.
- PE: Erythematous (atrophic) type-- Red, shiny, flat patches on the palate or dorsum of the tongue, associated with absence or decreased numbers of papillae.
- PE: Hyperplastic (hypertrophic) type--hard, white-yellowish plaques affecting the buccal mucosae, the sides and/or the dorsum of the tongue, resembling leukoplakia. Cannot be scraped off.
- PE: Angular cheilitis type (perleche)--red, fissured, sometimes ulcerated crusts on the corners of the mouth. Oral mucosal involvement may or may not be seen.
- Lab: KOH prep shows budding yeasts and pseudo-hyphae which are thicker and more irregularly shaped than true hyphae.

TREATMENT REGIMENS

Systemic therapy

- Recommended in cases of extensive oropharyngeal involvement with severe pain, refractory candidiasis, recurrent disease with evidence of extra oral involvement and when compliance is a problem.
- Fluconazole (Diflucan) 200mg PO on the first day, then 100mg PO qd x 14d
- Itraconazole (Sporanox) 200mg tablet PO qd x 14d; 200mg suspension PO qd x 14d
- Ketoconazole (Nizoral) 200mg PO qd x 14 d

Topical therapy

- Clotrimazole (Mycelex) 10mg troches - dissolve one troche slowly, without chewing 5x/d x 14d
- Nystatin (Mycostatin) 500000 U tablets PO tid-qid x 14d; cream or ointment applied to inner aspects of dentures after each meal x 14d
- Amphotericin oral suspension 100mg/mL - swish with 1mL for 3 min. qid and swallow.
- Angular cheilitis: nystatin/triamcinolone (Mycolog-II) cream or ointment topically qAM and qHS; clotrimazole/betamethasone (Lotrisone) cream topically qAm and qHS.
- Daily oral hygiene: wash dentures with chlorhexidine 0.12% oral rinse (Peridex); allow dentures to dry completely; brush affeced mucosa; oral antifungals to be used without the dentures in place.

DRUG-SPECIFIC COMMENTS

Ketoconazole: Not a good choice. Much less effective than fluconazole as a result of poor bioavailability (this drug requires low pH for better absorption). Additionally, it has significant drug interactions and higher potential for hepatotoxicity.

IMPORTANT POINTS

- These guidelines are based on the guidelines of care of the American Academy of Dermatology
- Candida yeasts are part of the normal flora of certain areas of the skin, mouth, intestinal tract and vagina. Multiple factors may cause the development of the clinical infection known as candidiasis.

- Non-albicans species of Candida have been isolated more frequently, especially in patients with advanced HIV disease. These are commonly intrinsically resistant to therapy with azole antifungals.
- Predisposing factors: age (infancy, old age), immunocompromised states (HIV, chemo Tx, corticosteroids), malignancies, dentures, antibiotics, endocrine (pregnancy, diabetes), smoking, drooling
- Differential diagnosis includes: other forms of leukoplakia (traumatic, oral hairy leukoplakia, malignant), lichen planus, geographic tongue (psoriasis), other forms of glossitis (pellagra, Moeller's)

SELECTED READINGS

Drake L.A., Dinehart S.M et. al. Guidelines of Care for Superficial Mycotic Infections of the Skin: Mucocutaneous Candidiasis. Dermatology World, American Academy of Dermatology, Guidelines of Care, Supplement, 15-21, April 1995

Martin M.V. The use of fluconazole and itraconazole in the treatment of Candida albicans infections: a review. Journal of Antimicrobial Therapy, 44:429-437, 1999

Siegel M.A. Strategies for Management of Commonly Encountered Oral Mucosal Disorders. CDA Journal, 27(3):210-19, MArch 1999

Akpan A, Morgan R. Oral Candidiasis: Review. Postgraduate Medical Jornal 2002; 78:455-59

ORBITAL CELLULITIS
Khalil G. Ghanem, M.D.

DIAGNOSTIC CRITERIA

- Preseptal cellulitis = anterior to orbital septum; hyperemia of eyelids, soft tissue edema and NO orbital congestion. Postseptal cellulitis = orbital cellulitis; acute infection of orbital contents.
- Etiology: (1) spread from ANY infected sinuses most common (2) direct inoculation: post-trauma (or surgery) (3) acute dacrocystitis; (4) bites (5) hematogenous (very rare).
- Symptoms: Early - fever, lid edema & rhinorrhea. Later: orbital pain, headaches and tenderness to palpation of lids; lids hyperemic; conjunctival hyperemia, chemosis & proptosis.
- PE/LAB: limited ocular motility; decreased visual acuity (later); decreased corneal sensation; congested retinal veins; WBC count~15,000; blood cx: variable yield; conjunctival cx may help.
- Scans: CT w/contrast initial study of choice: best to visualize bony changes; MRI useful for dx of cavernous sinus thrombosis. CT in preseptal cellulitis is normal +/- soft tissue edema.

COMMON PATHOGENS: Haemophilus influenzae ; Staphylococcus aureus ; Group A beta hemolytic strep ; Streptococcus pneumoniae ; Aspergillus ; Mucor

TREATMENT REGIMENS

Antimicrobials

- Begin immediately after cultures; do not wait for radiology results!
- Coverage for gram + bacteria in addition to anaerobes as initial regimen. Can be modified based on cx data.
- Unasyn 1-2g IV q6 (for adults)[see Bodenstein, et al]. Ceftriaxone 1g IVq12h +/- vancomycin 1g IVq12h [Mandell: Principles and Practice of Infectious Diseases, 5th Ed., 2000]
- Other choices: clindamycin 300mg IV q8h or cefuroxime 750mg-1.5g IV q8h.
- If stage I (preorbital): can use PO amox/clav or clindamycin for 10-14 days.

- Duration: 10-14 days usual unless bone changes suggestive of osteomyelitis; then 3-6 weeks.
- Initially, Rx with IV antibiotics if orbital cellulitis. Switching to PO feasible based on clinical judgment.
- Amphotericin B should be used for mucor or aspergillus (usually from sinus extension) in addition to mandatory & prompt surgical debridement.
- Voriconazole can be considered as an alternate to ampho B for aspergillus in view of its excellent activity & better toxicity profile [no prospective studies in this setting, however].

Surgical

- Orbital cellulitis requires close consultation with ophthalmology and ENT.
- Surgical debridement is warranted with abscesses or if medical management fails to lead to an improvement in the first 24-36 hours.
- Cultures should be obtained if surgical debridement is pursued; often have high yield.
- If fungal: surgical debridement immediately!

IMPORTANT POINTS

- Periorbital cellulitis: mean age 21 mos; trauma & bacteremia are most common causes. Orbital cellulitis: mean age 12 yrs; sinusitis most common cause.
- Posterior orbital cellulitis: profound visual loss AND ophthalmoplegia early & in absence of inflammatory signs; usually sphenoid or ethmoid spread. STAT CT; consider doppler imaging.
- In patients with DKA and visual sx, rhinocerebral mucormycosis should be suspected and IMMEDIATE surgical debridement obtained.
- Cavernous Sinus Thrombosis: suspect with internal and external ophthalmoplegia (CNs III, IV, V and VI involved)

SELECTED READINGS

Sobol SE, et al. Orbital complications of sinusitis in children. J Otolaryngol 2002 Jun;31(3):131-6

Dokmetas HS, et al. Diabetic ketoacidosis and rhino-orbital mucormycosis. Diabetes Res Clin Pract 2002 Aug;57(2):139-42

Starkey CR, Steele RW. Medical management of orbital cellulitis. Pediatr Infect Dis J 2001 Oct;20(10):1002-5

Ferguson MP, McNab AA. Current treatment and outcome in orbital cellulitis. Aust N Z J Ophthalmol 1999 Dec;27(6):375-9

Uzcategui N, et al. Clinical practice guidelines for the management of orbital cellulitis. J Pediatr Ophthalmol Strabismus 1998 Mar-Apr;35(2):73-9

Jayamanne DG, et al. Orbital cellulitis--an unusual presentation and late complication of severe facial trauma. Br J Oral Maxillofac Surg 1994 Jun;32(3):187-9

Kronish JW, et al. Orbital infections in patients with human immunodeficiency virus infection. Ophthalmology 1996 Sep;103(9):1483-92

Givner LB. Periorbital versus orbital cellulitis. Pediatr Infect Dis J 2002 Dec;21(12):1157-8

Donahue SP, Schwartz G. Preseptal and orbital cellulitis in childhood. A changing microbiologic spectrum. Ophthalmology 1998 Oct;105(10):1902-5

Ruttum MS, Ogawa G. Adenovirus conjunctivitis mimics preseptal and orbital cellulitis in young children. Pediatr Infect Dis J 1996 Mar;15(3):266-7

OSTEOMYELITIS, ACUTE

Eric Nuermberger, M.D.

DIAGNOSTIC CRITERIA

- Distinction between acute and chronic osteomyelitis is vague: "acute" includes first presentation of osteomyelitis, acute symptomatology (< 2 weeks), and absence of necrotic bone or sequestrum
- Acute symptoms and signs: fever/chills/night sweats, localizing pain/tenderness or swelling/erythema (more common with hematogenous infections)
- Chronic: Exposure of bone on visual inspection or by probing is diagnostic for osteomyelitis arising from a contiguous focus
- Lab: Isolation of pathogen from bone lesion (aspiration or bxp) or blood in setting of suggestive bony changes

COMMON PATHOGENS: Staphylococcus aureus ; Pseudomonas aeruginosa ; Enterobacteriaceae ; Staphylococcus species ; Salmonella species ; Serratia species ; Streptococcus species ; Enterococcus ; Eikenella corrodens ; Pasteurella multocida

TREATMENT REGIMENS

Hematogenous osteomyelitis (pathogen-directed)

- General recommendation is 4-6 wks parenteral therapy. Subsequent oral therapy does not clearly improve outcome.
- Staph (MSSA): nafcillin or oxacillin 2g IV q4h or cefazolin 2 IV q6-8h
- Staph (MSSA): ceftriaxone 2g IV qd (option for outpatient Rx)
- Staph (MSSA): clindamycin 600mg IV q6h or 900mg IV q8h
- MRSA: vancomycin 1g IV q12h (+/- rifampin 600mg IV or PO qd)
- MRSA: linezolid 600mg IV or PO q12h
- Strep: penicillin G 2-4 MU IV q4-6h or ampicillin 2g IV q6h (+/- gentamicin 1.0 mg/kg IV q8h for Streptococcus agalactiae or enterococcal species)
- GNB: ampicillin/sulbactam 3g (2g/1g respectively) IV q6h or ticarcillin/clavulanate 3.1g IV q4-6h or piperacillin/tazobactam 3.375 g IV q4-6h
- GNB: ciprofloxacin 400mg IV q12h (may make early transition to oral therapy: 750mg PO q12h). Other quinolones less potent, but probably adequate.
- GNB: ceftriaxone 2g IV qd or cefotaxime 2g IV q6-8h or ceftazidime 2g IV q8h or cefepime 2g IV q12h

Contiguous focus or inoculation osteomyelitis

- Leg/foot ulcer: orthopedic consult, consider vascular evaluation if signs of insufficiency present
- Decubitus ulcer: plastic surgery consult
- Osteomyelitis under chronic ulcer is often polymicrobial. If vascular insufficiency present, include anaerobic coverage.
- General recommendation is 6 or more weeks of abx (at least 2 wks of initial IV therapy) following surgical debridement
- Use regimens under hematogenous osteo when guided by culture data. Empiric regimens given below:
- Clindamycin 600mg IV q6h or 900mg IV q8h + ciprofloxacin 400mg IV or 750mg PO q12h or levofloxacin 750mg IV or PO qd
- Ampicillin/sulbactam 3g (2g/1g respectively) IV q6h or ticarcillin/clavulanate 3.1g IV q4-6h or piperacillin/tazobactam 3.375g IV q4-6h
- Ertapenem 1g IV qd or imipenem 500mg IV q6h or meropenem 1g IV q8h
- Ceftriaxone 2g IV qd or cefotaxime 2g IV q6-8h or ceftazidime 2g IV q8h or cefepime 2g IV q12h + metronidazole 500mg IV q6h

- Human or animal bite: ampicillin/sulbactam 3g (2g/1g respectively) IV q6h

Oral regimens (to follow parenteral therapy)

- Erratic oral bioavailability of penicillins and cephalosporins, plus lower vascular penetration of bone makes these agents less desirable. Use pathogen sensitivities to guide therapy.
- Staph (MSSA) or anaerobes: clindamycin 300-450mg PO q6h
- Staph (MSSA): minocycline 100mg PO qd (+/- rifampin 600 mg PO qd)
- Staph (MSSA): any fluoroquinolone (cipro least favored) + rifampin 600mg PO qd
- Staph (MSSA) or GNB: trimethoprim/sulfamethoxazole DS 2 tabs PO q6-8h
- GNB: ciprofloxacin 750mg PO q12h or levofloxacin 750 mg PO qd (add rifampin 600mg PO for Staph)
- Anaerobes: metronidazole 500mg PO q6-8h
- Mixed infection: clindamycin + fluoroquinolone
- MRSA or VRE: linezolid 600mg PO q12h
- Human or animal bite: amoxicillin/clavulanate 875-1000 mg PO bid

DRUG-SPECIFIC COMMENTS

Ampicillin + Sulbactam: Like other beta-lactam/lactamase inhibitor combinations, it provides broad coverage. A good choice for polymicrobial infections or infections with resistant nosocomial organisms.

Aztreonam: Broad activity against gram-negative bacilli, but no gram-positive or anaerobic activity. An alternative for resistant nosocomial pathogens.

Cefepime: Like ceftazidime, this agent's broad spectrum of activity, particularly against Pseudomonas, makes it an agent of choice for empiric treatment of nosocomial or iatrogenic infections.

Ceftazidime: Third generation cephalosporin with the greatest activity against Pseudomonas aeruginosa, though less active against Staphylococcus aureus. Therefore, a better choice when pseudomonas is suspected (diabetic foot, traumatic inoculation in a moist environment).

Ceftriaxone: A convenient option for outpatient parenteral therapy of susceptible Staph aureus infections.

Ciprofloxacin: Efficacy comparable to other parenteral regimens for susceptible organisms. Allows early conversion to oral therapy. Most potent quinolone for gram-negatives though levo-, gati- or moxifloxacin close, and latter are preferred for Staph infections (consider pairing with rifampin).

Daptomycin: New parenteral agent with bactericidal activity against many gram-positive organisms. However, it's unproven in osteomyelitis. Use in the absence of alternatives.

Levofloxacin: Fluoroquinolone with potency against gram-negatives approaching that of ciprofloxacin and potency against gram-positives approaching that of gatifloxacin or moxifloxacin, especially if 750mg dose is used. Good safety record.

Linezolid: Reliable activity vs. MRSA, VRE. Oral and parenteral forms - both very expensive. Less effective than cefazolin for S. aureus in animal model. Reserve for use when alternatives not available. Monitor blood counts with prolonged Rx--may see reversible anemia, thrombocytopenia with >2 wks therapy, low baseline hematocrit.

Piperacillin + Tazobactam: Like other beta-lactam/lactamase inhibitor combinations, it provides broad coverage. A good choice for polymicrobial infections or infections with resistant nosocomial organisms. More reliable anti-pseudomonal coverage than other penicillins.

Ticarcillin + Clavulanic Acid: Like other beta-lactam/lactamase inhibitor combinations, it provides broad coverage. A good choice for polymicrobial infections or infections with resistant nosocomial organisms.

IMPORTANT POINTS

- Acute hematogenous osteo: most common in children (usually S. aureus) and in adults over 50 or with IV drug use (S. aureus > GNB)
- Acute hematogenous osteo is usually monomicrobial; whereas contiguous-focus infections tend to be polymicrobial.
- Optimal management of acute osteo: establish pathogen(s) prior to antibiotic Rx.
- Indications for surgery: failure to respond to abx, soft tissue abscess, joint infection, and spinal instability
- Selected patients may be converted to oral agents after 2 weeks of IV therapy, if there are good oral options
- Acute osteomyelitis due to nail puncture wounds though sneaker are usually caused by Pseudomonas aeruginosa and often respond to aggressive surgical debridement and oral ciprofloxacin for two weeks

SELECTED READINGS

Lew DP, Waldvogel FA. Osteomyelitis. Lancet 2004;364:369

Darville T & Jacobs RF. Management of acute hematogenous osteomyelitis in children. Ped Infect Dis J 2004;23:255

Shuford JA & Steckelberg JM. Role of oral antimicrobial therapy in the management of osteomyelitis. Curr Opin Infect Dis 2003;16:515

Tice AD, Hoaglund PA, Shoultz DA. Outcomes of osteomyelitis among patients treated with outpatient parenteral antimicrobial therapy. Am J Med 2003;114:723.

Stengel D, Bauwens K, Sehouli J, et al. Systematic review and meta-analysis of antibiotic therapy for bone and joint infections. Lancet Infect Dis 2001;1:175.

Khatri G, Wagner DK, Sohnle PG . Effect of bone biopsy in guiding antimicrobial therapy for osteomyelitis complicating open wounds. Am J Med Sci 2001;321:367

Guglielmo BJ, Luber AD, Paletta D, et al. Ceftriaxone therapy for staphylococcal osteomyelitis: A review. Clin Infect Dis 2000;30:205.

Lew DP, Waldvogel FA. Use of quinolones in osteomyelitis and infected orthopedic prosthesis. Drugs 1999;58 Suppl.2:85

Gathe J, Harris R, Garland B, et al. Candida osteomyelitis: Report of 5 cases and review of the literature . Am J Med 1987;82:927

Sapico FL, Montgomerie JZ. Vertebral osteomyelitis in intravenous drug abusers: Report of three cases and review of the literature. Rev Infect Dis 1980; 2:196

OSTEOMYELITIS, CHRONIC   Eric Nuermberger, M.D.

DIAGNOSTIC CRITERIA

- "Chronic" infection may be defined by previous failed treatment, symptom duration >3 weeks, presence of bony destruction, persistent drainage or sinus tract; but the hallmark is necrotic bone.
- Exposure of bone on visual inspection or by probing with cotton swab is diagnostic for osteomyelitis arising from a contiguous focus
- Bony destruction should be present on plain x-rays.
- Confirmatory evidence is isolation of pathogen from bone or blood in setting of radiographic changes or acute inflammation on a pathologic specimen from bone biopsy

- Superficial cultures of ulcers or draining sinus tracts may not accurately reflect the organism(s) infecting bone.

COMMON PATHOGENS: Staphylococcus aureus ; Streptococcus species ; Enterococcus ; Enterobacteriaceae

TREATMENT REGIMENS

Parenteral therapy with curative intent

- 4-6 weeks of IV therapy after aggressive surgical debridement then >= 8 wks oral therapy.
- Staph (MSSA): nafcillin or oxacillin 2g IV q4h or cefazolin 2g IV q8h
- Staph (MSSA): ceftriaxone 2g IV qd (convenient for outpatient parenteral Rx)
- Staph (MSSA), strep, anaerobes: clindamycin 600mg IV q6h or 900mg IV q8h
- MRSA: vancomycin 1g IV q12h + rifampin 600mg IV or PO qd
- Strep: penicillin G 2-4 mU IV q4-6h or ampicillin 2g IV q6h (+/- gentamicin 1.0 mg/kg IV q8h for S. agalactiae or enterococcal species)
- GNB/anaerobes: ampicillin/sulbactam 2g IV q6h or ticarcillin/clavulanate 3.1g IV q4-6h or piperacillin/tazobactam 3.375g IV q4-6h
- GNB: ciprofloxacin 400mg IV q12h (may make early transition to oral therapy: 750mg PO q12h) or levofloxacin 750mg IV (then PO) qd
- GNB: ceftriaxone 2g IV qd or cefotaxime 2g IV q6-8h or ceftazidime 2g IV q8h or cefepime 2g IV q12h
- GNB, mixed infection: ertapenem 1g IV qd (convenient for outpatient parenteral therapy)

Oral regimens (consolidative or suppressive)

- Staph (MSSA): cephalexin 500mg PO q6h or cefadroxil 500mg PO q12h or dicloxacillin 500mg PO q6h (+/- rifampin 600mg PO qd)
- Staph (MSSA): minocycline 200mg PO qd (+/- rifampin 600mg PO qd)
- Staph (MSSA), Strep, GNB, Anaerobes: Amoxicillin/clavulanate 500mg PO q8h
- Staph (MSSA), anaerobes: clindamycin 300-450mg PO (+/- rifampin 600mg PO)
- Staph (MSSA), GNB: ciprofloxacin 750mg PO q12h or other quinolone (esp. if S.aureus) (+ rifampin 600mg PO qd for S.aureus)
- MRSA: Trimethoprim/sulfamethoxazole DS 2 tabs PO q6-8h or linezolid 600mg PO bid or clindamycin or minocycline (+/- rifampin 300mg PO bid)
- Anaerobes: Metronidazole 500mg PO q6-8h
- POLYMICROBIAL INFECTIONS MAY REQUIRE COMBINATION THERAPY

Adjunctive surgical therapy

- Drainage of infection and complete debridement of necrotic bone cannot be overemphasized
- Management of dead space by local tissue flap, free flap, or cancellous bone graft when necessary
- Antibiotic-impregnated beads to sterilize and temporarily fill dead space
- Local delivery of antibiotics to dead space via impregnated acrylic beads or implantable infusion pump
- Bone saucerization and grafting
- Revascularization
- Hyperbaric oxygen therapy - controversial role
- Amputation

DIAGNOSIS

DRUG-SPECIFIC COMMENTS

Ampicillin + Sulbactam: Like other beta-lactam/lactamase inhibitor combinations, it provides broad coverage. A good choice for polymicrobial infections or infections with resistant nosocomial organisms.

Aztreonam: Broad activity against gram-negative bacilli, but no gram-positive or anaerobic activity. An alternative for resistant nosocomial pathogens.

Cefepime: Like ceftazidime, this agent's broad spectrum of activity, particularly against Pseudomonas, makes it an agent of choice for empiric treatment of nosocomial or iatrogenic infections.

Ceftazidime: Third generation cephalosporin with the greatest activity against Pseudomonas aeruginosa, though less active against Staphylococcus aureus. Therefore, a better choice when pseudomonas is suspected (diabetic foot, intravenous drug use, traumatic inoculation in a moist environment).

Ceftriaxone: A convenient option for outpatient parenteral therapy of susceptible Staph aureus infections.

Ciprofloxacin: Efficacy comparable to other parenteral regimens for susceptible organisms. Allows early conversion to oral therapy. Most potent quinolone for GNB. Levo-, gati- or moxifloxacin probably preferred for Staph infections (pair with rifampin for Staph).

Daptomycin: Parenteral agent with bactericidal activity against many gram-positive organisms. However, it's unproven in osteomyelitis. Use in the absence of alternatives.

Ertapenem: More convenient for outpatient dosing (1g IV qd) than other carbapenems. However, not active against Pseudomonas or Acinetobacter species.

Imipenem/Cilastatin: Broad-spectrum, including anaerobes, make this agent (as well as meropenem) an attractive alternative for polymicrobial infections or infections with resistant organisms.

Linezolid: Reliable activity vs. MRSA, VRE. Oral and parenteral forms - both very expensive. Less effective than cefazolin for S.aureus in animal model. Reserve for use when alternatives not available. Monitor blood counts with prolonged Rx--may see reversible anemia, thrombocytopenia with >2 wks therapy, low baseline hematocrit.

Metronidazole: Exceptional anaerobic activity and excellent oral bioavailability make this a favored agent when anaerobic infection is suspected. No activity against anaerobes, though.

Minocycline: When combined with rifampin, this drug may be active against MRSA and MRSE isolates.

Piperacillin + Tazobactam: Like other beta-lactam/lactamase inhibitor combinations, it provides broad coverage. A good choice for polymicrobial infections or infections with resistant nosocomial organisms. More reliable anti-pseudomonal coverage than other penicillins.

Ticarcillin + Clavulanic Acid: Like other beta-lactam/lactamase inhibitor combinations, it provides broad coverage. A good choice for polymicrobial infections or infections with resistant nosocomial organisms.

IMPORTANT POINTS

- Guidelines are author's opinion
- Identification of pathogen(s) is essential; if possible, defer treatment until after bone biopsy
- Cultures of sinus tracts and contiguous ulcers are unreliable and should not guide therapy if bone biopsy is possible

- Following any surgical debridement, the remaining tissue bed is considered contaminated and treated with abx for at least 6 wks
- Usual reason for failure: inadequate debridement or abx noncompliance or host problem (e.g., immune suppression)
- Long-term suppressive therapy may be required when definitive surgery is not possible
- Revascularization is a necessary adjunct in attempts to salvage infection in limbs with vascular insufficiency

SELECTED READINGS

Lew DP, Waldvogel FA. Osteomyelitis. Lancet 2004;364:369

Rayner CR, Baddour LM, Birmingham MC, et al. Linezolid in the treatment of osteomyelitis: results of compassionate use experience. Infection. 2004;32:8

Senneville E, Legout L, Valette M, et al. Risk factors for anaemia in patients on prolonged linezolid therapy for chronic osteomyelitis: a case-control study. J Antimicrob Chemother 2004;54:798

Parsons B & Strauss E. Surgical management of chronic osteomyelitis. Am J Surg 2004;188(1A Suppl):57

Shuford JA & Steckelberg JM. Role of oral antimicrobial therapy in the management of osteomyelitis. Curr Opin Infect Dis 2003;16:515

Tice AD, Hoaglund PA, Shoultz DA. Outcomes of osteomyelitis among patients treated with outpatient parenteral antimicrobial therapy. Am J Med 2003;114:723

Khatri G, Wagner DK, Sohnle PG. Effect of bone biopsy in guiding antimicrobial therapy for osteomyelitis complicating open wounds. Am J Med Sci 2001;321:367

Stengel D, Bauwens K, Sehouli J, et al. Systematic review and meta-analysis of antibiotic therapy for bone and joint infections. Lancet Infect Dis 2001;1:175

Lew DP, Waldvogel FA. Use of quinolones in osteomyelitis and infected orthopedic prosthesis. Drugs 1999;58 Suppl.2:85

Gentry LO, Rodriguez GG. (1) Oral ciprofloxacin compared with parenteral antibiotics in the treatment of osteomyelitis and (2) Ofloxacin versus parenteral therapy for chronic osteomyelitis . (1) Antimicrob Agents Chemother 1990;34:40 and (2) Antimicrob Agents Chemother 1991;35:538

OTITIS EXTERNA

Daniel J. Lee, M.D.

DIAGNOSTIC CRITERIA

- Clinical: otalgia, esp. pinna, otorrhea, hx of local trauma (Q-tips) or water exposure ("swimmer's ear"), periauricular adenopathy
- Complications (common): conductive hearing loss, narrowing of external auditory canal. Rare: malignant otitis externa (MOE +/- cranial nerve involvement) seen in diabetics, immunocompromised state
- Indications for topical abx: otalgia, swelling, otorrhea. Add oral abxs for recurrent infections, severe sx's, diabetics, immunocompromise. Cx: only for chronic/recurrent infxn.
- Indication for biopsy: chronic infections resistant to aggressive topical/oral therapy, presence of granulation tissue (r/o aggressive fungal infxn/malignancy), pain, immunocompromised.
- Indications for labs: r/o immunocompromised state (diabetes, HIV, etc.) or autoimmune disease. Temporal bone CT only to r/o MOE, not for routine infxn.

COMMON PATHOGENS: Staphylococcus (coagulase-negative) ; Staphylococcus aureus ; Corynebacterium spp ; Candida ; P. aeruginosa

Diagnosis

Treatment Regimens

Uncomplicated bacterial infection: primary therapy
- Neomycin+polymixin+hydrocortisone (Cortisporin Otic) 4 drops TID x 7-10d (prescribe SUSPENSION, not solution that burns)
- Ciprofloxacin + steroid (Cipro HC) 3-4 drops TID x 7-10d
- Ofloxacin (Floxin) 10 drops BID x 7-10d (often used by PCPs in the setting of TM perforation or tympanostomy tube, but most otolaryngologists will use Cortisporin susp. or Cipro HC as well)
- Tobramycin (Tobradex ophth.) 3-4 drops TID x 7d (use only if TM intact)
- Gentamicin (Garamycin ophth.) 3-4 drops TID x 7d (use only if TM intact)
- Acetic acid+propylene glycol+hydrocortisone 1% (VoSol HC) 4-6 drops TID x 10d
- Ciprofloxacin 0.3%/dexamethasone 0.1% (CIP/DEX) 4 drops BID x 7-10d

Uncomplicated fungal infection: primary therapy
- Acetic acid+propylene glycol+hydrocortisone 1% (VoSol HC) 4-6 drops TID x 10d
- Acetic acid (Domeboro Otic) 4-6 drops QID x 10d
- Clotrimazole (Lotrimin solution) 3-4 drops BID x 7d
- DEBRIDEMENT AND DRY EAR HYGIENE CRUCIAL in otomycosis

Severe/recurrent bacterial infection
- Aggressive outpt debridement by otologist/otolaryngologitst essential for severe infxn, placement of ear wick for stenotic external canal to facilitate topical therapy
- Surgery not indicated for recurrent or chronic infection - controversial for malignant otitis externa
- Ciprofloxacin (Cipro) 500mg PO BID x 10-14d
- Ofloxacin (Floxin) 400mg PO BID x 10-14d
- In poorly responsive severe otitis externa, consider parenteral antipseudomonal therapy; use cx + sensitivities to guide selection.

Important Points
- Guidelines based on author's opinion and Current Therapy in Otolaryngology-Head and Neck Surgery (6th Edition, 1998, Gates, G., Editor)
- Pathophysiology: maceration of external canal skin (mechanical/chemical damage), allergy, diabetes, resulting in atrophy of sebaceous and cerumen glands, increase in canal pH
- Referral to otolaryngologist or otologist essential in severe otitis externa. Outpatient debridement using binocular otomicroscopy essential.
- Stenotic canals impairing administration of drops require temporary wick placement. Strict dry ear precautions while showering/bathing (use cotton ball/Vaseline/hair dryer).
- Diabetics: improved glucose control essential.

Selected Readings

Roland PS, Pien FD, Schultz CC, et al. Efficacy and safety of topical ciprofloxacin/dexamethasone versus neomycin/polymyxin B/hydrocortisone for otitis externa. Curr Med Res Opin. 2004 Aug;20(8):1175-83

van Balen FA, Smit WM, Zuithoff NP, et al. Clinical efficacy of three common treatments in acute otitis externa in primary care: randomised controlled trial . Evid Based Nurs. 2004 Apr;7(2):43

Roland, P. S. and Stroman, D. W. Microbiology of acute otitis externa. Laryngoscope 2002; 112(7 Pt 1): 1166-77

Berenholz, L., Katzenell, U. and Harell, M. Evolving resistant pseudomonas to ciprofloxacin in malignant otitis externa. Laryngoscope 112(9): 1619-22.

Barza, M. Use of quinolones for treatment of ear and eye infections. Eur J Clin Microbiol Infect Dis 10 (4): 296-303

Selesnick, S. H. Otitis externa: management of the recalcitrant case. Am J Otol 15(3): 408-12

Simpson, K. L. and Markham, A. Ofloxacin otic solution: a review of its use in the management of ear infections. Drugs 58(3): 509-31

OTITIS MEDIA
Daniel J. Lee, M.D.

DIAGNOSTIC CRITERIA

- Clinical: otalgia, aural fullness, decreased hearing (512 Hz tuning fork - lateralizes to involved ear); otoscopy-erythema, tympanic membrane (TM) bulging, or fluid/pus behind TM air bubbles
- Main indications for oral abx: pain, TM erythema, fever. Presence of middle ear fluid alone - not strict indication for abx. Abx-steroid ear drops for purulent otorrhea.
- Cultures not routine (and not obtainable) until spontaneous TM rupture or myringotomy performed - cultures may be helpful in chronic draining infection resistant to multiple therapies.
- Imaging: fine-cut temporal bone CT indicated for chronic infxn, concern for middle ear mass, retraction pocket, cholesteatoma, or if febrile +/- mastoid erythema, otalgia and OM.
- Complications (common): conductive hearing loss, mastoiditis, TM perforation; (rare): labyrinthitis/vertigo, facial palsy, meningitis, Gradenigo's (abducens palsy/retroorbital pain/OM)

COMMON PATHOGENS: S.pneumoniae ; Haemophilus influenzae

TREATMENT REGIMENS

Uncomplicated acute otitis media (adults)
- Amoxicillin 500mg PO tid x 7-10d
- Cefuroxime (Ceftin) 500mg PO bid x 7-14 d
- Ceftriaxone 1g IM (Rocephin) qod x 3 doses
- Alt (betalactam allergy or fails initial Rx): clindamycin 300mg PO tid/qid, gatifloxacin (Tequin) 400 mg PO qd, levofloxacin (Levaquin) 500mg PO qd, moxifloxacin (Avelox) 400mg PO qd --all x 7-10d.

Uncomplicated, recurrent/chronic otitis media
- Amoxicillin/clavulanate (Augmentin) 875mg PO bid (or 500mg PO TID) x 10-14 d
- Amoxicillin/clavulanate use as primary therapy for immunocompromised or diabetic patient
- Alt: clindamycin 300mg tid x 7-10 d (pen allergy)
- Referral to specialist to r/o chronic otomastoiditis or cholesteatoma in setting of chronic OM

Adjunctive therapy for otitis media
- Nasal decongestants: pseudoephedrine 120mg + topical vasoconstrictors - oxymetazoline nasal sprays 2 puffs tid x 3-4 days only (may use OTC preparations such as Afrin, Neosynephrine, Dristan)
- Antihistamines: loratadine (Claritin) 10mg PO qd or fexofenadine (Allegra) 60mg PO bid
- NSAIDs - ibuprofen (Motrin) 400mg PO tid x 5d, celecoxib (Celebrex) 200mg PO QD x 5d

DIAGNOSIS

- For persistent infection, intractable pain, or complications listed above, referral to specialist essential. Most adults tolerate myringotomy +/- tympanostomy tube placement in clinic setting.
- Severe vertigo/facial palsy/mastoid abscess/meningitis requires tympanstomy tube placement, hospital admission, temporal bone CT, cultures / LP, intravenous antibiotics, possible surgical drainage

IMPORTANT POINTS

- Guidelines based on author's opinion and Current Therapy in Otolaryngology-Head and Neck Surgery (6th Edition, 1998, Gates, G., Editor)
- Topical steroid / antibiotic ear drops not helpful in acute OM unless tympanic perforation +/- otorrhea
- Otorrhea and tenderness of pinna is otitis externa, not OM, which can be managed with topicals alone; oral abx not useful unless patient diabetic, immunocompromised
- "Muffled hearing" should not be treated w/ abx / decongestant unless obvious otitis media present & 512 hz tuning fork test (Weber test) lateralizes to problem ear (conductive hearing loss).
- "Muffled hearing," if acute, may represent sudden nerve deafness - an otologic emergency-requiring 60mg predisone/day and prompt referral to otologist
- Chronic effusion following antibiotic therapy w/o otalgia does not warrant abx's. Patient with muffled hearing and fluid (clear or amber) but no otalgia managed with decong./ nasal steroids/referral

SELECTED READINGS

Jang CH, Park SY. Emergence of ciprofloxacin-resistant pseudomonas in chronic suppurative otitis media. Clin Otolaryngol. 2004 Aug;29(4):321-3

Jang CH, Song CH, Wang PC. Topical vancomycin for chronic suppurative otitis media with methicillin-resistant Staphylococcus aureus otorrhoea . J Laryngol Otol. 2004 Aug;118(8):645-7.

Pichichero, M. E. and Casey, J. R. Otitis media. Expert Opin Pharmacother 2002 Aug 3(8): 1073-90

Sheahan, P., Donnelly, M. and Kane, R. Clinical features of newly presenting cases of chronic otitis media. J Laryngol Otol 2001 Dec 115(12): 962-6

Yung, M. W. and Arasaratnam, R. Adult-onset otitis media with effusion: results following ventilation tube insertion. J Laryngol Otol 2001 Nov 115(11): 874-8

Culpepper, L., Froom, J., Bartelds, A. I.,et al. Acute otitis media in adults: a report from the International Primary Care Network. J Am Board Fam Pract 1993 Jul-Aug 6(4): 333-9

Celin, S. E., Bluestone, C. D., Stephenson, J., et al. Bacteriology of acute otitis media in adults. JAMA 1991 Oct 266(16): 2249-52

PARONYCHIA
Spyridon Marinopoulos, M.D.

DIAGNOSTIC CRITERIA

- Acute: hx - tender/red perionychium +/- abscess. Rapid progression (days). PE: erythema/edema/tenderness along lateral nail fold, fluctuance (abscess). Etiology: bacterial
- Chronic: hx-tenderness/edema/erythema (< than in acute), no abscess,+onycholysis. Indolent course >6 wk. PE-erythema/edema/tenderness,boggy nail fold,no fluctuance. Etiology: fungal/inflam/mycobact/GNR
- Risk factors - Acute: nail biting, finger sucking, mani/pedicure, hangnails, trauma/ foreign body. Chronic: exposure to water/irritants (bartenders, dishwashers, housekeepers), psoriasis, DM, meds.

- Ddx: felon, skin Ca (SC/BC/melanoma), pemphigus vulgaris, pyogenic/foreign body granuloma, wart, syph. chancre, Reiter's, psoriasis, herpetic whitlow, mucous cyst, subungual fibroma, leukemia cutis
- Studies (serious/refractory cases): gram stain, cx, KOH prep, fungal cx, bx. X-ray if foreign body, trauma or suspect osteo. Check glucose r/o DM.

COMMON PATHOGENS: Staph aureus (acute) ; Streptococcus sp. (acute) ; Anaerobes (acute) ; Candida albicans (chronic) ; Atypical mycobacteria (chronic) ; Gram-negative rods (chronic)

TREATMENT REGIMENS

Topical/miscellaneous

- All cases: avoid irritants, manicures/pedicures, finger sucking, nail biting, exposure to moisture. Use protective gloves when necessary
- Acute paronychia: NOTE: topical abx penetrate nail plate poorly; not effective for Rx of acute paronychia; use PO abx instead
- Warm compresses/soaks w/ 1/2-strength hydrogen peroxide or w/ Burrow's soln (OTC aluminum acetate, Domeboro) tid - qid x 20 min may be effective
- Chronic paronychia: NOTE: topical Rx first line. If ineffective, consider PO and/or surgical Rx
- NOTE: if caused by meds - indinavir, lamivudine, isotretinoin - d/c meds & reassess
- Ciclopirox (Loprox) 0.77% cream to affected area bid x 6-12 wk (+ strict irritant avoidance) effective
- Alternative: betamethasone 0.05%-clotrimazole 1% (Lotrisone) cream to affected area bid x 2-4 wk
- Alternative: miconazole (Monistat-Derm) 2% cream bid to nail folds until resolved
- Alternative: econazole (Spectazole) 1% cream qd to nail folds until resolved

Oral antibiotics

- NOTE: mixed infections common in paronychia; cx may help determine appropriate Rx
- Acute paronychia: Note: PO abx alone not sufficient if abscess; I&D required. Most authorities support use of PO abx even w/ adequate I&D
- Preferred: amoxicillin-clavulanate 500mg PO tid or 875mg bid x 7d or until infection resolves
- Preferred (PCN allergy): clindamycin 300mg PO q6h x 7d or until infection resolves
- Alternative (ineffective if anaerobes suspected): dicloxacillin 250-500mg PO qid or cephalexin (Keflex) 500mg PO q6h x 7d or until infection resolves
- Chronic paronychia (PO second line, use topical rx first): fluconazole (Diflucan) 100-200mg PO qwk until normal nail anatomy restored
- Alternatives: itraconazole (Sporanox) 200mg PO bid x 1 wk x 3 consecutive mo or terbinafine (Lamisil) 250mg PO qd x 3 mo
- Chronic paronychia + suspected bacterial superinfection: Add abx as in acute paronychia

Surgical

- NOTE: consult hand surgeon if cellulitis, deep space infection, glomus tumor, mucous cyst, or osteomyelitis suspected
- Acute paronychia : I&D necessary if abscess & no drainage w/ soaks alone. Use anesthesia (digital block/ethyl chloride spray) unless skin yellow/white (infarcted nerve endings)
- Insert #11 surgical blade under affected cuticle margin & extend incision along lateral nail bed. Keep blade directed away from nail plate to avoid permanent nail growth abnormalities

- Alternative (superficial abscess): run large gauge needle along nail into abscess (no need for local anesthesia)
- Continue frequent warm soaks after I&D to assist wound drainage
- Follow up in 48h to remove packing, irrigate area & reevaluate wound
- NOTE: if subungual abscess (pus under nailbed), I&D alone not sufficient; must remove entire nail plate
- NOTE: I&D not indicated for herpetic whitlow, mucous cyst, glomus tumor, osteomyelitis (all may be confused for paronychia)
- Chronic paronychia (conservative Rx ineffective): refer hand surgeon for eponychial marsupialization (excision of 3-mm wide crescent-shaped piece of skin/thickened tissue from eponychium)
- Alternative: Remove entire nail & apply antifungal-steroid oint - i.e., betamethasone 0.05%-clotrimazole 1% (Lotrisone) - to affected area bid x 2-4 wk

Drug-Specific Comments

Amoxicillin + Clavulanate: Excellent coverage includes anaerobes. First line Rx for acute paronychia. Useful in pts w/ paronychia due to oral anaerobes contracted through nail biting/finger sucking.

Cephalexin: Adequate coverage unless anaerobes suspected. 10% cross reactivity if penicillin allergic. Inconvenient qid dosing.

Dicloxacillin: Narrow spectrum penicillin effective in most cases of paronychia, but not if anaerobes are suspected

Fluconazole: Useful in chronic paronychia when fungal etiology suspected. Risk of hepatotoxicity. Use second line after topical Rx fails

Miconazole: Topical antifungal. Topical use precludes hepatotoxicity risk.

Important Points

- Recommendations are author's opinion. If no response to rx in 4-5d, cx, bx +/- refer to hand surgeon. Complications: nail loss, osteomyelitis, flexor tendon septic tenosynovitis, felon
- Think felon if pain/erythema/edema in pad of fingertip. Refer to hand surgeon for urgent I&D to prevent osteomyelitis, permanent nail deformity, ischemic necrosis of fingertip
- Think CA if irregular border/surrounding tissue w/ irregular appearance. Think melanoma if brown/black nail lines & subungual pain. Refer Derm for bx
- Think mucous cyst if painless edema lateral to nail plate in pt w/ OA. Think glomus tumor if constant severe pain w/ nail plate elevation/bluish discoloration & blurring of lunula. Refer hand surgeon
- Think herpetic whitlow if vesicles, ulceration, crusting, intense pain. Tzanck smear: multinucleated giant cells. I&D contraindicated (risks hematogenous viral dissemination). Rx HSV

Selected Readings

Daniel CR 3rd, Daniel MP, Daniel J, et al. Managing simple chronic paronychia and onycholysis with ciclopirox 0.77% and an irritant-avoidance regimen. Cutis. 2004 Jan;73(1):81-5.

Tosti A, Piraccini BM, Ghetti E, et al. Topical steroids versus systemic antifungals in the treatment of chronic paronychia: an open, randomized double-blind and double dummy study. J Am Acad Dermatol. 2002 Jul;47(1):73-6.

Cahali JB, Kakuda EY, Santi CG, et al. Nail manifestations in pemphigus vulgaris. Rev Hosp Clin Fac Med Sao Paulo. 2002 Sep-Oct;57(5):229-34.

Rockwell PG. Acute and chronic paronychia. Am Fam Physician. 2001 Mar 15;63(6):1113-6.

Tosti A, Piraccini BM, D'Antuono A, et al. Paronychia associated with antiretroviral therapy. Br J Dermatol. 1999 Jun;140(6):1165-8

Roberge RJ, Weinstein D, Thimons MM. Perionychial infections associated with sculptured nails. Am J Emerg Med. 1999 Oct;17(6):581-2.

Jebson PJ. Infections of the fingertip. Paronychias and felons. Hand Clin. 1998 Nov;14(4):547-55, viii.

Daniel CR 3rd, Daniel MP, Daniel CM, et al. Chronic paronychia and onycholysis: a thirteen-year experience. Cutis. 1996 Dec;58(6):397-401.

Hochman LG. Paronychia: more than just an abscess. Int J Dermatol. 1995 Jun;34(6):385-6.

Brook I. Paronychia: a mixed infection. Microbiology and management. J Hand Surg [Br]. 1993 Jun;18 (3):358-9.

PAROTITIS

John G. Bartlett, M.D.

DIAGNOSTIC CRITERIA

- Hx for bacterial parotitis: severe pain, tenderness, erythematous swelling--pre-auricular to angle of jaw
- PE: fever, toxicity, tender swelling along the mandible with purulent drainage from parotid duct
- Lab: blood cx +/- cx and gram stain of drainage (Stenson's duct) or aspirate
- Anatomic studies for stone: CT, ultrasound or sialography
- Ddx: Sjogren's, sarcoid, HIV-related, TB, tumor. Evaluate by CT/US & aspirate/bxp.

COMMON PATHOGENS: Staphylococcus aureus ; Mumps

TREATMENT REGIMENS

Antibiotics

- Principles: Cause - stone in duct, dehydration or viral; empiric abx for S. aureus if bacterial (often unilateral, while viral = bilateral); surgical drainage usually unnecessary.
- Staph (preferred): nafcillin or oxacillin 2g IV q4-6h
- Staph: cefazolin 0.75-1.5g IV q6-8h
- Staph (MRSA or beta-lactam allergy): vancomycin 1g IV q12h
- Anaerobes or Staph: clindamycin 600mg IV q8h
- Anaerobes or Staph: ampicillin-sulbactam (Unasyn) 1.5-3.0g IV q6h

Surgery

- May probe duct or get CT, US or sialogram to detect stone
- Acute suppurative parotitis rarely requires surgery for drainage and decompression.
- The main indication is failure to respond to medical management; main concern with surgery: facial nerve palsy

Miscellaneous

- Warm compresses, analgesics
- Prevention: Increase oral fluid intake, chew hard candy
- Prevention: Discontinue predisposing medications--anticholinergics such as tricyclics, Benadryl, etc.
- Artificial saliva--expensive and doesn't last
- Oral pilocarpine 5-10mg PO TID
- Recurrent/chronic - usually obstruction or reduced saliva (xerostomia). Need sialogram +/- siladenoscopy. ?surgery-ligate duct, ductoplasty, parotidectomy

Diagnosis

Drug-Specific Comments

Clindamycin: Active vs most community acquired S. aureus and virtually all oral microbes including anaerobes and strep. Major concern is GI side effects and inducible resistance by S. aureus (positive D test).

Gatifloxacin: Risky without bacteriology to justify use without basis using in vitro sensitivity tests.

Linezolid: Should be reserved for cases involving methicillin-resistant S. aureus in patients with a contraindication or non-response to vancomycin. Need to monitor platelet counts while on this drug - expensive.

Nafcillin: This oxacillin or cefazolin are the preferred agents for parenteral treatment of serious MSSA infections. None are adequate for anaerobes.

Piperacillin + Tazobactam: Good regimen for all anticipated pathogens except methicillin-resistant S. aureus. Could add vancomycin for empiric treatment of serious nosocomial infections.

Ticarcillin + Clavulanic Acid: Good regimen for all anticipated pathogens except methicillin-resistant S. aureus. Could add vancomycin for empiric treatment of serious nosocomial infections.

Important Points

- Guidelines are author's opinion
- Predisposing: elderly, dehydration, anticholinergic, Sjogren's syndrome, duct stones or duct atresia, diabetes, immunosupp, HIV/AIDS [DILS-diffuse infiltrative lymphocytic syndrome]
- Ddx for tender submandibular swelling: cervical adenitis, perimandibular space infections & actinomycosis. Ddx enlarged parotid: sarcoid, Sjogren's, tumor (CA, benign, lymphoma), TB, HIV.
- S. aureus the major cause of suppurative parotitis--usually unilateral & causes severe toxicity. Empiric therapy should cover S. aureus.
- Suppurative (bacterial) usually unilateral + predisposing cause. Pain is intense and aggressive, analgesic therapy is needed.

Selected Readings

Berker M, et al. Acute parotitis following sitting position neurosurgical procedures: review of five cases. J Neurosurg Anesthesiol 2004;16:29-31

Behzatoglu K, et al. Five needle aspiration biopsy of the parotid gland. Acta Cytol 2004;48:149-54

Marioni G, Rinaldi R, deFilippis C, et al. Candidal abscess of the parotid gland associated with facial nerve paralysis. Acta Otolaryngol 2003;123:661-3

Vargas PA, Mauad T, Bohon GM, et al. Parotid gland involvement in advanced AIDS. Oral Dis 2003;9:55-61

Motamed M, et al. Management of chronic parotitis: A review. J Laryngol Otol 2003;117:521-6

Ahai S, Mandel L. Chronic parotitis. NY State Dental J 2003;69:21-3

Flaitz CM. Parotitis as the initial sign of juvenile Sjogren's syndrome. Pediatr Dent 2001;23:140

Patel S, Mandel L. Parotid gland swelling in HIV diffuse infiltrative CD8 lymphocytosis syndrome. NY State Dental J 2001;67:22

Handa U, Kumar S, Punia RS, et al. Tuberculosis parotitis: a series of five cases diagnosed on fine needle aspiration cytology. J Laryngol Otol 2001;115:235

Mandel L. Ultrasound findings in HIV-positive patients with parotid gland swellings. J Oral Maxillofac Surg 2001;59:283

PELVIC INFLAMMATORY DISEASE (PID)

Noreen A. Hynes, M.D., M.P.H.

DIAGNOSTIC CRITERIA

- Minimal criteria in sexually active female (1 or both): (1) uterine/adnexal tenderness OR (2) cervical motion tenderness AND no other cause for illness identified
- This is a CLINICAL diagnosis, not a laboratory-based diagnosis.
- Most specific criteria for diagnosing PID: a) Histopathologic evidence of endometritis on endometrial biopsy; b) Transvaginal sonography or other imaging techniques showing thickened, fluid filled tubes with or without free pelvic fluid or tubo-ovarian complex; c) Laparoscopic abnormalities consistent with PID
- Additional criteria supporting the clinical diagnosis: a) Oral temperature > 101degrees Fahrenheit (>38.3 degrees Celsius); b) Abnormal cervical or vaginal discharge; c) Elevated erythrocyte sedimentation rate; d) Elevated C-reactive protein; e) Laboratory documentation of cervical infection with N. gonorrhoeae or C. trachomatis

COMMON PATHOGENS: Chlamydia trachomatis ; Neisseria gonorrhoeae ; Vaginal bacterial flora

TREATMENT REGIMENS

Oral/outpatient treatment of PID

- Ofloxacin 400mg PO BID x 14 d with or without Metronidazole 500mg PO BID x 14 d (Preferred)
- Levofloxacin 500mg PO qd with or without Metronidazole 500mg PO bid x 14 d (Preferred)
- Ceftriaxone 250mg IM x 1 PLUS Doxycycline 100mg PO BID x 14d with or without Metronidazole 500mg PO BID x 14d
- Cefoxitin 2g IM PLUS probenecid 1g PO x 1 PLUS Doxycycline 100mg PO BID x 14 d with or without Metronidazole 500mg PO BID x 14d
- Other parenteral 3rd generation cephalosporin PLUS Doxycycline 100mg PO BID x 14 d with or without Metronidazole 500mg PO BID x 14 d.

Recommended inpatient/parenteral regimens for PID

- Cefotetan 2g IV q12h or cefoxitin 2g IV q6h PLUS Doxycycline 100mg IV or PO q12h for at least 24h after clinical improvement, then outpatient regimen to complete 14 d.
- Cefoxitin 2g IV q6h PLUS Doxycycline 100mg IV or PO q12h for at least 24 hours after clinical improvement, then outpatient regimen to complete 14 d
- Clindamycin 900mg IV q8h PLUS gentamicin loading dose IV/IM(2mg/kg), then 1.5mg/ kg q8h or 5mg/kg qd for at least 24h after clinical improvement; then change to outpatient regimen to complete 14d.

Alternative regimens (limited data)

- Ofloxacin 400mg IV q12h or Levofloxacin 500mg IV qd with or without Metronidazole 500mg IV q8h, for at least 24h after clinical improvement, then change to outpatient regimen to complete 14 d
- Ampicillin/sulbactam 3g IV q6h PLUS Doxycycline 100mg IV or PO q12h for at least 24 hrs after clinical improvement; then change to outpatient regimen to complete 14 d
- Amoxicillin/clavulanic acid 500/125mg PO TID x 14d PLUS Doxycycline 100mg PO BID x 14d
- INDICATIONS FOR HOSPITALIZATION: lack of response after 72h of Rx; pregnant women (could see PID in 1st trimester) because of high risk of maternal mortality, fetal wastage, preterm delivery.

Diagnosis

Drug-Specific Comments

Amoxicillin + Clavulanate: At least one clinical trial has demonstrated that when amoxicillin/clavulanate is combined with doxycycline it is effective in treating PID. However, gastrointestinal symptoms might limit the use of this regimen as well as the TID for one arm of treatment (axox/clav) and BID dosing for the other (doxy).

Ampicillin + Sulbactam: Ampicillin + sulbactam when combined with doxycycline provides good coverage for C. trachomatis, N. gonorrhaeae, and anaerobes and appears to be effective for patients who have tubo-ovarian abscess.

Cefotetan: May provide better anaerobic coverage than ceftriaxone-based outpatient regimen.

Ceftriaxone: Ceftriaxone demonstates excellent acivity against N. gonorrhea but must be combined with doxycycline to provide needed treatment of C. trachomatis. Ceftriaxone has limited activity against anaerobes which leads many experts to recommend the addition of metronidazole to the PID regimen.

Doxycycline: Because of the pain associated with infusion, this agent should be given PO whenever possible, even when the patient is hospitalized. Both PO and IV doxycycline have similar bioavailability. If must give IV, use of lidocaine or other short-acting anesthetic, heparin, or steroids with a steel needle or extension of infusion time may reduce infusion complications.

Gentamicin: Single daily dose gentamicin has not been evaluated for the treatment of PID. However, it is efficacious in analogous situations.

Levofloxacin: Preliminary data suggest that levofloxacin is as effective as ofloxacin and may be substituted for it. Fluoroquinolones (FQ) should not be used to treat PID patients who acquired disease in CA, HI, MA, NY City, or the Pacific Basin due to high rates of FQ resistant gonorrhea.

Metronidazole: In combination with ofloxacin, this regimen is the preferred, albeit most expensive, regimen. Ofloxacin provides excellent coverage for GC, CT, Gram negative rods and anerobes which may be involved in PID. Increasingly anaerobes are believed to play a significant role in PID. Some clinicians, who wish to provide less expensive Rx treat with Ceftriaxone, doxycycline AND metronidazole. Use of this agent will also treat concurrent bacterial vaginosis or trichomoniasis.

Important Points

- Based on CDC's 2002 STD Rx Guidelines (MMWR 2002; 51 (RR-6); CDC 2004 revised recommendations for gonorrhea treatment (MMWR 2004 53:335-338).
- The International-Infectious Disease Society for Obstetrics and Gynecology-USA has published concerns about the CDC Rx guidelines. Prefer use of different terms and emphases.
- PID comprises a spectrum of disorders of the upper female genital tract; an STD is implicated in approximately 2/3 of cases, especially GC and CT
- Clinical diagnosis is imprecise: predictive value depends on clinical setting. Empiric therapy is unlikely to impair dx and mngmt of other causes of lower abd pain
- Ectopic pregnancy, acute appendicitis, and functional pain must always be in differential diagnosis of PID
- Hospitalization if surgical emergency cannot be excluded, patient is pregnant, patient does NOT respond to outpatient therapy, severe illness (nausea/vomiting/high fever), tubo-ovarian abscess present, HIV with low CD4 count, other cause of immunodeficiency.

- Some cases asymptomatic or without clinical diagnostic triad but have nonspecific symptoms or signs
- Long term adverse outcomes include ectopic pregnancy, infertility, chronic pelvic pain.
- Risk factors for PID: young age, douching, bacterial vaginosis, gynecologic surgery, smoking, HIV
- There may be extragenital intraabdominal spread of GC or CT PID leading to perihepatitis or periappendicitis

SELECTED READINGS

Hall MN et al. Which blood tests are most useful in evaluating pelvic inflammatory disease?. J Fam Pract 2004 53: 330-331.

Dunbar-Jacob J et al. Adherence to oral therapies in pelvic inflammatory disease. J Womens Health (Larchmt) 2004 13:285-291.

Centers for Disease Control and Prevention. Sexually transmitted diseases treatment guidelines 2002. MMWR; 2002; 51 (RR-6).

Hemsel DL et al. Concerns regarding the Centers for Disease Control's published guidelines for pelvic inflammatory disease. Clin Infect Dis 2001; 32:103-7.

Jackson SL and Soper De. Pelvic inflammatory disease in the postmenopausal woman. Infect Dis Obstet Gynecol. 7(5):248-52. 1999.

Merchant JS et al. Douching: a problem for adolescent girls and young women. Arch Pediatr Adolesc Med 153(8):834-7. 1999.

Paavonen J and Eggert-Kruse W. Chlamydia trachomatis: impact on human reproduction. Hum Reprod Update 5(5):443-7. 1999.

Pavletic AJ et al. Infertility following pelvic inflammatory disease. Infect Dis Obstet Gynecol 7(3):145-52. 1999.

Korn AP and Landers DV. Gynecologic disease in women infected with human immunodeficiency virus type 1. J Acquir Immune Defic Syndr Hum Retrovirol 9(4):361-70. 1995.

Westrom L. Consequences of pelvic inflammatory disease. In Pelvic Inflammatory Disease, GS Berger and L Westrom (eds). New York, Raven Press, pp 100-110. 1992.

PEPTIC ULCER DISEASE, H. PYLORI-RELATED

Paul Auwaerter, M.D.; Arjun Srinivasan, M.D.

DIAGNOSTIC CRITERIA

- Direct histologic demonstration of the organism on endoscopic biopsy specimens (>90% sensitive and specific)
- Positive urease test on endoscopic biopsy specimens (>90% sensitive and specific)
- Positive results from labeled urea breath test (>95% sensitive and specific). This technology is becoming more available.
- Positive IgG serum antibody (>95% sensitive and specific) BUT cannot distinguish active from remote infection.
- Culture of H. pylori is actually the least sensitive diagnostic test (70-80% sensitive).

COMMON PATHOGENS: Helicobacter pylori

TREATMENT REGIMENS

Three-drug regimens

- Proton pump inhibitor (PPI) bid + clarithromycin 500mg bid + amoxicillin 1g bid [Available as Prevpac using PPI lansoprazole]. Eradication 85-90%. Duration 10-14 days*

- Bismuth subsalicylate 525mg QID + tetracycline 500mg QID + metronidazole 400-500mg tid-QID Duration=14 days*. Cheapest option (about $15), but efficacy reduced without PPI.
- * denotes FDA approved regimens. PPI's = omeprazole 20mg, lansoprazole 30mg, pantoprazole 40mg, rabeprazole 20mg, esomeprazole 40mg ALL PO bid.
- Proton pump inhibitor bid + clarithromycin 500mg bid + metronidazole 500mg bid. Duration 10-14 days [for PCN allergic pts]
- Ranitidine bismuth citrate 400mg bid + clarithromycin 500mg bid + amoxicillin 1g bid Duration= 7-10 days
- PPI bid + amoxicillin 500mg bid-tid + metronidazole 500mg bid-tid x 10-14d
- Ranitidine bismuth citrate 400mg bid + clarithromycin 500mg bid + metronidazole 500mg bid. Duration= 7 days
- Metronidazole containing regimens may have reduced efficacy due to common resistance.
- Specific diagnosis and tests of cure are NOT necessary in patients who only have duodenal ulcers.

Two-drug regimens (FDA-approved)

- Dual therapy well-studied, but lower eradication rates (60-85%) make them second tier options. Potential use for the pt intolerant of clari or metronidazole.
- PPI + either clarithromycin 500mg tid OR Amox 1g bid for 2 weeks then PPI for 2 more weeks (PPI = omeprazole 40mg QD or lansoprazole 30mg tid)
- Ranitidine bismuth citrate (RBC) 400mg bid + clarithromycin 500mg tid OR bid for 2 weeks then RBC for 2 more weeks

Four-drug regimen

- Proton pump inhibitor bid + Bismuth subsalicylate 525mg QID + Tetracycline 500mg QID + Metronidazole 500mg tid-QID. Duration 2 weeks

Drug-Specific Comments

Amoxicillin: Standard drug to employ in regimen since resistance rare. Use unless PCN-allergic.

Metronidazole: Higher rates of resistance mean lower eradication rates in dual or triple regimens.

Rifabutin: Studied with PPI and amoxicillin for 10d "rescue" regimen showing better efficacy in small studies than standard second regimens.

Tetracycline: Described resistance rare.

Important Points

- Multiple regimens exist, optimal therapy not defined. Main treatment indication is PUD.
- H. pylori does not appear to cause GERD or non-ulcer dyspepsia. Treatment in these conditions (without ulcers) is controversial.
- Note that H. pylori infection is common in the population and of uncertain significance. No evidence supports routine screening and treatment in order to reduce the risks of gastric cancer.
- NIH consensus panel recommends testing & Rx all pts with sx peptic ulcer disease even if other risks for PUD present. Also Rx for gastric CA and mucosal-associated lymphoid tissue (MALT) lymphoma.
- Testing and treatment also recommended for those with atrophic gastritis and 1st degree relatives of pts with gastric cancer.

SELECTED READINGS

Ford A, Delaney B, Forman D, et al. Eradication therapy for peptic ulcer disease in Helicobacter pylori positive patients. Cochrane Database Syst Rev 2003; (4): CD003840

McMahon BJ, Hennessy TW, Bensler JM et al. The relationship among previous antimicrobial use, antimicrobial resistance, and treatment outcomes for Helicobacter pylori infections. Ann Intern Med. 2003 Sep 16;139(6):463-9

Chi CH, Lin CY, Sheu BS et al. Quadruple therapy containing amoxicillin and tetracycline is an effective regimen to treat failed triple therapy by overcoming the antimicrobial resistance of Helicobacter pylori. Aliment Pharmacol Ther. 2003 Aug 1;18(3):347-53

Suerman, Sebastian and Michetti, Pierre. Helicobacter pylori Infection. New England Journal of Medicine, October 2002;347(5):1175-86

Malfertheiner P, Megraud F, O'Morain C et al. Current concepts in the management of Helicobacter pylori infection--the Maastricht 2-2000 Consensus Report. Aliment Pharmacol Ther. 2002 Feb;16 (2):167-80

Fendrick, Mark. Who Should be Treated for H. pylori infection?. Hippocrates. April 2000. Page 29.

de Boer, Wink and Tytgat, Guido. Treatment of Helicobacter pylori infection. British Medical Journal. 1 January 2000. Volume 320 page 31.

Fendrick, Mark et.al. Symptom Status and the Desire for Helicobacter pylori Confirmatory Testing after Eradication Therapy in Patients with Peptic Ulcer Disease. The American Journal of Medicine. August 1999. Volume 107 page 133.

NIH consensus panel on H. pylori. Helicobacter pylori in Peptic Ulcer Disease. Journal of the American Medical Association. July 6, 1994. Volume 272, number 1, page 65.

PERICARDITIS
Richard Nettles, M.D.

DIAGNOSTIC CRITERIA

- Sx: acute fulminant onset of high fevers, shaking chills, dyspnea, chest pain/pleuritic, arthralgia, myalgia. Can be more insidious.
- PE: tachycardia, friction rub, muffled heart sounds, jugular venous distention and pulsus paradoxus.
- Radiographic: increased cor silhouette, +/- pleural effusion or wide mediastinum; Echo: pericardial effusion or cardiac tamponade; CT- pericardial effusion or thickening.
- EKG: sinus tach, diffuse ST/T wave changes , or electrical alternans from tamponade.
- Dx cornerstone: pericardial fluid gram stain & culture of organism. Increased PMNs or pus = pyogenic purulent pericarditis.

COMMON PATHOGENS: VIRUSES: HIV; Enteroviruses (Coxsackievirus, Echovirus), Influenza, Mumps, Varicella, Epstein Barr; Fungi: Histoplasma capsulatum, Coccidioides immitus; AIDS-ASSOCIATED Pericarditis; IMMUNOSUPPRESSED Patients: Candida sp, Aspergillus spp, Cryptococcus; Consider NONINFECTIOUS causes: post-MI/Dressler's syndrome, uremia, neoplasm, irradiation, dissecting aortic aneurysm, sarcoidosis, collagen vascular disease, drug induced

TREATMENT REGIMENS

Antibiotic therapy

- Empiric: vancomycin + [ceftriaxone or cefotaxime] x 14-42d
- S. pneumoniae (pen sens): penicillin G, cefotaxime, or fluoroquinolone x 14-42 d
- S. pneumoniae (pen resist): fluoroquinolone, vancomycin, linezolid x 14-42 d
- S. aureus (MSSA): nafcillin, oxacillin, cefazolin, vancomycin (if PCN allergic), clindamycin x 14-42 d
- S. aureus (MRSA): vancomycin, linezolid x 14-42 d
- N. meningitidis: penicillin G., ceftriaxone, cefotaxime x 14-42 d

- GNB: fluoroquinolone, cefepime x 14-42d.
- anaerobes: clindamycin, metronidazole, beta lactam - betalactamase inhibitor x 14-42d.
- Mycoplasma pneumoniae: doxycycline, macrolide x 14-42d.
- Legionella pneumophila: : fluoroquinolone, azithromycin x 14-42d.

Surgical intervention

- Pericardiotomy with biopsy increases diagnostic yield (esp TB, fungal) compared to pericardiocentesis .
- Surgical drainage essential for moderate to severe tamponade or purulent pericarditis
- Pericardial drain prevent reaccumulation.
- Pericardial window: if thick purulent drainage or reaccumulation.
- Intrapericardial streptokinase if drainage incomplete.
- Pericardiectomy for severe constrictive pericarditis.

Special considerations

- Enteroviral Pericarditis: treatment includes supportive care and NSAIDs. Avoid steroids in early disease. Unclear if steroids later in disease course prevent recurrence.
- AIDS Pericarditis: often asymptomatic. Invasive dx questionable if asymptomatic. Symptomatic cases warrant aggressive dx infection and neoplasm.
- Meningococcal Pericarditis: test complement deficiency. Prophylaxis for very close contacts: Rifampin 600mg PO q12h 3 day OR ciprofloxacin 500mg PO x1 OR ceftriaxone 250 IM x1.
- Vaccinia-related myopericarditis: incidence after smallpox vaccination is about 1:15,000. In certain cases, steroids or vaccinia immune globulin (CDC,404-639-3670) may be useful.

Drug-Specific Comments

Clarithromycin: (Biaxin)Only available orally, not parenterally. Otherwise, good therapy for atypical organisms. Oral agents not recommended for acute pericarditis.

Doxycycline: Used primarily for Lyme disease with 1st degree block. IV and PO formulations, well tolerated, experience with Lyme disease is extensive and good.

Gatifloxacin: (Tequin) Active vs S. pneumoniae, atypicals, most MSSA, and many GNB. Oral and parenteral formulations, once daily dosing, few side effects; concern for abuse.

Piperacillin + Tazobactam: (Zosyn) Option for S. pneumoniae, MSSA, anaerobes and GNB. Coverage can be narrowed if pathogen cultured.

Ticarcillin + Clavulanic Acid: (Timentin) Option for gram negative bacilli pericarditis. Broad coverage good for empiric coverage of MSSA, gram negative and anaerobic bacteria but is not advocated for S. pneumoniae. Coverage can be narrowed if organism cultured and identified.

Important Points

- Guidelines are author's opinions.
- Classic symptoms and signs of pericarditis are often absent. High index of suspicion is necessary, pt with fever and ECG changes.
- Predisposing conditions: prior pericardial effusions, renal failure, thoracic surgery, diabetes, myeloproliferative disorders, local/distant infections (endocarditis/pneumonia)+ PPD.
- NSAIDS and steroids should probably be avoided in those with signs of myocarditis.
- Patients with recurrent idiopathic or viral pericarditis, colchicine at 1mg/d may be effective for reducing recurrent episodes

SELECTED READINGS

Sagrista-Sauleda J, Angel J, Sanchez A, et al. Effusive-Constrictive Pericarditis. N Engl J Med. 350. 2004. pp 469-75.

Task force on the diagnosis and management of pericardial diseases of European Society of Cardiology. Guidelines on the diagnosis and management of pericardial diseases executive summary. European Heart Journal. 25. 2004. pp 587-610

Halsell JS, Riddle JR, Atwood JE, et al. Myopericarditis following smallpox vaccination among vaccinia-naive US military personnel. JAMA. 289 (24). June 25 2003. pp. 3283-9

Hakim JG, Ternouth I, Mushangi E, et al. Double blind randomized placebo controlled trial of adjunctive prednisolone in the treatment of effusive tuberculous pericarditis in HIV seropositive patients. Heart, Vol 84(2), 2000, pp. 183-8.

Adler Y, Finkelstein Y, Guindo J, et al. Colchicine . Treatment for recurrent pericarditis A decade of experience. Circulation, Vol 97, 1998, pp.2183-2185

Dooley DP, Carpenter JL, Rademacher S. "Adjunctive Corticosteroid Therapy for Tuberculosis: A Critical Reappraisal of the Literature". CID, vol 25, 1997, pp. 872-77.

Corey GR, Campbell, PT, Van Trigt et al. Etiology of large pericardial effusions. Am J Med. Vol.95, 1993, pp. 209-13

Go C, Asnis DS, Saltzman H. "Purulent Pericarditis Since 1980". CID, vol. 27, Nov, 1988, pp. 1338-40.

Strang JI, Kakaza HH, Gibson DG, et al. Controlled trial of prednisolone as adjunctive treatment for tuberculous constrictive pericarditis in Transkei. Lancet, 1987 pp1418-22

Permanver-Miralda G, Sagrista-Sauleda J, Soler-Soler J. Primary acute pericardial disease: a prospective series of 231 consecutive patients. Am J Cardiol. Vol 56(10). 1985. pp. 623-30

PERITONITIS, SPONTANEOUS BACTERIAL AND SECONDARY
Pamela A. Lipsett, M.D.; Chris Carpenter, M.D.

DIAGNOSTIC CRITERIA

- Patients with ascites, fever (may be low-grade or absent) and/or abdominal pain should be evaluated for spontaneous bacterial peritonitis (SBP = primary peritonitis) or other forms of peritonitis.
- Other signs/symptoms (e.g., encephalopathy) may be the only clues of SBP. Abdomen SBP often has mild diffuse discomfort but rarely is it consistent with classic findings of peritonitis.
- Diagnostic criteria for SPB include > 250 PMN cells/mL with positive ascites cultures and no surgically treated intraabdominal source of infection.
- Variant forms of primary peritonitis include culture-negative neutrophilic (PMN>250) ascites (CNNA - up to 40%) and monomicrobial non-neutrophilic (PMN<250) bacterioascites (MNB).
- Secondary peritonitis = peritonitis with a surgically amenable source (e.g., appendicitis, diverticulitis; polymicrobial); tertiary peritonitis = peritonitis/abscess following secondary peritonitis.
- The possibility of SBP should be considered in 1) all cirrhotic patients on admission to hospital; 2) all patients with ascites who develop hepatic encephalopathy, renal impairment, or altered GI motility; and 3) all patients with ascites with a GI bleed (empirical treatment/prophylaxis may be indicated).

COMMON PATHOGENS: Enterobacteriaceae ; Escherichia coli ; Klebsiella species ; Enterobacter species ; Enterococcus ; Streptococcus species ; Polymicrobial (secondary peritonitis) ; Anaerobes (secondary peritonitis) ; S.pneumoniae

DIAGNOSIS

TREATMENT REGIMENS

SBP prophylaxis
- Authors' opinion form basis of recommendations.
- Prophylaxis recommended after first episode of SBP; benefits for other indications (variceal bleeding, low ascitic fluid protein, etc.) controversial, especially with concerns of resistance promotion.
- Trimethoprim-sulfamethoxazole 1 DS qd
- Norfloxacin 400mg qd
- ciprofloxacin 750mg qwk

SBP Treatment
- Cefotaxime 2.0g IV q8h or ceftriaxone 1.0g IV qd
- Duration of 5-7 days likely adequate; traditional 10-14 days is likely longer than needed unless complicated patients or positive blood cultures.
- Repeated paracentesis may be considered; PMN's < 250 with negative culture support an abbreviated course (< 5 days)
- Recent single center report of effectiveness of cefotaxime + albumin in reducing mortality and irreversible renal impairment
- Ciprofloxacin 400mg IV q12h or levofloxacin 500mg IV qd or gatifloxacin 400mg IV qd or moxifloxacin 400mg IV qd
- Ofloxacin has been reported effective as an oral alternative at 400mg PO bid.
- Ticarcillin-clavulanate 3.1g IV q6h or piperacillin-tazobactam 3.375g IV q6h or 4.5g IV q8h or ampicillin-sulbactam 3.0g IV q6h
- Imipenem 0.5g IV q6h, meropenem 1.0g IV q8h, or ertapenem 1.0g IV qd

Secondary peritonitis treatment
- Supportive therapy
- Operative management is indicated to eliminate the source of contamination, reduce the bacterial load, and prevent recurrence
- Empiric antimicrobial coverage - should include coverage of gram-negative aerobes, gram-positive cocci, and anaerobes
- Upper tract source (e.g., perforated ulcer) usually predominantly gram-positive infections; lower tract (distal small bowel or colon) generally results in anaerobic and gram-negative aerobes
- Duration is generally 5 to 7 days, longer if leukocytosis/left shift and fever are slow to resolve or source control inadequate
- Cefoxitin 1-2g IV q6h or cefotetan 1-2g IV q12h
- Ticarcillin-clavulanate 3.1g IV q6h or piperacillin-tazobactam 3.375g IV q6h or 4.5g IV q8h or ampicillin-sulbactam 3.0g IV q6h
- Imipenem 0.5g IV q6h or meropenem 1.0g IV q8h or ertapenem 1.0g IV qd
- Metronidazole/clindamycin plus aminoglycoside/3rd generation cephalosporin/fluoroquinolone/aztreonam

DRUG-SPECIFIC COMMENTS

Ampicillin + Sulbactam: Good single agent for primary or secondary peritonitis, lacks Pseudomonas aeruginosa coverage but covers enterococci better that piperacillin-tazobactam or ticarcillin-clavulanate.

Aztreonam: Excellent gram-negative coverage, use in combination with gram-positive (primary, secondary) and anaerobe (secondary) empiric coverage, would reserve for seriously ill patients with no other reasonable alternatives.

Cefotaxime: Primary treatment choice for SBP.

Ceftriaxone: Appropriate empirical choice for SBP; biliary sludging may be a concern.

Ertapenem: Carbapenem with gram-positive, gram-negative, and anaerobic coverage; does not cover enterococci, Pseudomonas, etc.

Gatifloxacin: Excellent broad spectrum coverage but clinical data limited on anaerobe coverage; would use other agents first while clinical data accumulates on its use in serious infections.

Imipenem/Cilastatin: Excellent broad spectrum coverage (anaerobes, gram-positives, gram-negatives), would reserve for seriously ill patients.

Levofloxacin: Excellent gram-positive and gram-negative coverage

Meropenem: Excellent broad spectrum coverage (anaerobes, gram-positives, gram-negatives), would reserve for seriously ill patients.

Piperacillin + Tazobactam: Good single agent for primary or secondary peritonitis.

Ticarcillin + Clavulanic Acid: Good single agent for primary or secondary peritonitis.

IMPORTANT POINTS

- Patients with cirrhosis and ascites have a one year risk of SBP as high as 29%
- Peritonitis associated with chronic ambulatory peritoneal dialysis (CAPD) requires coverage of Staphylococcus aureus, coagulase-negative staphylococci, rarely Enterobacteriaceae, P. aeruginosa, yeast
- Treat CAPD-associated peritonitis empirically with vancomycin plus gram-negative coverage; catheter may need removal (especially for yeast, Pseudomonas)
- Culture-negative neutrophilic ascites (CNNA) has clinical, prognostic, and therapeutic characteristics similar to spontaneous bacterial peritonitis (SBP) and should be treated in a similar fashion
- Patients with monomicrobial non-neutrophilic bacterioascites (MNB) typically respond similar to CNNA and SBP if the patient is symptomatic; asymptomatic patients usually do not need antibiotics

SELECTED READINGS

Gines et al. Management of Cirrhosis and Ascites. The New England Journal of Medicine 2004 Apr 15;350(16):1646-54

Solomkin et al. Guidelines for the Selection of Anti-Infective Agents for Complicated Intra-abdominal Infections. Clin Infect Disease 2003 October 15;37:997-1005

Mazuski JE, Sawyer RG, Nathans AB. THE SURGICAL INFECTION SOCIETY GUIDELINES ON ANTIMICROBIAL THERAPY FOR INTRA-ABDOMINAL INFECTIONS: AN EXECUTIVE SUMMARY . Surgical Infections 2002, Vol 3

Soares-Weiser K, Brezis M, Leibovici L. Antibiotics for spontaneous bacterial peritonitis in cirrhotics. Cochrane Library 2002, Issue 4

Mowat C Stanley AJ. Review article: spontaneous bacterial peritonitis-diagnosis, treatment and prevention. Aliment Pharmacol Ther 2001;15:1851-859

Rimola A, Garcia-Tsao G, Navasa M et al. Diagnosis, treatment and prophylaxis of spontaneous bacterial peritonitis: a consensus document . J Hepatology 2000: 32: 141-53

Sort P, Navasa M, Arroyo V et al. Effect of intravenous albumin on renal impairment and mortality in patients with cirrhosis and spontaneous bacterial peritonitis. N Engl J Med 1999:341:443-4

Runyon BA. Management of adult patients with ascites caused by cirrhosis. Hepatology 1998:27:264-72

PHARYNGITIS, ACUTE

John G. Bartlett, M.D.

DIAGNOSTIC CRITERIA

- Clinical: pharyngeal pain +/- dysphagia, URI symptoms, cough (if present suggests viral not bacterial cause), fever, & other constitutional sx
- PE: red throat +/- purulent exudate (exudative tonsillitis)
- Strep pharyngitis: microbial detection w/positive rapid antigen test or throat culture. Clinical criteria of Centor: fever, tonsillar exudate, no cough, & tender cervical adenopathy
- Other treatable agents: gonococcal: throat cx for GC; influenza: rapid test or clinical (epidemic + typical sx); acute HIV: plasma HIV RNA + risk; EBV: mono spot + atypical lymphs
- Ddx of sore throat: epiglottitis, peritonsillar abscess, retropharyngeal abscess, thyroiditis, oropharyngeal or laryngeal tumor.

COMMON PATHOGENS: Most common: Streptococcus pyogenes (Group A) ; Influenza ; Parainfluenza virus ; Rhinovirus ; Coronavirus ; Neisseria gonorrhoeae ; HIV ; Epstein-Barr Virus ; TREATABLE VIRUSES: influenza, HSV, and HIV; UNTREATABLE VIRUSES: rhinovirus, RSV, parainfluenza, EBV; RARE: gonococci, diphtheria; Arcanobacterium haemolyticum: can mimic S. pyogenes in college age females, pharyngitis + rash.

TREATMENT REGIMENS

Streptococcal pharyngitis

- Principles: 90% are viral; give pen/erythro if: 1) (+) strep Ag or 2) (+) throat culture
- Lab tests GAS: rapid antigen tests (80-90% sensitive & available in minutes) or throat culture (90% sensitive, but delays treatment 24-48 hrs.) No test-of-cure required.
- Preferred: penicillin VK 250mg PO qid or 500-1000mg PO bid x 10d or penicillin benzathine 1.2 mU IM x 1
- Pen allergy: erythromycin estolate 500mg bid or tid x 10 d or azithromycin - (Z-pack) or clarithromycin (Biaxin) 1g XR or 500mg bid x 5d
- Cefpodoxime (Vantin) 200mg bid x 5d
- Cefadroxil 500mg bid x 5 d
- Loracarbef (Lorabid) 200mg x 5 d

Gonococcal pharyngitis

- Preferred (CDC-MMWR 2002;55:RR-6): ceftriaxone 125mg IM + doxycycline 100mg PO bid x 7d
- Ciprofloxacin (Cipro) 500mg PO x 1 + doxycycline 100mg PO bid x 7d
- Azithromycin (Zithromax) 2g PO x 1

Miscellaneous agents

- Influenza (within 48h): rimantadine 100mg PO bid, zanamivir (Relenza) 10mg bid inhaled, oseltamivir (Tamiflu) 75mg PO bid, ea x 5d; must start when sx < 48 hrs.
- Acute HIV: See HIV/AIDS--acute retroviral syndrome
- HSV: acyclovir (Zovirax) 400mg PO tid x 5-10d; valacyclovir (Valtrex) 1g PO bid x 5-10d; famciclovir (Famvir) 250mg PO bid x 5-10d
- Diphtheria: erythromycin 500mg PO qid x 14d; TMP-SMX 1 DS BID x 14d

DRUG-SPECIFIC COMMENTS

Amoxicillin: An acceptable substitute for penicillin V, which is also always active against Strep; well tolerated, & cheap. There is more diarrhea with amoxicillin & a risk of rash, which is magnified if the patient really has mononucleosis. It appears that a single daily dose of 1g works as well as Pen V 2-4x/d

Cefixime: It works & has possible advantages along with other oral cephalosporins--Strep eradication rates are higher than they are with penicillin & treatment can be 5-7 days instead of the customary 10 days. Disadvantages are possible abuse of broad spectrum agents & cost.

Cefpodoxime Proxetil: It works & has possible advantages along with other oral cephalosporins--Strep eradiction rates are higher than they are with penicillin & treatment can be 5-7 days instead of the customary 10 days. Disadvantages are possible abuse of broad spectrum agents & cost.

Clarithromycin: Should work as well as erythromycin with advantage of better GI tolerance, but higher cost. Also, 5%+ of strep are resistant.

Doxycycline: No. No. No. A New York Times editorial found 20% of physicians (mostly surgeons) thought doxycycline was a good strep drug & the author lamented the sorry state of medical knowledge among our colleagues. The problem is high rates of resistance & poor strep eradication rates.

Penicillin: Consensus choice as preferred agent even though cephalosporins have a better track record in eradicating strep

IMPORTANT POINTS

- Source: CDC guidelines (Ann Intern Med 2001;134:506&509), ACP (AIM 2001;134:506), and Bisno (NEJM 2001: 344: 205); IDSA (CID 2002;35:113)
- Recent meta-analysis shows cephalosporins superior to penicillin (CID 2004;38:1526) but experts still like penicillin best
- Some experts treat strep based on Centor clinical criteria (ACP) but others treat only with lab-proven strep (IDSA)
- Dx: (Centor criteria) Hx of fever, exudative tonsillitis, no cough, tender cervical LN. Some recommend empiric Rx when 3 of 4 are present but others think strep Ag detection helps prevent ABX abuse
- Reasons to treat: prevent rheumatic fever (rare) & peritonsillar abscess (rare), reduce spread (usually non-contagious in 48 hrs), relieve suffering (modest benefit).
- -Greatest concern about spread is with pediatric patients

SELECTED READINGS

Casey JR. Meta-analysis of cephaolosporins vs. penicillin for the treatment of Group A streptococcal tonsillopharyngitis in adults. Clin Infect Dis 2004;38;1526

Bisno AL, Gerber MA, Gwaltney JM, et al. Diagnosis and management of group a streptococcal pharyngitis: a practice guideline. Acute Pharyngitis Guideline Panel, IDSA. Clin Infect Dis 1997;25:574

Zwart S, et al. Penicillin for acute sore throat in children: randomized, double blind trial. BMJ 2003;327:1324

Snow V, Mottur-Pilson C, Cooper RJ. Principles of appropriate antibiotic use for acute pharyngitis in adults. Ann Intern Med 2001;134:506.

Cooper RJ, Hoffman JR, Bartlett JG. Principles of appropriate antibiotic use for acute pharyngitis in adults: Background. Ann Intern Med 2001;134:509.

Bisno AL, Gerber MA, Gwaltney JM Jr., et al. Practice guidelines for the diagnosis and management of group A streptococcal pharyngitis:Infectious Diseases Society of America . Clin Infect Dis 2002:35:113-25

Casey JR, Pichichero ME. Meta-analysis of cephalosporins versus penicillin for treatment of Gr A tonsillopharyngitis in adults. Clin Infect Dis 2004;38;1526

Stollerman GH. Commentary: Penicillin therapy for streptococcal pharyngitis--what have we learned in 50 years?. Infect Dis Clinc Pract 1995;4:54

Bisno A. Group A streptococcal infection and acute rheumatic fever . N Engl J Med 1991;325:783

Centor RM, Witherspoon JM, Dalton, HP, et al. The diagnosis of strep throat in adults in the emergency room. Med Decis Making 1981;1:239

PNEUMOCYSTIS JIROVECI PNEUMONIA

John G. Bartlett, M.D.

DIAGNOSTIC CRITERIA

- Clinical: cough (no sputum), fever & dyspnea over 2-4wks (AIDS), over 5-14days (non-AIDS). Formerly P. carinii (PCP).
- Always in a compromised host: AIDS, organ tx, cancer chemo Rx, steroids.
- Studies: CXR bilateral interstitial infiltrates, hypoxemia or oxygen desaturation w/ exercise, elevated LDH, CD4 count <250/mm^3 (AIDS).
- Definitive dx: demonstration of P. jiroveci cysts on induced sputum or bronchoscopy specimen.
- Up to 20% have negative CXR

COMMON PATHOGENS: Pneumocystis jiroveci

TREATMENT REGIMENS

Antibiotics

- Principles: HOST: CD4 <250; DX: induced sputum +/or bronch; RX: Multiple options +/- prednisone; expect slow response
- Preferred: TMP-SMX 5mg/kg q 8h (trimethoprim) PO or IV x 21 days.
- Alternative: Dapsone 100mg/d PO + trimethoprim 5mg/kg q8h PO x 21 days.
- Clindamycin 1.8-2.4g/d PO or IV + primaquine 30mg base/d PO x 21 days.
- Atovaquone 750mg (5 mL) PO w/food bid x 21 days
- Pentamidine IV 3-4 mg/kg/day x 21 days
- Trimetrexate 45mg/m2 IV QD + leucovorin 20mg/mg q 6h (last resort)

Prednisone

- Indications for prednisone: pO2 <70 mm/Hg or A-a gradient >35mm Hg)
- Steroid regimen: prednisone 40mg PO bid x 5d, then 40mg PO qd x 5d, then 20mg PO qd x completion of therapy.

Failure to respond/adverse drug reaction

- Drug failure: Failure to improve or progression at 5d
- Oral regimens: TMP-SMX; Dapsone + TMP; Clind-prim considered equally effective & w/o cross reactions
- IV regimens TMP-SMX and pentamidine considered equally effective; pent - expect serious side effects
- Switch therapy: Usually works w/change for drug toxicity, often fails if prompted by "failure" of initial Rx
- Clindamycin-primaquine: May be optimal oral regimen for switch therapy due to Rx failure (Arch Int Med 2001;161:1529)

DRUG-SPECIFIC COMMENTS

Atovaquone: Oral therapy that is very expensive compared to alternatives

Dapsone: When combined with trimethoprim, a highly effective combination for mild to moderate PCP. This is an alternative to TMP-SMX.

Pentamidine: This requires parenteral administration and is a major alternative to TMP-SMX in patients who are seriously ill. Serious side effects are common (~50%) including renal failure, hypoglycemia, hypotension, GI intolerance.

Primaquine: When combined with clindamycin, a highly effective combination for mild to moderate PCP. This is an alternative to TMP-SMX.

Trimethoprim: When combined with dapsone, highly effective combination for mild to moderate PCP. This is an alternative to TMP-SMX.

Trimethoprim + Sulfamethoxazole: Clearly preferred for prophylaxis due to high rate of efficacy, low cost and benefit in preventing many other infections including pneumonia, sinusitis, listeria, GNB, legionella, etc. Main problem is high rate of intolerance with rash and GI side effects.

IMPORTANT POINTS

- Guidelines from CDC/IDSA (MMWR 2004;53:RR-15)
- PCP is always fatal if untreated. Hospitalized patients w/PCP have 15-20% mortality despite recommended Rx.
- Rate of reactions to TMP-SMX in AIDS pts is 30-40%, esp fever, pruritis, rash, GI intol; less common--hepatitis, neutropenia
- Data provided are based on experience with PCP in AIDS; PCP in other settings is similar in clinical features, diagnosis, and treatment but course is more rapid, diagnostic yield with bronchoscopy is somewhat less sensitive, and mortality is higher.

SELECTED READINGS

Thomas CF and Limper AH. Pneumocystis pneumonia. N Engl J Med 2004;350:2487

Larsen HH, et al. A prospective, blinded study of quantitative touch-down polymerase chain reaction using oral wash samples for diagnosis of Pneumocystis pneumonia in HIV infected patients. JID 2004;189:1679-83

Kovacs JA & Masur H. Prophylaxis against opportunistic infections in patients with HIV infection. NEJM 2000;342:1416

Safrin S, Finkelstein DM, Feinberg J. A double blind, randomized comparison of oral TMP-SMX, dapsone-trimethoprim & clindamycin-primaquine for treatment of mild to moderate PCP in patients with AIDS. Ann Intern Med 1996;124:792

Gagnon S, Boota AM, Fischl MA, et al. Corticosteroids as adjunctive therapy for severe P. carinii pneumonia in AIDS: A double blind, placebo controlled trial. NEJM 1990;323:1444

Stansell JD, Osmond DH, Charlebois E, et al. Predictors of Pneumocystis carinii pneumonia in HIV-infected persons. Am J Respir Crit Care Med 1997;155:60

Wachter RM, Luce JM, Safrin S, et al. Cost and outcome of intensive care for patients with AIDS, Pneumocystis carinii pneumonia and severe respiratory failure. JAMA 1995;273:130

Bozzette SA, Sattler FR, Chin J, et al. A controlled trial of early adjunctive treatment with corticosteroids for Pneumocystis carinii pneumonia in AIDS. NEJM 1990;323:1451

Masur H, Shelhamer J. Empiric outpatient management of HIV-related pneumonia. Ann Intern Med 1996;111:451

Osmond DH. Impact of bacterial pneumonia and P. carinii pneumonia on HIV progression. Clin Infect Dis 1999;29:536

PNEUMONIA, ASPIRATION   John G. Bartlett, M.D.

DIAGNOSTIC CRITERIA

- Three forms based on aspirate: bacteria (infection), acid (chem. pneumonia) or water/vegetal (obstruction)
- Infection: Pt aspiration prone (dysphagia, consciousness), fever, cough, infiltrate (10-15% community-acq pneumonia)
- Acid pneumonia: Sudden dyspnea +/- cyanosis, fever, wheezing, often ARDS
- Obstruction: Vegetal (peas & beans, etc), water (drowning)

Diagnosis

- Lab: X-ray - no infiltrate = no disease. Culture - useless

Treatment Regimens

Infection

- Principles: Suspect with aspiration prone pt + infiltrate + cough/fever - Abx empiric vs anaerobes - community-acq or GNB - nosocomial
- Preferred vs anaerobes: clindamycin 600mg IV q 8h or 300mg qid PO (+/- fluoroquinolone) x 10d
- Alt. PO: amox-clav (Augmentin) 875mg PO bid x 10d or amp-sub (Unasyn) 1.5-3g IV q 6h
- Alt. IV: pip-tazo (Zosyn) 3.375g IV q 6h; imipenem 0.5-1g IV q 6h x 10d
- CAP with ? aspiration: fluoroquinolone + clindamycin (IDSA guidelines)
- Gatiflox (Tequin), moxiflox (Avelox), clarithro (Biaxin), azithro (Zithromax), erythro
- Nosocomial case: See nosocomial pneumonia - for anaerobes use imipenem, pip-tazo (Zosyn) or clind + GNB coverage

Chemical/acid

- Guidelines from: Marik PE (NEJM 2001;344:665)
- Principles: Fulminant w/dyspnea, decreased O2, infiltrate +/- wheezing - suction + support
- Suction: To remove particles, fluid, etc
- Support: IV fluids, ventilatory support (ARDS)
- Controversial: Pos pressure vent, colloids, steroids & abx
- Steroids: Not useful in 2 controlled trials
- ABX: Not necessary, but usually given

Obstruction/prevention

- Obstruction foreign body: bronch
- Obstruction laryngeal level: Heimlich maneuver
- Obstruction fluids: Tracheal suction
- Prevention: Upright or semi-upright position (documented benefit)
- Controversial: Trach, N-G tube, PEG, gastric pH increase
- Gastric paresis: Postpyloric feeding tube
- Nutrition: Feeding tubes/gastroscopy tubes may be necessary - don't lower aspiration risk

Important Points

- Guidelines - infection: IDSA 2003 (CID 2003;37:1405); chemical: Marik (NEJM 2001;344:665)
- Three different syndromes: Infection (pneumonia), acid (chemical burn), food/water (obstruction)
- Infection: 10-15% community acquired pneumonia, pathogen: Anaerobes/strep; RX: Clindamycin, betalactam - BLI
- Nosocomial cases: Bacteriology & Rx completely different - GNB + S. aureus +/- anaerobes
- Chemical pneumonitis: 3 courses - rapid recovery, ARDS, superinfection
- Rx anaerobes: Clind, imipenem, pip-tazo, amp-sulbac, POSSIBLE: gati, moxi, macrolides

Selected Readings

Marik PE. Aspiration pneumonitis and aspiration pneumonia. NEJM 2001;344:665

Mendelson CL. The aspiration of stomach contents into the lungs during obstetric anaesthesia. Am J Obstet Gyn 1946;52:191

Bynum LJ, Pierce AK. Pulmonary aspiration of gastric contents. Am Rev Respir Dis 1976;114:1129

Wolfe JE, Bone RC, Ruth WE. Effects of corticosteroids in the treatment of patients with gastric aspiration. Am J Med 1977;63:719

Bartlett JG, O'Keefe P, Tally FP, et al. The bacteriology of hospital-acquired pneumonia. Arch Intern Med 1986;146:868

Bartlett JG. Anaerobic bacterial infections of the lung and pleural space. Clin Infect Dis 1993;4:S248

Levison ME, Mangura CT, Lorber B, et al. Clindamycin compared with penicillin for the treatment of anaerobic lung abscess. Ann Intern Med 1983;98:446

Drakulovic MB, Torres A, Bauer TT, et al. Supine body position as a risk for nosocomial pneumonia in mechanically ventilated patients. Lancet 1999;354:1851

DeToledo JC, Lowe MR, Gonzalez J, Haddad H. Risk of aspiration pneumonia after an epileptic seizure: a retrospective analysis of 1644 adult patients. Epilpsy Behav 2004;5:593-5

Allewelt M, Schuler P, Boleskei PL, et al. Ampicillin + sulbactam vs clindamycin +/- cephalosporin for the treatment of aspiration pneumonia and primary lung abscess. Clin Microbiol Infect 2004;10:163-70.

PNEUMONIA, COMMUNITY-ACQUIRED

John G. Bartlett, M.D.

DIAGNOSTIC CRITERIA

- Hx: cough, fever & sputum production +/- GI symptoms, or pleurisy
- PE: fever, tachypnea, rales
- Chest XR always shows infiltrate; PCP an occasional exception
- Site of care--use judgment + PORT (see Tables 5a-5c) or CURB -65 score (decreased consciousness, increased BUN, respiratory rate >30/min and BP <90 systolic plus age >65 years)

COMMON PATHOGENS: S. pneumoniae ; Haemophilus influenzae ; Chlamydia pneumoniae ; Legionella species ; Influenza ; Parainfluenza ; Mycoplasma ; RSV

TREATMENT REGIMENS

Outpatient (empiric)
- Outpatient and uncomplicated: doxycycline or macrolide
- Doxycycline 100mg bid x 7-10d
- Azithromycin 500mg PO qd x 3d (tri-pak)
- Clarithromycin 1g PO qd x 7d
- Outpatient and comorbidity (COPD, diabetes, CHF, etc) and/or recent abx: above drugs or fluoroquinolone or ketolide
- Telithromcyin 800mg qd x 7-10d
- Fluoroquinolone: levofloxacin 750mg/d x 5d, gatiflox 400mg/d, or moxiflox 400mg/d x 7d

Hospitalized patient (empiric)
- Preferred (IDSA guidelines), either: 1. fluoroquinolone (alone); or 2. [ceftriaxone OR cefotaxime] AND [erythro, azithro, OR clarithro] as dosed below
- Levofloxacin (Levaquin) 750mg IV/PO qd OR gatifloxacin (Tequin) 400mg IV/PO qd or moxiflox (Avelox) 400mg PO/IV qd x 7-10d
- Ceftriaxone (Rocephin) 1g IV qd OR cefotaxime 1g IV q8h, each with macrolide
- Azithromycin 500mg IV/PO qd x 3d usually with ceftriaxone or cefotaxime
- Clarithromycin XL (Biaxin) 500mg PO bid OR erythromycin 500mg - 1g IV q6h or 500mg PO qid, each x 7-10d with cefotaxime or ceftriaxone

- Aspiration: clindamycin 600mg IV q8h + fluoroquinolone

Pathogen-specific

- S pneumo (pen-sens): amox, ceftriaxone, cefotaxime, cefpodoxime, cefprozil, macrolide, until afebrile 3 days
- Mycoplasma or chlamydia: macrolide, doxycycline x 7d
- Legionella: azithromycin x 3-5d or fluoroquinolone x 7d
- H. flu: doxycycline, 2nd or 3rd gen. cephalosporin, fluoroquinolone x 1-2w
- Influenza: rimantadine, zanamivir, oseltamivir x 5d
- Anaerobes: clindamycin or amoxicillin-clavulanate (Augmentin) or ampicillin-sulbactam (Unasyn) or piperacillin-tazobactam (Zosyn)
- S. pneumo (pen-resistant): gati/Levo/moxifloxacin, vancomycin, linezolid, telithromycin

Drug-Specific Comments

Amoxicillin: Often considered the drug of choice for oral treatment of infections caused by S. pneumoniae, even in the era of escalating penicillin resistance. The major disadvantage is lack of activity against atypical agens and 30-40% of H. influenzae. A good choice, in fact the preferred agent, for oral treatment of pneumococcal pneumonia unless the strain is likely to show high level penicillin resistance.

Amoxicillin + Clavulanate: All the advantages of amoxicillin with the additional activity against H. influenzae, but it is far more expensive than amoxicillin, and like amoxicillin, lacks activity against atypical agents. A good choice, especially if common bacteria (S. pneumoniae and H. influenzae) are predicted but relatively expensive.

Ampicillin + Sulbactam: Good activity against S. pneumoniae and H. influenzae, but poor activity against atypical agents. This is a rational choice, but a macrolide or fluoroquinolone should be added if atypical agents are likely or if the patient is seriously ill.

Cefaclor: Relatively inactive against S. pneumoniae and totally inactive against atypical agents.

Cefepime: Good activity against S. pneumoniae and H. influenzae, but no activity against atypical agents. This is a rational choice for bacterial pneumonia, but a macrolide or fluoroquinolone should be added if the patient is seriously ill or atypical agents are likely.

Ceftriaxone: A preferred agent for S. pneumoniae, but inactive against atypical strains and questionable activity against S. pneumoniae strains with MIC values above 4mcg/mL (6% of strains in US). This is a rational choice, but should be combined with a macrolide or fluoroquinolone in patients who are seriously ill.

Clarithromycin: Advantages are activity against atypical strains, better tolerance than with erythromycin, and convenience of once- or twice-daily dosing. Disadvantages are lack of an IV formulation and resistance by 30-40% of S. pneumoniae. A good choice.

Daptomycin: Do not use for pneumonia, as study employing agent had high failure rate.

Doxycycline: Active against atypical strains including Legionella, dirt cheap, generally well tolerated, convenience of twice-daily dosing, and good activity in clinical trials despite its reputation as a "wimpish antimicrobial". The main disadvantage is variable rates of resistance by S. pneumoniae. This is a rational choice.

Gatifloxacin: Active against nearly all treatable agents of community-acquired pneumonia except influenza, including atypical agents, S. pneumoniae, H. influenzae, etc. Other advantages include convenience of once-daily dosing, good tolerance, IV and oral formulations, and good performance in multiple clinical trials. The main disadvantage is relatively high cost and a concern that this may promote fluoroquinolone resistance. All the advantages of levofloxacin with slight differences - gatifloxacin has not been tested or FDA approved for treatment of pneumonia caused by PCN-resistant strains of S. pneumo.

Imipenem/Cilastatin: Good activity against S. pneumoniae and H. influenzae, but no activity against atypical agents. This is a rational choice for bacterial pneumonia, but a macrolide or fluoroquinolone should be added if the patient is seriously ill or atypical agents are likely.

Levofloxacin: Active vs all major treatable agents including 99% of S. pneumoniae, H. flu and the three atypical agents. Sometimes criticized for interiority compared to moxifloxacin and gatifloxacin based on PK/PD data but this was largely corrected by the higher dose of 750mg/d.

Moxifloxacin: Active against nearly all treatable agents of community-acquired pneumonia except influenza, including atypical agents, S. pneumoniae, H. influenzae, etc. Other advantages include convenience of once-daily dosing, good tolerance, IV & oral formulations, and good performance in multiple clinical trials. The main disadvantage is relatively high cost and a concern that this may promote fluoroquinolone resistance. All the advantages of levofloxacin with slight differences - moxifloxacin has not been tested or FDA approved for treatment of pneumonia caused by PCN-resistant strains of S pneumonia.

Telithromycin: New drug of the ketolide class, available only orally. Treats nearly all drug-resistant pneumococci. Has good activity against H. influenzae and atypical agents.

Ticarcillin + Clavulanic Acid: Ticarcillin is relatively inactive against S. pneumoniae as well as lacking activity against atypical agents. This is a bad choice.

IMPORTANT POINTS

- Source: IDSA Guidelines (CID 2003; 37:1405)
- Patients with cough and abnormal vital signs should have a chest x-ray. If negative--no abx; if infiltrate--abx
- Hospitalized patients should receive abx within 4hr of arrival; earlier is better
- IV to PO switch: clinically improving, pO2>92, T<38C, p <100, RR <24, able to take pills, GI tract works
- Admission: Two CURB 65 criteria - consciousness, Urea, RR >30, BP <90, >65yrs
- Major debate: Role of Mycoplasma and Chlamydia, and need for fluoroquinolones.
- See http://www.journals.uchicago.edu/CID/journal/issues/v37n11/32441/32441. web.pdf for IDSA Guidelines on CAP.

SELECTED READINGS

Mandell L, Bartlett JG, Dowell SF, et al. Update of practice guidelines for the management of pneumonia in immunocompetent adults. Clin Infect Dis 2003;37:1405-33

Centers for Disease Control. Effect of susceptibility breakpoints on reporting of resistance in Streptococcus pneumoniae, United States, 2003. MMWR 2004;53:152

Musher DM, Montoya R, Wanahita A. Diagnostic value of microscopic examination of gram-stained sputum and sputum cultures in patients with bacteremic pneumococcal pneumonia. Clin Infect Dis 2004;39:165-9

Nuermberger EL, Bishai WR. The clinical significance of macrolide-resistant Streptococcus pneumoniae. Clin Infect Dis 2004;38:99-103

Karlowsky JA, Thornsberry C, Critchley IA, et al. Susceptibilities to levofloxacin in Streptococcus pneumoniae, Haemophilus influenzae and Moraxella catarrhalis clinical isolates from children: results from 2000-01, 2001-02 TRUST studies in the U.S. Antimicrobial Ag Chemother 2003;47:1790-7

Houck P, Bratzler DW, Nsa W, et al. Timing of antibiotic administration and outcomes for medicare patients with community-acquired pneumonia. Arch Intern Med 2004;164:637-44

Lim WS, van der Eerden MM, Laing R, et al. Defining community-acquired pneumonia severity on presentation to hospital: an international derivation and validation study. Thorax 2003;58:377-82

Marrie TJ, Lau CY, Wheeler SL, et al. A controlled trial of a critical pathway for treatment of community-acquired pneumonia. J Amer Med Assoc 2000;283:749-55

Marrie T et al. Predictors of Symptom Resolution in Patients with Community-Acquired Pneumonia. Clin Infect Dis 2000; 31:1362

Whitney CG. Increasing prevalence of multidrug-resistant Streptococcus pneumoniae in the United States . New Engl J Med 2000; 343:1917

PNEUMONIA, HOSPITAL-ACQUIRED

John G. Bartlett, M.D.

DIAGNOSTIC CRITERIA

- Clinical: pneumonia symptoms (fever, purulent respiratory secretions +/- dyspnea) + pulmonary infiltrate on CXR acquired >48-72 hrs after hospitalization.
- Lab: culture of blood, sputum, endotracheal aspirate, bronchoscopic specimen.
- Legionella: urinary antigen, sputum PCR or sputum culture.
- Preferred micro study is bronch with quantitative culture - but need is controversial.
- Organisms to ignore: Staphylococcus epidermidis, enterococcus, all gram positive rods other than Nocardia and B. anthracis, candida species.

COMMON PATHOGENS: Enterobacteriaceae ; Pseudomonas aeruginosa ; Staphylococcus aureus ; Legionella species

TREATMENT REGIMENS

Antibiotics - empiric

- Empiric abx based on risk of multiply-resistant (MDR) pathogens.
- Risk of MDR: hospitalization > 4 d, admitted from chronic care facility, abx Rx within past 90 d, immunosuppression, high rates of abx resistance in region or facility.
- Low risk of MDR: ceftriaxone 2 gm/d IV, levofloxacin 750mg or moxifloxacin 400 mg/d IV, ampicillin-sulbactam 2gm IV q6h, or ertapenem 1 gm IV qd.
- High risk of MDR: Rx for P. aeruginosa, other GNB, S. aureus (MRSA) using 1) beta-lactam and 2) fluoroquinolone or aminoglycoside and 3) vancomycin or linezolid.
- Antipseudomonal betalactams (IV): cefepime 1-2 gm q 8-12h or ceftazidime 2 gm q8h or imipenem 0.5-1.0 g q6h or meropenem 1 gm q8h or piperacillin-tazobactam 4.5 gm q6h --PLUS
- Levofloxacin 750 mg IV qd or ciprofloxacin 400 mg IV q8h --OR
- Gentamicin 7 mg/kg/d, tobramycin 7 mg/kg/d or amikacin 20 mg/kg/d IV (goal toughs: gent/tobra < 1 ug/mL, amikacin < 4-5 ug/mL)--PLUS
- Vancomycin 15 mg/kg IV q12h or linezolid 600 mg IV q12h.
- Follow-up at 48-72h (clinically improved): cx negative - consider stopping abx; if cx positive - de-escalate, treat for 7-8d.
- Follow-up at 48-72h (clinically unimproved): cx negative - look for alternative causes; cx positive - adjust abx.

Pathogen specific

- Pseudomonas: use sensitivity tests to guide-ceftaz, cipro, cefepime, aztreonam, imipenem, pip +/- aminoglycoside (tobramycin or amikacin). Some treat longer (10-14d) for Pseudomonas pneumonitis.
- Coliforms: in vitro tests needed.
- Anaerobes (aerobic GNB usually more important in mixed infections): amp-sulbactam, ticar-clav, pip-tazo, clindamycin, imipenem, ertapenem.

- S. aureus: oxacillin or nafcillin; MRSA or pen allergy: vancomycin or linezolid.
- Legionella: levofloxacin 750 mg/d, gatifloxacin 400mg/d, moxifloxacin 400mg/d x 7-10d or azithromycin 500mg/d x 5d.

Prevention

- Recommendations based on 2003 meta-analysis (Ann Int Med 2003;138:494).
- Semi-recumbent position - if possible
- Sucralfate instead of H2 blocker or proton pump inhibitor in order to preserve gastric acidity.
- Subglottic aspiration - use if available
- Decontamination of gut - works but not recommended.

DRUG-SPECIFIC COMMENTS

Amikacin: (Used as amikacin + ceftazidime)--Amikacin is the most predictably active aminoglycoside vs. GNB. It is also the most expensive. Watch for nephrotoxitity (check daily creatinine) and otoxicity (audiologic, vestibular).

Aztreonam: Monobactam with gram-negative coverage that can be used in patients with penicillin allergies. Coverage against Pseudomonas aeruginosa and Acinetobacter spp. is variable, hence should not be relied upon for empiric therapy alone.

Cefepime: (Maxipime) Goal is to cover major pathogens including GNB and S. aureus (MRSA requires vancomycin or linezolid). Cefepime has ceftazidime-like activity vs P. aeruginosa and cefotaxime-like activity vs GPC. Not active against MRSA, S. maltophilia, and anaerobes.

Ceftazidime: Usually used in combination with tobramycin--intent is broad-spectrum coverage vs. coliforms and Pseudomonads. Ceftazidime is not active vs MRSA, enterococcus, S. maltophilia may be combined with vancomycin--goal is to cover major pathogens including GNB and S. aureus (vancomycin). Need for "double coverage" of P. aeruginosa is debated.

Imipenem/Cilastatin: (Primaxin) With or without adding vancomycin--goal is to cover major pathogens including coliforms, anaerobes, and S. aureus (vancomycin for MRSA). May cause seizures if dose adjustment is not made with renal failure. This is the most predictably active drug vs nosocomial GNB in many reports.

Linezolid: (Zyvox) Active vs nearly all GPC including MRSA. IV or po well tolerated, achieves excellent penetration into lung tissues and fluids. Expensive.

Piperacillin + Tazobactam: (Zosyn) The intent is coverage of coliforms, anaerobes and Pseudomonas. This is a logical choice due to good activity against most GNB & many GPC other than MRSA.

Ticarcillin + Clavulanic Acid: (Timentin) The intent is coverage of coliforms and pseudomonads.

Tobramycin: Used in combination with antipseudomonal betalactam to get synergy vs. coliforms and Pseudomonas. Tobramycin + piperacillin +/- vancomycin--goal is coverage of P. aeruginosa. With tobramycin - watch for nephrotoxicity (daily creatinine) and ototoxicity.

Vancomycin: Drug employed to cover the possibility of MRSA. Poor lung penetration means that dosing should be greater than the routine 1 gm IV q12h, so recommended dosing for pneumonia is 15 mg/kg q12h.

IMPORTANT POINTS

- Frequency is 0.5% of all hospitalized pts, 15-20% of ICU pts and 20-60% of ventilated pts.

- Usual dx criteria are fever, infiltrate & purulent respiratory secretions. Many patients w/ these findings have other conditions--pulmonary infarcts, CHF, atelectasis, etc.
- Major pathogens are GNB (50-70%), S. aureus (15-30%), Legionella (4%), or viral (10-20%).
- Role of bronchoscopy (protected brush catheter or BAL) for bacterial studies is controversial--some love it, some hate it. If used, the methodology must be precise for specimen collection & micro.
- If patient fails to respond: 6 possible reasons--
- 1) wrong diagnosis (not pneumonia)
- 2) need drainage (empyema)
- 3) inadequate host response (most common)
- 4) wrong antibiotic (change coverage)
- 5) complication of antibiotic (drug fever)
- 6) inadequate dose (aminoglycoside).
- Need for double coverage of GNB is unclear; best supported with synergy between aminoglycoside + betalactam for P. aeruginosa, but controversial here as well.

SELECTED READINGS

American Thoracic Society; Infectious Diseases Society of America. Guidelines for the management of adults with hospital-acquired, ventilator-associated, and healthcare-associated pneumonia. Am J Respir Crit Care Med. 2005;171:388

Dezfulian C, Shojania K, Collard HR, et al. Subglottic secretion drainage for preventing ventilator-associated pneumonia: a meta-analysis. Am J Med. 2005;118:11

Gibot S, Cravoisy A, Levy B, et al. Soluble triggering receptor expressed on myeloid cells and the diagnosis of nosocomial pneumonia. N Engl J Med 2004;350:451-8

Srinivasan A, Wolfenden LL, Song X, et al. An outbreak of Pseudomonas aeruginosa associated with flexible bronchoscopes. N Engl J Med 2003;348:221-7

Collard HR, Saint S, Matthay MA. Prevention of ventilator-associated pneumonia: An evidence-based systematic review. Ann Intern Med 2003;138:494-501

deJonge E, Schultz MG, Spanjaard L, et al. Effects of selective decontamination if digestive tract on mortality and acquisition of resistant bacteria in intensive care: A randomized controlled trial. Lancet 2003;362:1011-6

Wunderink RG, Rello J, Cammarata SK. Linezolid vs vancomycin: Analysis of two double-blind studies of patients with methicillin-resistant Staphylococcus aureus nosocomial pneumonia. Chest 2003;124:1789-97

Ost DE, Hall CS, Joseph. Decision analysis of antibiotic and diagnostic strategies in ventilator-associated pneumonia. Am Rev Respir Crit Care Med 2003;168:1060-7

Chastre J, Wolff M, Fagon JY, et al. Comparison of 8 vs 15 days of antibiotic therapy for ventilator-associated pneumonia in adults; a randomized trial. JAMA 2003;290:2588-98

Zanetti G, Bally F, Gieub G, et al. Cefepime vs Imipenem - cilastatin for treatment of nosocomial pneumonia in intensive care unit patients: A multi-center, evaluator-blind, prospective, randomized study. Antimicrob Ag Chemother 2003;47:3442-7

PRION DISEASES
Khalil G. Ghanem, M.D.

DIAGNOSTIC CRITERIA

- Classification: familial [fatal familial insomnia (FFI) & Gerstmann-Straussler Scheinker disease (GSS)]; sporadic (85% of cases) [Creutzfeld-Jakob disease (sCJD) .
- Acquired from suspected agent [variant-CJD (vCJD)]; iatrogenic CJD (iCJD) [kuru]. All forms universally fatal.

- sCJD: rapidly progressive dementia with 2 or more of: (startle) myoclonus, cortical blindness, pyramidal signs, cerebellar signs, extrapyramidal signs, or mutism.
- Age 45-75 years; CT/MRI normal or with atrophy; EEG-pseudoperiodic complexes is diagnostic; CSF profile bland but protein 14-3-3 usually +; brain biopsy if dx unclear.
- vCJD: depression, anxiety, withdrawl, peripheral sensory symptoms; then ataxia, chorea, athetosis; then dementia. Onset in young (20's) adults; incubation ~10yrs;

TREATMENT REGIMENS

Prevention

- Universal system of precautions currently in place is adequate for dealing w/patients: gloves in handling bodily fluids, masks, eyewear, & gowns for extensive blood or fluid exposures.
- Sterilization controversial: suggested methods include steam autoclaving at 132CX1 hr; immersion in 1 N NaOH X 1hr; concentrated (>3M) guanidine thiocyanate;
- Others have suggested 4.5 hrs of steam autoclaving at 121C & 15lbs pressure.
- Banning feeding of ruminant proteins to ruminants yields control of the BSE epidemic?
- Three cases of transfusion-associated prion disease described. Red Cross and FDA restrict importation of European blood products.

Treatment

- Treatment with agents such as idoxuridine, acyclovir, amphotericin, & interferon have been unsuccessful.
- There are no FDA licensed treatments for any of the human TSE.
- There have been case reports of stabilization w/ various agents including amantadine & vidarabine, but no trials have been performed.
- Several new investigational agents are being evaluated (see references).

IMPORTANT POINTS

- Not thought to contain DNA/RNA. Prions cause disease in both humans and animals; resistant to radiation, heat, nucleases, & alcohols. Annual rate of sCJD is 1.5 per million.
- Exact number of cases of vCJD in Europe (especially U.K.), although limited, may still increase as exact duration of incubation period unknown.
- Epidemiological studies suggest that the number of new cases should remain relatively low in view of the recent decline in the number of cases.
- Negative CSF 14-3-3 should not rule-out CJD in pts with compatible clinical syndrome.
- Transmission of TSE: ingestion of contaminated foods, iatrogenic (equipment/organs contaminated with neural tissue from infected source: dura mater grafts & human growth hormone most common sources), genetic (familial variants). No documented transmission w/ blood transfusions to date, although theoretical risk w/ vCJD.
- BSE epidemic in U.K. (late 1980s to early 1990s), a result of rendering process used (1970s-1980s) that did not inactivate BSE agent, transferring it from bovine to bovine (practice of feeding cattle the waste of other cattle); thought to have resulted in the human cases of vCJD seen in Britain, France and Germany (late 1990s-2000s) via ingestion of contaminated meat.Exact number of cases of vCJD in Europe (especially U.K.), although limited, may still increase as exact duration of incubation period unknown. Epidemiological studies suggest that the number of new cases should remain relatively low in view of the recent decline in the number of cases.

SELECTED READINGS

White AR, et al. Monoclonal antibodies inhibit prion replication and delay the development of prion disease. Nature. 2003 Mar 6;422(6927):80-3.

Diagnosis

Spencer MD, et al. First hundred cases of variant Creutzfeldt-Jakob disease: retrospective case note review of early psychiatric and neurological features. BMJ. 2002 Jun 22;324(7352):1479-82.

Montagna P, et al. Familial and sporadic fatal insomnia. Lancet Neurol. 2003 Mar;2(3):167-76.

Geschwind MD, et al. Challenging the clinical utility of the 14-3-3 protein for the diagnosis of sporadic Creutzfeldt-Jakob disease. Arch Neurol. 2003 Jun;60(6):813-6.

Smith PG. The epidemics of bovine spongiform encephalopathy and variant Creutzfeldt-Jakob disease: current status and future prospects. Bull World Health Organ. 2003;81(2):123-30

Ramasamy I, et al. Organ distribution of prion proteins in variant Creutzfeldt-Jakob disease. Lancet Infect Dis. 2003 Apr;3(4):214-22

Zanusso G, et al. Detection of pathologic prion protein in the olfactory epithelium in sporadic Creutzfeldt-Jakob disease. N Engl J Med. 2003 Feb 20;348(8):711-9.

Hunter N, Houston F. Can prion diseases be transmitted between individuals via blood transfusion: evidence from sheep experiments. Dev Biol (Basel). 2002;108:93-8.

Croes EA, et al. Creutzfeldt-Jakob disease 38 years after diagnostic use of human growth hormone. J Neurol Neurosurg Psychiatry. 2002 Jun;72(6):792-3.

Weber DJ, Rutala WA. Managing the risk of nosocomial transmission of prion diseases. Curr Opin Infect Dis. 2002 Aug;15(4):421-5.

PROCTITIS [SEXUALLY TRANSMITTED]

Noreen A. Hynes, M.D., M.P.H.

Diagnostic Criteria

- Proctitis: Limited to rectum i.e., above the anorectal line to 15cm on sigmoidoscopy
- Clinical: recent anal receptive intercourse; anorectal pain; tenesmus with or without constipation; mucopurulent discharge with or without hematochezia
- Lab: >4 PMNs/hpf on gram stain of anorectal secretions; collect specimens for CX and gram stain using anoscope (GC, CT, syphilis); syphilis serology

Common Pathogens: Neisseria gonorrhoeae ; Chlamydia trachomatis ; Herpes Simplex Virus ; Chlamydia trachomatis, LGV serovars

Treatment Regimens

Initial Empiric Therapy

- Ceftriaxone 125mg IM once PLUS doxycycline PO bid x 7d

HSV proctitis, first clinical episode

- Acyclovir 400mg 5 x per d x 10d
- Valacyclovir 1g PO bid x 7-10d
- Famciclovir 250mg PO tid x 7-10d

HSV proctitis suppression after 4 bouts/yr

- No HIV infection: acyclovir 400mg PO bid or famciclovir 250mg PO bid or valacyclovir 1g PO qd
- HSV proctitis in AIDS: acyclovir 5-10mg/kg IV q8h until clinical resolution, then acyclovir 400-800mg PO bid-tid or famciclovir 500mg PO bid or valacyclovir 500mg PO bid

Drug-Specific Comments

Acyclovir: Randomized trials indicate that acyclovir, valacyclovir, and famciclovir provide clinical benefit in treatment. Although the greatest amount of clinical data is available for acyclovir, its dosing frequency makes it less acceptable to patients.

Cefixime: Should not be used if patient has had oro-genital contact as agent does not attain adequate penetration of Waldyer's ring.

Ceftizoxime: Has been shown to be highly effective against uncomplicated urogenital and anorectal gonococcal infections. Ceftizoxime offers no advantage in comparison to ceftriaxone.

Ceftriaxone: A single 125mg injection provides sustained, high bactericidal levels in the blood. Extensive clinical experience indicates that ceftriaxone is safe and effective for the Rx of uncomplicated GC at all sites, curing 99.1% of uncomplicated urogenital and anorectal infections in published studies.

Ciprofloxacin: Effective against most strains of N. gonorrhoeae in the US (excluding Hawaii, New York City, MA and CA). A dose of 500mg provides sustained bactericidal levels in the blood. In published clinical trials, it has curred 99.8% of uncomplicated urogenital and anorectal infections. Ciprofloxacin is safe, relatively inexpensive, and can be given PO.

Doxycycline: Doxycyline is a highly effective agent against chlamydia trachomatis, including the LGV serovars. However, LGV requires at least 21d of therapy compared with 7d for non-LGV chlamydia proctitis. Doxycycline can be used to treat early syphilis in penicillin-allergic patients. It is NOT as efficacious as penicillin. Therefore, patients need close follow-up to detect treatment failures.

Famciclovir: No available data regarding efficacy in treatment of HSV proctitis

Penicillin: Parenteral penicillin is the treatment of choice for ALL stages of syphilis and is the only treatment for pregnant women. Desensitization is necessary for penicillin allergic pregnant women. Ideally, HIV-infected persons with syphilitic proctitis should only be treated with penicillin.

Spectinomycin: Spectinomycin is expensive and must be injected. However, it has been effective in published clincal trials curing 98.2% of uncomplicated urogenital and anorectal gonococcal infections. Therefore, it is a good alternative therapy for Rx of patients who can not tolerate either cephalosporins or fluoroquinolones.

IMPORTANT POINTS

- Recommendations based on CDC's 2002 STD Rx Guidelines; MMWR 2002; 51(RR-6); CDC 2004 revised recommendations for gonorrhea treatment (MMWR 2004 53:335-338)
- Proctitis potentially increases risk of HIV acquisition by up to 9-fold
- Immunocompromised patients may have severe HSV proctitis
- Must distinguish proctitis from proctocolitis and enteritis because suspect organisms differ.
- If inflammation seen above 15cm on sigmoidoscopy, then proctocolitis more likely & more classic foodborne & waterborne pathogens are seen; sx of both proctitis & colitis seen, including diarrhea
- On presentation anoscopy for specimen collection should be performed.
- Gram stain of exudate or rectal mucosa should be performed on initial visit
- Cultures for GC should be obtained from rectum, urethra, pharynx; rectal culture for CT
- Serologic test for syphilis in ALL cases; if ulcer or condylomata lata seen, darkfield microscopy of expressed serous secretions indicated; HSV diagnostic test also if ulcers present.
- If proctocolitis indicated by symptoms or findings on sigmoidoscopy, then cultures for Campylobacter, Salmonella, Shigella and stool exam for E. histolytica and Giardia lamblia indicated.
- Urinary retention with rectal pain and constipation suggests HSV proctitis in the right historical context.

SELECTED READINGS

Klausner JD et al. Etiology of clinical proctitis among men who have sex with men. Cln Infect Dis 2004 38:300-302.

Renzi C et al. Safety and acceptability of the Reality condom for anal sex among men who have sex with men. AIDS 2003 17:727-731.

Centers for Disease Control and Prevention. Sexually transmitted diseases treatment guidelines 2002. MMWR 2002; 51(No. RR-6).

Rompalo AM. Diagnosis and treatment of sexually acquired proctitis and proctocolitis: an update. Clin Infect Dis 1999; 28 (Suppl 1):S84-90.

Law C. Sexually transmitted diseases and enteric infections in the male homosexual population. Semin Dermatol 1990; 9(2):178-84.

Mirdel A et al. Primary and secondary syphilis, 20 years' experience: clinical features. Genitourin Med 1989; 65:1-3.

Goodell SE et al. Herpes simplex virus proctitis in homosexual men: clinical, sigmoidoscopic, and histopathologic features. N Engl J Med 1983; 308:868-871.

Quinn TC, et al. The etiology of anorectal infections in homosexual men. Am J Med 1981; 71(3):395-406.

Hansfield HH et al. Correlation of auxotype and penicillin susceptibility for Neisseria gonorrheoeae with sexual preference and clinical manifestations of gonorrhea. Sex Trans Dis 1980; 7:1-4.

PROSTATITIS, ACUTE BACTERIAL

Noreen A. Hynes, M.D., M.P.H.

DIAGNOSTIC CRITERIA

- Acute bacterial prostatitis (ABP) = Category I prostatitis by NIH classification; Only 5% of all prostatitis is ABP!
- Symptoms: (1) SX of UTI-dysuria, freq, urgency PLUS (2) SX of prostatitis-low back pain, perineal/penile/rectal pain +/- (3) SX of bacteremia--fever, rigors; arthralgia, myalgia
- Signs: (1) Localized to prostate-extremely tender, tense, swollen gland; warm to touch [DO NOT MASSAGE!] +/- (2) Bacteremia: fever, tachycardia
- Bacteriuria and pyuria on midstream urine; if sterile cx, acute bacterial prostatitis unlikely; also obtain blood cultures for bacteria and antibiotic sensitivities.
- Presents dramatically and is essentially a CLINICAL diagnosis.

COMMON PATHOGENS: E. coli ; Other Enterobacteriaceae

TREATMENT REGIMENS

Outpatient therapy

- Preferred PO Rx (UK Guidelines 2001): ciprofloxacin 500 mg PO bid x 28d OR ofloxacin 200mg bid x 28d
- Allergy to quinolones: TMP-SMX 1 DS PO BID x 28d OR TMP 200mg bid x 28d

Intravenous therapy

- Ceftriaxone 1-2g IV q12-24h (depending on severity) PLUS gentamicin 1.7mg/kg q8h depending upon renal function) until can tolerate PO regimen and afebrile for 48h; then PO regimen to complete 28d Rx
- Cefotaxime 1-2g q6-8h (up to 12g/d) PLUS gentamicin 1.7 mg/kg q8h depending upon renal function) until can tolerate PO regimen and afebrile for 48h; then PO regimen to complete 28d Rx

Supportive therapies and modalities

- Bed rest often needed

- Antipyretics/antiinflammatory for fever, myalgia, arthralgia
- Foley catheter may be needed to relieve bladder outlet obstruction due to prostatic edema
- Stool softeners
- Hydration
- Sitz bath

IMPORTANT POINTS

- Recommendations based on 2001 UK Guideline for Management of Prostatitis (www. mssvd.org.uk).
- Indications for hospitalization/IV RX: febrile with toxicity; concomitant illness; debilitated by age; immunosuppressed.
- Good antibiotic penetration into all areas of prostate achieved due to intense inflammation; antibiotics should be continued or changed according to sensitivity results.
- DO NOT perform prostatic massage! Extremely painful and of little benefit as pathogens almost always isolated from urine; persistent fever after 48h of ABX requires transrectal US to look for abscess.
- After full recovery, investigate urinary tract to exclude structural cause for prostatitis.
- Acute prostatitis can be hard to treat. Follow-up required for at least 3 months.
- In middle-aged men, Prostate Specific Antigen (PSA) levels may be elevated for 3 to 6 months after acute phase of inflammation.
- If transurethral ultrasound done, hypoechoic areas in prostate peripheral zone may persist for many months; use color Doppler ultrasound to differentiate these areas from prostatic cancer.

SELECTED READINGS

Kravchick S et al. Acute prostatitis in middle-aged men: a prospective study. BJU International 2004; 93:93-96.

Clinical Effectiveness Group. National guideline for the management of prostatitis (Association of Genitourinary Medicine and the Medical Society for the Study of Venereal Diseases). www.mssvd. org.uk June 2001 update.

Lloyd GL and Schaeffer AJ. The new age of prostatitis. Current Infect Dis Reprt 2001;3:354-9.

Mawhorter SD, et al. Prostatic and central nervous system histoplasmosis in an immunocompetent host: case report and review of prostatic histoplasmosis literature. Clin Infect Dis 2000 30(3):595-8

Stevermer JJ, Easley SK. Treatment of prostatitis. Am Fam Physician 2000; 61(10):3015-22; 3025-6.

Krieger JN et al. NIH consensus definition and classification of prostatitis. JAMA 1999;282;236-7.

Lipsky BA. Prostatitis and urinary tract infection in men: what's new; what's true?. Am J Med 1999 106 (3):327-34

Mitsumori K, et al. Virulence characteristics of Escherichia coli in acute bacterial prostatitis. J Infect Dis 1999; 180(4):1378-81

Nickel JC. Prostatitis: evolving management strategies. Urol Clin North Am 1999;26(4):737-51.

Schaeffer AJ. Prostatitis: U.S. perspective. Int J Antimicrob Agents 1999; 11:205-11;213-6

PROSTATITIS, CHRONIC BACTERIAL

Noreen A. Hynes, M.D., M.P.H.

DIAGNOSTIC CRITERIA

- Chronic bacterial prostatitis = Category II prostatitis by NIH classification

- Presents with vague symptoms which are not specific to chronic bacterial prostatitis. THE MAJORITY W/THESE SX WILL NOT HAVE INFECTIOUS CAUSE OF PROSTATITIS SYNDROME.
- SX: perineal pain, lower abdominal pain, penile pain (esp the tip), testicular pain, post ejaculatory pain, rectal or lower back pain, dysuria. Fever, prostration, bacteremia is NOT a feature.
- SIGNS: few objective signs; gland may or may not be locally or diffusely tender to palpation
- Localization test=Definitive DX modality: LAB-based gold std uses 4-glass method-- sequential cx of urine and expressed prostatic secretions. Some experts use only glass 1 and 4.

COMMON PATHOGENS: Enterobacteriaceae

TREATMENT REGIMENS

Recommended regimens
- Ciprofloxacin 500mg PO bid x 28d
- Norfloxacin 400mg PO bid x 28d
- Ofloxacin 200mg PO bid x 28d

Quinolone allergy regimens
- Doxycycline 100mg PO bid x 28d (less toxicity than minocycline regimen)
- Minocycline 100mg PO bid x 28d
- Trimethoprim-Sulfamethoxazole 1 double-strength tablet PO bid x 28d
- Trimethoprim 200mg PO bid x 28d

DRUG-SPECIFIC COMMENTS

Ciprofloxacin: The greatest amount of information in treating chronic bacterial prostatitis exists for the fluoroquinolones although there are no RCT for the treatment of bacterial prostatitis. It appears to be the quinolone of choice when Pseudomonas is the cause because it is more active than the other fluoroquinolones.

Doxycycline: Can be used in the treatment of chronic bacterial prostatitis (CBP) in fluoroquinolone-allergic patients because of its activity against Enterobacteriaceae. However, antimicrobial sensitivities are critical prior to use.

Minocycline: The side effect profile is high and most practitioners prefer to use doxycycline or TMP-SMX to treat chronic bacterial prostatitis in fluoroquinolone allergic patients. Antimicrobial sensitivities are critical if this drug is to be used due to resistance of Pseudomonas spp and many Enterobacteriaceae.

Norfloxacin: The greatest amount of information in treating chronic bacterial prostatitis exists for the fluoroquinolones although there are no RCT for the treatment of bacterial prostatitis.

IMPORTANT POINTS

- This module is based on the 2001 U.K. National Guideline for the Management of Prostatitis and published information from U.S. experts. There is no published U.S. guideline.
- The 4-glass localization test, although time consuming is key to differentiating this condition from non-bacterial causes.
- Before localization test: (1) no antibiotics for at least 1 mo, (2) no ejaculation for 2 days, (3) full, non-distended bladder. DO NOT perform if evidence of urethritis or UTI. RX acute problem first.

- Prostatic calculi suggested as source of recurrent infection. Very common radiologic finding. Radical TURP or total prostatectomy may be effective in carefully selected patients.

SELECTED READINGS

Schneider H et al. The 2001 Giessen Cohort Study on patients with prostatitis syndrome--an evaluation of inflammatory status and search for microorganisms 10 years after a first analysis. Andrologia 2003 35; 258-262.

Choe W, et al. Imaging prostatitis with Tc-99m ciprofloxacin. Clin Nucl Med 2002; 27(7):527-9

Clinical Effectiveness Group. National guideline for the management of prostatitis (Association of Genitourinary Medicine and the Medical Society for the Study of Venereal Diseases); . www.mssvd.org. uk. June 2001.

Nickel JC et al. Prevalence of prostatitis-like symptoms in a population-based study using the National Institutes of Health chronic prostatitis symptom index. J Urol 2001; 165:842-845.

Lipsky BA. Prostatitis and urinary tract infection in men: what's new; what's true. Am J Med 1999; 106 (3):327-34

Litwin MS et al. The National Institutes of Health chronic prostatitis symptom index: development and validation of a new outcome measure. Chronic Prostatitis Research Netork. J Urol 1999; 162:369-375.

Nickel JC. Prostatitis: evolving management strategies. Urol Clin North Am 1999; 26(4):737-51.

Nickel JC, et al. Prostatitis unplugged? Prostatic massage revisited. Tech Urol 1999; 5(1):1-7

Nickel JC, et al. Research guidelines for chronic prostatitis: consensus report from the first National Institutes of Health International Prostatitis Collaborative Network. Urol 1999; 54(2):229-33

Bjerklund JTE, et al. The role of antibiotics in the treatment of chronic prostatitis: a consensus statement. Eur Urol 1998; 34(6):457-66.

PYELONEPHRITIS, ACUTE UNCOMPLICATED

Noreen A. Hynes, M.D., M.P.H.

DIAGNOSTIC CRITERIA

- History: No hx of urologic abnormalities; other dx have been excluded.
- Clinical: fever, chills, flank pain; may or may not have sx of lower tract UTI; nausea/vomiting may be present; pathognomonic = tenderness to palpation/percussion over 1/both CVA.
- Lab: Urine Cx-- >100,000 CFU/mL of etiologic agent; Spun urine-- >9 WBC/HPF
- Ddx: PID, appendicitis, urolithiasis, biliary tract disease, acute pancreatitis, basal pneumonia
- Essentially all cases in women 18-40 years; risk factors: sexually active; diaphragm user

COMMON PATHOGENS: Escherichia coli ; Proteus species

TREATMENT REGIMENS

Oral regimens

- Ciprofloxacin 500mg PO bid x 14d
- TMP-SMX 1 double strength tablet PO bid x 14d (Only where local TMP-SMX resistant E. coli <20%)
- Ampicillin-clavulanate 500/125mg PO bid x 14d
- Ofloxacin 200mg PO bid x 14d
- Levofloxacin 500mg PO qd x 14d
- Norfloxacin 400mg PO bid x 14d

Intravenous regimens

- Ciprofloxacin 400mg IV q12h. Treat IV x 48h; then PO to complete 14d

- Gentamicin, tobramycin, 2 mg/kg loading dose IV, then 1.5-3.0 mg/kg/day or divided dose, until afebrile 48h , then PO Rx to complete 14d
- Amikacin 7.5mg/kg IV loading dose; then 15mg/kg/day or divided dose, until afebrile x 48h, then PO Rx to complete 14d
- Ampicillin/sulbactam 1-2g ampicillin/1g sulbactam IV q6h until afebrile x 48h, then PO cephalosporin to complete 14d
- Cefotaxime 1 or 2g IV q8h until afebrile x 48h, then give PO cephalosporin to complete 14d
- Ceftriaxone 1g IV qd until afebrile x 48h, then give PO cephalosporin to complete 14d
- Ceftazidime 1 - 2g IV q8-12h until afebrile x 48h, then give PO cephalosporin to complete 14d
- Levofloxacin 500mg IV qd until afebrile x 48h, then give PO levofloxacin to complete 14d

Drug-Specific Comments

Amoxicillin: Problem is high rates of resistance by E. coli. If E. coli sensitive to this agent it is a good choice for RX---inexpensive, good urine levels, and good safety profile in pregnancy.

Amoxicillin + Clavulanate: Use for Rx of mild acute uncomplicated pyelonephritis when the etiologic agent is KNOWN to be gram-positive cocci or to complete a 14d course of therapy for same which began with parenteral ampicillin+sulbactam.

Ampicillin + Sulbactam: If gram-positive cocci are the causative agent, then this parenteral agent with or without and aminoglycoside can be used for more severe cases of acute uncomplicated pyelonephritis. Use of PO amoxicillin-clavulanate to complete a 14d course of RX should follow.

Ceftazidime: Active agains most gram-negative organisms including P. aeruginosa. Attains good levels in urine.

Moxifloxacin: This FQ is not a good choice for Rx of UTIs as it attains poor urine levels.

Important Points

- Recommendations based on IDSA Guidelines (CID 1999; 29:745); these Rx guidelines endorsed by the European Soc Clin Micro Infect Dis and Amer Urol Assn.
- Mild case = low grade T; normal or sl elev peripheral WBC without nausea or vomiting. Oral Rx indicated. Rx in outpatient setting remains controversial despite oral RX.
- Criteria for hospitalization: high T, high peripheral WBC, vomiting, volume depletion, or evidence of sepsis OR failure to improve in 48 hours after initiation of oral RX. IV RX indicated initially.
- High risk for complications: Diabetes, pregnancy, immunocompromised, previous pyelonephritis, sx >14 days, structurally abn urinary tract--begin Rx for these in hospital regardless of sx
- Some experienced clinicians have successfully treated mild cases with 5- to 7-day Rx of aminoglycosides, beta-lactams, or fluoroquinolones.
- Less frequent pathogens: S. saprophyticus, Grp B streptococci, enterococci
- Route of infection is ascending: organisms enter urethra, colonize bladder, ascend to the renal pelvis and ultimately invade renal parenchyma.
- More virulent forms of E. coli cause uncomplicated acute pyelonephritis than cause cystitis but are more susceptible to antimicrobial therapy.

Selected Readings

Fihn SD. Acute uncomplicated urinary tract infections in women. N Engl J Med 2003 349:259-266.

Nickel JC. The management of acute pyelonephritis in adults. Can J Urol 2001;8(Suppl 1):29-38

Warren JW, et al. Guidelines for antimicrobial treatment of uncomplicated acute bacterial cystitis and acute pyelonephritis in women. Clin Infect Dis 1999; 29:745-58

Stamm WE, Stapleton AE. Approach to the patient with urinary tract infection. In Gorbach SL et al (eds). Infectious Diseases,1998, 2nd ed. W.B. Saunders, Philidelphia, PA, pp 943-1138.

Niclau DP, et al. Experience with a once-daily aminoglycoside program administered to 2184 adult patients. Antimicrob Agents Chemother 1995; 39:650-60.

Barclay ML, et al. What is the evidence for once-daily aminoglycoside therapy?. Clin Pharmacokinet 1994; 27:32-38

Rubin RH, et al. Evaluation of new ant-infective drugs for the treatment of urinary tract infection. Clin Infect Dis 1992; 15(Suppl 1):S216-27

Hooper DC, Wolfson JS. Fluoroquinolone antimicrobial agents. N Engl J Med 1991; 324:384-392

Talan DA, et al. Comparison of ciprofloxacin (7 days) and trimethoprim-sulfamethoxazole (14 days) for acute uncomplicated pyelonephritis in women. JAMA 200; 283:1583.

PYOMYOSITIS

John G. Bartlett, M.D.

DIAGNOSTIC CRITERIA
- Clinical: painful, tender, localized swelling over muscle + fever
- Lab: CT scan or MRI demonstrates muscle abscess
- Aspiration of abscess (by surgery or CT/US guided) yields pus, usually with S. aureus
- May be single or multiple sites and may result from trauma or occur spontaneously
- Most common sites are large leg mm (quadriceps & gluteus mm) and psoas mm.

COMMON PATHOGENS: Staph aureus

TREATMENT REGIMENS

Treatment based on gram stain/culture of aspirate
- Principles: risk - IDU, AIDS, penetrating trauma, tropics. Dx: CT/MRI - muscle abscess; cx - usually S. aureus; Rx: Abx +/- drainage
- Preferred: S. aureus--nafcillin/oxacillin 2g IV q6h x 14-28d
- S. aureus--cefazolin 500mg-1g IV q8h x 14-28d
- S. aureus- (MRSA) vancomycin 1g IV bid or linezolid 600mg bid PO/IV x 14-28 d or daptomycin 6mg/kg/d IV
- S. aureus (Meth sens) & pen allergy: clindamycin, TMP-SMX, fluoroquinolone
- Staph, Strep, or anaerobes--clindamycin 600mg IV q8h x 14-28d
- Anaerobes: ampicillin-sulbactam (Unasyn) 1.5-3g IV q6h

Surgery
- Open drainage or CT/US-guided aspirate with drainage
- Complicated cases may require fasciotomies and debridement
- Some respond to empiric antibiotic treatment vs. S. aureus without drainage

Abx modified when GS & cult results available
- S. aureus--sensitivity to methicillin will dictate use of alternatives to beta-lactams, usually vancomycin but sometimes clindamycin, TMP-SMX, linezolid, fluoroquinolone. Determine by in vitro testing
- Anaerobes (putrid or consistent gram-stain or cx)-clindamycin, Unasyn, Zosyn, Timentin, Imipenem

DRUG-SPECIFIC COMMENTS

Amoxicillin + Clavulanate: A good drug for oral use in outpatient component of care. Active vs methacillin sensitive S. aureus and all anaerobes

Ceftazidime: Not a good choice for S. aureus

Cefuroxime and Cefuroxime axetil: Reasonable alternative to nafcillin or oxacillin that may be given orally or parenterally

Dicloxacillin: A good choice for oral agent for outpatient component of care

Gatifloxacin: Use only if in vitro sensitivity data show activity--15-30% of S. aureus are now resistant. Main interest is oral form for outpatient component of care.

Imipenem/Cilastatin: More drug than necessary, in most cases, but active vs. most meth-sensitive S. aureus. Best justification is setting where broad spectrum activity is necessary because infection is serious, cause is unknown, and process is unknown.

Linezolid: Good choice for the unusual case that combines meth-resistant S. aureus & contraindication to vancomycin. Oral & parenteral. Expensive--very expensive.

IMPORTANT POINTS

- Guidelines are author's opinion
- S. aureus is most common pathogen
- Predisposing conditions: HIV, IDU, penetrating trauma, tropical exposure ("tropical pyomyositis"), diabetes, steroids, cirrhosis
- Differential dx: necrotizing fasciitis, gas gangrene, cellulitis, carbuncle, streptococcal myositis, phlebitis

SELECTED READINGS

Chauhan S, et al. Tropical pyomyositis: current perspective. Postgrad Med J 2004;80:267-70

Ebright JR, Pieper B. Skin and soft tissue infections in injection drug users. Infect Dis Clinics N. Amer 2002;16:697-712

Lawn SD, et al. Pyomyositis and cutaneous abscesses due to Mycobacterium avium: an immune reconstitution manifestation in a patient with AIDS. Clin Infect Dis 2004;38:461-3

Fan HC, Lo WT, Wang CC. Clinical characteristics of Staphylococcal pyomyositis. J Microbiol Immunol Infect 2002;35:121

Yusufu LM, Sabo SY, Nmadu PT. Pyomyositis in adults: a 12 year review. Trop Doc 2001;31:154

Medical Letter Consultants. Choice of antibacterial drugs. Medical Ltr 2001;43:69

Hossain A.; Reis E.D.; Soundararajan K et al. Nontropical pyomyositis: Analysis of eight patients in an urban center. Am Surg 2000; 66:1064

Cone LA, Lamb RB, Graff-Radford A. Pyomyositis of the anterior tibial compartment. Clin Infect Dis 1997;25:146.

Harbarth SJ, Lew DP. Pyomyositis as a nontropical disease. Current Clinical Topics in Infect Dis. Remington J, Swartz MN (Eds), Blackwell Science Publ. 1997;37-50.

Rogers WB, Yodlowski ML, Mintzer CM. Pyomyositis in patients who have the human immunodeficiency virus. J Bone Join Surg 1993;75:588.

RETROVIRAL SYNDROME, ACUTE

John G. Bartlett, M.D.

DIAGNOSTIC CRITERIA

- Definition: HIV infection prior to seroconversion or within 6 months of seroconversion
- Clinical features: fever, pharyngitis, weight loss, adenopathy, GI symptoms, +/- rash or neurologic symptoms, oral or genital ulceration
- Consider when typical symptoms, enigmatic fever in patient at risk, or "mono-spot negative mononucleosis"
- Lab: HIV serology usually neg or indeterminant or positive (seroconversion at 3 wks-6 mos. post-transmission)

- Plasma HIV RNA by PCR testing is pos @ >10,000 copies/mL (false-positives at low levels in 3-5%); confirm seroconversion, other labs--lymphopenia, elevated transaminases.
- Signs and symptoms of acute retroviral syndrome: Fever: 96%; Lymphadenopathy: 74%; Pharyngitis: 70%; Rash: 70% (maculopapular face, trunk, ext.; mucosal ulceration); Myalgias/arthralgias: 54%; Diarrhea; 32%; Headache: 32%; Nausea +/- vomiting: 27%; Hepatosplenomegaly:14%; Neurologic sx: 12%

TREATMENT REGIMENS

Treatment

- Principle: benefit of early Rx is unclear. Refer to trial if possible
- If Rx - Preferred: 2 NRTIs + 1-2 PIs or NNRTI
- Benefit of HAART: reduce symptoms, limit viral heterogenicity, preserve immune function
- Disadvantages to HAART: no documented benefit with early use
- HAART = 2 NRTIs (usually AZT/3TC or TDF/FTC) plus boosted PI or NNRTI (see below)
- Invirase 1000mg BID + Ritonavir 100mg BID
- Kaletra 400/100mg BID
- Efavirenz (Sustiva) 600mg hs or NVP 200mg qd x 2 wks, then 200mg bid
- Atazanavir 300mg qd + ritonavir 100mg
- Resistance (genotype) testing: indicated for immediate use (if treated) or future use

Treatment - counseling

- Prevention: acute retroviral syndrome associated with the highest VL in blood and genital secretions - WARN patient of transmission risk
- Adherence - must take >95% of prescribed pills
- Risks of drugs including lipodystrophy
- Standard evaluation: CD4, VL, CBC, chem panel, toxo serology, VDRL, Hep B & C, PPD, lipids

DRUG-SPECIFIC COMMENTS

Abacavir (ABC): (Ziagen) This is the most potent nucleoside vs. HIV, usually paired with 3TC. Must be aware of a serious hypersensitivity reaction with fever >38C + GI symptoms, rash or cough + dyspnea, usually within 6 weeks.

Atazanavir (ATV): A potent PI with several advantages given once daily, boosts well, and no lipid effect. Main problem is need for food and gastric acide for optimal absorption.

Delavirdine (DLV): (Rescriptor) NNRTI that is infrequently used due to inconvenient dosing regimen & limited published experience. Sometimes combined with PIs because DLV inhibits P450 pathway. Main toxicity is rash usually in first 6 weeks.

Didanosine (ddI): Usually paired with AZT; must be taken on empty stomach. Main toxicities are pancreatitis, peripheral neuropathy, lactic acidosis, and GI intolerance.

Efavirenz (EFV): NNRTI class with good potency, good clinical trial results even with baseline viral load >100,000/mL. Warn patient of CNS toxicity in first 2-3 weeks with "disconnected" feeling & bad dreams.

Fosamprenavir (FPV): A potent PI that is usually combined with ritonavir to improve tolerance and reduce pill burden, also improve PK parameters

Indinavir (IDV): (Crixivan) Usually combined with ritonavir for BID dosing which can be given without regard to meals but dose regimen is arbitrary: Indinavir 800 + ritonavir 100-200mg bid--more nephrolithiasis; indinavir 400 + ritonavir 400 bid--more GI intolerance.

Lamivudine (3TC): (Epivir) Very popular nucleoside due to good tolerance; usually paired with AZT, ABC or d4T; unlike other nucleosides, a single mutation (at codon 184) confers high level resistance & this has occurred within 3 weeks with 3TC monotherapy.

Lopinavir (LPV): (Kaletra) A potent combination of two PIs (lopinavir/ritonavir) which has an excellent record in trials as initial or salvage treatment.

Nelfinavir (NFV): (Viracept) The only PI that is not boosted with RTV. Potency is suboptimal but may be better with care to take with fatty meal. Main side effect is diarrhea, which usually responds to loparamide.

Nevirapine (NVP): (Viramune) A potent NNRTI that has early potentially serious reactions rash and hepatotoxicity and a one step "knock-out" resistance mutation, but good efficacy & excellent record for preventing perinatal transmission with single intrapartum dose.

Ritonavir (RTV): (Norvir) Potent PI, but few patients can tolerate the GI side effects with standard dose. Main use now is with a second PI to exploit drug interactions of the second PI--usually saquinavir, indinavir, fosamprenavir, atazanavir or lopinavir.

Saquinavir (SQV): (Fortovase) Invirase is now the preferred formulation due to better GI tolerance compared to fortovase.

Stavudine (d4T): Commonly used nucleoside based on good tolerance usually paired with 3TC; should not be paired with AZT or ddI. Main toxicity is peripheral neuropathy, pancreatitis, lactic acidosis, lipoatrophy, hyperlipidemia and lactic acidosis.

Tenofovir (TDF): A nucleotide often given with FTC (coformulated) or 3TC. Generally well tolerated.

Zalcitabine (ddC): Nucleoside that was previously used in combination with AZT; now rarely used due to toxicity.

IMPORTANT POINTS

- Guidelines for antiretroviral agents in adults & adolescents from the DHHS (11/04 www. hivatis.org) & IAS-USA (JAMA 2004;292:251).
- Resistance testing advocated for drug selection
- Benefit of early treatment is unproven, but this may be the optimal time to start Rx
- IAS-USA and DHHS guidelines recommend HIV resistance testing to help regimen selection. Resistance test results and antiretrovirals in source may help initial decision.

SELECTED READINGS

Pilcher CD, et al. Brief but efficient: Acute HIV infection and the sexual transmission of HIV. J Infect Dis 2004;189:1785

Pilcher CD, et al. Acute HIV revisited: New opportunities for treatment and prevention. J Clin Invest 2004;113:937

Vanhems P, et al. Incubation and duration of specific symptoms at acute retroviral syndrome as independent predictors of progression to AIDS. J AIDS 2003;32:542

Smith DE, Walker BD, Cooper DA, et al. Is antiretroviral treatment of primary HIV infection clinically justified on the basis of current evidence. AIDS 2004;18:709

Fidler S, et al. Virologic and immunologic effects of short course antiviral therapy in primary HIV infection. AIDS 2002;16:2049

Kahn JO, Walker BD. Acute human immunodeficiency virus type 1 infection. N Engl J Med 1998;339:33

Daar ES et al. Diagnosis of primary HIV infection. Ann Intern Med 2001; 134:25

Vanhems P et al. Comparison of clinical features, CD4 and CD8 responses among patients with acute HIV infection from Geneva, Seattle and Sydney. AIDS 2000; 14:375

Schacker T, Collier AC, Hughes J, et al. Clinical and epidemiologic features of primary HIV infection. Ann Intern Med 1996;125:257

Rich JD, Merriman NA, Mylonakis E, et al. Misdiagnosis of HIV infection by HIV-1 plasma viral load testing: A case series. Ann Intern Med 1999;130:37

RHEUMATIC FEVER, ACUTE   Paul Auwaerter, M.D.

DIAGNOSTIC CRITERIA

- Syndromic immunologic (non-suppurative) aftermath of Group A strep (GAS) pharyngitis, average latent period following sore throat 19d but range 1-5wks.
- Most frequent in 6-15yr. children, in US now rare w/ attack rate declining (likely well <0.4%) after GAS pharyngitis, but more common in developing world.
- Major Criteria: carditis, polyarthritis, chorea, subcut. nodules, erythema marginatum.
- Minor Criteria: fever, arthralgia, heart block, elevated ESR/CRP or wbc. Supportive: recent positive GAS throat cx, rising ASO titer.
- ARF likely by Am. Heart Assoc. criteria = 2 major, or 1 major and 2 minor. Recurrences of ARF unlikely to meet full criteria.

COMMON PATHOGENS: Group A beta hemolytic strep

TREATMENT REGIMENS

Prevention

- Duration rather than dose believed important for GAS eradication from oropharynx.
- Parenteral: PCN G benzathine 1.2 millionU IM (single dose), if wt. < 60lb dose 600,000 mU IM.
- Oral: PCN VK 250mg PO tid (children), 500mg tid (adolescents, adults) for FULL 10 days. Amoxicillin liquid often preferred w/young children, dose 25-50 mg/kg/day PO q8h for FULL 10d.
- PCN allergic: erythromycin 40mg/kg/d 2-4 times daily (max. 1g/d) for FULL 10 days.
- Treatment of strep throat even 9d after onset is still effective in prevention of ARF.

Treatment of ARF

- Arthralgia or mild arthritis, no carditis: analgesia only e.g., codeine or propoxyphene.
- Mod. or severe arthritis, no carditis or carditis w/o CHF: ASA 90-100mg/kg 2-6wks.
- Carditis w/CHF +/- arthritis: prednisone 40-60mg qd with subsequent taper. Steroid recommendation is not based on good, prospective randomized trial data.
- If throat GAS (+), treat with benzathine PCN G 1.2mU.

Secondary prevention of ARF

- To prevent recurrent attacks, exact role controversial.
- Benzathine PCN G 1.2mU IM q4wk (or q3wk if high risk) or PCN VK 250mg bid. Emycin 250mg bid if PCN allergic.
- Duration of secondary prevention uncertain, many discontinue by late teenage/early adult years OR 10 yrs after last attack if adult.

DRUG-SPECIFIC COMMENTS

Clarithromycin: May be effective for GAS pharyngitis, but more expensive than PCN or erythromycin AND macrolide resistance may be prevalent in the US.

Erythromycin: Often prescribed for GAS infection in PCN allergic patients; however, macrolide resistance common in Europe, and may approach 20-25% in some US cities.

Penicillin: Treatment of choice for prevention of ARF.

IMPORTANT POINTS

- Source recommendations: Dakamo AS, Circ 1993; 87:302 and Bisno A, Princ. Prac. Inf. Dis, 5th ed, 2000 Chap.187.

- Hx of prior ARF significantly elevates risk of future bouts of ARF and rheumatic heart disease.
- Only long-term sequelae of ARF is rheumatic heart disease (valvular). Only 6% risk if no carditis at initial ARF, climbs to 40-65% w/ murmurs or CHF at initial disease.
- Chorea tends to be a late finding. Carditis more common in younger children, rates of arthritis tend to increase w/age.
- SQ nodules (assoc. w/ severe carditis) and EM (trunk and extremities) occur <10%.

SELECTED READINGS

McDonald M, Currie BJ, Carapetis JR. Acute rheumatic fever: a chink in the chain that links the heart to the throat?. Lancet Infect Dis. 2004 Apr;4(4):240-5

Bisno AL, Brito MO, Collins CM. Molecular basis of group A streptococcal virulence. Lancet Infect Dis. 2003 Apr;3(4):191-200

Mert A, Ozaras R, Tabak F. Fever of unknown origin: a review of 20 patients with adult-onset Still's disease. Clin Rheumatol. 2003 May;22(2):89

Cilliers AM, Manyemba J, Saloojee H. Anti-inflammatory treatment for carditis in acute rheumatic fever. Cochrane Database Syst Rev 2003;(2):

Stollerman GH. Rheumatic fever in the 21st century. Clin Infect Dis. 2001 Sep 15;33(6):806

Aviles RJ, Ramakrishna G, Mohr DN, Michet CJ Jr. Poststreptococcal reactive arthritis in adults: a case series. Mayo Clin Proc. 2000 Feb;75(2):144

Dakamo AS. Ayoub E, Bierman EZ et al. Guidelines for the diagnosis of rheumatic fever. Jones criteria, updated 1992. Circ 1993; 87:302

SARS [SEVERE ACUTE RESPIRATORY SYNDROME]

Yukari C. Manabe, M.D. and Trish Perl, M.D.

DIAGNOSTIC CRITERIA

- CRITERIA FOR SUSPECTED AND PROBABLE CASES:
- Clinical criteria: asymptomatic/mild resp illness; Moderate: T>100.4 F plus resp illness; Severe: Temp>100.4 F and resp illness and radiographic evidence of pneumo, ARDS or an autopsy w/ ARDS or pneumo
- Epidemiologic: Travel w/in 10 days of onset of symptoms to a SARS area, previously documented or suspected transmission community transmission of SARS/close contact w/in 10 days of onset of SARS case.
- Laboratory Criteria: Confirmed = Detection of SARS-CoV Ab (acute or convalescent), isolation of SARS-CoV, or positive RT-PCR (confirmed with 2nd PCR with different primers)
- "Probable" = meets clinical criteria for severe resp illness of unknown etiology, and epi criteria of exposure; w/ or lab criteria or undetermined "Suspect" = as above x moderate resp illness.
- Close contact is defined as having cared for, having lived with, or having direct contact with respiratory secretions and/or body fluids of a patient known to be or suspected SARS case.
- Travel (including transit and being at an airport) within 10 days of onset of symptoms to an area with current or recently documented or suspect community transmission of SARS.
- Suspect cases are defined as above.
- Probable cases are suspect cases plus x-ray evidence of pneumonia or ARDS, or autopsy consistent with otherwise unexplained ARDS

SARS [Severe Acute Respiratory Syndrome]

- As of Jan. 13, 2004, 3 new SARS cases have been documented. In 2003, over 8,000 suspected and/or probable SARS cases had been reported to WHO from 37 countries, including the United States (28 cases). The reported SARS cases include deaths (case-fatality proportion). http://www.who.int/csr/sarscountry/en/

Treatment Regimens

Treatment

- Cover with 3rd generation cephalosporin and macrolide or fluoroquinolone to cover community-acquired pneumonias esp. with atypical features.
- High dose corticosteroids have been used in some patients, although data is not controlled.
- Interferon has been used in uncontrolled case series.
- Insufficient data to firmly recommend either steroids and/or interferon.
- Ribavirin is contraindicated.

Infection control

- Contact the infection control practitioner immediately.
- Management Guidelines: screening in ambulatory care and emergency rooms for possible cases should be done. Suspect cases should wear a surgical mask and be evaluated in a separate room.
- Personnel should wear gowns, gloves, and a N95 respirator.
- Diagnostic evaluation includes CXR, pulse oximetry, blood cultures, sputum GS and culture, tests for influenza and RSV, and urinary antigens for pneumococcus and Legionella.
- Testing: Acute and convalescent sera can be sent to state health dept for testing at CDC. RT-PCR detection of the now-sequenced coronavirus is available through the CDC.
- Hand hygiene, N95 repirators, goggles, gown and gloves. Transmission occurs by direct contact with infectious material including large respiratory droplets.
- Healthcare workers: only workers not wearing appropriate precautions and exposed to high-risk (aerosol generating procedures), unprotected encounters need be furloughed.
- Since airborne wear goggles, PAPR. Isolation recommended by CDC.
- All others protected & unprotected low risk should have 2x daily temp. Check. (www.hopkins-heic.org).
- Laboratory: Viral cell culture and initial characterization of recovered viral agents should be conducted under BSL-3 conditions. http://www.cdc.gov/ncidod/sars/sarslabguide.htm

Important Points

- As of July 2005, no cases of SARS described in >1 year.
- Clinical features have included fever, non-productive cough, dyspnea that rapidly progresses to ARDS. Fatigue, anorexia, diarrhea are prominent. Most series suggest coryza is rare.
- The illness is triphasic with a prodrome lasting 2-6 days; a febrile phase and finally a respiratory phase. Most cases that decompensate develop decreased 02 saturation 7-10 days into their illness.
- Mortality has ranged from 5-19% and is higher in documented cases. Mortality is much higher in patients >60 yrs.
- Laboratory features include elevated LDH, liver transaminases, creatinine kinase and leukopenia and thrombocytopenia.

- Suspect cases should be reported immediately to infection control; local and state public health authorities.
- Updates are available from the CDC http://www.cdc.gov/ncidod/sars

Selected Readings

CDC. Outbreak of Severe Acute Respiratory Syndrome ---Worldwide, 2003. MMWR 2003;52:226-8.

Tsang KW, Ho PL, Ooi GC, et al. A cluster of cases of severe acute respiratory syndrome in Hong Kong. N Eng J Med 2003

Poutanen SM, Low DE, Henry B, et al. Identification of severe acute respiratory syndrome in Canada. N Eng J Med 2003

CDC. Interim guidance on infection control precautions for patients with suspected severe acute respiratory syndrome (SARS) and close contacts in households. http://www.cdc.gov/ncidod/sars/ic-closecontacts.htm

Johns Hopkins. Plan for healthcare facilities; infection control procedures; temperature screening forms and flow sheets. www.hopkins-heic.org

CDC Specimen collection and laboratory diagnosis. specimen collection. http://www.cdc.gov/ncidod/sars/guidance/f/pdf/app4.pdf

CDC. Serum antibody tests. www.cdc.gov/ncidod/sars/lab/eia

CDC. RT-PCR. www.cdc.gov/ncidod/sars/lab/rtpcr

World Health Organization. Severe acute respiratory syndrome (SARS). http://www.who.int/csr/sars/en

CDC. Severe acute respiratory syndrome (SARS) updated interim case definition. http://www.cdc.gov/ncidod/sars/casedefinition.htm

SEPSIS - UNKNOWN SOURCE   John G. Bartlett, M.D.

Diagnostic Criteria

- Sepsis syndrome: Infection + Temp > 38.3C or < 35.6C + pulses >90 + RR > 20 + either - altered mental status, pO2 <75, increased lactate or oliguria
- Severe sepsis: Sepsis + organ failure, decreased perfusion (lactic acidosis, oliguria, altered mental status) OR low BP
- Septic shock: hypotension despite fluids + lactic acidosis, oliguria, altered mental status
- Systemic inflammatory response syndrome (SIRS): Sepsis + non-infectious processes - burns, pancreatitis
- Sepsis - SIRS + infection
- Systemic inflammatory response syndrome (SIRS); 2 or more of the following:
- Fever (T>38C or hypothermia (T<36C)
- Tachycardia (HR>90)
- Tachypnea (RR>20)
- Leukocytosis (WBC>12,000;or diff>10% bands)

Common Pathogens: Most common: Enterobacteriaceae ; Escherichia coli ; Staphylococcus aureus ; Streptococcus species ; N. Meningitidis ; OTHER CAUSES: Salmonella enteritidis, S. typhi, Plasmodium falciparum, Listeria monocytogenes.; SPECIAL POPULATIONS: NEONATAL (< 1 week): Group B streptococci, E. coli. ; HIV with CD4< 50-100: MAC, CMV, TB, line sepsis, ABC hypersensitivity, Cryptococcus. ; INJECTION DRUG USERS: Staph aureus, esp. MRSA ; SPLENECTOMIZED: Streptococcus pneumoniae, Haemophilus influenzae, Neisseria meningitidis ; NEUTROPENIC: GNB, Aspergillus.; TRAVELER: Malaria, salmonellosis; HEALTHY YOUNG ADULT: Toxic shock (S. aureus or group A strep), N. meningitidis, RMSF, bioterrorism, hantavirus.; DIAGNOSTIC CLUES: Ecthyma gangrenosum: Pseudomonas aeruginosa; petechiae or purpura: Neisseria meningitidis; traveler: Salmonella typhi, Plasmodium falciparum.

TREATMENT REGIMENS

Treatment: antibiotic selection (all IV)

- Guideline: Medical Letter (2004;2:13)
- Empiric: aminoglycoside + betalactam +/- vancomycin
- Aminoglycoside: gentamicin or tobramycin 5mg/kg/d or amikacin 15mg/kg/d all IV.
- Betalactam (IV, choose one): cefotaxime 2g q6h, ceftriaxone 1g q12h, cefepime 2g q12h, ceftazidime 2g q8h, imipenem 0.5-1g q6h, meropenem 1g q8h or piperacillin-tazobactam 3.375g q6h
- Vancomycin 1g q 12h
- Neutropenia: ceftazidime, imipenem or cefepime +/- aminoglycoside
- Intra-abdominal sepsis: ticarcillin-clavulanate, piperacillin-tazobactam, imipenem, +/- aminoglycoside

Treatment: tissue perfusion

- Resuscitation: IV fluids, then packed RBC to Hct >30% and/or dobutamine <20 ug/kg/min.
- Resuscitation goals: CVP 8-12mm Hg; mean arterial pressure >65, urine output >0.5 mL/kg/hr; venous O2 sat >70%.
- Cultures: blood x 2 (1 via each access device), + urine, + other suspect sources.
- Fluids: Colloids and crystalloids equally effective
- Vasopressors: norepinephrine (usual adult: 0.1mg/kg/min then 0.05mcg/kg/min) or dopamine (2-25mcg/kg/min)
- Inotropic agent: dobutamine to increase cardiac output
- Steroids: hydrocortisone 200-300mg/d x 7d; D/C if >9ug/dl response to 250mg ACTH (Cosyntropin) stimulation test.
- Blood: transfuse if Hgb <7, target goal Hgb >7-9
- Activated protein C (drotrecogin): APACHE >25 (see APACHE tables in appendix II), septic shock, >1 organ dysfunction and no bleeding risks. Dose 24mcg/kg/hr continuous IV infusion x 96h.
- Hypoxemia: PEEP (but concern for barotrauma)

DRUG-SPECIFIC COMMENTS

Amikacin: The most broad spectrum aminoglycoside vs gram-neg bacilli, but the disadvantages in terms of toxicity, underdosing and need for monitoring levels is the same.

Cefepime: Called a 4th generation cephalosporin because it has activity against GNB like ceftazidime and activity vs GPC like cefotaxime/ceftriaxone. Good choice for empiric treatment of sepsis with or without an aminoglycoside (for increased GNB spectrum) clindamycin/metronidazole (for anaerobes) or vancomycin (for S. aureus, S. epidermidis, enterococcus)

Ceftazidime: A favored 3rd generation cephalosporin when P. aeruginosa is established or suspected. Reduced activity vs. GPC compared to ceftriaxone/cefotaxime and poor activity vs. enterococci, anaerobes and S. aureus.

Ceftriaxone: Good, broad spectrum 3rd generation cephalosporin with activity against most GNB other than P. aeruginosa. Activity vs. anaerobes is not well established.

Ciprofloxacin: Good drug for sepsis according to in vitro activity vs most GNB and many clinical trials. Concerns are declining activity vs. P. aeruginosa, poor activity vs many S. aureus including nearly all MRSA and virtually no activity against anaerobes.

Drotrecogin alpha : FDA approved for sepsis with APACHE II score >25. Bleeding diathesis or recent bleed is contraindication. $8,000 per course.

Gentamicin: Recommended here as the Medical Letter choice for empiric treatment of sepsis, but many authorities are willing to use aminoglycoside alternatives such as betalactams & fluoroquinolones to avoid the risk of aminoglycoside nephrotoxicity. Gent + betalactams are synergistic in vitro, but in vivo synergy has not been convincingly shown. A major concern with this class is the "tight" toxic therapeutic ratio, the high rate of ototoxicity as well as nephrotoxicity, the tendency to underdose & the need to monitor levels.

Imipenem/Cilastatin: A favored drug for serious infections which require a broad spectrum agent and extensive clinical experience to assure effectiveness. Concerns are dose related seizure protential, need to reduce dose in renal failure and lack of activity vs. VRE, S. epidermidis, MRSA.

Meropenem: Very similar to imipenem in activity. Probably less seizure potential.

Piperacillin + Tazobactam: (Zosyn): A favored drug for empiric treatment of sepsis with good activity vs. most GNB, all anaerobes and most GPC other than VRE, MRSA and S. epidermidis.

Ticarcillin + Clavulanic Acid: A favored drug for empiric treatment of sepsis with good activity vs most GNB, all anaerobes and most GPC other than VRE, MRSA and S. epidermidis.

Tobramycin: Recommended for combination with a betalactam for empiric treatment of sepsis with unknown pathogen by Med Letter. Many authorities avoid aminoglycoside due to ototoxicity and nephrotoxicity. If used monitor hearing, balance, and renal function.

IMPORTANT POINTS

- Guidelines: Abx - Med Letter (2004;2-13) septic shock (Crit Care Med 2004; 32:858)
- Classic signs sepsis: fever, chills & hypotension
- Septic shock (persistent hypotension): blood cx pos in 50%, mortality is 30%-50%
- Sepsis mortality increased: wrong abx, increased age, nosocomial, resp>abd>urine, underlying dis, complications (decreased BP, decreased temp, anuria), shock
- Complications: bleeding, leukopenia, thrombocytopenia, acidosis, oliguria, jaundice, DIC, CHF, ARDS

SELECTED READINGS

Wispingloff H. Nosocomial bloodstream infections in US Hospitals: Analysis of 24,179 cases in a nationwide surveillance study. Clin Infect Dis 2004;39:309

MacArthur RD. Adequacy of early empiric antibiotic treatment and survival in severe sepsis. Clin Infect Dis 2004;38:284

The Med Letter. Treatment guidelines for the Medical Letter. The Med Letter 2004;2:13

Dellinger RR. Surviving sepsis campaign: guidelines for management of severe sepsis and septic shock. Crit Care Med 2004;32:858

Bernard GR. Efficacy and safety of recombinant human activated protein C for severe sepsis. N. Engl J. Med 2001;344:699

Annane D. Effect of treatment with low doses of hydrocortisone and fludrocortiosne on mortality in patients with septic shock. JAMA 2002;288:862

Wheeler AP, Bernard GR. Treating patients with severe sepsis. NEJM 1999;340:207

Cohen J, Guyatt G, Bernard GR, et al. New strategies for clinical trials in patients with sepsis and septic shock. Crit Care Med 2001;29:880

(No authors). Guidelines for the management of severe sepsis and septic shock. The International Sepsis Forum. Intensive Care Med 2001;27:Suppl 1: S1-134

Annane D. Corticosteroids for septic shock. Crit Care Med 2001;29: Suppl 7:S117

SEPSIS, VASCULAR CATHETER-ASSOCIATED

John G. Bartlett, M.D.

DIAGNOSTIC CRITERIA

- Bacteremia: Fever + no alternate source + same pathogen peripheral blood & significant growth from cath tip
- Cath colonization: Significant growth cath tip only (>15 colonies)
- Phlebitis: Hot, red, tender cath exit site.
- Tunnel infection: Hot, red tender >2cm exit site.
- Sites of infection: 1. blood = bacteremia; 2. cath insertion site: phlebitis (chemical or infection); 3. Pocket 4. Complicated: septic, phlebitis, abscess
- DX: BC - 2 sets (1 periph), CVC - roll tip

COMMON PATHOGENS: Staph aureus ; Enterobacteriaceae ; Enterococcus ; Candida

TREATMENT REGIMENS

Treatment : Removable central venous cath (CVC)

- Guidelines from IDSA (CID 2001;32:1249)
- DX: 2 BC (1 periph cx): D/C CVC, cult cath tip, insert new line or guidewire placement
- Empiric abx Rx: If seriously ill - low BP, organ failure
- Peripheral blood culture(PBC) & CVC cult neg: seek another source
- PBC neg & CVC >15 CFU: monitor for infx and blood culture if heart valve dis, neutropenia, Candida or S. aureus
- PBC + CVC pos + S. epi: D/C CVC + Abx 7d OR keep CVC + Abx IV + lock x 10-14d
- PBC & CVC pos + Complicated (endocarditis, osteo, septic phlebitis): D/C CVC + Abx 4-8 wks
- PBC & CVC pos + GNB or Candida: D/C CVC + Abx 14d
- PBC & CVC pos + S. aureus: D/C CVC + TEE + Abx 14d

Treatment: Tunneled CVC

- Tunnel infect/port abscess: D/C line + Abx x 10-14d
- Septic phlebitis, endocarditis, osteo: D/C line + Abx 4-8 wks
- Candida: D/C line + Abx 14d post last pos BC
- S. epid.: Keep line + Abx & lock Rx x 10-14d
- GNB: D/C line + Abx 10-14d OR keep line + Abx IV + lock Rx 14d
- S. aureus: TEE is neg. for endocarditis, D/C line + Abx 14d OR keep line + Abx IV + lock Rx 14d

Treatment: miscellaneous/lock Rx

- Permanent line removed: replace after bacteremia clears.
- Empiric abx: vancomycin + ceftazidime or cefepime
- Periph line: remove
- CVC cult: roll tip - >15 CFU or sonicate >10(2) = infection
- Hemodialysis cath: colonization 10-55% OR endocarditis, osteo, septic phlebitis
- Septic thrombophlebitis: D/C line, remove vein, abx 4-6wks
- Lock Rx: 1-5mg/mL Abx + heparin 50-100u OR saline to fill lumen cath (2-5mL)

DRUG-SPECIFIC COMMENTS

Cefepime: Good agent for empiric choice due to activity vs most gram-negative bacteria. Must be combined with vancomycin for assurance of activity against likely pathogens including S. epidermidis & S. aureus

Ceftazidime: Good agent for empiric use due to excellent activity vs gram-negative bacteria including P. aeruginosa

Imipenem/Cilastatin: Good agent for empiric choice due to activity vs most gram-negative bacteria. Must be combined with vancomycin for assurance of activity against likely pathogens including S. epidermidis & S. aureus

Linezolid: Rational alternative to vancomycin for S. epidermidis, Meth-resistant S. aureus and Enterococcus - virtually all gram-positive bacteria

Tobramycin: Good activity vs GNB but must be combined with agent for gram-positive bacteria when used empirically. Main use is in combination with a betalactam for relatively resistant or refractory infection involving GNB. Monitor for nephrotoxicity (daily creatinine) and ototoxicity (Rhomberg)

IMPORTANT POINTS

- Main dx issue: matching blood cult & cath tip cultures
- Main Rx issues: 1) line removal: peripheral-D/C line; CVC-line salvage option best with Coag-neg Staph; 2) duration abx - usually 7-14d
- Feared complications: S. aureus - endocarditis, septic phlebitis & osteo.; Candida - endophthalmitis; GNB-septic shock
- Guidelines from IDSA for line management (CID 2001;32:1249)

SELECTED READINGS

Jernigan JA, Farr B. Short course therapy for catheter-related Staphylococcus aureus bacteremia: a meta-analysis. Ann Intern Med 1993;119:304

Fowler VG, Li J, Corey GR, et al. Role of echocardiography in evaluation of patients with Staphylococcus aureus bacteremia: experience in 103 patients. J Am Coll Cardiol 1997;30:1072

Rose HD. Venous catheter - associated candidemia. Am J Med Sci 1978;275:265

Rex JH, Bennett JE, Sugar AM, et al. A randomized trial comparing fluconazole with amphotericin B for the treatment of candidemia in patients without neutropenia. NEJM 1994;331:1325

Radd II, Sabbagh MF. Optimal duration of therapy for catheter-related Staphylococcus aureus bacteremia: a study of 55 cases & review. CID 1992;14:75

Mermel LA, Farr BM, Sherertz J, et al. Guidelines for the management of intravascular catheter-related infections. CID 2001;32:1249

Christensen GB, Bisnoi AL, Parisi JT, et al. Nosocomial septicemia due to multiply resistant Staphylococcus epidermidis. Ann Intern Med 1982;96:1

Anaissie E, Rex JH, Uzun O, et al. Prognosis and outcome of candidemia in cancer patients. Am J Med 1998;104:238

Kite P, Dobbins BM, Wilcox MH, et al. Rapid diagnosis of central-venous-catheter-related bloodstream infection without catheter removal. Lancet 1999;354:1504

Sheretz RJ, Heard SO, Raad II. Diagnosis of triple lumen catheter infection: comparison of roll plate, sonification and flushing methodologies. J Clin Micro 1997;35:641

SHUNT INFECTIONS   Paul Auwaerter, M.D.

DIAGNOSTIC CRITERIA

- Hx: Fever (variable), abdominal pain, shunt malfunction causing raised intracranial pressure (headache, nausea or vomiting, altered mental status); meningeal symptoms less common
- PE: Erythema and tenderness of skin over tubing; Ventriculoperitoneal (VP) shunts: abdominal pain, focal or generalized peritonitis, intraabdominal abscess, perforated viscus

- For ventriculoatrial shunts: sepsis, positive blood cultures, right-sided endocarditis, shunt nephritis, hepatosplenomegaly
- Lab: Shunt tap revealing CSF leukocytosis (cells > 10/mm3) (may see eosinophilia) +/- elevated protein and/or positive CSF gram stain or culture

COMMON PATHOGENS: S.aureus ; Coagulase-negative staphylococci ; Propionibacterium species ; Enterobacteriaceae ; Streptococcus species ; Candida species

TREATMENT REGIMENS

Shunt revision

- Complete favored over partial shunt removal with temporary external ventricular drain. Partial revisions usually with high failure rates (up to 80%).
- Monitor CSF for up to 3 days off antibiotics before placement of permanent shunt to document CSF sterility
- Timing/need for new shunt or continued external drainage based on neurosurgical considerations.
- Antibiotic treatment for 3-14d (exact duration not well studied)
- IV antibiotics may be continued for an additional 7-14d from shunt revision.

Parenteral therapy (empiric)

- Vancomycin 1g IV q6-12h [15mg/kg q6h pediatric] + Ceftazidime 2g IV q8h [ceftriaxone (if not suspecting Pseudonomas) 2g IV q12 [50mg/kg q12h pediatric]
- Vancomycin 1g IV q12h + cefepime 2g IV q12h
- For PCN allergic, consider ciprofloxacin 400mg IV q 12h to replace cephalosporin choice.

Parenteral therapy (organism known)

- Use antimicrobial sensitivities to guide therapy.
- S. epid or S. aureus (MRSA): vancomycin 1g IV q12h +/- rifampin 600mg IV or PO qd
- S. aureus (MSSA): nafcillin or oxacillin 2g IV q4h +/- rifampin 600mg IV or PO qd
- S. aureus: TMP/SMX 4-5mg/kg/d (of trimethoprim component) q8h
- GNB: ceftriaxone 2g IV q12h or cefepime 2g IV q12h or Meropenem 2g IV q8h or aztreonam 2g IV q6h. Choose on sensitivities. Intrathecal aminoglycosides rarely required for shunt-related infections.
- P. acnes, Strep: Penicillin G 4mU or ampicillin 2g IV q4h +/- gentamicin 1-1.7mg/kg q8h (add gentamicin for Group B streptococcal and enterococcal infections)
- Fungi: Amphotericin B 0.6-1.0mg/kg IV qd (exact recommendation based on recovered organism)

DRUG-SPECIFIC COMMENTS

Aztreonam: Beta-lactam with broad activity against gram-negative bacilli, including Pseudomonas; but no activity against gram-positive organisms. Given lack of cross-sensitivity with other beta-lactam, aztreonam is a good choice for patients with gram-negative bacillary meningitis and history of severe allergic reaction to penicillins and/or cephalosporins.

Cefepime: Like ceftazidime, this agent's broad spectrum of activity, particularly against Pseudomonas, makes it an agent of choice for empiric treatment of nosocomial or iatrogenic infections.

Ceftazidime: Treatment of choice (with an active aminoglycoside) for pseudomonal meningitis. Administration with an aminoglycoside may help to reduce the risk of development of resistance to the beta-lactam while on therapy.

Meropenem: Broad spectrum of activity. Good CSF penetration in the presence of inflamed meninges. Improved CSF penetration and possible lower risk of seizures favors meropenem over imipenem. Should be used only when antimicrobial susceptibility testing shows organism to be resistant to cephalosporins.

IMPORTANT POINTS

- Guidelines are author's opinions
- Obtain CSF (aspirate directly from shunt or reservoir), blood (VA shunt), peritoneal fluid (VP shunt), distal shunt tip (roll on plate do not put in broth)
- Parenteral abx therapy and complete replacement of shunt is successful in > 90% of cases versus 36% for abx alone or partial revision of shunt
- CSF cultures are generally negative within 2 days of externalization and appropriate abx therapy.
- Failure to improve: remove temporary drain, change abx or increase dose, add rifampin (for GPC) or give intraventricular abx
- Antibiotics should be selected for bactericidal activity and ability to penetrate the CSF space to exceed the MIC of the infecting organism.

SELECTED READINGS

Tuli S, Tuli J, Drake J, Spears J. Predictors of death in pediatric patients requiring cerebrospinal fluid shunts. J Neurosurg Spine. 2004 May;100(5):442-6

Morris A, Low DE. Nosocomial bacterial meningitis, including central nervous system shunt infections. Infectious Disease Clinics of North America 1999; 13(3):735-751

Dunbar SA, Eason RA, Musher DM, et al. Microscopic examination and broth culture of cerebrospinal fluid in diagnosis of meningitis . J Clin Micro 1998;36:1617

Thompson TP, Albright AL. Propionibacterium [correction of Proprionibacterium] acnes infections of cerebrospinal fluid shunts. Childs Nerv Syst. 1998 Aug;14(8):378-80

Quagliariello VJ and Scheld WM . Treatment of bacterial meningitis . N Engl J Med 1997;336:708

Langley JM, LeBlanc JC, Drake J, et al. Efficacy of antimicrobial prophylaxis in placement of cerebrospinal fluid shunts: Meta-analysis . Clin Infect Dis 1993;17:98

Wen DY, Bottini AG, Hall WA, et al. Infections in neurologic surgery. The intraventricular use of antibiotics . Neurosurg Clin NA 1992;3:343

Kim JH, van der Horst C, Mulrow CD, et al. Staphylococcus aureus meningitis: Review of 28 cases . Rev Infect Dis 1989;11:698

Fong IW and Tomkins KB . Review of Pseudomonas aeruginosa meningitis with special emphasis on treatment with ceftazidime . Rev Infect Dis 1985;7:604

Levitz RE and Qunitiliani R . Trimethoprim-sulfamethoxazole for bacterial meningitis . Ann Intern Med 1984;100:881

SINUSITIS, ACUTE   John G. Bartlett, M.D.

DIAGNOSTIC CRITERIA

- Clinical: purulent nasal drainage +/- maxillary or frontal pain/tenderness or decreased transillumination (PE is usually not helpful)
- Complications: orbital infection or cavernous sinus thrombosis--both very rare
- Only 0.2-10% clinical sinusitis are bacterial; cultures are not useful unless taken from sinuses
- Recommended test with routine case - no culture, no CT scan and no x-ray

COMMON PATHOGENS: Rhinovirus ; S.pneumoniae ; Haemophilus influenzae ; Less common pathogens are M. catarrhalis, S. aureus, and anaerobes

TREATMENT REGIMENS

Antibiotics

- Principles: most sinusitis is viral or allergic; usual indication for Abx-symptoms >7d, preferred Abx = amoxicillin
- Indications for Abx: Nasal pus + symptoms are severe, persists 10 days or worse at 7 days
- Preferred abx: amoxicillin 0.5-1g tid x 7 d; doxy 100 mg bid x 10 d or TMP-SMX DS bid x 3 or 10 d
- Alt: Augmentin XR 2000/125mg bid x 10 d or 500/125 mg tid x 7 d
- Alt: azithro 500mg qd x 3 d, clarithromycin 500mg bid x 14 d
- Telithromycin (Ketek) 800mg qd x 5 d
- Alt: cipro 500mg bid po, gatifloxacin (Tequin) 400 mg/d, levofloxacin (Levaquin) 500 mg/d, moxifloxacin (Avelox) 400 mg/d - all 5-10 d

Adjunctive

- Abx cost (above regimens, 2004): amoxicillin $9-20, doxy $9 amox-clav $55, TMP-SMX $3-12, azithro $45, telithromycin $54, cefprozil $21, other cephalosporins $100-170, cipro $24, other FQ $91-100.
- Complicated sinusitis: periorbital edema, erythema, face pain +/- mental status change. CT scan & ceftriaxone, fluoroquinolone, amox-clav, azithro
- Endoscopy +/- drainage by an otolaryngologist (reserved for refractory and complicated infections)
- Systemic decongestant - pseudoephedrine 120mg + sedating antihistamine PO bid x 1-2wks (OTC preps as Actifed, Advil, Allerest, Contac, Dristan, etc) ASA, acetaminophen, or ibuprofen.
- Topical nasal spray; oxymetazoline nasal spray 2 sprays bid x 5d (OTC preps available as Afrin, Dristan, Vicks, Sinex nasal sprays); avoid use > 5 d.
- Allergic rhinitis: loratadine (Claritin) 10mg PO qd & flunisolide spray (Flonase) 2 sprays each nostril/d
- Not proven effective: vit C, inhaled steam, nasal steroids

DRUG-SPECIFIC COMMENTS

Amoxicillin: Considered to be the drug of choice by the Cochrane Library Agency for Health Care Research, IDSA, CDC, Am College Phys. This impression is based in part on two recent meta-analyses of trials showing no antibiotic to be superior. A theoretical concern is resistance by 10-15% of S. pneumoniae, 30-50% of H. influenzae, and >90% of M. catarrhalis. May need high dose (1g TID).

Amoxicillin + Clavulanate: (Augmentin) Sometimes advocated over amoxicillin due to improved activity vs. H. influenzae and M. catarrhalis. Much more expensive than amoxicillin and high rates of diarrhea.

Cefixime: (Suprex) Weak activity against S. pneumoniae. Don't use it unless it is combined with amoxicillin or clindamycin - a recommend "salvage" regimen in the ENT guidelines.

Cefpodoxime Proxetil: (Vantin) Good activity against major pathogens including most S. pneumoniae and virtually all H. influenzae and M. catarrhalis. This is a preferred oral cephalosporin due to activity vs. S. pneumoniae. Expensive compared to amoxicillin.

Cefprozil: (Cefzil) This is one of the 3 favored oral cephalosporins for S. pneumoniae (cefpodoxime & cefuroxime are the others).

Cefuroxime and cefuroxime axetil: (Ceftin) Reasonably good activity vs S. pneumoniae and reasonable choice for this indication.

DIAGNOSIS

Clarithromycin: (Biaxin) Clinical trials show results comparable to other drugs including fluoroquinolones. More expensive than amoxicillin or TMP-SMX. New 1g extended-release dose permits once-daily dosing.

Gatifloxacin: (Tequin) FDA approved for sinusitis, active vs. all likely treatable pathogens, well tolerated, and convenience of once-daily treatment. Major concern is perception of abuse with risk of resistance to fluoroquinolones and cost. Usually reserved for moderately severe cases with recent abx exposure, betalactam allergy or failure with alternative agent.

Levofloxacin: Active against treatable pathogens, but usually reserved for patients with refractory cases.

Moxifloxacin: (Avelox) FDA approved for sinusitis, active vs. all likely treatable pathogens, well tolerated, and convenience of once-daily treatment. Major concern is perception of abuse with risk of resistance to fluoroquinolones and cost. Usually reserved for moderately severe cases with recent abx exposure, betalactam allergy or failure with alternative agent.

Telithromycin: (Ketek) Member of new class (ketolide) related to macrolides; effective against drug-resistant S. pneumoniae, H. influenzae and Morexella.

IMPORTANT POINTS

- Most colds are complicated by viral sinusitis and do not respond to abx
- Dx is clinical - no routine x-ray, CT scan or culture
- If abx Rx - amoxicillin is usual first choice, but may need high dose (3g/d)
- Unresponsive to abx at 72hrs - image & change abx to fluoroquinolone or amox-clavulanate
- Guidelines based on CDC & ACP (Ann Int Med 2001;134:495,498) also Piccirillo J. NEJM 2004;351:902

SELECTED READINGS

Piccirillo JR. Acute Bacterial sinusitis . N.Engl J. Med 2004;351:902-10

Snow V, Mottur-Pilson C, Hickner JM. Principles of appropriate antibiotic use for acute sinusitis. Ann Intern Med 2001;134:495.

Hickner JM, Bartlett JG, Besser R, et al. Principles of acute antibiotic use for acute rhinosinusitis in adults: Background. Ann Intern Med 2001;134:498.

Piccirillo JF, et al. Impact of first-line vs second-line antibiotics for the treatment of acute uncomplicated sinusitis. JAMA 2001;286:1849

Anvand, VK. Epidemiology and economic impact of rhinosinusitis. Ann Otol Rhinol Laryngol Suppl 2004;193:3-5

Parilch SL, et al. Invasive fungal sinusitis: a 15 year review from a single institution. Amer J. Rhinol 2004;18-75-81

Taj-Aldeen SJ, et al. Allergic fungal sinusitis: a report of 8 cases. Am J. Otolaryngol 2004;25:213-8

Silberstein SD. Headaches due to nasal and paranasal sinus disease. Neurol Clin 2004;22:1-19

Gwaltney JM Jr, Phillips CD, Miller RD, et al. Computed tomographic study of the common cold. N Engl J Med 1994;330:25.

Williams JR Jr. et al. Cochrane Database Sys. Rev.2003;2:CD000243www.cochrane.org/cchrane/revabstr/AB000243;accesed 9/1/04

SINUSITIS, SUBACUTE CHRONIC

Raj Sindwani, M.D., F.R.C.S.C., and Ralph Metson, M.D.

DIAGNOSTIC CRITERIA

- Sinusitis definitions: inflamed sinonasal mucosa; acute - symptoms lasting for up to 4 weeks, subacute - lasting between 4 and 12 weeks, chronic - longer than 12 weeks.
- Pathophysiology: obstruction of ventilation and drainage of ostiomeatal complex and sinus outflow tracts causing retained secretions and subsequent infection.
- Clinical: facial pain, nasal blockage, nasal discharge, postnasal drip, hyposmia, fatigue; inflamed mucosa, purulent secretions; transillumination not helpful, endoscopy helpful but not required.
- Tests: Initial - no x-rays or CT scans. Culture - not needed and difficult to access, Others only for alternative diagnoses; allergy, cystic fibrosis, Wegener's.
- Imaging: Obtained only after maximal medical therapy trial has failed. CT best modality, necessary for preoperative work-up. Plain x-ray insufficient bony detail.

COMMON PATHOGENS:

Streptococcus pneumoniae ; Haemophilus influenzae ; Moraxella catarrhalis ; Bacteriology of chronic sinusitis less well defined than acute. Chronic sinusitis - polymicrobial, increased gram negatives and possibly anaerobes. Pseudomonas aeruginosa, Staphylococcus aureus more common in nosocomial and immunocompromised infections. Controversy exists over role of fungi in chronic sinusitis. Suggestion that fungal elements may be inciting an eosinophil-mediated immune response in sinonasal mucosa. Use of antifungal agents for chronic sinusitis unproven and not currently recommended.

TREATMENT REGIMENS

Adjuvant pharmacotherapy

- Intranasal steroid sprays: Fluticasone (Flonase), Mometasone (Nasonex), Triamcinolone (Nasacort) - 2 sprays each nostril/d for prolonged period.
- Systemic Decongestant - Pseudoephedrine 120mg + sedating antihistamine PO bid (OTC preparations - Actifed, Contac, Dristan).
- Topical decongestant spray: oxymetazoline nasal spray 2 sprays bid x 4d only (OTC preparations - Afrin, Dristan, Vicks, Sinex nasal sprays).
- Antihistamine (systemic or topical): loratadine (Claritin) 10mg PO qd or fexofenadine (Allegra) 60mg po bid; astelin - only topical antihistamine available
- Pain relief: ASA, acetaminophen, ibuprofen.
- Others: nasal saline irrigation, inhaled steam.
- Immunotherapy: specific allergy treatment if appropriate.
- Systemic Steroids: in selected patients - allergy, polyps, asthma.
- Leukotriene antagonists: Used in some severe patients, particularly those with comorbid asthma - uncertain benefit at present.

Antibiotics

- Principles: Prolonged antibiotic therapy for 3 to 6 weeks with appropriately selected agent (similar to those used for acute infections).
- First Line: Amoxicillin/Clavulanate (Augmentin) 875mg po bid x 3-6 weeks
- Alternatives:
- Clindamycin (Cleocin) 300mg PO tid x 3-6 weeks
- Cefuroxime axetil (Ceftin) 500mg PO bid x 3-6 weeks
- Cefprozil (Cefzil) 500mg PO bid x 3-6 weeks
- Clarithromycin (Biaxin) 500mg PO bid x 3-6 weeks
- Gatifloxacin (Tequin) 400mg PO qd x 3-6 weeks

- Levofloxacin (Levaquin) 500mg PO qd x 3-6 weeks
- Moxifloxacin (Avelox) 400mg PO qd x 3-6 weeks

Surgery

- Goal of "functional endoscopic sinus surgery" (FESS) to restore physiologic ventilation and drainage of sinuses.
- Indications: recurrent/chronic infection not responsive to medical therapy with demonstrated abnormalities on endoscopy and/or CT scan, and orbital or intracranial complications of sinusitis.
- Risks of sinus surgery: bleeding, infection, orbital injury, intracranial injury or CSF leak, and risks of general anesthesia - major complications are rare
- Ongoing medical therapy often still required.
- Important role in management.
- Computer-aided sinus surgery using surgical navigation systems may improve efficacy and safety of procedure

Drug-Specific Comments

Amoxicillin: Poor choice in chronic sinusitis patients. Resistant S. pneumonia, H. influenzae and M. catarrhalis a major concern.

Amoxicillin + Clavulanate: Our first line agent for chronic sinuistis. Prefered over just amoxicillin to capture resistent strains (especially H. influenzae). We actually use Augmentin 500mg PO bid, instead of the recommended tid dose, and it appears to be better tolerated (GI side effects) by patients. We also prefer to treat for 3 weeks. there is no good evidence to suggest that treating for longer is better.

Cefuroxime and Cefuroxime axetil: (Ceftin). Reasonable choice for chronic sinuistis, fairly broad coverage.

Cephalexin: Reasonable first line agent. fairly broad spectrum coverage.

Clarithromycin: Good choice, especially for pen-allergic patients. Some studies suggest anti-inflammatory mechanism of action of macrolides may also improve their efficacy for inflammatory conditions such as sinusitis.

Gatifloxacin: (Tequin) Usually reserved for nonresponders. Well tolerated, convenient once-daily dosing, but expensive. Concern over abuse and development of resistance to fluoroquinolone class.

Levofloxacin: (Levaquin). Convenient once-daily dosing and well tolerated, but expensive. Concern over abuse and development of resistance to fluoroquinolone class.

Metronidazole: (Flagyl). Maybe added to cover anaerobes. Role of anaerobic organisms somewhat controversial in chronic sinusitis.

Moxifloxacin: (Avelox). Convenient once daily dosing and well-tolerated, but expensive. Concern over abuse and development of resistance to fluoroquinolone class.

Important Points

- Mainstay of medical therapy is prolonged course of antibiotics. Duration required uncertain, most recommend 3-6 weeks.
- Most common adjuvant therapy: intranasal steroid spray and saline irrigation.
- Important to address predisposing factors: allergies, nasal foreign body (NG tube, packing), anatomic abnormalities (septal deviation), illnesses (asthma, cystic fibrosis).
- Chronic sinusitis often requires surgical intervention.
- Guidelines based on Report of Rhinosinusitis Task Force Committee of American Academy of Otolaryngology-Head and Neck Surgery (Sept, 1997) and J Otolaryngol Head Neck Surg 2000 recommendations.

- Indications for ENT referral: recurrent or chronic infection not responsive to medical management, suspected anatomic abnormality (eg. deviated nasal septum, polyps), concern over underlying disease (eg. sinonasal malignancy, granulomatous diseases) or complications of sinusitis.

SELECTED READINGS

Sindwani R, Metson R. The Impact of Image-Guidance on Frontal Sinus Obliteration Surgery. Otolaryngol Head Neck Surgery. 2004. 131:150-5.

Subramanian HN, Schechtman KB, Hamilos DL . A retrospective analysis of treatment outcomes and time to relapse after intensive medical treatment for chronic sinusitis. Am J Rhinol 2002;Nov-Dec;16 (6):303-12

Metson, RB, Gliklich RE . Clinical outcomes in patients with chronic sinusitis. Laryngoscope 2000;110 (3 Pt 3):24-8

Zinreich SJ. Imaging of chronic sinusitis in adults: x-ray, computed tomography and magnetic resonance imaging. J Allergy Clin Immunol 1992;90(3):445-451

Doyle PW, Woodham JD. Evaluation of the microbiology of chronic ethmoid sinusitis. J Clin Microbiol 1991;29:2396-400

Kennedy DW, Zinreich J, Rosenbaum AE, et al. Functional endoscopic sinus surgery. Arch Otolaryngol 1985;111:576-82

Lanza DC, Kennedy DW . Adult rhinosinusitis defined; Task Force on Rhinosinusitis Research. Otolaryngol Head Neck Surg.

SMALLPOX
John G. Bartlett, M.D.

DIAGNOSTIC CRITERIA
- Hx: exposure - incubation period: 7-17d
- Sx: prodrome - sudden fever over 39C + HA x 2-3d, then rash - maculopapular, nodular, pustules @ 7d
- Lab: EM of vesicle fluid in BL4 lab. PCR confirms.
- Dx: Scrapings, pustule fluid, blood & tonsil swab - to BSL4 lab after notifying health dept

TREATMENT REGIMENS

Treatment
- Principles: Any case of smallpox = bioterrorism; HIGHLY CONTAGIOUS - consider everyone susceptible; Rx: Vaccine <3-4d contact; PREVENTION: isolation + vaccine
- Cidofovir active in vitro; no clinical experience
- Prevention: Vaccination within 3-4 days of exposure. Prior vaccination may result in amnestic response.
- Antibacterial agents to treat secondary bacterial infections of skin.
- Contact health dept, infection control, warn lab, call CDC 770-488-7100

Prevention
- Transmission - airborne after onset of rash
- Isolate all suspected cases immediately
- Preferred site of care: Home or non-hospital facility
- Hospital: Neg pressure room with HEPA filtration
- Contacts: Daily temp from exposure to 17d; any unexplained temp over 38C suggests smallpox: isolate & vaccinate
- Contacts (defined as face-to-face contact after onset of fever): Vaccinate within 3-4d of contact
- Vaccinate health care workers; furlough those w/vaccine contraindications

- Lab tests: need BSL4 facility

Treatment/prevention - vaccination

- Bifurcated needle - reconstitute vaccine - droplet held by capillary between needle tines - 15 perpendicular strokes that draw trace blood in 5mm area - cover
- Primary take: red papule day 3, vesicle day 5, pustule day 7 +/- adenopathy + fever - crusts - falls off at 3 wks
- Vaccine complications: postvaccinial encephalitis (1/300,000); prog. vaccinia: local spread (VIG Rx); eczema vac (spread to prior eczema area); gen. vaccinia (disseminated lesions); myopericarditis.
- VIG (for progressive vaccinia, eczema vaccinations, severe gen vaccinia): 0.6mL/kg IM, divided doses over 24-36hrs
- Prior vaccination: partial protection 5-10yrs, possibly longer
- Vaccine contraindications: immune comp esp reduced CMI & hx eczema; these are relative

IMPORTANT POINTS

- Guidelines from Johns Hopkins Center for Bioterrorism (JAMA 1999;281:2127) & DA Henderson (NEJM 2002;346:1300)
- Smallpox was eradicated in 1977; any case now means bioterrorism
- 3 vaccine strategies: 1) 1st responders; 2) ring vaccination (contacts); 3) everybody
- Vesico-pustular rash: Differential is chickenpox, Coxsackie, Herpes, impetigo, molluscum, monkeypox, SJS, drug reaction, pemphigus
- Main Ddx: chickenpox - VZV, Ab neg, rash superficial, various stages, centripetal
- Smallpox: spread person-to-person by aerosol droplets; pt - infectious at onset of rash.
- Priorities: Confirm dx, notify public health & infection control, isolate cases, vaccinate exposed.
- GUIDELINES RECOMMENDATIONS (from reference 1)
- Transmission - person to person by droplets or aerosols from oropharynx; most infectious from onset rash to rash d 7-10.
- Clinical features - incubation period: 7-17d, M-P rash face & forearms, then trunk & legs - vesicles - pustules - crusts (3 wks total).
- Rash - all lesions evolve as a single crop. Rash legions day 2-4 of prodrome, palms & soles involved. Papules to vesicles in 3-4d, vesicles to pustules in 5-6d, slough crusts d 18-20. Lesions may be confluent or discrete.
- Mortality - 30%.
- Dx - EM of vesicle fluid in BL4 lab
- Immunity with vaccination - declines substantially within 5-10 yrs.
- Postexposure vaccination "first few days after exposure and perhaps as late as 4 days" to prevent or attenuate disease.
- Hospital transmission is serious problem - prefer home or non-hospital facility for cases.

SELECTED READINGS

Henderson DA, Inglesby TV, Bartlett JG, et al. Smallpox as a biological weapon. JAMA 1999;281:2127

Downie AW, McCarthy K. The antibody response in man following infection with viruses of the pox group. III: Antibody response in smallpox. J Hyg 1958;56:479

Dixon CW. Smallpox in Tripolitania, 1946; an epidemiological and clinical study of 500 cases including trials of penicillin treatment. J Hyg 1948;46:357

Lance JM, Ruben FL, Neff JM, et al. Complications of smallpox vaccination 1968; national surveillance in the U.S. NEJM 1969;281:1201

Alibek K. "Biohazard". Random House, Inc. NY, NY 1999

World Health Organization. WHO declaration of global eradication of smallpox. Wkly Epidemiol Rec 1980;55:145

Noble J. Smallpox. Chapter 110 IN: Infectious Diseases, Gorbach S, Bartlett JG, Blacklow N, Eds. 1st Ed. WB Saunders, Phil 1992, pg 1112

Centers for Disease Control and Prevention. Vaccinia (Smallpox) Vaccine. MMWR 2001;50 (No. RR-10;1): pp 1-22

Henderson DA, Fenner F. Recent events and observations pertaining to smallpox virus destruction in 2002. CID 2001;33:1057

LeDuc JW, Jahrling PB. Strengthening national preparedness for smallpox. Emerg Infect Dis 2001;7:155

SURGICAL PROPHYLAXIS

Paul Auwaerter, M.D.; Arjun Srinivasan, M.D.

DIAGNOSTIC CRITERIA

- Surgical prophylaxis refers to the administration of antibiotics in patients with no signs of infection to reduce the risk of post-operative wound infections.
- Antibiotics should be given prior to procedures where the risk of contamination is high (e.g., gastrointestinal surgery) or the consequences of infection would be very serious (e.g., cardiac surgery).
- Antibiotics should cover the predominant flora of the operative site. Staph and strep for most cases, Anaerobes and enterobacteriaceae for GI cases.
- In general, clean cases (most plastic surgery and dermatologic surgery) DO NOT require pre-operative prophylaxis.

COMMON PATHOGENS: Coag neg staph (esp cardiac surg and hardware) ; Streptococcus species ; Staphylococcus aureus

TREATMENT REGIMENS

General surgery

- For procedures not listed here and for important dosing information, see Table 9 in Appendix I.
- Colon surgery/whipple procedure: neomycin & erythromycin (or metronidazole), 1g each PO at 1, 2 & 11pm day before surgery. IV: cefotetan 2g pre-op. [Some combine PO & IV]
- Colon surgery/whipple procedure - PCN allergy: clindamycin 600mg IV + gentamicin 5mg/kg IV pre-op
- Cholecystectomy open or laparoscopic - cefotetan 2g IV pre-op recom. for: pt age > 60, previous biliary surgery, acute symptoms, jaundice. PCN allergy: clindamycin 600mg IV +/- gentamicin 5mg/kg
- Appendectomy (uncomplicated - if complicated or perforated treat as peritonitis) - cefotetan 2g IV pre-op; PCN allergy: clindamycin 600mg IV pre-op
- Penetrating abdominal trauma - cefotetan 2 IV pre-op; continue 2g IV Q12H for 24H. PCN allergy: clindamycin 600mg IV + gentamicin 5mg/kg IV
- Inguinal hernia repair - uncomplicated: prophylaxis not recommended. Complicated, recurrent or emergent: cefotetan 2g IV; PCN allergy: clindamycin 600mg IV +/- gentamicin 5mg/kg
- Esophageal cases - cefotetan 2g IV pre-op; PCN allergy: clindamycin 600mg IV pre-op
- Mastectomy - no abx recommended

Gynecologic surgery

- Cesarean section - uncomplicated: no prophylaxis needed. Complicated: cefazolin 2g IV after cord clamping OR metronidazole 500mg IV after clamping

- Hysterectomy (abdominal or vaginal) - cefotetan 2g IV pre-op or cefazolin or cefoxitin. PCN allergy: clindamycin 600mg IV pre-op or metronidazole 500mg IV
- Repair of cystocele or rectocele - cefotetan 2g IV pre-op; PCN allergy: clindamycin 600mg IV pre-op
- Dilation and curettage - uncomplicated: no prophylaxis needed. Complicated: cefotetan 2g IV pre-op; PCN allergy: clindamycin 600mg IV pre-op

Orthopedic surgery

- Open reduction of fracture - cefazolin 2g IV pre-op, continue 72h for closed hip fractures (open fractures should be treated as infected, use cefazolin 2g IV q8h x 10d)
- Open reduction of fracture - PCN allergy: vancomycin 1g IV pre-op and at 12 hours
- Joint replacement-cefazolin 2g IV pre-op; PCN allergy: vancomycin 1g IV pre-op or clindamycin 600mg IV. Infuse before inflation of tourniquet. Cefuroxime also recommended for total hip arthroplasty.
- Lower limb amputation - cefotetan 2g IV pre-op PCN allergy: gentamicin 5mg/kg IV + clindamycin 600mg IV pre-op
- Spinal fusion - cefazolin 2g IV pre-op; PCN allergy: vancomycin 1g IV pre-op
- Arthroscopic surgery, laminectomy - no data support prophylaxis

DRUG-SPECIFIC COMMENTS

Ampicillin-sulbactam: With unavailability of cefotetan, some institutions are recommending ampicillin-sulbactam instead, especially given shortages of cefoxitin.

Cefotetan: Normal dosing 1-2g IV; drug currently not available in the U.S.

Cefoxitin: Cefoxitin 1-2g IV may be substituted for suggested cefotetan

Cefuroxime and Cefuroxime axetil: May be substituted in cardiothoracic and vascular surgical cases at 1.5g IV

IMPORTANT POINTS

- Studies indicate antibiotics should be given no more than 2h prior to case, with newer guidelines suggesting 1h for optimal efficacy.
- The entire infusion of the antibiotic must be complete when the incision is made.
- Abx must be redosed during procedures. Cefazolin should be re-dosed q 1500mL blood loss. Optimal redosing time of all agents is not known but general guidelines are given in treatment table.
- Preoperative antibiotics should not be continued beyond 24h of surgery, and no data exist that post-op doses are efficacious in infection prevention.

SELECTED READINGS

Bratzler DW, Houck PM et al. Antimicrobial prophylaxis for surgery: an advisory statement from the National Surgical Infection Prevention Project. Clin Infect Dis. 2004 Jun 15;38(12):1706-15

Zanetti G, et al. Improvement of intraoperative antibiotic prophylaxis in prolonged cardiac surgery by automated alerts in the operating room. Infection Control Hospital Epidemiology 2003;24:13-6.

Zanetti, G. Clinical consequences and cost of limiting use of vancomycin for perioperative prophylaxis: example of coronary artery bypass surgery. Emerging Infectious Diseases 2001;7:820-7.

Barie, Philip. Modern surgical antibiotic prophylaxis and therapy- less is more. Surgical Infections 2000;1:23-29.

Swaboda, SM et al. Does intraoperative blood loss affect antibiotic serum and tissue concentration?. Archives of Surgery 1996;131:1165-72.

Classen, DC et al. The timing of prophylactic administration of antibiotics and the risk of surgical wound infection. New England Journal of Medicine 1992;326:281-6.

SURGICAL WOUND INFECTIONS

Pamela A. Lipsett, M.D.; Chris Carpenter, M.D.

DIAGNOSTIC CRITERIA

- Surgical site infection = wound infection; types include superficial, deep, or organ space infection
- Risk factors: pre-existing medical illnesses e.g., diabetes, prolonged operation (site specific), wound contamination, and contaminated or dirty wounds.
- Traditional wound classification (clean, clean-contaminated, contaminated, and dirty-infected) alone does not adequately predict infection risk.
- Most postoperative SSI's occur a median of 12 days (3-28d, 25-75%) after surgery; more rapid presentations suggest toxin producing pathogens, e.g., Clostridium spp., Streptococcus pyogenes
- PE: erythema, tenderness, drainage, fluctuance, +/- fever

COMMON PATHOGENS: Staphylococcus aureus ; Coagulase-negative staphylococci ; Streptococcus species ; Enterococcus ; Enterobacteriaceae ; Other gram-negative bacilli

TREATMENT REGIMENS

Surgical site infections or dirty wound coverage

- For dirty wounds, antimicrobial coverage should be considered treatment, not prophylaxis.
- The length of treatment for dirty wounds is controversial; durations as short as 24 hours have been recommended.
- Coverage for SSI and dirty wounds should include gram -positive organisms, and in special circumstances gram- negative and anaerobic coverage (e.g., perforated viscus).
- For general wound infections, cefazolin 1-2g IV q8h is often adequate; vancomycin, linezolid, or daptomycin may be required in patients with or at risk of resistant gram-positive pathogen infections
- Vancomycin should also be considered for patients with serious B-lactam allergies or evidence of MRSA.
- Coverage for wounds infections with increased risk GNR/anaerobic infection: beta-lactam beta-lactamase inhibitor combination, cefotetan, cefoxitin, cefazolin + metronidazole, clindamycin + gentamicin

Clean-contaminated wound prophylaxis

- Antimicrobial prophylaxis indicated. See "Surgical Prophylaxis"
- Cefazolin 1-2g IV sufficient for majority of surgeries
- Vancomycin 1g IV in patients with serious beta-lactam allergies or at high risk for methicillin resistant Staphylococcus aureus infection.
- Cefotetan 1-2g IV or cefoxitin 1-2g IV or a beta-lactam beta-lactamase inhibitor combination should be considered in patients at high risk for anaerobic SSI, e.g., colorectal operations.
- Cefazolin 1-2g IV plus metronidazole 750mg IV may be an alternative.
- Mechanical bowel preparation with oral antibiotics may be considered in colorectal operations, e.g., neomycin plus erythromycin base, 1g each, at 1, 2, and 11 pm the day prior to an 8 am surgery.

Clean wound prophylaxis

- In general, antimicrobial prophylaxis is not recommended in clean wound operations. See "Surgical Prophylaxis" for more details.

DIAGNOSIS

- Exceptions: include operations where infection outcome can be drastic, such as craniotomy or cardiac surgery
- Cefazolin 1-2g IV within 60 minutes prior to surgical incision
- Vancomycin 1g IV in patients with serious B-lactam allergies or at high risk for methicillin-resistant Staphylococcus aureus infection.
- Intranasal mupirocin may reduce S aureus infections in colonized pts.

DRUG-SPECIFIC COMMENTS

Cefazolin: Recommended prophylaxis for most surgeries

Daptomycin: Excellent coverage of resistant gram-positive cocci (MRSA, VRE, etc.).

Linezolid: May be required for resistant GPC infections

IMPORTANT POINTS

- Primary treatment is to open/drain the wound. Antibiotics not indicated unless cellulitis is present or fascia involved
- Optimal prevention involves appropriate choice of antibiotic (usually cefazolin), timing (within 60 minutes of incision) and duration (< 24 hrs). SSI surveillance decrease rates of infection.
- Rapidly developing wounds on postoperative day 1 or 2, either with or without systemic toxicity, should raise suspicion of infection with Clostridium species or Streptococcus pyogenes.
- Hair removal should be performed using clippers and not razor blades because the latter is associated with an increase in SSI's.
- Temperature control, glucose control, wound space oxygenation, and smoking cessation decrease SSI

SELECTED READINGS

National Surgery Infection Prevention Project. Antimicrobial prophylaxis for surgery: an advisory statement from the National Surgical Infection prevention Project. Clin Infect Dis 2004 June 15;38(12):1706-15

The Medical Letter - Treatment Guidelines. Antimicrobial prophylaxis in surgery. Treatment Guidelines 2004 April;19:13-26

Zelenitsky SA, Ariano RE, Harding GK, et al. Antibiotic pharmacodynamics in surgical prophylaxis: an association between intraoperative antibiotic concentrations and efficacy. Antimicrob Agents Chemother 2002;46:3026-30

Perl TM, Cullen JJ, Wenzel RP et al. Intranasal mupirocin to prevent postoperative Staphylococcus aureus infections. N Engl J Med 2002 346:1871-7

de Lalla F. Surgical Prophylaxis in practice. J Hosp Infect 2002;50 Suppl A:S9-12

Leaper DJ Melling AG. Antibiotic prophylaxis in clean surgery: clean non-implant wounds. J Chemotherapy 2001;13 Spec No1:96-101

Gyssens IC. Preventing Postoperative Infections. Drugs, February 1999, vol. 57(2):175-85

Sawyer RG and Pruett TL. Wound Infections. Surgical Clinics of North America, June 1994, vol. 74(3):519-36

Page CP, Bohnen JM, Fletcher JR, et al. Antimicrobial prophylaxis for surgical wounds: Guidelines for clinical care. Archives of Surgery, 1993, vol. 128:79-88

Horan TC, Gaynes RP, Martone WJ, et al. CDC definitions of surgical site infections, 1992: A modification of CDC definitions of surgical wound infections. Amer J Infect Control, 1992, vol. 20:271-274

TINEA CORPORIS/TINEA CRURIS

Ciro R. Martins, M.D.

DIAGNOSTIC CRITERIA

- PE: Well-circumscribed patches or plaques of skin. Usually single, may be multiple.
- PE: Typical lesions are round to oval shaped, with elevated, erythematous, scaly borders and central clearing, giving them an annular ("ring-like") shape - hence the term "ring worm."
- PE: Atypical lesions are also common, especially in immunocompromised patients (flat, with ill-defined borders, eczematous, vesicular, pustular, bullous, psoriasiform or papular).
- Clinical: Pruritus is usually present, especially in tinea cruris. Pain varies with intensity of inflammation or secondary bacterial infection.
- Lab: KOH prep of scales obtained from the active border is positive for septated hyphae of dermatophytes. Cultures in dermatophyte-specific media are more sensitive, but not as practical.

COMMON PATHOGENS: Trichophyton rubrum

TREATMENT REGIMENS

Topical therapy

- Recommended for localized, uncomplicated non-inflammatory lesions
- Terbinafine 1% (Lamisil) cream qd x 3-4w; Naftifine 1% (Naftin) cream qd, gel bid x 3-4w; Butenafine 1% (Mentax) cream qd x 2w
- Econazole 1% (Spectazole) cream qd-bid x 2-4w
- Ketoconazole 2%(Nizoral) cream, shampoo qd-bid x 2-4w
- Clotrimazole 1% (Lotrimin, Mycelex) cream,lotion, solution bid x 2-4w
- Oxiconazole 1% (Oxistat) cream, lotion bid x 2-4w
- Miconazole 2% (Monistat-Derm, Micatin) cream, powder, spray bid x 2-4w
- Sulconazole 1% (Exelderm) cream, solution qd-bid x 3-4w
- Ciclopirox 1% (Loprox) cream bid x 2-4w; Haloprogin 1% (Halotex) cream, solution bid x 2-4w
- Tolnaftate 1% (Tinactin) cream, gel, powder, spray bid x 2-4w

Systemic therapy

- Indications: failure of adequate topical therapy, intolerance to topical medications, extensive and/or disabling, multifocal or inflammatory disease, deeper infection with hair follicle involvement
- Terbinafine (Lamisil) 250mg PO qd x 2-4w
- Itraconazole (Sporanox)200mg PO qd x 2-4w or 200mg bid x 7d
- Ketoconazole (Nizoral) 200mg PO qd x 2-4w
- Griseofulvin microsize (Grifulvin V) 500mg PO qd, griseofulvin ultramicrosize (Gris-Peg) 375mg PO qd x 2-4w

General measures

- Avoidance of tight fitting clothes/underwear
- Drying agents such as aluminum acetate or diluted acetic acid solutions may be used as soaks tid-qid on intertriginous areas when maceration and oozing are present
- If secondary bacterial infection is suspected, obtain bacterial cultures and start adequate oral antibiotic coverage
- Avoidance and proper treatment of infected animals/people

DRUG-SPECIFIC COMMENTS

Griseofulvin: Potential side-effects and adverse reactions as well as difficulty finding this drug on the market makes of it a less than optimal choice.

Ketoconazole: Not a good choice. The risks of liver toxicity and drug interactions are not justified by the benign nature of this diagnosis.

Terbinafine: This is my first choice. Very few drug interactions. Very well tolerated. No blood tests are needed if there is no h/o liver disease and when used for less than 4 weeks.

IMPORTANT POINTS

- These guidelines are based on the Guidelines of Care of the American Academy of Dermatology
- Predisposition to acquiring a dermatophyte infection varies significantly. Not every exposed individual will acquire it, even in cases of prolonged and intimate contact with infected persons
- Peak prevalence of dermatophyte infections of the skin occurs after puberty. This is especially true for tinea pedis, manuum and cruris. T. corporis and faciei can occur in the pre-adolescent period
- Recurrences are common, especially in tinea cruris. This may be due to premature discontinuation of topical therapy when the symptoms subside after a few days.
- Differential diagnosis includes: numular dermatitis, asteatotic eczema, psoriasis, parapsoriasis, figurate erythemas, candidiasis, contact dermatitis, erythrasma

SELECTED READINGS

Lesher, JL. Oral therapy of common superficial fungal infections of the skin. J.Am.Acad. Dermatol. 40 (6)Part2:S31-4, 1999

Smith EB. The treatment of dermatophytosis: Safety considerations. J.Am.Acad.Dermatol.43(5):S113-9, 2000

Adams B. Tinea Corporis Gladiatorum. Journal of the American Academy of Dermatology 2002; 47(2): 286-90

TINEA PEDIS
Ciro R. Martins, M.D.

DIAGNOSTIC CRITERIA

- PE (non-inflammatory type): Hyperkeratosis and scaling of the soles and/or interdigital spaces where maceration and fissuring may be noticed. The sides of the foot may be affected ("mocassin" pattern).
- PE (inflammatory type): acute onset of clustered deep seated vesicles and/or blisters on an erythematous, edematous base. Oozing and crusting develops. Vesicles rapidly spread by peripheral extension.
- Clinical: Pruritus is common in the dry, non-inflammatory type. Pain and discomfort which can be debilitating are common in the inflammatory type. Hyperhydrosis and bad odor are frequently associated.
- Lab: KOH prep of scales or vesicle roof shows septated hyphae of dermatophytes.
- Lab: Fungal culture may be helpful in cases when KOH prep is repeatedly negative, which is not uncommon in inflammatory cases. Speciation does not influence the therapeutic decisions.

COMMON PATHOGENS: Trichophyton rubrum ; Trichophyton mentagrophytes

Treatment Regimens

Topical therapy

- Terbinafine 1% (Lamisil) cream qd x 2w; Naftifine 1% (Naftin)cream qd, gel bid x 2w; Butenafine (Mentax)cream qd x 2w.
- Ketoconazole 2% (Nizoral), econazole 1% (Spectazole), clotrimazole 1% (Lotrimin), oxiconazole 1%(Oxistat), miconazole 2% (Micatin), sulconazole 1%(Exelderm) cream, lotion, gel, powder, spray bid x 3-4w
- Ciclopirox 1% (Loprox) cream bid x 3-4w; Haloprogin (Halotex) cream, solution bid x 3-4w; Tolnaftate 1% (Tinactin) cream, gel, powder, spray bid x 3-4w.

SYSTEMIC THERAPY

- Terbinafine (Lamisil) 250mg PO qd x 2w
- Itraconazole (Sporanox) 200mg PO qd x 3w or 400mg PO qd x 1w
- Fluconazole (Diflucan) 150mg PO qw x 4w
- Griseofulvin ultramicrosize (Gris-Peg) 250mg PO bid, griseofulvin microsize (Grifulvin V) 500mg PO bid X 4-8w

Adjunctive therapy

- Keratolytic agents such as urea 20-40% (Carmol cream) or salicylic acid 3-5% preparations can be used in cases with severe hyperkeratosis of the soles
- Drying agents such as aluminum acetate, potassium permanganate or diluted acetic acid can be used as soaking solutions bid in cases of wet interdigital tinea and in cases of G(-)toe web infection
- Topical or systemic corticosteroids may be needed in cases of extensive or severe inflammatory tinea pedis
- Topical or systemic antibiotics are needed in cases of secondary Gram-negative toe web infection
- Topical antifungals used in conjunction with systemic antifungals may speed up mycologic cure.

Drug-Specific Comments

Griseofulvin: Potential side-effects and adverse reactions as well as longer duration of therapy makes this drug less desirable than the other antifungals

Terbinafine: Excellent choice. Very effective, qd regimen of short duration. Very well tolerated and no major drug interactions. Fungicidal.

Important Points

- Tinea pedis caused by T. rubrum is more chronic, persistent, recalcitrant to therapy and recurrences occur in up to 70% of cases.
- Causes of recurrences: increased susceptibility of the affected individual, premature discontinuation of therapy, re-exposure to fungus and presence of a fungal "reservoir" such as infected nails.
- Prophylaxis of recurrences: correction of hyperhydrosis, wearing absorbant socks, thorough drying of the toes after showers, use of an antifungal powder applied to feet, socks and shoes regularly.
- Differential diagnosis includes: contact dermatitis, psoriasis, atopic dermatitis, erythrasma, intertrigo, palmo-plantar keratoderma.
- These guidelines are based on the Guidelines of Care of the American Academy of Dermatology.

SELECTED READINGS

Drake L.A., Dinehart S.M. et. al. Guidelines of Care for Superficial Mycotic Infections of the Skin: Tinea Corporis, Tinea Cruris, Tinea Faciei, Tinea Manuum and Tinea Pedis. Dermatology World - American Academy of Dermatology, Guidelines of Care, Supplement, 22-6, April 1995

Lesher J.L. Oral therapy of common superficial fungal infections of the skin. Journal of the American Academy of Dermatology, 40(6) Part 2, S31-4, June 1999

Del Rosso J.Q., Gupta A.K. The use of intermittent itraconazole therapy for superficial mycotic infections: a review and update on the "one week" approach. International Journal of Dermatology, 38 (Suppl.2), 28-39, 1999

Rich P. Onychomycosis and Tinea Pedis in Patients with Diabetes. Journal of the American Academy of Dermatology 2000; 43(5): S130-S134

TINEA VERSICOLOR
Ciro R. Martins, M.D.

DIAGNOSTIC CRITERIA

- PE: hypopigmented and/or hyperpigmented scaly patches (non-elevated or minimally elevated) affecting mainly the trunk, neck and proximal extremities
- PE: lesions are usually multiple, small, round or oval in shape or coalescent into large, irregularly shaped patches
- PE: Woods lamp examination aids in revealing the true extent of involvement by showing yellowish fluorescence of the lesions
- Clinical: Usually asymptomatic, but may be mildly to moderately pruritic
- Lab: KOH prep of scales show short, stubby, blunt-ended interlaced hyphae with clusters of spores and yeast cells ("spaghetti and meat balls" appearence)

COMMON PATHOGENS: Malassezia furfur (Pityrosporum ovale)

TREATMENT REGIMENS

Topical therapy

- Topical therapy alone is indicated as first line regimen and is effective in most cases.
- Selenium sulfide 2.5% (Selsun), ketoconazole (Nizoral) or zinc pyrithione shampoo scrubbed onto the affected areas using a mildly abrasive sponge and rinsed off in 3-5 minutes qd x 1w or qod x 2w.
- Selenium sulfide 2.5% lotion applied to the affected areas and rinsed-off after 10 minutes qd x 7d or left overnight and rinsed off in the morning as a single application (repeat in 1w).
- Econazole 1%(Spectazole), ketoconazole 2% (Nizoral), clotrimazole 1% (Lotrimin), oxiconazole 1% (Oxistat), miconazole 2% (Micatin), sulconazole 1% (Exelderm) cream, lotion or solution, qd x 1-2w
- Terbinafine (Lamisil) 1% spray or cream or butenafine 1% cream (Mentax) qd X 1-2w
- Ciclopirox 1% (Loprox)cream qd x 1-2w
- Miscelaneous: benzoyl peroxide 5-10% lotion, gel, cream or wash, sulfur and salicilic acid preparations, propylene glycol 50% solution, sodium thiosulfate 25% with salicilic acid 1%applied qd x 1-2w

Systemic therapy

- Ketoconazole (Nizoral) 400mg PO single dose repeated in 1 wk or 200mg PO qd x 7-10d.
- Oral treatment is recommended in cases with extensive involvement, with frequent recurrences, when topical treatment failed or when patient is sensitive to or unable to apply topical medications.
- Fluconazole (Diflucan) 300mg PO single dose repeated in 1 week
- Itraconazole (Sporanox) 200mg PO qd x 7d

- Exercise with sweating two hours after taking the oral medication improves drug delivery to the skin. Showers should be avoided for 12 hours.
- Topical medications can be used in association with systemic treatment.

DRUG-SPECIFIC COMMENTS

Ketoconazole: Safe, inexpensive and effective as a single dose or for a short (<7days) course.

Terbinafine: Not an effective oral agent against P. ovale.

IMPORTANT POINTS

- These guidelines are based on the guidelines of care of the American Academy of Dermatology.
- Tinea versicolor is a superficial infection of the stratum corneum caused by a yeast that is part of the normal cutaneous flora in 90-100% of individuals, therefore it is not a contagious process.
- People of all age groups are affected, but more frequently seen in adults. More common in geographic areas with warm and humid tropical climate. More common in the summer months.
- Individual predisposition is needed for development of the clinical infection but multiple other factors contribute to its pathogenesis. Recurrences are common in predisposed individuals.
- Differential diagnosis includes: pityriasis rosea, seborrheic dermatitis, pityriasis alba, secondary syphilis, hypopigmented variant of cutaneous T-cell lymphoma and Hansen's disease.

SELECTED READINGS

Drake L.A., Dinehart S.M., et. al. Guidelines of Care for Superficial Mycotic Infections of the Skin: Pityriasis (Tinea) Versicolor. Dermatology World, American Academy of Dermatology, Supplement, 36-8, April 1995

Montero-Gei F, Robles ME, Suchil P. Fluconazole vs. Itraconazole in the treatment of tinea versicolor. International Journal of Dermatology, 38:601-3, 1999.

Savin R. Diagnosis and treatment of tinea versicolor. Journal of Family Practice, 43: 127-32, 1996

Sunenshine PJ, Scwartz RA, Janniger CK. Tinea Versicolor - Review. International Journal of Dermatology 1998, 37:648-55

TOXIC SHOCK SYNDROME, STAPHYLOCOCCAL

Joel Blankson, M.D., Ph.D.

DIAGNOSTIC CRITERIA

- Fever: T > 38.9C. Hypotension: SBP < 90 in adults or < 5th percentile for children <16 years. Orthostatic hypotension. (See Table 6 in Appendix I)
- Rash: diffuse macular erythorderma. Desquamation: palms and soles usually involved, 1-2 weeks after onset of illness.
- Multisystem involvement (3 or > of following) a.) GI: vomiting, diarrhea at onset; b.) musculoskeletal: CPK > 2X nl or severe myalgia; c.) renal: BUN/creatinine > 2X nl or sterile pyuria; d.) hepatic: Bilirubin, AST or ALT > 2X nl; e.) hematologic: plts < 100 000/mm3; f.) CNS: altered mental status without focal neurologic signs.
- Negative Cx for other explanation e.g., blood, throat or CSF cultures (Cx can be positive for S. aureus). There should not be an increase in titer to Rocky Mountain spotted fever, leptospira, rubeola.

TREATMENT REGIMENS

Treatment
- Clindamycin 900mg IV q 8hrs + oxacillin 2g IV q 4 hrs for methicillin sensitive S. aureus.
- Clindamycin 900mg IV q 8hrs + vancomycin 1g IV q 12 hrs for methicillin resistant S. aureus.
- Consider IVIG: 2gm/kg IV X 1, repeat in 48hrs if pt remains unstable
- Supportive Case/ ICU monitoring

IMPORTANT POINTS
- S. aureus produces the enterotoxins, TSST-1, SEB and SEC. These toxins are superantigens capable of activating up to 25% of T cells.
- Therapy guided at stopping toxin production. Clindamycin inhibits protein synthesis and is the drug of choice.
- Most patients with Staph TSS have been shown to lack antibodies to the toxin, IVIG contains these antibodies to this common antigen.
- No controlled studies exist for this therapy in S. aureus TSS, but a small study showed a decrease in mortality in Streptococcal TSS.
- A mortality rate of 3 -5 % is generally quoted for S. aureus TSS
- Tampon use is a risk factor
- Tampons are infrequent cause following withdrawal of Rely brand

SELECTED READINGS
Darenberg J, Soderquist B, Normark BH, Norrby-Teglund A. Differences in potency of intravenous polyspecific immunoglobulin G against streptococcal and staphylococcal superantigens: implications for therapy of toxic shock syndrome. Clin Infect Dis vol 38. Mar 2004 p.836-42

Darenberg J, Ihendyane N, Sjolin J, Aufwerber E, Haidl S, Follin P, Andersson J, Norrby-Teglund A; S. Intravenous immunoglobulin G therapy in streptococcal toxic shock syndrome: a European randomized, double-blind, placebo-controlled trial. Clin Infect Dis. Vol 37 Aug 2003 p. 333-40

Russell NE, Pachorek RE. Russell NE, Pachorek RE. Ann Pharmacother. Vol. 34 Jul-Aug 2000 p. 936-9.

Kaul R, McGeer A, Norrby-Teglund A, Kotb M, Schwartz B, O'Rourke K, Talbot J. Intravenous immunoglobulin therapy for streptococcal toxic shock syndrome,a comparative observational study. The Canadian Streptococcal Study Group. Clin Infect Dis vol 28. April 1999. p. 800-7

Bergdoll MS, Crass BA, Reiser RF, Robbins RN, Davis JP. A new staphylococcal enterotoxin, enterotoxin F, associated with toxic-shock-syndrome Staphylococcus aureus isolates. Lancet. May 1981 p 1017-21

Reingold AL, Hargrett, NT, Shands KN, Dan BB, Schmid GP, Strickland BY Broome CV. Toxic Shock Syndrome Surveillance in the United States, 1980-1981. Ann Intern Med vol 96 June 1982 , p. 875-880

TOXIC SHOCK SYNDROME, STREPTOCOCCAL

Joel Blankson, M.D., Ph.D.

DIAGNOSTIC CRITERIA
- Isolation of S. pyogenes [Group A Streptococci] A. from a normally sterile site (e.g., blood, CSF) B. from a non sterile site (e.g. throat, superficial skin lesion)
- Clinical signs of severe disease (see Table 7 in Appendix I) A.) Hypotension SBP <90 or < 5th percentile in children AND B. Multisystem involvement: 2 or more of the following systems:
- Renal. 1.) Creatinine > 2X baseline 2.) Hematologic: Plts < 100 000/mm3 or diss. intravascular coagulopathy 3. Hepatic: bilirubin, AST/ALT >2x nl. 4. Pulm: ARDS
- 5. Generalized erythematous rash that may desquamate. Soft tissue necrosis, including necrotizing fasciitis, myositis, or gangrene.

- Ddx includes: S. aureus (toxic shock syndrome), RMSF, Leptospira interrogans, Neisseria meningitidis, Streptococcus pneumoniae

COMMON PATHOGENS: Streptococcus pyogenes (Group A)

TREATMENT REGIMENS

Treatment
- Surgical debridement essential for GAS associated necrotizing fasciitis or myositis
- Clindamycin 900mg IV q 8hrs + PCN G 4 mU IV q 4 hrs for GAS
- Consider IVIG: the studied dose in RCT is 1g/kg (day 1) and 0.5g/kg (days 2 and 3)
- Supportive Cases/ICU monitoring

DRUG-SPECIFIC COMMENTS

Clindamycin: Routinely recommended due to its protein synthesis (and therefore toxin) inhibition properties in addition to pencillin for the treatement of streptococcal toxic shock syndrome.

Penicillin: Frequently used in conjunction with clindamycin. PCN is rapidly bacteriocidal, and there has been no documented resistance to date with GAS.

IMPORTANT POINTS
- S. pyogenes produces exotoxins SPEA, SPEB, and SPEC. These toxins are superantigens capable of activating up to 25% of T cells. Therapy guided at stopping toxin production.
- Clindamycin inhibits toxin synthesis and is the drug of choice.
- A small comparative observational study showed a decrease in mortality in Streptococcal TSS associated with IVIG tx.
- A follow up double blind, placebo controlled study found decreased mortality (but did not reach statistical significance) in Streptococcal TSS associated with IVIG tx
- Early surgical intervention is crucial for fasciitis or myonecrosis. Suspect when pain is out of proportion to exam.

SELECTED READINGS

Stevens DL. Dilemmas in the treatment of invasive Streptococcus pyogenes infections. Clin Infect Dis vol 37. Aug 2003 p.341-3

Darenberg J, Ihendyane N, Sjolin J et al. Intravenous immunoglobulin G therapy in streptococcal toxic shock syndrome: a European randomized, double-blind, placebo-controlled trial. Clin Infect Dis vol 37. Aug 2003.p.333-40

Russell NE, Pachorek RE. Clindamycin in the treatment of streptococcal and staphylococcal toxic shock syndromes. Ann Pharmacother. Vol. 34 Jul-Aug 2000 p. 936-9.

Kaul R, McGeer A, Norrby-Teglund A, et al. Intravenous immunoglobulin therapy for streptococcal toxic shock syndrome, a comparative observational study. The Canadian Streptococcal Study Group. Clin Infect Dis vol 28. April 1999. p. 800-7

Breiman et al. Defining the Group A Streptococcal toxic shock syndrome. JAMA vol 269. January 1993 p. 390-391

Eagle H. Experimental approach to the problem of treatment failure with penicillin. Am J Med vol 13 Oct 1952 p. 389-399

TUBERCULOSIS, ACTIVE   Timothy Sterling, M.D.

DIAGNOSTIC CRITERIA
- Hx: Pulmonary TB = cough > 2 wks, fever, night sweats, weight loss, hemoptysis, shortness of breath. Disseminated TB = fevers, weight loss, organ involvement. See also "Meningitis, TB"

Diagnosis

- CXR: upper lobe infiltrate classic (may be cavitary); atypical presentations if HIV+; adenopathy
- Sputum AFB smear--50% sensitive
- AFB culture--80% sensitive
- PCR: best for sputum with pos AFB smear +, expensive
- Typically 4 drugs used for 8 wks, then using susceptibilities 2 or 3 drugs are used for balance of duration

Common Pathogens: Mycobacterium tuberculosis; M. bovis (part of MTb complex, 30 recent cases in U.S.)

Treatment Regimens

Adults

- Initial therapy: INH 5mg/kg (300mg max) + RIF 10mg/kg (600mg max) + PZA 15-30mg/kg (2g max) + EMB 15-25mg/kg (1.6g max) + vit B6 50mg--All PO qd
- Can use rifabutin in place of rifampin in persons on HIV treatment protease inhibitors, NNRTI, methadone. Dose adjustments necessary, TB always treated first unless patient already on HAART.
- Check drug susceptibilities; treat with at least 2 drugs to which M. tb is susceptible
- Rx duration determined by site of disease, response to therapy
- Refer to health department so pt. can receive directly-observed therapy (DOT).
- Dosing less frequently than daily is possible, but must be done via DOT.
- Usual duration 6 mos, but 9 mos if cavitary disease and cx (+) after 2 mos.
- For meningitis, see "Meningitis, TB"

Infection control

- TB isolation: cough > 2 weeks + abnormal CXR
- Can discontinue if 3 expectorated or 1 induced sputum is AFB smear-neg
- If AFB smear-pos or on TB treatment, can discontinue after 2 weeks of Rx, clinical improvement, and AFB smear-neg

Drug-Specific Comments

Rifabutin: Can be used in place of rifampin; drug interactions to lesser extent than with rifampin (e.g., less likely to precipitate methadone withdrawal)

Important Points

- Guidelines based on ATS/CDC Guidelines. (Am J Respir Crit Care Med 2003;167:603-62.) This includes a new recommendation to extend treatment to 9 mos if cavitary disease plus cx + after 2 months
- Refer all cases to local health dept for treatment and contact investigation
- Directly-observed therapy (DOT) preferred for both adults and children
- TB Rx in HIV-infected patient: concern re: drug interactions, paradoxical worsening

Selected Readings

CDC. Updated guidelines for the use of rifamycins for the treatment of tuberculosis among HIV-infected patients. Updated January 20, 2004. http://www.cdc.gov/nchstp/tb/TB_HIV_Drugs/PDF/tbhiv.pdf

Frieden TR, Sterling TR, Munsiff SS et al. Tuberculosis. Lancet 2003;362:887-99

ATS/CDC/IDSA. Treatment of tuberculosis. Am J Respir Crit Care Med 2003;167:603-62

Burman WJ, Jones BE. Treatment of HIV-related tuberculosis in the era of effective antiretroviral therapy. Am J Respir Crit Care Med 2001;164;7-12

Small PM, Fujiwara PI. Management of tuberculosis in the United States. N Engl J Med 2001;345:189-200.

Havlir DV, Barnes PF. Tuberculosis and HIV. N Engl J Med 1999;340:367-73

TUBERCULOSIS, LATENT
Timothy Sterling, M.D.

DIAGNOSTIC CRITERIA

- Evidence of latent infection (and indication to treat) based on mm induration on tuberculin skin test, TB risk. Unless risk factors present, routine PPD not advocated.
- 5mm: HIV+, close contact of TB case, fibrosis on chest x-ray, or immunosuppressed (e. g., prednisone > 15 mg/d for >1 month)
- 10 mm: recent immigrant; injection drug user; resident/employee of prison, jail, nursing home, hospital, shelter; DM, renal failure, leukemia/lymphoma, weight loss, gastrectomy; child <4 years
- Recent converter: >10 mm increase in induration within 2 years
- If meet above high-risk criteria, treat regardless of age.

COMMON PATHOGENS: Mycobacterium tuberculosis

TREATMENT REGIMENS

HIV-seronegative Adults

- Pref: isoniazid 5mg/kg (300mg max)PO qd x 9 months. Pyridoxine (vit B6) 50mg qd may decrease neuropathy risk
- Alt: rifampin 10mg/kg (600mg max) qd x 4 months
- Monitoring for toxicity: INH - baseline LFTs in pts at increased risk of hepatotoxicity (HIV+, liver disease, EtOH, pregnant or < 3 mos post-partum).
- RIF/PZA 2 mos. no longer recommended by CDC due hepatotoxicity

HIV-seropositive Adults

- Isoniazid 5mg/kg (300mg max)PO qd x 9 months. Pyridoxine (vit B6) 50mg qd may decrease neuropathy risk.

Children < 18 Yrs.

- Isoniazid 10-20mg/kg (300mg max) qd x 9 months. Pyridoxine (vit B6) generally not necessary.

IMPORTANT POINTS

- Guidelines based on ATS/CDC guidelines. (Am J Resp Crit Care Med 2000;161:S221-S247.) Revised recommendation re: monitoring for toxicity in MMWR 2001;50:733-5.
- Must exclude active TB before treatment of latent infection (TLI)
- Obtain CXR if skin test +; sputum AFB if CXR abnormal and/or symptomatic
- If HIV+, eligible for TLI if close contact of TB case even if skin-test negative, or prior TLI.
- Interactions with rifampin: antiretrovirals, methadone, oral contraceptives, anticoagulants, steroids, etc.

SELECTED READINGS

CDC. Tuberculosis associated with blocking agents against tumor necrosis factor-alpha. MMWR 2004;53:683-6.

Horsburgh CR. Priorities for the treatment of latent tuberculosis infection in the United States. N Engl J Med 2004;350:2060-7

CDC. Update: Adverse event data and revised American Thoracic Society/CDC recommendations against the use of rifampin and pyrazinamide for treatment of latent tuberculosis infection--United States, 2003. MMWR 2003;52:735-9

American Thoracic Society, Centers for Disease Control and Prevention. Targeted tuberculin testing and treatment of latent tuberculosis infection. Am J Resp Crit Care Med 2000;161:S221-S247.

Comstock GW. How much isoniazid is needed for prevention of tuberculosis among immunocompetent adults?. Int J Tuberc Lung Dis 1999;3:847-50.

UPPER RESPIRATORY INFECTIONS

John G. Bartlett, M.D.

Diagnostic Criteria
- Acute infection, usually of viral origin, involving the upper airways & often sinuses, pharynx, larynx, or bronchi, i.e., sinusitis, laryngitis, pharyngitis & bronchitis.
- PE: Red throat, nasal pus (yellow or green), etc.
- Dx: clinical syndrome. No cultures
- R/O pneumonia, epiglottitis, space infection, thrush (HIV)

Common Pathogens: Rhinovirus ; Coronavirus ; Parainfluenza virus ; Adenovirus ; Enteroviruses ; RSV

Treatment Regimens
Common cold
- Principles: Viral infection - symptomatic Rx +/- antiflu agent vs allergy. For allergy - topical steroids, and non-sedating antihistamines (claritin, etc.)
- Preferred (Irwin NEJM 2000; 343:1715): Nasal decongestants, sedating antihistamines, anticholinergic and antiinflammatory agents (see below)
- Decongestants: Pseudoephedrine & sedating antihistamine such as dexbrompheniramine, brompheniramine chlorpheniramine, diphenhydramine carbinoxamine--OTC as Actifed, Atrofed, Cardec, etc
- Anticholinergic: Ipratropium bromide nasal spray (Atrovent 0.6%) 2 sprays each nostril 3-4x/day
- Oral decongestant: Pseudoephedrine, 120mg PO bid (available OTC)
- Nasal sprays: Oxymetazone nasal solutions (0.05%)--Afrin, Allerest, Dristan, Neo-Synephrine, 2-3 qtts/nostril BID. Otrivin, Vicks vapor inhaler, etc: 2-6 sprays/nostril no more than q2-10h
- Anti-inflammatory agents: ASA, acetaminophen, naproxen (Aleve)(not ibuprofen)
- Antihistamines - sedating 1st generation: preferred - Benadryl, hydroxyzine (Atarax)
- Heated humidified air

Allergic basis
- Nasal steroids such as fluticasone (Flonase) flunisolide (Nasalide), beclomethasone (Beconase), triamcinolone (Nasacort), budesonide (Rhinocort) - all 2 sprays bid
- Antihistamine - 2nd generation nonsedating such as Fexofenadine (Allegra) 60mg PO bid or Loratadine (Claritin) 10mg PO qd
- Avoid allergen

Controversial/prevention
- Zinc gluconate lozenges 13-23mg Zn, 1 q 2h while awake: conflicting data
- Vitamin C: probably no benefit
- Humidified hot air
- Prevention: avoid hand contact and aerosol; flu vaccine or anti-influenza agents (flu); fresh air in office (rhinovirus)
- MISCELLANEOUS:
- Naproxen (Aleve) 220 mg--2, then 1 q8-12h
- Zinc gluconate lozenges (Cold-Eze) 13.3-23.0mg Zn lozenge q2h while awake--studies are variable with 6 positive trials & 5 negative trials. Must be taken frequently & have noxious taste.
- Intranasal ipratropium demonstrated benefit in controlled trials in terms of nasal discharge & reduced sneezing

- Ibuprofen may increase rhinovirus replication--use alternative such as acetominophen for symptomatic treatment
- Vitamin C--great hype, but not much science. Clinical trial studies are variable.
- Antihistamine--2nd generation preferred for allergic rhinitis. First generation (sedating) antihistamines preferred for common cold.
- Antibiotics--no proven benefit--major source of antibiotic abuse
- Humidified hot air--rationale is to heat rhinovirus which grows best at 33 degrees C. Trials have not shown benefit.

IMPORTANT POINTS

- Recommendations from the CDC (Ann Intern Med 2001;134:487) and Irwin RS (NEJM 2000; 343:1715)
- Probably not effective Rx: Zinc, Vit C, humidified hot air
- Antihistamines - sedating 1st gen may help cold; non-sedating 2nd gen - work only for allergy
- Viral URIs are a major cause of sinusitis, otitis, bronchitis, laryngitis, exacerbations of bronchitis & asthma
- URI does not benefit from antibiotics, but is a major cause of antibiotic abuse
- Drainage often yellow or green with viral infection.
- Viral URIs are a major cause of hospitalization in pts with cold, asthma, diabetes, elderly age etc.
- Purulent or green nasal discharge or cough does NOT mean bacterial infection in most cases (although suspicion of sinusitis increases if nasal discharge occurs >7d and is associated with unilateral sinus or tooth pain.

SELECTED READINGS

Myatt TA, et al. Detection of airborne rhinovirus and its relation to outdoor air supply in office environments. Am J Crit Care Med 2004;169:1187.

Sperber SJ, Shah LP, Gilbert RD, et al. Echinacea purpurea for prevention of experimental rhinovirus colds. Clin Infect Dis 2004;38:1367-71

Hong CY, et al. Acute respiratory symptoms in adults in general practice. Fam Pract 2004;21:317-23

Cochrane Database Syst Rev. Cochrane Database System Review. 2004;CD001728

Stevens MM, Naselsky J. Do inhaled beta-agonists control cough in URI's or acute bronchitis?. J Fam Pract 2004;53:662

Rutschmann OT, Domino ME. Antibiotics for upper respiratory tract infection in ambulatory practice in the U.S. 1997:99: does physician specialty matter. J Am Board Fam Pract 2004;17:196

Cohen S, Tyrrell DAJ, Smith AP. Psychological stress and susceptibility to the common cold. N Engl J Med 1991;325:606

Hall WJ, Hall CB. Alterations in pulmonary function following respiratory viral infection. Chest 1979;76:458

Gadomski A. A cure for the common cold. JAMA 1998;279:1999

Mainous AG, Hueston WJ, Eberlein C. Colour of respiratory drainage and antibiotic use. Lancet 1997;350:1077

URETHRITIS [MEN]

Noreen A. Hynes, M.D., M.P.H.

DIAGNOSTIC CRITERIA

- Rapid dx: gram stain of urethral secretions >4 WBCs/oil immersion averaged over 5 fields w/ greatest concentration of PMNs.
- Gonococcal urethritis = gram negative intracellular diplococci (GNID) and + Rapid dx test; non-gonococcal urethritis (NGU)=no GNIDs and + Rapid dx test.

- Other Lab: Positive leukocyte esterase test on first void urine (FVU); >9 WBCs/HPF on microscopic exam of FVU.
- Symptoms: urethral discharge; dysuria; penile irritation; OR asymptomatic.
- Signs: urethral discharge which may only be present after milking the urethra. Some may be without discharge with findings only on laboratory testing.

COMMON PATHOGENS: Chlamydia trachomatis ; Neisseria gonorrhoeae ; Trichomonas vaginalis ; Ureaplasma urealyticum ; Mycoplasma genitalium

TREATMENT REGIMENS

Gonococcal urethritis

- Cefixime 400mg PO x 1 PLUS azithromycin 1g PO x 1 OR doxycycline 100mg PO bid x 7 d if chlamydia infection has not been ruled out
- Ceftriaxone 125mg IM x 1 PLUS azithromycin 1g PO x 1 OR doxycycline 100mg PO bid x 7 d if chlamydia infection has not been ruled out
- Ciprofloxacin 500mg PO x1 PLUS azithromycin 1g PO x 1 OR doxycycline 100mg PO bid x 7 d if chlamydia infection has not been ruled out
- Ofloxacin 400mg PO x 1 PLUS azithromycin 1g PO x 1 OR doxycycline 100mg PO bid x 7 d if chlamydia infection has not been ruled out
- Levofloxacin 250mg PO x 1 PLUS azithromycin 1g PO x 1 OR doxycycline 100mg PO bid x 7d if chlamydia infection has not been ruled out
- Alternative regimens: Spectinomycin 2g IM x 1 OR Gatifloxacin 400mg PO x 1; Norfloxacin 800mg PO x 1; Lomefloxacin 400 PO x 1

Non-gonococcal urethritis

- Azithromycin 1g PO x 1
- Doxycycline 100mg PO bid x 7d

Recurrent or persistent urethritis

- Metronidazole 2g PO OR Tinidazole 2g PO once PLUS erythromycin base 500mg PO qid x 7d
- Metronidazole 2g PO OR Tinidazole 2g PO once PLUS erythromycin ethylsuccinate 800mg PO qid x 7d

DRUG-SPECIFIC COMMENTS

Cefixime: Has an antimicrobial spectrum similar to ceftriaxone but the 400mg PO dose does not provide as high nor as sustained a bactericidal level as that provided by the 125-mg dose of ceftriaxone. In published trials, 400-mg dose cured 97.1% of uncomplicated urogenital gonococcal infections. The advantage of cefixime is it can be administered PO. It is more expensive than ciprofloxacin.

Ceftizoxime: Ceftizoxime is safe and highly effective against uncomplicated urogenital and anorectal gonococcal infections. However, it offers no advantage in comparison with ceftriaxone.

Ciprofloxacin: Ciprofloxacin is effective against most strains of N. gonorrheae in the U.S., excluding Hawaii. At a dose of 500 mg, ciprofloxacin provides sustained bactericidal levels in blood. In published trials, it ahs cured 99.8% of uncomplicated urogenital and anorectal infections. It is safe, relatively inexpensive, and can be administered as a single oral dose in directly observed therapy.

Gatifloxacin: Gatifloxacin appears to be safe and effective for the treatment of uncomplicated gonorrhea, but data regarding its use are limited and it does not offer any advantage over ciprofloxacin, ofloxacin, or levofloxacin.

Lomefloxacin: Lomefloxacin appears to be safe and effective for the treatment of uncomplicated gonorrhea, but data regarding its use are limited and it does not offer any advantage over ciprofloxacin, ofloxacin, or levofloxacin.

Metronidazole: In RCTs, the recommended regimens cured 90%-95% of infections. Ensuring Rx of sexual partners may increase this rate of efficacy. Pts with cultured-confirmed infection who do not respond to this agent and in whom reinfection has been excluded should be managed in consultation with an expert.

Norfloxacin: Norfloxacin appears to be safe and effectie for the treatment of uncomplicated gonorrhea, but data regarding its use are limited and it does not offer any advantage over ciprofloxacin, ofloxacin, or levofloxacin.

Spectinomycin: Spectinomycin is expensive and must be injected; however, it has been effective in published clinical trials, curing 98.2% of uncomplicated urogenital and anorectal GC infections. It is useful for Rx of patients who cannot tolerate cephalosporins AND quinolones.

Tinidazole: The adverse effects of tinidazole are similar to those seen with metronidazole, but a single dose of tinidazole is better tolerated than a single dose of metronidazole. It may be effective in patients with metronidazole-resistant trichomoniasis. Do not use in patients in metronidazole allergic patients.

Important Points

- Recommendations based on CDC 2002 STD Rx Guidelines (MMWR 2002; 51 (RR-6). Tinidazole approved in July 2004 by FDA for Rx of trichomoniasis.
- GC urethritis requires concurrent Rx for chlamydia (CT) due to high rates of coinfection unless CT is ruled out by the time Rx is given.
- Chlamydia probably most common etiology in most locations (30-50% of NGU); GC has high frequency in some US urban areas and is increasing in certain high risk groups including young MSM
- T. vaginalis accounts for up to 17% of NGU depending on overall prevalence in community; U. urealyticum and M. genitalium together may cause up to 20% of NGU.
- COMPLICATIONS OF URETHRITIS: epididymitis; sexually acquired reactive arthritis/Reiter's syndrome(esp after chlamydia NGU); urethritis has been shown to facilitate the transmission of HIV infection.

Selected Readings

Deguchi T et al. Association of Ureaplasma urealyticum (Biovar 2) with nongonococcal urethritis. Sex Transm Dis 2004 31:192-195

Kaydos-Daniels SC et al. The use of specimens from various genitourinary sites in men, to detect Trichomonas vaginalis infection. J Infect Dis 2004 v189 p1926 to 1931.

Kane BG et al. Compliance with the Centers for Disease Control and Prevention recommendations for the diagnosis and treatment of sexually transmitted diseases. Acad Emerg Med 2004 11:371-377.

Crowell AL et al. In vitro metronidazole and tinidazole activities against metronidazole-resistant strains of Trichomonas vaginalis. Antimicrob Agents Chemother 2003 47:1407-1409.

Centers for Disease Control and Prevention. Sexually Transmitted Diseases Treatment Guidelines 2002. MMWR 2002(No. RR-6)

Gift TL et al. A cost-effectiveness evaluation of testing and treatment of Chlamydia trachomatis infection among asymptomatic women infected with Neisseria gonorhoeae. Sex Transm Infect 2002; 29(9):542-551

Lau C-Y and Qureshi AK. Azithromycin versus doxycycline for genital chlamydial infections: a meta-analysis of randomized clinical trials. Sex Transm Dis 2002; 29(9): 497-502

Centers for Disease Control and Prevention. Alternatives to spectinomycin for the treatment of Neisseria gonorrhoeae. MMWR 2001; 50(22):470.

Horner P et al. Role of Mycoplasma genitalium and Ureaplasma urealyticum in acute and chronic nongonococcal urethritis. Clin Infect Dis 2001;32:995-1003.

Taylor-Robinson D and Horner PJ. The role of Mycoplasma genitalium in non-gonococcal urethritis. Sex Transm Inf 2001;77:229-31

URINARY TRACT INFECTION, RECURRENT [WOMEN]

Noreen A. Hynes, M.D., M.P.H.

DIAGNOSTIC CRITERIA

- Recurrent infection: >2 symptomatic UTIs within a 12-month period following clinical resolution of each previous UTI after treatment with antimicrobial agents.
- Reinfection: a type of recurrent UTI caused by a different pathogen strain at any time or the original infecting strain >13d after Rx of the original UTI
- Relapse: a type of recurrent UTI caused by the same species as that causing the original UTI within 2 weeks after Rx.
- Recurrent cyctitis: Investigation for urinary tract abnormalities unlikely to be beneficial; subgroups who would clearly benefit from investigation NOT adequately defined.
- Recurrent pyelonephritis/relapsed infection: Investigate for structural abnormalities; refer to a specialist for proper diagnostic and Rx approach.

COMMON PATHOGENS: Escherichia coli ; Staphylococcus saprophyticus

TREATMENT REGIMENS

Continuous prophylaxis

- TMP-SMX 1/2 SS tab (40mg/200mg) PO qhs or TMP 100mg PO qhs, if E. coli resistance locally to these agents <20% x 6-12 mo
- Nitrofurantoin 100mg PO qhs x 6-12 mo
- Ciprofloxacin 125mg PO qd x 6-12 mo
- Norfloxacin 200mg PO qhs x 6-12 mo
- Cefaclor 250mg PO qhs x 6-12 mo
- See "Urinary Tract Infections in Pregnancy"
- Long-term antibiotic prophylaxis (>12 months): Has not been adequately evaluated in randomized controlled clinical trials and may be of benefit although is likely to have a significant side effect profile.
- Cranberry juice and cranberry-containing products for prophylaxis: There is some evidence from 2 RCTs that cranberry juice may decrease the number of UTIs over a 12-mo period in child-bearing aged women. Data for children or elderly men and women not clear. The optimal dose is also uncertain.

Postcoital regimens

- TMP-SMX 1/2 single strength tab (40mg/200mg) PO postcoitally x 1 (if TMP-SMX-resistant E. coli prevalence locally <20%)
- Ofloxacin 100mg PO or norfloxacin 200mg PO or ciprofloxacin 125mg PO --- postcoitally x 1
- Nitrofurantoin 50-100mg PO postcoitally x1.

• See "Urinary Tract Infections in Pregnancy"

Self-treatment

• TMP-SMX 1/2 SS tab (40mg/200mg) PO x1 at the onset of sx (if TMP-SMX-resistant E. coli prevalence locally <20%)
• See "Urinary Tract Infections in Pregnancy"

Drug-Specific Comments

Cefaclor: Shown to be an effective agent against recurrent bacterial cystitis when given as a once per day dose. No clinical trials reported to determine its effectiveness as a post-coital prophylaxis option.

Ciprofloxacin: Consistent evidence from randomized-controlled clinical trials shows that antibiotic prophylaxis (either continuous or postcoital) using nitrofurantoin, a quinolone, TMP or TMP-SMX reduces infection rates in women with high rates of recurrent UTI.

Nitrofurantoin: Consistent evidence from randomized-controlled clinical trials shows that abx prophylaxis (either continuous or postcoital) using nitrofurantoin, a quinolone, TMP or TMP-SMX reduces infection rates in women with high rates of recurrent UTI. Nitrofurantoin provides the lowest cost option.

Norfloxacin: Consistent evidence from randomized-controlled clinical trials shows that antibiotic prophylaxis (either continuous or postcoital) using nitrofurantoin, a quinolone, TMP or TMP-SMX reduces infection rates in women with high rates of recurrent UTI.

Important Points

• No published national guidelines; recommendations based on Clinical Evidence 2000;3:961-8, literature review, and author's opinion.
• 80-90% of recurrent UTIs are reinfections; 1/3 with original strain; recurrent acute uncomplicated cystitis occurs in 12-27% with previous UTI; ratio of recurrent cystitis to recurrent pyelo = 18:1.
• Women >54 years old are more likely to have a recurrence after an initial UTI than younger women.
• <5% of women with recurrent UTI have an underlying anatomical or functional abnormality as the cause; in absence of abnormalities associations include maternal hx of UTI, blood-group secretor status.
• Other possible associations: 1) sexual intercourse, esp w/ new partner, 2) use of spermicidal creams, 3) use of a diaphragm, 4) post-menopausal status

Selected Readings

Finh SD. Acute uncomplicated urinary tract infection in women, N Engl J Med 2003 349:259-266.

Johnson JR et al. Clonal relationships and extended virulence genotypes among Escherichia coli isolates from women with first or recurrent episode of cystitis. J Infect Dis 2001;183:1508-17

Jepson RG et al. Cranberries: preventing urinary tract infections. Cochrane Database Syst Rev 2000; 66(2):CD001322.

Melekos MD, et al. Post-intercourse versus daily ciprofloxacin prophylaxis for recurrent urinary tract infections in premenopausal women. J Urol 1997; 157:935-9.

Brumfitt W and Hamilton-Miller JMT. A comparative trial of low-dose cefaclor and macrocrystalline nitrofurantoin in the prevention of recurrent urinary tract infection. Infection 1995; 23:98-102.

Brumfitt W et al. Cefaclor as a prophylactic agent for recurrent urinary infections: a comparative trial with macrocrystalline nitrofurantoin. Drugs Exp Clin Res 1992; 18:239-44.

Nikel JC et al. Value of urologic investigation in a targeted group of women with recurrent urinary tract infections. Can J Surg 1991; 34:591-4.

Stamm WE, et al. Natural history of recurrent urinary tract infections in women. Rev Infect Dis 1991; 13:77-84.

DIAGNOSIS

Raz R and Boger S. Long-term prophylaxis with norfloxacin versus nitrofurantoin in women with recurrent urinary tract infection. Antimicrob Agents Chemother 1991; 35:1241-2.

Nicolle LE, et al . Prospective, randomized, placebo-controlled trial of norfloxacin for the prophylaxis of recurrent urinary tract infection in women. Antimicrob Agents Chemother 1989; 33:1032-5.

URINARY TRACT INFECTIONS IN PREGNANCY

Noreen A. Hynes, M.D., M.P.H.

DIAGNOSTIC CRITERIA

- Asymptomatic bacteriuria: >100,000 cfu/mL of urine with same organism identified in a pregnant woman (some experts say 2 consecutive samples) with NO clinical signs or symptoms of a UTI
- Acute bacterial cystitis: Clinical--urgency, frequency, superpubic discomfort, no fever, no flank pain. Lab-- 100,000 cfu/mL or higher on midstream clean-catch urine culture; >9 WBCs/HPF on spun urine
- Acute bacterial pyelonephritis: Clinical--fever, flank pain, with or without signs/sx of lower tract UTI; nausea/vomiting may be present; pathognomonic=tenderness to palpation/percussion over CVA

COMMON PATHOGENS: Enterobacteriaceae ; Escherichia coli

TREATMENT REGIMENS

Asymptomatic bacteriuria and cystitis

- Cephalexin 200-500mg PO qid x 3-7d
- Nitrofurantoin 100mg PO qid x 3-7d
- Ampicillin 250mg PO qid x 3-7d (NOT for empiric Rx; use only for known sensitive organisms)

Acute pyelonephritis

- Single dose IV in emergency department then home with oral an option for clinically stable patient
- Ampicillin 2g IV q6h + gentamicin 3-5mg/kg/d IV in 3 divided doses until afebrile x 48h, then change to PO to complete 14d (use for known sensitive organisms only, NOT for empiric Rx)
- Cefazolin 1g IV q8h until afebrile x 48h, then change to PO to complete 14d
- Ceftriaxone 1g IV or IM q24h until afebrile x 48h, then change to PO to complete 14d
- Mezlocillin 1-3g IV q6h until afebrile x 48h, then change to PO to complete 14d
- Piperacillin 4g IV q8h until afebrile 48h, then change to PO to complete 14d

DRUG-SPECIFIC COMMENTS

Ceftriaxone: An excellent choice for the initial parenteral treatment of pyelonephritis in the pregnant woman. A RCT comparing ampicillin + gentamicin, IV cefazolin, and IM ceftriaxone among 179 pregnant women with acute pyelonephritis demonstrated no differences in clincal response to antimicrobial therapy or birth outcomes.

Cephalexin: Cephalexin and nitrofurantoin have been shown to be equally efficacious in eradicating bacteriuria in pregnancy. Single dose therapy should be avoided for asymptomatic bacteriuria pending further study as studies have demonstrated that 50% of cases are renal in origin suggesting longer therapy may be better.

Gentamicin: At least one study has demonstrated that the pregnant women treated for pyelonephritis with standard doses of gentamicin (2mg/kg loading dose, followed by 1.5mg/ kg q8h) do not achieve therapeutic levels. This drug should be avoided in all but very severe infections. There have been no studies examining the use of once daily dosing in pregnant women with pyelonephritis.

Mezlocillin: 96% of women treated with this agent become afebrile within 96h of commencement of Rx. However, this was slower than for that observed with ceftrixone use.

Nitrofurantoin: Demonstrated equal efficacy with cephalexin in treating asymptomatic bacteriuria and acute cystitis in pregnancy. Note that this agent can cause hemolysis in patients or a fetus with glucos-6-phosphate dehydrogenase deficiency. Consider continuing prophylaxis/suppression with 50mg PO q hs in pregnant women following a full course of therapy for pyelonephritis (with a sensitive organism).

Piperacillin: 96% of women treated with this agent become afebrile within 96h of commencement of Rx. However, this was slower than for that observed with ceftriaxone.

Sulfisoxazole: A study published in late 2000 demonstrated that trimethoprim and other agents, including sulfonamides, which inhibit folic acid metabolism increase the risk for congenital malformations. Additionally, sulfonamides should be avoided in the 3rd trimester as they are transplacentally transmitted and compete with bilirubin-binding sites on plasma albumin, increasing the risk of kernicterus.

Trimethoprim: Trimethoprim is a potent folic acid antagonist and must be avoided in the first 3 months of pregnancy during the formation of vital organs. This agent should only be used in pregnancy if the potential benefits outweigh the risk. If used, it should be administered with a supplemental multivitamin containing folic acid.

IMPORTANT POINTS

- Low socioeconomic status increases risk of bacteriuria in pregnancy 5-fold. Women with sickle cell trait have a 2-fold increase in risk.
- Acute pyelo is one of most common serious medical complications of preg; seen in 1-2% of pregnant women; majority in 2nd, 3rd trimester; increase in premature labor; hospitalize initially for Rx.
- There are no published consensus guidelines for the treatment of UTIs in pregnant women. This module is based upon expert opinion cited in the peer-reviewed literature.
- Contraindicated abx in treating UTI during pregnancy: tetracyclines, trimethoprim, sulfa-containing agents. Can cause congenital cardiac and cleft defects.
- Asymptomatic bacteriuria in pregnancy has been associated with pyelonephritis, preterm labor, hypertension in pregnancy, and early pregnancy loss. Therefore, treatment is a must!
- Prevalence of bacteriuria in pregnancy ranges from 4%-7%; may be as high as 11% in indigent women; pyelonephritis occurs in 25-40% of pregnant women with untreated asymptomatic bacteriuria; usual onset of asymptomatic bacteriuria is between wk 9 and 17 of pregnancy; all women should be screening for bacteriuria at 1st prenatal visit and at the 28th week of pregnancy.
- Avoid urinary catheterization during pregnancy; may increase risk of subsequent infection.
- Hydroureters of pregnancy is a physiological change of pregnancy. Extends to level of pelvic brim. Dilatation begins by the 7th week of pregnancy and progresses until term. Both mechanical and hormonal changes contribute. Right ureter is more affected than the left. Post-partum ureters return to normal in most patients by 2 months.
- In 3rd trimester bladder changes to become an abdominal rather than pelvic organ and has decreased tone secondary to hormonal changes.
- After pyelonephritis, some experts recommend daily suppressive therapy with nitrofurantoin until delivery.

DIAGNOSIS

- Test of cure is required one week after completion of Rx.

SELECTED READINGS

Nicolle LE. Asymptomatic bacteriuria: when to screen and when to treat. Infect Dis Clin North Am 2003; 17:367-394

Hillebrand L, et al. Urinary tract infections in pregnant women with bacterial vaginosis. Am J Obstet Gynecol 2002; 186(5):916-7

Ovalle A and Levancini M. Urinary tract infections in pregnancy. Curr Opin Urol 2001; 11:55-9

Czeizel AE et al. A population-based case-control teratologic study of furazidine, a nitrofuran-derivative treatment during pregnancy. Clin Nephrol 2000; 53:257-63.

Delzell JE and LeFevre ML. Urinary tract infections during pregnancy. Am Fam Phy 2000; 61:713

Hernandez-Diaz, et al. Folic acid antagonists during pregnancy and the risk of birth defects. N Engl J Med 2000; 343:1608-14.

MacLean AB. Pregnancy. In Stanton SL and Dwyer PL (eds). 2000. Urinary Tract Infection in the Female, Martin Dunitz, Ltd, London, pp 145-160.

Sobel JD and Kaye D. Urinary Tract Infections (Ch 62). In Mandell GL et al (eds). 2000. Principles and Practice of Infectious Diseases, 5th Ed, Vol 1, Churchill Livingstone, Philadelphia, PA, pp790-1.

Gilstrap III JC and Faro S. Urinary-tract infection in pregnancy. in Infections in Pregnancy, 2nd ed, 1997. John Wiley & Sons, New York, NY, pp 21-38.

Miller LK, Cox SM. Urinary tract infections complicating pregnancy. Inf Dis Clin N Amer 1997; 11:13-26.

VAGINAL DISCHARGE   Noreen A. Hynes, M.D., M.P.H.

DIAGNOSTIC CRITERIA

- 1) Characterize discharge, 2) pH of vaginal fluid, 3) Microscopy (saline and KOH mounts) for epithelial and clue cells, white cells, motile trichomonads, or fungal elements, 4) Whiff test
- Bacterial vaginosis (BV): 3 of 4--> 1) malodorous, homogeneous, white, non-inflammatory d/c coating vag walls, 2) vag pH >4.5, 3) clue cells, 4) + whiff test. (See "Bacterial Vaginosis")
- Candida: 1) scant-mod white, clumped discharge; adherent vag plaques; 2) pH <4.6; 3) yeast/ pseuodhyphae on wet prep/gram stain ; 4) neg whiff test; 5) vag/vulvar erythema/ pruritis common
- Trichomoniasis: 1) profuse, yellow, homogeneous discharge; colpitis macularis is pathognomonic but infrequent; 2) pH usually >4.9; 3) motile trich on saline wet mount; 4) + whiff test common
- Cervicitis due to gonorrhea, chlamydia, HSV can lead to yellow vaginal discharge.

COMMON PATHOGENS: Trichomonas vaginalis ; Chlamydia trachomatis ; Neisseria gonorrhoeae ; Candida species ; Disruption of vaginal flora ecology

TREATMENT REGIMENS

Pathogen-specific in nonpregnant women

- BV (Non-pregnant preferred therapies) metronidazole 500 mg PO bid x 7d OR metronidazole gel 0.75%, 1 applicatorful (5g) intravag qd x 5d OR clindamycin cream 2%, 1 applicatorful (5g) intravag hs x 7d
- BV in non-preg: (Alternative Therapies) metronidazole 2g PO x 1 OR clindamycin 300mg PO bid x 7d OR clindamycin ovules 100mg intravag hs x 3d
- Trichomonas vaginalis: metronidazole or tinidazole 2 g PO x 1 (preferred); metronidazole 500mg PO bid x 7d (alternative)

- Uncomplicated vulvovaginal candidiasis (14 different intravaginal agents many OTC given 1, 3 or 7 days depending upon dose or fluconazole 150mg PO x 1)
- Recurrent vulvovaginal candidiasis [VVC] (>3 episodes/yr). Give same intravaginal agents as for uncomplicated VVC but longer or fluconazole 150mg PO x 1 and repeat again in 3d
- Severe vulvovaginal candidiasis [VVC] (extensive vulvar erythema, edema, excoriation, fissures). Give same intravag agents as uncomplicated VVC but longer or Fluconazole 150mg PO x1, repeat in 72h
- Chlamydia (non-pregnant): Azithromycin 1g PO x 1 OR Doxycycline 100mg PO bid x 7d
- Gonorrhea: cefixime 400mg PO x 1 OR ceftriaxone 125mg IM x 1 (see "Cervicitis") PLUS therapy for chlamydia (the STANDARD OF CARE is to treat for both) if chlamydia not ruled out.

Pathogen-specific in pregnancy

- Bacterial Vaginosis: metronidazole 250mg PO tid x 7d (preferred); clindamycin 300mg PO bid x 7 d (alternative)
- Candida vulvovaginal: Only topical azoles recommended; give 7 d of Rx (terconazole, clotrimazole and miconazole are 3 d depending upon dose).
- Trichomonas vaginalis: metronidazole 2 g PO x 1
- Chlamydia: erythromycin base 500mg PO qid x 7d (preferred)
- Gonorrha: cefixime 400mg PO x 1 or ceftriaxone 125 mg IM (preferred) PLUS an antichlamydial agent if chlamydia infection not ruled out. Do not use fluoroquinolones or tetracyclines.

DRUG-SPECIFIC COMMENTS

Cefixime: Does not attain adequate penetration of the Waldeyer's ring and should not be used to treat gonorrhea in anyone with orogenital exposure. Probenicid increases concentration.

Metronidazole: Must abstain from alcohol during Rx and for 24-48 hours thereafter to avoid disulfiram-like effect. Side effects much lower with gel form of drug. A recent meta-analysis does NOT suport teratogenicity in humans, hence CDC recommends can be used the treat pregnant women with certain indications.

Spectinomycin: Expensive, must be injected. Effective in curing 98.2% of uncomplicated urogenital and anorectal gonococcal infections. Test of cure required if used to treat patient with orogenital exposure. Use in patients with gonorrhea who cannot tolerate quinolones or cephalosporins.

Tinidazole: The adverse effects of tinidazole are similar to those seen with metronidazole, but a single dose of tinidazole is better tolerated than a single dose of metronidazole. It may be effective in patients with metronidazole-resistant trichomoniasis. This drug is not approved for use in bacterial vaginosis. Do not use during the 1st trimester of pregnancy or in metronidazole allergic patients.

IMPORTANT POINTS

- Recommendations based on CDC's 2002 STD Treatment Guidelines. (MMWR 2002; 51 (RR-6); CDC 2004 revised recommendations for gonorrhea treatment (MMWR 2004; 53:335-338)
- Presenting signs and symptoms are NOT sufficiently sensitive or specific to guide therapy. Some laboratory aids to diagnosis are needed.
- Directly-observed, single dose therapy is preferred whenever possible to ensure treatment and to decrease ongoing transmission

- BV and candidiasis are considered sexually-associated rather than sexually transmitted diseases. However, in women who have sex with women BV has been shown to be sexually transmitted.
- Initial Rx: use best available evidence provided by point-of-care tests AND a risk assessment of the cause for discharge in each pt. NO one agent is available to treat all of the likely causes.
- Gonococcal, chlamydial and herpes virus infections of the cervix may present as vaginal discharge and must be considered if these organisms are circulating in a community. The absence of mucopus does not rule out these infections
- Other non-infectious causes of vaginal discharge must also be considered
- The 3 most common causes of vaginal discharge in women are BV, trichomoniasis, and vulvovaginal candidiasis.
- Differential includes: desquamative inflammatory vaginitis, retained foreign body (e.g., tampon), allergic vaginitis, invasive CA of cervix

Selected Readings

Hager WD. Treatment of metronidazole-resistant Trichomonas vaginalis with tinidazole. Sex Transm Dis 2004; 31:343-345

Holley RL et al. A randomized, double-blind clinical trial of vaginal acidification versus placebo for the treatment of symptomatic bacterial vaginosis. Sex Transm Dis 2004 31:236-238.

Kane BG et al. Compliance with the Centers for Disease Control and Prevention recommendations for the diagnosis and treatment of sexually transmitted diseases. Acad Emerg Med 2004; 11:371-377

Rylander E et al. Vulvovaginal candida in a young sexually active population: prevalence and association with oro-genital sex and frequent pain at intercourse. Sex Transm Infect 2004; 80:54-57.

Centers for Disease Control and Prevention. Sexually transmitted diseases treatment guidelines 2002. MMWR. 2002; 51 (RR-6)

Barousse MM et al. Growth inhibition of Candida albicans by human vaginal epithelial cells. J Infect Dis 2001;184:1489-93

El-Din SS et al. An investigation into the pathogenesis of vulvo-vaginal candidiasis. Sex Transm Inf 2001;77:179-183

Guise JM et al. Screening for bacterial vaginosis in pregnancy. Am J Prev Med 2001;20(3 Suppl):62-72

Schwebke JR and Lawing LF. Prevalence of Mobiluncus spp among women with and without bacterial vaginosis as detected by polymerase chain reaction. Sex Transm Dis 2001;28:195-9

Antonelli NM, et al. A randomized trial of intravaginal nonoxynol 9 versus oral metronidazole in the treatment of vaginal trichomoniasis. Am J Obstet Gynecol 2000; 182:1008-10.

WARTS (NON-GENITAL)

Ciro R. Martins, M.D. and David Kouba, M.D.

Diagnostic Criteria

- Diagnosis: Clinical examination in most instances; histopathology (biopsy) in atypical cases
- Etiology: Human papillomaviruses (HPV), a diverse group of non-enveloped, ds DNA tumor viruses. At least 130 genotypes have been identified. HPV typing not recommended
- Common warts: exophytic, hard, rough papules; may coalesce to form larger plaques. Black dots (thrombosed capillaries) may be seen
- Plantar warts: thick, usually flat, endophytic, yellowish colored rough plaques. Black dots may also be seen. Pain may be present. Resemble calluses.

- Other variants: Flat warts (minimally elevated, usually light-colored, small papules), filiform warts (pedunculated, firm papules, often with finger-like projections; may resemble a small "horn")

COMMON PATHOGENS: HPV 3,10 - Flat warts ; HPV 1 - Palmar and plantar warts ; HPV 2,4 - Common warts ; HPV 16 - Digital squamous cell carcinoma ; HPV 5 - squamous cell carcinoma in EV ; HPV 3,5,8 - Epidermodysplasia verruciformis (EV)

TREATMENT REGIMENS

Verruca Vulgaris (common warts)
- Cryotherapy q3-4 weeks followed by OTC salicylic acid plasters and/or paring of lesions
- 70-90% trichloroacetic acid (TCA) applied by the physician preceded by paring of lesions q week or q 2 weeks.
- 5-Fluorouracil cream (5%) applied under occlusion qHS - local irritation common
- Sensitization in the office with 2% squaric acid (SADBE) followed by application of 0.2% to warts, 2 weeks later
- Cantharadin (blister beetle extract) applied by physician q3-4 wks
- Imiquimod cream qHS x4-6 weeks
- Intralesional injection of 1% cidofovir or bleomycin in extensive, recalcitrant cases

Verruca palmares et plantares (plantar warts)
- Regular paring and use of keratolytic plasters between visits is critical to ensure treatment success
- Combination modalities help to increase therapeutic success rates
- Combination 1: Cryotherapy followed by patient applied imiquimod under occlusion (duct tape) qHS
- Combination 2: Cryotherapy followed by patient applied podophyllotoxin cream or gel under occlusion (duct tape) qHS
- Combination 3: 5 fluoro-uracil cream qoHS alternating with imiquimod cream qoHS under occlusion (duct tape)

Peri-ungual verruca
- Verrucae around the nail are often recalcitrant to treatment and often cause nail dystrophy
- Topical therapies often do not get under the nail fold
- Laser therapy with Flashlamp pulsed dye (585 nm) may be effective
- Squaric acid (SADBE) sensitization, cidofovir or bleomycin injections are alternatives

IMPORTANT POINTS
- Infection occurs through personal contact or fomites
- Intact cell-mediated immunity appears critical to eradication of HPV by host
- Defects in cell-mediated immunity make treatment more difficult and strict patient compliance is required for HPV containment
- Podophyllin and podophyllotoxin are TERATOGENIC
- High concentrations of trichloroacetic acid may cause permanent scarring

SELECTED READINGS

Koutsky LA, Ault KA, Wheeler CM, et al. A controlled trial of a human papillomavirus type 16 vaccine. N Engl J Med. 2002 Nov 21;347(21):1645-51

Majewski S, Jablonska S. Do epidermodysplasia verruciformis human papillomaviruses contribute to malignant and benign epidermal proliferations?. Arch Dermatol. 2002 May;138(5):649-54

Del Mistro A, Chieco Bianchi L. HPV-related neoplasias in HIV-infected individuals. Eur J Cancer. 2001 Jul;37(10):1227-35

DIAGNOSIS

Carr J, Gyorfi T. Human papillomavirus. Epidemiology, transmission, and pathogenesis. Clin Lab Med. 2000 Jun;20(2):235-55

Zabawski EJ Jr. A review of topical and intralesional cidofovir. Dermatol Online J. 2000 Sep;6(1):3

PATHOGENS

BACTERIA

ACINETOBACTER BAUMANNII John G. Bartlett, M.D.

CLINICAL RELEVANCE & DIAGNOSIS
- Common in environment (water, soil) and hospital (catheters, lotions, ventilation equipment)
- Emerging as important global-pan resistant GNB nosocomial pathogen
- May cause nosocomial epidemics from contaminated common sources - ventilation equipment, catheters, etc
- Clearly pathogenic when recovered from blood and normally sterile body sites
- Often insignificant in wounds, sputum, etc, especially if seen polymicrobially or at low concentrations
- Aerobic gram-neg coccobacilli or rods, often mistaken for Neisseria or Moraxella on GS; grows on standard agar media
- A. baumannii is major clinical isolate of Acinetobacter; others - A. calcoaceticus, A. lwoffii, A. junii, A. johnsonii

SITES OF INFECTION
- NOSOCOMIAL INFECTIONS
- Pneumonia - especially ventilator associated
- Septicemia - may be catheter associated
- Wounds - burns, and war wounds acquired in Iraq
- Community-acquired pneumonia (one major report)
- Rare: meningitis (post neurosurgery), liver abscess, endocarditis, urinary tract infections, brain abscess

TREATMENT REGIMENS

Antibiotics
- Antibiotic selection guided by in vitro sensitive tests - most active: imipenem, pip/tazo, amp/sulbactam, ceftriaxone, cefepime, cefotaxime, amikacin, cipro/levo/moxi/gatifloxacin, TMP-SMX
- Imipenem (Primaxin): 0.5-1g IV q6h (Preferred - Med Letter 2004;2:21)
- Amp/sulbactam (Unasyn) 2-3g IV (amp) q6h
- Ceftriaxone (Rocephin): 1-2g IV qd
- Cefotaxime: 2-3g IV q6-8h
- Ciprofloxacin (Cipro): 400mg IV q12h or 750mg PO bid (or, levo, gati or moxi)
- Cefepime (Maxipime): 1-2g IV q12h
- TMP-SMX: 15-20mg (TMP)/kg/d IV divided 3 or 4 doses/d or 2 DS PO tid
- Amikacin: 7.5mg/kg q12h IV or 15mg/kg/d IV
- Pan-resistant isolate: colistin 2.5-5 mg/kg/d IV +/- imipenem or ampicillin/sulbactam

Outbreaks
- Notify infection control
- Emphasize barrier precautions and hand washing
- Identify common source - water, ventilators, catheters, endoscopes, feeding tubes, etc.

IMPORTANT POINTS
- Has become major nosocomial pathogen, especially as a multiply resistant GNB.
- Major clinical sources; blood, respiratory secretions and urine

BACTERIA

- Nosocomial pathogen - colonizes skin, dry surfaces & water, including hand lotion, ventilation equip, catheters.
- Nosocomial outbreaks, esp in ICUs usually multiple-resistant.
- Lab isolations often meaningless unless from normally sterile site, dominant pathogen, outbreak &/or good clinical correlations.

SELECTED READINGS

Markou N, Apostolakos H, Koumoudiou C, et al. Intravenous colistin in the treatment of sepsis from multi-resistant gram-negative bacilli in critically ill patients. Crit. Care 2003;R78-83

Jain R, Danziger LH. Multidrug resistant acinetobacter infections: an emerging challenge to clinicians. Ann Pharmacother 2004;38:1449-59

Rhomberg PR, Jones RN, Sader HS, et al. Antimicrobial resistance rates and clonality results from the Meropenem yearly susceptibility test information collection (MYSTIC) Programme: Report of year 5 (2003). Diag Microbial Infect. Dis. 2004;49:273-81

Higgins, PG, Wisplingogg J, Stefanik D & Siefert H. In vitro activities of the beta-lactamase inhibitors clavulanic acid, sulbactam & tazobactam alone or in combination w/ beta-lactams against epidemiologically characterized multidrug-resistant Acin.. Antimicrob Ag Chemother 2004;48:1586-92

Yoon J Urban C Terzian C, et al. In vitro double and triple synergistic activities of polymyxin B, imipenem and rifampin against multidrug resistant Acinetobacter baumannii. Antimicrob Ag Chemother 2004;48:753-7

ACTINOMYCES   John G. Bartlett, M.D.

CLINICAL RELEVANCE & DIAGNOSIS

- Thin, branching Gram pos bacilli, microaerophilic, grow best anaerobically, VERY fastidious
- Recovery important only if from uncontaminated source - tissue, needle aspirates, sulfur granules, etc
- Characteristic gram stain in tissue or sulfur granule with radiating GPR
- Nearly always mixed infection - esp w/Actinobacillus actinomycetemcomitans, Eikenella, Bacteroides, Strep
- Characteristic lesion - dense fibrosis ("woody"), draining fistulae, "sulfur granules", infection advances thru tissue planes
- Agents: A. israelii, A. gerencseriae, A. naeslundii, A. odontolyticus, A. viscosus, A. meyer & P. propionicum

SITES OF INFECTION

- Oral cervico-facial ("lumpy jaw")
- Pelvic infection (IUD-associated)
- Thoracic - pneumonia, mass lesion
- Intra-abdominal - abscess or mass lesion
- Musculoskeletal
- Disseminated (rare)
- CNS meningitis, encephalitis, brain abscess
- Endocarditis

TREATMENT REGIMENS

Antibiotics

- Guidelines from author
- Preferred: Pen G 18-24mU IV/d x 2-6wks, then amoxicillin 500-750mg PO tid/qid x 6-12mo; oral therapy may be adequate

- Alt: Doxycycline 100mg bid IV x 2-6wks, then 100mg PO bid x 6-12mo; erythromycin 500mg PO qid.
- Clindamycin 600mg IV q 8h x 2-6wks, then clind 300mg PO qid x 6-12mo
- Other agents (limited data): clari, azithro, imipenem, cefotaxime/ceftriaxone
- Not active: metronidazole, TMP/SMX, ceftazidime, aminoglycoside, oxacillin

Miscellaneous

- Surgery: Usually reserved for abscess drainage, lesion in vital area (epidural, CNS, etc), or unresponsive to abx
- Surgical procedures: Debulking, excision of fistula tracts, abscess drainage

IMPORTANT POINTS

- Guidelines from author
- Disease is "Actinomycosis" caused by one of 6 agents, most commonly A. israelii
- Suspect: Characteristic lesion (hard, chronic inflam mass (+/- sinus tracts) passing thru tissue planes) and micro (gram stain ID culture often negative)
- ABX: High dose & long duration justified by tradition & perceived need for penetration into dense fibrotic tissue to dense fibrotic lesion
- Main differential is Nocardia - looks same on gram stain but Nocardia is weakly AFB & usually disease of immunocompromised host

SELECTED READINGS

Christodoulou N, et al. Actinomycotic liver abscess. Case report and review of the literature. Chir Ital 2004;56:141-6

Sudhakar SS, Ross JJ. Short-term treatment of actinomycosis: two cases and a review. Clin Infect Dis 2004;38:444-7

Kramer J. Instant Replay: The Green Bay Diary of Jerry Kramer. The World Publishing Co 1968; pg 48-50

Holm P. Studies on etiology of human actinomycosis. Acta Pathol Microbio Scand 27:736, 1950 and 28:391, 1951

Harvey J, Cantrell J, Fisher A. Actinomycosis: its recognition and treatment. Ann Intern Med 1957;46:868

BACILLUS SPECIES

Paul Auwaerter, M.D.

CLINICAL RELEVANCE & DIAGNOSIS

- Facultative anaerobe or aerobic spore-forming usually gram-positive rods. For anthrax, please see "Anthrax" in Diagnoses section
- Ubiquitous in decayed organic matter & soil. Some species are part of normal flora.
- B. cereus capable of producing enterotoxins causing emesis & diarrhea.
- Actual infection rare, most isolates considered culture contaminates. Risk factors for actual infection: IDU, sickle cell, intravascular catheters, cancer, AIDS, immune suppression, neutropenia.
- Potential human pathogens include B. cereus, B. subtilis, B. megaterium, B. circulans, B. sphaericus.

SITES OF INFECTION

- Food poisoning: B. cereus w/ 2 forms. Emetic: 1-6h after ingestion contam. food, e.g., fried rice. Diarrheal: 10-12h after eating e.g., tainted meats w/watery diarrhea, tenesmus lasting <2-10d.
- Bacteremia: Uncommon, may complicate mixed infections including surgical wounds or infected necrotic tumors. Source of pseudobactermia: contam. blood cx, gloves, syringes etc.

- Meningitis, brain abscess: uncommon presentations, may complicate otitis, mastoiditis, neurosurg. procedures & shunts.
- Ocular: A primary pathogen of post-traumatic endophthalmitis, risk factor also IV drug use. May also cause keratitis, orbital abscess, conjunctivitis, dacryocystitis.
- Endocarditis: rare complication in IVDU population. TV endocarditis mostly indolent in nature.
- Soft tissue: rare reports of fasciitis.
- Pneumonia: Rare pathogen of compromised host. May mimic anthracis-type presentation.

TREATMENT REGIMENS

Serious Bacillus infections

- First consider if isolate a contaminate or part of significant infection.
- Most species sensitive to penicillins, cephalosporins, FQ and AG. Except B. cereus often resistant to beta-lactams. Antibiotic sensitivities extremely variable for Bacillus spp.
- B. cereus most common isolate in significant infections. Vancomycin 1g IV q 12h drug of choice based on in vitro case reports. Clindamycin (600mg IV q8h) an alternative reported w/successful outcomes

B. cereus food poisoning

- Self-limited, no antibiotics necessary.
- Supportive therapy, hydration & anti-emetics.
- Prevention: fried/boiled rice should be maintained >60C or rapidly cooled <8C. to avoid room temperature germination of spores and toxin.

Bacillus endophthalmitis

- Rapid, massive destruction of vitreous/retina in IDAs or posttraumatic w/ ring abscess within 48h ~pathognomic B. cereus panophthalmitis.
- Early ophthamological consultation, culture ocular fluids. Early vitrectomy and intravitreal abx advocated.
- Intravitreal clindamycin 450mcg & gentamicin 400mcg. Some advocate intravitreal dexamethasone. Prognosis for sight retention poor.
- Intravitreal abx combined with systemic antibiotics (see choices under Serious Bacillus Infections).

Bacillus endocarditis

- Well-described but rare complication of IDU. Most blood cx's in IDU positive for bacillus are contaminates or represent transient bacteremia.
- Evidence of valvular involvement should be sought by echocardiography to prove endocarditis. Tricuspid valve most common. Course indolent.
- Successful treatment reported with either vancomycin (1g IV q12h) or clindamycin (600mg IV q 8h).

IMPORTANT POINTS

- Recommendations based upon author's opinion and C. Tuazon (Princ. Prac. Infect Dis 2000, 5th ed, Chap 197:2222)
- Blood culture isolates are mostly contaminates until proven otherwise especially in IDU population.
- Ocular infections devastating and require quick intervention.
- Gram stain similarity may stoke concern in pneumonia, meningitis and soft-tissue presentations until culture results rule-out B. anthracis.

SELECTED READINGS

Tuazon CU, Hill R, Sheagren JN. Microbiologic study of street heroin and injection paraphernalia. J Infect Dis. 1974 Mar;129(3):327-9

Sliman R, Rehm S, Shlaes DM. Serious infections caused by Bacillus species. Medicine (Baltimore). 1987 May;66(3):218-23

Mahler H, Pasi A, Kramer JM et al. Fulminant liver failure in association with the emetic toxin of Bacillus cereus. N Engl J Med. 1997 Apr 17;336(16):1142-8

Reynolds DS, Flynn HW Jr. Endophthalmitis after penetrating ocular trauma. Curr Opin Ophthalmol. 1997 Jun;8(3):32-8

Gigantelli JW, Torres Gomez J, Osato MS. In vitro susceptibilities of ocular Bacillus cereus isolates to clindamycin, gentamicin, and vancomycin alone or in combination. Antimicrob Agents Chemother. 1991 Jan;35(1):201-2

BACTEROIDES FRAGILIS   John G. Bartlett, M.D.

CLINICAL RELEVANCE & DIAGNOSIS

- Small, pleomorphic gram-neg anaerobic bacillus; easily grown relative to other anaerobes
- Colonizes virtually all human colons
- Most common agent of anaerobic bacteremia
- Usually part of polymicrobial infection
- Most common pathogen in intra-abdominal sepsis except biliary infections and spontaneous bacterial peritonitis
- Infrequent above diaphragm except otogenic brain abscess
- Abscessogenic - causes abscesses
- Detection: rarely cultured - suspect with mixed flora on gram stain, intra abdominal/pelvic infection, putrid pus
- Culture only uncontaminated specimens: blood, peritoneal specimens etc

SITES OF INFECTION

- Intra-abdominal: Peritonitis, abscess, appendicitis, diverticulitis, post-op wound infection, liver abscess, cholangitis
- Gynecologic infections: PID, tubo-ovarian abscess, post gynecologic surgery wound infection, endometritis, pelvic cellulitis, pelvic abscess
- Toxigenic diarrhea (peds only)
- Bacteremia
- Abscesses: Otogenic brain abscess, intra-abdominal abscess, pelvic abscess, soft tissue abscess below waist, perirectal abscess

TREATMENT REGIMENS

Empiric abx, mixed infection

- Recommendations assume polymicrobial infection and empiric Rx of B. fragilis
- Monotherapy: Imipenem (Primaxin) 0.5g q6h, pip-tazo (Zosyn) 3.375g q6h; amp-sulbactam (Unasyn) 1-2g q6h
- Combo Rx: Metronidazole 0.75-1.0g IV q12h + cefotaxime 1.5-2g q6h, aztreonam 1-2g q 8h or ceftriaxone 1g q12h

Surgery

- Drain abscesses. Exceptions - most tubo-ovarian abscess; some brain and liver abscesses respond to abx alone
- Repair - anastamotic leaks, perforations, appendicitis

IMPORTANT POINTS

- Guidelines from IDSA for intra-abd sepsis (CID 2003;37:997).
- Abx for intra-abdominal sepsis-Rx B. fragilis and E. coli; this covers everything common and important
- B. fragilis is most common cause of anaerobic bacteremia - "sepsis for surgeons"
- B. fragilis is often suspected (intra-abd or pelvic sepsis), sometimes seen (gram stain w/mixed flora), occasionally smelled (putrid) and rarely cultured
- Abx always active against B. fragilis: metronidazole, imipenem (Primaxin), pip-tazo (Zosyn); Increasing resistance: clindamycin, cefoxitin and cefotetan

SELECTED READINGS

Wilson WR, Martin WM, Wilkowski CJ, et al. Anaerobic bacteremia. Mayo Clin Prac 1972;47:639

Chow AW, Guze LP. Bacteroidaceae bacteremia: Clinical experience with 112 patients. Medicine 1974;53:93

Aldridge KE, et al. Bacteremia due to Bacteroides fragilis group: distribution of species, betalactamase production and antimicrobial susceptibility patterns. Antimicrob Ag Chemother 2003;47:148

Solomkin JS, Mazuski JE, Baron EJ, et al. Guidelines for selection of anti-infective agents for complicated intra-abdominal infections. Clin Infect Dis 2003;37:997-1005

Schaumann R, Blatz R, Beer J, et al. Effect of moxifloxacin versus imipenem/cilastatin treatment on the mortality of mice infected intravenously with different strains of Bacteroides fragilis and E. coli. J Antimicrob Chemother 2004;53:318-24

BARTONELLA SPECIES   John G. Bartlett, M.D.

CLINICAL RELEVANCE & DIAGNOSIS

- Curved gram-neg rod; best seen with Warthin-Starry silver stain
- Hard to grow - fresh chocolate agar & CO_2
- Most human disease: B. henselae from cats with chronic bacillemia; B. bacilliformis - Oroya fever (Peru); B. quintana (louse borne) - urban trench fever; SBE and chronic bacteremia in homeless
- Most common diseases - cat scratch fever (healthy host) and bacillary angiomatosis (AIDS)
- Dx: Warthin-Starry stain tissue & serology (IFA). Other: hard to culture (only early, low yield); PCR - experimental; skin test - useless and risky

SITES OF INFECTION

- Skin nodule +/- regional adenopathy: Cat Scratch disease (CSD)
- Conjunctivitis + preauricular node: Parinaud oculoglandular syndrome
- Liver +/- spleen: peliosis hepatitis
- CNS: encephalitis, myelitis, aseptic meningitis
- Skin nodules: bacillary angiotomatosis
- Endocarditis: culture negative
- FUO: esp in homeless & alcoholics
- Eye: neuroretinitis

TREATMENT REGIMENS

Treatment

- Based on Raoult D, et al AAC 2004;48:1921
- Cat scratch disease: no abx; extensive adenopathy-azithromycin 500mg x 1
- Bacillary angiomatosis: erythromycin 500mg PO qid or doxy 100 bid x >3 mos
- Retinitis: doxycycline 100mg bid & rifampin 300 mg bid all PO x 4-6 wks

- Peliosis hepatitis: erythro 500mg qid or doxy 100mg po x 4 mos
- Oroya fever: cipro 500mg bid x 10d
- Endocarditis: gentamicin 3mg/kg/d divided q 8h x 14d & ceftriaxone 2g/d IV x 6 weeks +/- doxy 100mg bid x 6 weeks

IMPORTANT POINTS

- Recommendations are author's opinion.
- Most common: 1) cat scratch disease = cat injury - nodule + node & 2) bacillary angiomatosis seen w/AIDS - skin nodule like KS.
- Most serious: endocarditis (mortality 25%), CNS, neuroretinitis
- Epidemiology: cats (cat owners w/CSD), lice (homeless w/fever) & AIDS pts with BA
- Dx: silver stain tissue or serology (>1:256 w/ acute infection, >1:800 correlates with chronic infection)

SELECTED READINGS

Chia JK, Nakata MM, Lami JL, et al. Azithromycin for the treatment of cat-scratch disease. CID 1998;26:193

Kordick DL, Papich MG, Breitschwerdt EB. Efficacy of enrofloxacin or doxycycline for treatment of Bartonella henselae or Bartonella clarridgeiae infection in cats. AAC 1997;41:2448

Holley HP. Successful treatment of cat-scratch disease with ciprofloxacin. JAMA 1991;265:1563

Williams A, Sheldon CD, Riordan T. Cat scratch disease. Brit Med J 2002;324:1199

Margileth AM. Cat scratch disease. Adv Paedr Infect Dis 1993;8:1

BORDETELLA SPECIES

David Zaas, M.D. and Paul Auwaerter, M.D.

CLINICAL RELEVANCE & DIAGNOSIS

- Typical infection lasts several weeks and consists of 3 stages.
- Catarrhal stage: rhinorrhea and mild cough
- Paroxysmal stage: increased cough with spells of repetitive cough, followed by sudden inspiratory effort (whoop) and post-tussive emesis.
- Convalescent stage: decreasing frequency and severity of coughing episodes.
- Bordetella are small aerobic gram-negative coccobacilli. B. pertussis is most comon etiology of whooping cough, B. parapertussis leads to less severe but similar sx.
- Clinical manifestations vary, highest mortality in infancy, often under-recognized in adolescents and adults, prior immunization can lead to atypical presentations.
- In adults, B. pertussis most commonly presents as a chronic dry cough that is misdiagnosed as bronchitis. Average duration of cough approximately 50 days.
- Adult incidence is estimated to be 1-2 cases/1,000 adults per year. Highest incidence reported in adult healthcare workers.
- 20% of people with acute pertussis may develop radiographic infiltrates.
- 20-30% of adolescents and adults with cough for greater than 1 week may be due to pertussis. Adults primary source of transmission to >60% of infants hospitalized with pertussis.

SITES OF INFECTION

- Respiratory Disease: laryngobronchitis, pneumonia (less common) usually B. pertussis; B. parapertussis less common cause of whooping cough.
- B. bronchiseptica (kennel cough), B. holmesii rarely been implicated to cause human respiratory disease.
- B. trematum is rarely found in wounds and ear infections.

- B. avium is a pathogen identified only in birds.
- B. hinzii, B. homesii uncommon cause of sepsis in immunocompromised hosts.

TREATMENT REGIMENS

B. pertussis and B. parapertussis

- In vitro, most strains are sensitive to both macrolides and fluoroquinolones, but resistant to beta-lactams.
- Rarely, strains of B. pertussis resistant to erythromycin have been identified.
- Macrolides are the first line of therapy. Most experience has been with erythromycin, but a placebo controlled trial found clarithromycin to be equally effective and better tolerated.
- Recommended treatment regimen: clarithromycin 500mg PO BID or erythromycin base 250mg PO QID or erythromycin ethylsuccinate 400mg PO QID
- The recommended treatment duration: 7-14 days.
- Trimethoprim-sulfamethoxazole is a second-line treatment option for patients who are intolerant of macrolides.
- Although azithromycin and fluoroquinolones have excellent in vitro sensitivity profiles, clinical experience for B. pertussis is limited.
- Antibiotic treatment is only indicated for acute infections, helpful in limiting spread.
- ABX not generally considered to shorten symptoms or decrease transmission when given to adults since chronic cough due to B. pertussis likely to have been present for wks at time of dx consideration.

IMPORTANT POINTS

- Gold standard for the dx of pertussis is culture of nasopharyngeal secretions. Nasal aspirates have greater yield than swabs. Cultures should be plated on Bordet-Gengou medium for 7 days.
- Due to the low sensitivity of culture dx often clinical. PCR based assays have been developed for respiratory secretions.
- Most sensitive test is standardized serological assays, usually for research epi. Enzyme immunoassays performed in acute and convalescent serum can detect IgG AB against pertussis antigens.
- The classic lymphocytosis associated with acute B. pertussis is more common in children than adults.
- Increasing incidence in adults may be due to waning immunity. The role of adult booster vaccinations in controversial and currently not recommended.

SELECTED READINGS

Lebel MH, Mehra S. Efficacy and safety of clarithromycin versus erythromycin for the treatment of pertussis: a randomized, single blind trial. Pediatric Infectious Disease Journal 2001; 20: 1149-1154.

Heininger U. Recent progress in clinical and basic pertussis research. European Journal of Pediatrics 2001; 160: 203-213.

Mortensen JE, Rodgers GL. In vitro activity of gemifloxacin and other antimicrobial agents against isolates of Bordetella pertussis and Bordetella parapertussis. Journal of Antimicrobial Chemotherapy 2000; 45(Suppl S1): 47-49.

Hoppe Je. Neonatal pertussis. Pediatric Infectious Disease 2000; 19: 244-247.

Hoppe JE, Halm U, Hagedorn HJ, Kraminer-Hagedorn A. Comparison of erythromycin ethylsuccinate and co-trimoxazole for the treatment of pertussis. Infection 1989; 17(4): 227-231.

BORRELIA SPECIES

Paul Auwaerter, M.D.

CLINICAL RELEVANCE & DIAGNOSIS

- Epidemic relapsing fever, person-person transmission (like typhus) by human body louse (Pediculus humanus)
- Worldwide infection (ex. S. Pacific), spirochete, helical 5-40um long with 3-10 spirals
- Sporadic endemic relapsing fever [RF] is tick-borne (Ornithodoros soft ticks), reservoirs include rodents & small animals
- B. recurrentis only causes epidemic LBRF, but >15 Borrelia spp. cause endemic TBRF.
- Dx: Wright-stained blood smear w/ spirochetemia; 4x serologic rise (reference labs only)
- Epidemic RF occurs usually in poor socioeconomic settings, war, famine. Louse-borne RF (LBRF) occurs endemically in parts Central/East Africa, Peru & Bolivia
- Tick-borne RF (most often acquired in warm climates, w/ 1,500-6,000 ft. elevation preferred by Ornithodoros soft ticks. In US, mostly in Cascades, Sierra Nevadas, Rockies and limestone caverns of Texas.
- Ddx: includes Colorado tick fever, yellow & dengue fever, African hemorrhagic fevers, lepto, LCMV, malaria, bartonella, enterovirus, rat bite fever
- Mortality greater in untreated LBRF than TBRF. Even w/ rx, LBRF has 5% mortality compared to only rare deaths due to TBRF.

SITES OF INFECTION

- General: fever - initially lasts 3-6d, may be associated w/ shock (esp louse-borne). After remittance, fever may return in 7-10d, usually less severe. Louse-borne single relapse; tick-borne multiple.
- General: fevers associated with headache, myalgia/arthralgia. Relapse episodes tend to be shorter, ~2-3d.
- Heme: DIC, thrombocytopenia
- GI: abd pain, n/v, diarrhea, jaundice (10%); hepatosplenomegaly (LBRF>>TBRF)
- Cutaneous: rash (25%), may turn petechial. Eschar at tick bite site rare
- CNS: altered mental status/photophobia (common); cranial nerve palsy, other focal neurologic deficits or frank meningitis (rare)
- Pulmonary: dry cough
- TBRF and LBRF tend to have similar clinical characteristics; however, LBRF tends to be more severe. LBRF cases typically have more liver/CNS bleeding complications and extensive petechiae.

TREATMENT REGIMENS

Tick-borne relapsing fever

- Majority of RF cases likely self-limited, without requiring abx rx.
- Preferred: doxycycline 100mg PO bid x 5-10d
- Alt: erythromycin 500mg PO qid 5-10d
- If meningitis/encephalitis present, use ceftriaxone 1-2g IV q 12h x 14d
- Untreated tick-borne infection mortality ~5%
- Jarisch-Herxheimer rxn (severe rigor, fever, low BP) may occur post-abx. More common w/ louse-borne infection.
- J-H may be life-threatening. 2hr post-initial abx observation period recommended.

Louse-borne relapsing fever

- Preferred: single dose tetracycline 500mg po
- Alt: erythromycin 500mg PO x 1

- Single dose therapy effective with few cases of relapse.
- Untreated louse-borne infection mortality ~40%
- Jarisch-Herxheimer rxn (severe rigor, fever, low BP) may occur post-abx
- J-H may be life-threatening. 2hr post-initial abx observation period recommended.

Prevention

- Avoid rodent and tick-infested dwellings and infested natural sites, such as animal burrows or caves. Many cases in US acquired by sleeping in tick-infested cabins.
- Avoid arthropod vectors; DEET sprays of uncertain help; tick inspection generally not helpful since soft ticks are nocturnal biters, leaving host by morning.
- De-lousing, good personal hygiene or insect sprays in dwellings may help control epidemic RF.

Important Points

- In US, TBRF generally only west of Mississippi. Suspect if febrile illness with rural, mountainous exposure esp. sleeping in primitive cabins, or rodent exposure.
- Epidemic RF clinically similar and confused with epidemic typhus (Rickettsia prowazekii) as both spread by body louse.
- Relapsing nature has been attributed to antigenic variation in spirochetes.
- High-level spirochetemia characteristic of RF w/ > 10,000 organisms/hpf; however, during afebrile/asx stages they're undetectable.
- Recommendations based upon Med Clin North Am. 2002 Mar;86(2):417-33 and Principles & Practice Inf Dis, 5th ed Chap 230, 2000.

Selected Readings

Brouqui P, Stein A, Dupont HT et al. Ectoparasitism and vector-borne diseases in 930 homeless people from Marseilles. Medicine (Baltimore). 2005 Jan;84(1):61-8

Centers for Disease Control and Prevention (CDC). Tickborne relapsing fever outbreak after a family gathering--New Mexico, August 2002. MMWR Morb Mortal Wkly Rep. 2003 Aug 29;52(34):809-12

Dworkin MS, Shoemaker PC, Fritz CL, et al. The epidemiology of tick-borne relapsing fever in the United States. Am J Trop Med Hyg. 2002 Jun;66(6):753-8

Dworkin MS, Schwan TG, Anderson DE Jr. Tick-borne relapsing fever in North America. Med Clin North Am. 2002 Mar;86(2):417-33, viii-ix

Dworkin MS, Anderson Jr DE, Schwan TG, et al. Tick-borne relapsing fever in the northwestern United States and southwestern Canada. Clin Infect Dis 26:122;131, 1998

BRUCELLA SPECIES
Joseph Vinetz, M.D.

Clinical Relevance & Diagnosis

- Aerobic, gram-neg coccobacilli causing brucellosis
- Zoonotic disease; most important species: B. abortus (cattle); B. melitensis (goat)
- Presentation varies: Acute febrile disease is systemic, non-focal; relapsing/"undulant form" (Malta fever) arthritis, hepatic; chronic may be cyclic or localized
- Lab cultures readily aerosolizable, potential weaponizable as bioterror agent (Category B)
- In developed countries, rare, may be in immigrants who ingest raw goat milk/cheese; abattoir workers/vets; potential from bison in Yellowstone and other areas
- Major endemic regions: Mediterranean (Spain, Portugal, Italy, Greece); Middle East; Latin America (Peru, Mexico, Argentina)

Sites Of Infection

- Systemic: fever, generalized myalgia/arthralgia, chills, night sweats, anorexia, lethargy

- Bone/joint: arthritis, often severe & disabling; involvement of back, hips; spondylitis; psoas abscess, etc.
- GU: epididymo-orchitis
- Renal: pyelonephritis, glomerulonephritis
- Neuro: Cerebral (papilledema, cranial neuritis, meningoenceph); Spinal (polio-like, cord compression (abscess), cauda equina syndrome, myelopathy, transverse myelitis); Peripheral
- Musculoskeletal: sacroiliitis, can clinically mimic acute pyogenic spondylodiskitis
- Psychiatric: depression, chronic fatigue, especially during chronic brucellosis and during convalescence

TREATMENT REGIMENS

First-line combination therapy

- Doxycycline 100mg bid x 45 d PLUS streptomycin 1g/IM/d for first 14 d or gentamicin for first 7 d; total duration of therapy 6 wks or longer

Second-line combination therapy

- Doxycycline 100mg bid PLUS rifampin 600-900mg/d x 6wks
- Ciprofloxacin 500mg/bid PLUS rifampin 600mg/d x 30 d
- Cipro + doxy 30 d regimen suggested to be equivalent to Doxy + rif 45 d regimen in open, randomized trial of 40 patients.

Third-line combination therapy

- Trimethoprim-sulfamethoxazole 160/800mg tid PLUS gentamicin (240mg IM/d or 5mg/kg IM/d for pts <50kg) for first 5 days

Treatment of children

- 7 years or older: same as adults
- 6 years or younger: Rifampin 10mg/kg/d x 4 wk PLUS streptomycin 30mg/kg/day IM (max: 1g) (14 d) or gentamicin 2.5mg/kg qd (7 d) IM OR PLUS TMP-SMX (5 mg/kg TMP component) x 4 wk

Pregnancy

- Rifampin 900mg qd OR Rifampin 600mg qd PLUS streptomycin or gentamicin as above

IMPORTANT POINTS

- Laboratory data: low or normal hemoglobin; WBC<4000/ul in 1/5 of cases with lymphocytosis in 1/2; AST/ALT/Alk Phos elev.
- Dx: blood culture (15-30% of cases pos); pos cx differentiates acute from chronic infection
- Neuropsychiatric illness, particularly depression, has been noted after microbiological cure and with dropping antibody titers. Retreatment without active infxn not effective in reducing psych sxs.
- Serological diagnosis: agglutination, titer 1/160 or greater considered diagnostic; titers can be lower; 2-mercaptoethanol Rx of serum destroys IgM-if agglutination titer decline post-2Me, acute infxn dx
- Serological diagnosis: may miss B. canis infection (which is nonetheless rare in humans).

SELECTED READINGS

Bayindir Y, Sonmez E, Aladag A, et al. Comparison of five antimicrobial regimens for the treatment of brucellar spondylitis: a prospective, randomized study. J Chemother. 2003 Oct;15(5):466-71

El Miedany YM, El Gaafary M, Baddour M, et al. Human brucellosis: do we need to revise our therapeutic policy?. J Rheumatol. 2003;30:2666-72.

Casao MA, Smits HL, Navarro E, et al. Clinical utility of a dipstick assay in patients with brucellosis: correlation with the period of evolution of the disease. Clin Microbiol Infect 2003;9:301-305

Solera J, Beato JL, Martinez-Alfaro E et al. Azithromycin and gentamicin therapy for the treatment of humans with brucellosis. Clin Infect Dis 2001;32:506-9

Solera J, Espinosa A, Martinez-Alfaro E, et al. Treatment of human brucellosis with doxycycline and gentamicin. Antimicrob Agents Chemother 1997;41:80-4

BURKHOLDERIA CEPACIA
John G. Bartlett, M.D.

CLINICAL RELEVANCE & DIAGNOSIS
- Nonfermenting aerobic gram-neg rod; easily grown on standard media
- Waterborne, nosocomial, opportunistic pathogen
- Ubiquitous - water, soil, plants
- Predisposed: cystic fibrosis, chronic lung dis, chronic granulomatous dis, sickle cell disease, burns, oncology pts
- Formerly Pseudomonas cepacia

SITES OF INFECTION
- Pneumonia
- Bacteremia +/- shock & DIC
- Cystic fibrosis: colonization /pneumonia/necrotizing pneumonia
- Post lung transplant pneumonia
- Ecthyma gangrenosum
- Burn wound sepsis
- Endocarditis - esp heroin addicts
- Bronchiectasis

TREATMENT REGIMENS

Treatment
- Sensitivities may further guide therapy.
- Preferred: TMP-SMX 15-20mg/kg/d (trimethoprim) divided q8h
- Alternative: ceftazidime 2g IV q8h, imipenem 1g IV q6h
- Alt #1: minocycline 100mg IV/PO bid
- Alt #2: chloramphenicol 1g IV q 6h

IMPORTANT POINTS
- Abx guidelines: Med Letter (2001;43:69)
- Opportunistic - esp cystic fibrosis, CGD and sickle cell disease
- Cystic fibrosis - usually colonizes; may cause pneumonia or fulminant infection w/sepsis
- Resistant to abx commonly used empirically for sepsis. Appears usually resistant to cefepime.

SELECTED READINGS
Woods CW, et al. Virulence associated with outbreak-related strains of Burkholderia cepacia complex among a cohort of patients with bacteremia. Clin Infect Dis 2004;38:1243

McDowell A, et al. Epidemiology of Burkholderia cepacia complex species recovered from cystic fibrosis patients: issues related to patient segregation. J Med Microbiol 2004;53:663-8

Moore JE, et al. Infection control and the significance of sputum and other respiratory secretions from adult patients with cystic fibrosis. Ann Clin Microbiol Antimicrob 2004;3:8

Bell JM, Turnidge JD et al. The Cefepime Study Group. Multicentre Study of the in vitro activity of cefepime, compared to other broad spectrum agents. Path 2001; 33:53

Matrician L, Ange G, Burns S, et al. Outbreaks of nosocomial B. cepacia infection and colonization associated with intrinsically contaminated mouthwash. Infect Control Hosp Epidemiol 2000;21:737

CAMPYLOBACTER AND RELATED SPECIES

Paul Auwaerter, M.D.

CLINICAL RELEVANCE & DIAGNOSIS

- Gram-negative bacteria w/ C. jejuni [see "Campylobacter jejuni"] most common member. Other members include C. coli, C. fetus, C. lari described in THIS module. Worldwide zoonosis.
- Non-jejuni spp. tend to cause extra-intestinal illness. C. fetus subsp. fetus most human common pathogen of this type. Infections acquired from ingesting infected animal excreta contaminating meat.
- Typical extra-intestinal Campylobacter infection affects debilitated hosts. Can infect normal hosts, but less common.
- Homosexual men appear at increased risk probably due to sexual practices.
- Dx: Blood culture isolate may take 4-14d to grow. IF attempting to culture C. fetus from feces [rarely achieved], alert micro lab for 37°C requirements and media without cephalosporins.
- Helicobacter spp. closely related (e.g., H.pylori formerly C. pylori) H. cinaedi, H. fennelliae, H. pullorum, H. westmeadii, H. canadensis--all reported cause enteritis & septicemia.

SITES OF INFECTION

- Bactermia: may be prolonged, w/ relapsing fever. Source inapparent.
- Endovascular: may cause endocarditis, mycotic aneursym esp. abdominal aorta. Predilection to cause septic thrombophelbitis.
- Meningoencephalitis: seen in neonates and adults.
- GI: diarrheal disease can occur with "atypical campylobacter" spp., but generally less severe and self-limited.
- Cellulitis: Described especially in immune suppressed with Helicobacter spp.

TREATMENT REGIMENS

Gastrointestinal

- Uncommon, usually self-limited in normal hosts [non-C. jejuni infections].
- Supportive care, rehydration (oral or IV).
- Antibiotics rarely needed in normal hosts, but in very ill or if sx persist >7d may choose from agents listed below.
- Erythromycin 250mg PO qid x 7d or clarithromycin 500mg bid or azithromycin 500mg qd [would NOT use for severe or systemic illness because of resistance concerns].
- Ciprofloxacin 500mg bid PO an alternative and may be preferred due to increasing resistance reports in non-C. jejuni spp.

Extra-intestinal infections

- If possible susceptibility tests should guide choices due to increasing resistance. Agents listed generally sensitive except as noted.
- Generally resistant to pencillins and cephalosporins; exceptions amoxicillin, ampicillin and ticarcillin/clav (but not sulbactam or tazobactam).
- Serious infections: gentamicin 5mg/kg/d IV or imipenem 1mg IV q6h or ceftriaxone 2g IV q12h.

- Endovascular infections prefer aminoglycoside (4-6 wk). CNS prefer ceftriaxone or chloramphenicol (2-3 wk).
- Atypical campylobacter or H. cinaedi infections acquired in developing countries often resistant to erythromcyin, tetracycline.

IMPORTANT POINTS

- C. fetus and related infections may be fatal in cirrhotics, diabetics or severely compromised patients.
- Survival in the very ill probably dependent on the timeliness of initating proper antibiotic.
- Systemic campylobacter infections deserve parenteral therapy. Erythromycin NOT always effective and should be avoided.

SELECTED READINGS

Francioli P, Herzstein J, Grob JP et al. Campylobacter fetus subspecies fetus bacteremia. Arch Intern Med. 1985 Feb; 145(2): 289-92

Tremblay C, Gaudreau C, Lorange M. Epidemiology and antimicrobial susceptibilities of 111 Campylobacter fetus subsp. fetus strains isolated in Quebec, Canada, from 1983 to 2000. J Clin Microbiol. 2003 Jan; 41(1): 463-6

Ichiyama S, Hirai S, Minami T et al. Campylobacter fetus subspecies fetus cellulitis associated with bacteremia in debilitated hosts. Clin Infect Dis. 1998 Aug; 27(2): 252-5

Andersen LP. New Helicobacter species in humans. Dig Dis. 2001; 19(2): 112-5

Kiehlbauch JA, Tauxe RV, Baker CN, Wachsmuth IK. Helicobacter cinaedi-associated bacteremia and cellulitis in immunocompromised patients. Ann Intern Med. 1994 Jul 15; 121(2): 90-3

CAMPYLOBACTER JEJUNI   Jeremy Gradon, MD

CLINICAL RELEVANCE & DIAGNOSIS

- Major cause of diarrhea. For non-C. jejuni infections, see "Campylobacter and Related Species"
- Rare cause of bacteremia, meningitis and endocarditis
- Guillain-Barre syndrome is preceded by Campylobacter infection in 20-50% of cases
- Dx: stool cx, special media and 42°C required to grow Campylobacter; lab notification may be required when considering this organism
- Campylobacter enteritis: ~8% w/ visible blood in stool, ~52% occult blood +, 59% w/ fever and 45% had abdominal tenderness

SITES OF INFECTION

- GI tract - diarrhea, colitis, acute abdominal pain/pseudo-appendicitis
- Systemic - (rare) bloodstream, meninges, focal abscesses

TREATMENT REGIMENS

GI

- Rehydration; most patients do not require antibiotics--exceptions: high fevers, bloody stools, prolonged illness (sx >1 wk), pregnancy, HIV and other immunosuppressed states
- Erythromycin stearate 500mg PO q12h x 5d (preferred)
- Ciprofloxacin 500mg PO q12h x 5d

• Campylobacter species also are generally susceptible to aminoglycosides, chloramphenicol, clindamycin and carbapenems as considerations for parenteral therapy if required

Prevention

• Poultry stocks nearly universally contaminated with Camplyobacter sp.
• Handwashing, thorough cooking of food esp. poultry
• Use of poorly cleaned cutting boards, food preparation utensils that cross-contaminate other foods are common ways of causing infection
• Avoid unpasteurized milk

IMPORTANT POINTS

• Most infections self-limited, not requiring abx. In US, the most common cause of bloody diarrhea is not Campylobacter but E. coli O157:H7 infection
• Fluoroquinolone resistance increasingly common (animal husbandry use of FQ driving resistance), so erythromycin preferred with lower rates
• Increasing quinolone resistance to C. jejuni especially in overseas travelers
• Certain clones of Campylobacters appear to be associated with Guillain-Barre syndrome (LPS-019+) but are often no longer present enterically at neurological presentation
• Campylobacter fetus blood stream infections are more common among immune-compromised hosts

SELECTED READINGS

Guerrant RL, et al. Practice guidelines for the management of infectious diarrhea. Clin Infect Dis 2001; 32: 331-350

Smith KE, et al. Quinolone-resistant Campylobacter jejuni infections in Minnesota, 1992-1998. N Engl J Med 1999; 340: 1525-1532

Rees JH, et al. Campylobacter jejuni infection and Guillain-Barre syndrome. N Engl J Med 1995; 333: 1374-1379

Peterson MC, et al. Prosthetic hip infection and bacteremia due to Campylobacter jejuni in a patient with AIDS. Clin Infect Dis 1993; 16: 439-440

Kuroki S, et al. Campylobacter jejuni strains from patients with Guillain-Barre syndrome belong mostly to Penner serogroup 19 and contain beta-N-acetylglucosamine residues. Ann Neurol 1993; 33: 243-247

CAPNOCYTOPHAGA CANIMORSUS

Paul Auwaerter, M.D.

CLINICAL RELEVANCE & DIAGNOSIS

• Facultatively anaerobic gram-negative rod, part of nl oral flora of dogs and cats. Previously known as DF-2 bacillus (dysgonic fermenter).
• May cause fulminant sepsis following dog > cat bites, particularly in asplenic patients, alcoholics or immune suppressed.
• Organism has a long, fusiform appearance on gram stain, making it distinctive enough to consider morphologic identification pending cx results. Organisms considered fastidious by micro lab.
• Many patients have hx of dog/cat bite or scratch.
• Infection may be mild to severe, including shock, DIC, acral gangrene, disseminated purpura, renal failure, meningitis and pulmonary infiltrates.

SITES OF INFECTION

• Soft tissue: dog > cat bites, cellultis
• Bacteremia/sepsis: risk of severe infection increased in asplenics, alcoholics

- CNS: meningitis
- Cardiac: endocarditis (rare)

TREATMENT REGIMENS

Mild cellulitis/dog or cat bites
- Preferred: amoxicillin/clavulanate 500mg tid or 875 mg bid PO, or amoxicillin 500mg PO tid. Since pathogen of bites usually not known, empiric amox/clav usually selected.
- Alt: clindamycin 300mg PO qid, doxycycline 500mg PO bid or clarithromycin 500mg PO bid

Severe cellulitis/sepsis
- Preferred: penicillin G 2-4 mU q 4h IV or clindamycin 600mg IV q 8h
- Alt: ceftriaxone 1-2q IV qd, ciprofloxacin 400mg IV q12h or meropenem 1g IV q8h
- Note that resistance to aztreonam described, and variable susceptibility reported to TMP-SMX and aminoglycosides.

Prevention
- Although no firm data supports this recommendation, many clinicians prophylax dog/cat bites in asplenic patients with amoxicllin/clavulanate for 7-10d.

IMPORTANT POINTS
- Consider C. canimorsus in all dog bite infections, or any fulminant infection in asplenics.
- Cx results or in vitro susceptibilities may be delayed due to slow growth of organism in the lab.
- All asplenic patients after a dog bite should be considered to undergo antibiotic prophylaxis, e.g., amox/clav.

SELECTED READINGS

Sandoe JA. Capnocytophaga canimorsus endocarditis. J Med Microbiol. 2004 Mar;53(Pt 3):245-8

Bobo RA, Newton EJ. A previously undescribed gram-negative bacillus causing septicemia and meningitis. Am J Clin Pathol. 1976 Apr;65(4):564-9

Pers C, Gahrn-Hansen B, Frederiksen W. Capnocytophaga canimorsus septicemia in Denmark, 1982-1995: review of 39 cases. Clin Infect Dis. 1996 Jul;23(1):71-5

Kullberg BJ, Westendorp RG, van 't Wout JW, Meinders AE. Purpura fulminans and symmetrical peripheral gangrene caused by Capnocytophaga canimorsus (formerly DF-2) septicemia--a complication of dog bite. Medicine (Baltimore). 1991 Sep;70(5):287-92

Bremmelgaard A, Pers C, Kristiansen JE, Korner B, et al. Susceptibility testing of Danish isolates of Capnocytophaga and CDC group DF-2 bacteria. APMIS. 1989 Jan;97(1):43-8

CHLAMYDOPHILA PNEUMONIAE

John G. Bartlett, M.D.

CLINICAL RELEVANCE & DIAGNOSIS
- Obligate intracellular bacteria - grows like a virus (cell cultures) but is a bacterium with RNA and DNA
- Asymptomatic carriage in pharynx reported, but uncommon
- Dx: most common is MIF serology - technically hard & poor interobserver correlation. Best dx is 4-fold or > titer rise.
- Culture with tissue culture best but (research labs only) and PCR (experimental)
- Seroprevalence is 50% by 20 yrs, 75% by 60 yrs
- Major cause respiratory infections: pharyngitis 1%, sinusitis 5%, bronchitis 5-10%, community-acquired pneumonia 5-15%

• Controversial role in coronary artery disease, stroke, Bechets, MS, Alzheimer's

SITES OF INFECTION
• Pharynx: pharyngitis
• Sinuses: sinusitis
• Larynx: laryngitis
• Bronchi: bronchitis
• Lung: pneumonia
• Asthma: exacerbations asthma (children & adults)
• Otitis
• Rare: endocarditis, erythema, nodosum, Guillian-Barre
• Coronary artery disease and carotid plaques; role in disease is uncertain

TREATMENT REGIMENS

Pneumonia
• Guidelines from IDSA
• Macrolide: erythro 250-500mg PO qid x 10-14d, clarithromycin (BiaxinXL) 1g qd or (Biaxin) 500mg bid x 10-14d or azithro (Zithromax) 500mg then 250mg qd x 4, or 500mg qd x3d
• Doxycycline: 100mg bid x 10-14d
• Fluoroquinolone: levofloxacin (Levaquin) PO/IV 500mg qd, moxifloxacin (Avelox) PO/IV 400mg qd, gatifloxacin (Tequin) PO/IV 400mg qd, all 10-14d

URI/sronchitis
• Guidelines from American College of Physicians and CDC
• URI (sinusitis, pharyngitis): no antibiotic
• Bronchitis: no antibiotic

IMPORTANT POINTS
• Guidelines - IDSA for pneumonia (CID 2003;37:1405) and ACP/CDC for bronchitis, sinusitis
• Clinician rarely knows C. pneumoniae is cause - must Rx empirically
• Common cause (5-15%) of URIs, bronchitis & pneumonia, but abx indicated only for pneumonia
• Role in coronary artery disease - supported by serologic studies, antigen in plaque 40-100%, mouse & rabbit models but abx trials are not supportive of role

SELECTED READINGS
Jackson LA, Grayston JT. Chlamydia pneumonia. Chapter 170 IN: Principles & Practice of Infectious Diseases. Mandell J, Bennett J, Dolin R, 5th Ed. Churchill, Livingston, 2000; pg 2007

Schneeberger PM, et al. Diagnosis of atypical pathogens in patients hospitalized with community-acquired respiratory infection. Scand J. Infect Dis 2004;36:269-73

Apfalter P, et al. No evidence of involvement of Chlamydia pneumoniae in severe cerebrovascular atherosclerosis by means of quantitative real-time polymerase chain reaction. Stroke 2004;(in press)

Littman AJ, et al. Interlaboratory reliability of immunofluorescence test for measurement of Chlamydia pneumoniae-specific immunoglobulin A and G antibody titers. Clin Diag Lab Immunol 2004;11:615-17

Apfalter P, et al. Reliability of nested PCR for detection of Chlamydia pneumoniae DNA in atheromas: results of a multicenter study applying standardized protocols. J. Clin Microbiol 2002;40:4428

CHLAMYDOPHILA TRACHOMATIS

Noreen A. Hynes, M.D., M.P.H.

CLINICAL RELEVANCE & DIAGNOSIS

- D-K biovars: Can cause mucopurulent cervicitis (MPC), dysuria-pyuria syndrome, PID, and perihepatitis in women. 70% of perihepatitis due to CT. Can cause adverse outcome in newborn.
- D-K biovars: Leading cause of PID; believed to cause "silent salpingitis" therefore must screen for CT; thought to be leading cause of infertility in women.
- 3 subsets: 1) D-K biovars--worldwide STD causing cervicitis, urethritis, PID, epididymitis, 2) L-serovars causing LGV, 3) A-C biovars causing trachoma.
- A-C biovars: cause hyperendemic blinding trachoma, usually in third world children.
- L serovars: cause the STD lymphogranuloma venereum (LGV) associated w/ genital ulcer-adenopathy syndrome and proctocolitis. Seen mostly in the developing world and among men who have sex with men.
- The STD forms (biovars D-K and L-serovars) enhance the acquisition and transmission of HIV.
- Genital CT infection, particularly those caused by serotype G and LGV L2 strain appear to be linked to cancer. Serotype G and infection over time with multiple serotypes linked to cervical SCC
- Nucleic acid amplification tests (NAAT) and similar tests are more sensitive (85%) than most previous tests but specificity less than culture. Hence, if CT prevalence in area <2% must confirm + NAAT.
- D-K biovars: Up to 70% infections in women are asymptomatic; up to 40% of men are asymptomatic

SITES OF INFECTION

- Eye: conjunctivitis, trachoma
- Rectum: proctitis
- Colon: colitis and proctocolitis.
- Genito-urinary tract: urethritis, cervicitis, PID, epididymitis, prostatitis (rare).

TREATMENT REGIMENS

CT cervicitis/urethritis (D-K biovars)

- Recommended regimen: azithromycin 1g PO x 1 (preferred if adherence is an anticipated problem)
- Recommended regimen: doxycycline 100mg PO bid x 7d
- Alternative regimen (2nd line): erythromycin base 500 mg PO qid x 7d
- Alternative regimen (2nd line): erythromycin ethylsuccinate 800mg PO qid x 7d
- Alternative regimen (2nd line): ofloxacin 300mg PO bid x 7d. Not for use in HI, CA, MA, New York City, Pacific Basin, where rates of fluoroquinolone resistant gonorrhea is high unless gonorrhea ruled out.
- Alternative regimen (2nd line): Levofloxacin 500mg PO qd x 7d. Not for use in HI, CA, MA, New York City, Pacific Basin, where rates of fluoroquinolone resistant GC is high unless gonorrhea ruled out.

CT cervicitis in pregnant women (D-K biovars)

- Recommended regimen: erythromycin base 500mg qid x 7d (Test of cure required 3 wks after end of Rx)
- Recommended regimen: amoxicillin 500mg PO tid x 7d (Test of cure required 3 wks after end of Rx)

- Alternative regimen (2nd line): azithromycin 1g PO x 1 (Test of cure required 3 wks after end of Rx)
- Alternative regimen (2nd line): erythromycin base 250 mg PO qid x 14d (Test of cure required 3 wks after end of Rx)
- Alternative regimen (2nd line): erythromycin ethylsuccinate 800mg qid x 7d (Test of cure required 3 wks after end of Rx)
- Alternative regimen (2nd line): erythromycin ethylsuccinate 400mg qid x 14d (Test of cure required 3 wks after end of Rx)

Other GU-related infections
- Epididymitis: See notes below or separate "Epididymitis" in the Diagnoses section
- Pelvic inflammatory diseases: See notes below or separate "Pelvic Inflammatory Disease" in the Diagnoses section
- Proctitis: See notes below or separate "Proctitis/Proctocolitis" in the Diagnoses section for proper management
- Lyphogranuloma venereum: Recommended regimen = Doxycycline 100mg PO BID X 21d; Alternative regimen = Erythromycin base 500mg PO qid x 21d

HIV-infected persons (D-K biovars)
- Treat same as HIV-uninfected persons

Ocular Infections
- Acute inclusion conjunctivitis: same as non-LGV genital CT Rx outlined above
- Trachoma: Azithromycin 1g PO X 1

IMPORTANT POINTS
- STD-related component of module based on 2002 CDC STD Rx Guideline (MMWR 2002; 51 (RR-6), 2000 AAP Red Book, p.139; ocular infection Rx based literature review).
- When rectal involvement suspected, culture or DFA only (inhibitors obscure other tests). Severe proctitis always consider LGV. Requires longer therapy.
- Screening recommended annually or more frequently, as needed for all sexually active women; biannually for sexually active adolescents; all pregnant women in 1st trimester & later, if needed.
- Counsel patients to refrain from sexual activity for sexually transmitted CT infections for 7 days after completion of Rx; TREAT PARTNERS!
- Test of cure not needed if RECOMMENDED (as opposed to alternative)regimens used (EXCEPT in pregnant women---test of cure needed in all pregnant women).

SELECTED READINGS
Dean D et al. Evidence for long-term cervical persistence of Chlamydia trachomatis by omp1 genotyping. J Infect Dis 2001;182:909-16

Jacobson GF et al. A randomized controlled trial comparing amoxicillin and azithromycin for the treatment of Chlamydia trachomatis in pregnancy. Am J Obstet Gynecol 2001;184:1352-6

Bauer GR and Welles SL. Beyond assumptions of negligible risk: Sexually transmitted diseases and women who have sex with women. Am J Public Health 2001;91:1282-6.

Clark KL et al. Hospitalization rates in female US Army recruits associated a screening program for Chlamydia trachomatis. Sex Transm Dis 2002;29:1-5

Andersen B et al. Population-based strategies for outreach screening of urogenital Chlamydia trachomatis infections: A randomized, controlled trial. J Infect Dis 2002;185:252-8

CITROBACTER SPECIES

Paul Auwaerter, M.D.

CLINICAL RELEVANCE & DIAGNOSIS

- Enteric gram-negative bacilli. Normal part of gut flora. May be mistakenly identified as Salmonella; colonies on plates resemble E. coli.
- Species associated w/ infection most commonly C. amalonaticus, C. koseri (previously known as C. diversus) & C. freundii.
- Mostly a nosocomial pathogen found in compromised hosts, patients aged >60 years, and neonates: UTIs, pneumonia, line infections.
- Beta-lactamases frequently expressed. Nosocomial isolates may be highly-resistant to multiple abx.

SITES OF INFECTION

- GU: UTI
- CNS: meningitis, brain abscess (mostly C. koseri in newborns)
- Pulmonary: nosocomial pneumonia (must distinguish from colonization)
- Bacteremia: frequently polymicrobial
- Endocarditis: rare reports
- Soft tissue: associated with superficial and deep infections, post-op wound infections
- GI: intraabdominal infection, usually part of polymicrobial flora

TREATMENT REGIMENS

General principles

- UTI's may be treated by monotherapy, hopefully an oral fluoroquinolone or TMP-SMX.
- More serious infections empirically should be treated at least initially with either cefepime or carbapenem if Citrobacter suspected.
- Aminoglycosides generally have activity and may be selected in combination, especially if ESBL suspected and using cephalosporin-based beta-lactam.
- For meningitis (adult recommendations only given in this guide), would employ third/fourth generation cephalosporin or meropenem.
- Susceptibility results should guide therapy; potential for multiple drug resistance, including ESBL.

Citrobacter koseri

- Preferred: ceftriaxone 1-2g IV q 12-24, cefotaxime 1-3g IV q6h or cefepime 1-2 IV q12h
- Alt: ciprofloxacin 400mg IV q 12h (or 500mg PO q12h for UTI), imipenem 1g IV q 6h, meropenem 1-2g IV q8h, aztreonam 1-2g IV q6h, or TMP-SMX 5mg/kg q6h IV (or DS PO bid for UTI).

Citrobacter freundii

- More resistance generally identified with this species.
- Preferred: meropenem 1-2g IV q8h or imipenem 1g IV q6h, cefepime 1-2g IV q12h, ciprofloxacin 400mg IV q12h (or 500mg PO bid for UTI), or aminoglycoside (eg gentamicin 5mg/kg/d)
- Alt: piperacillin/tazobactam 3.375mg q6h IV, aztreonam 1-2g IV q6h or TMP-SMX 5mg/kg q6h IV (or DS PO bid for UTI).

IMPORTANT POINTS

- Source of recommendations: author opinion
- Usually a nosocomial pathogen. Has been described as cause of outbreaks in healthcare facilities.
- Bacteremia often polymicrobial in ~50% of patients.

- Brain abscesses are rarely a complication of meningitis, with the exception of C. koseri infections in neonates with rates of ~70%.

SELECTED READINGS

Doran TI. The role of Citrobacter in clinical disease of children: review. Clin Infect Dis. 1999 Feb;28 (2):384-94

Drelichman V, Band JD. Bacteremias due to Citrobacter diversus and Citrobacter freundii: incidence, risk factors, and clinical outcome. Arch Intern Med 145 (1985), pp. 1808-1810

Tellez I, Chrysant GS, Omer I, et al. Citrobacter diversus endocarditis. Am J Med Sci. 2000 Dec;320(6): 408-10

Gupta N, Yadav A, Choudhary U, et al. Citrobacter bacteremia in a tertiary care hospital. Scand J Infect Dis. 2003;35(10):765-8

Rhomberg PR, Jones RN, Sader HS; MYSTIC Programme (US) Study Group. Results from the Meropenem Yearly Susceptibility Test Information Collection (MYSTIC) Programme: report of the 2001 data from 15 United States medical centres. Int J Antimicrob Agents. 2004 Jan;23(1):52-9

CLOSTRIDIUM BOTULINUM
John G. Bartlett, M.D.

CLINICAL RELEVANCE & DIAGNOSIS

- Gram-positive spore-forming, anaerobic rod that produces neurotoxin; found worldwide
- Dx: toxin in sera, stool, food; cx - wound, stool
- Forms: foodborne (outbreaks), infant ("floppy baby"), wound (IDU), inhalation (bioterrorism), unclassified
- US: 100 cases/yr - infant 71, foodborne 24, wound 3. Types A&B; E in Alaska.
- Clinical: 1) 4-D's (diplopia, dysarthria, dysphoria, dysphagia); 2) afebrile; 3) alert; 4) descending flaccid paralysis, 5) normal CSF & MRI, EEG = fasciculations
- Ddx: myasthenia, Eaton-Lambert; tick paralysis, Guillain-Barre, magnesium intoxication, CVA, paralytic shellfish toxins, nerve gas, CO poisoning, organophosphates
- Wound botulism causes regional (limb) paralysis; US seen mainly in IDU skin poppers.

SITES OF INFECTION

- Neurologic system (only)

TREATMENT REGIMENS

Treatment

- Principles: Suspect (cranial nerve palsy, descending symmetrical paralysis, alert, afebrile); obtain botulin toxin assay of stool, vomit, blood; Rx w/antitoxin & report.
- Preferred Rx (CDC): trivalent antitoxin (A 7,500IU, B 5,000IU & E 5,000IU) 1 vial diluted 1:10, IV infusion over 30 min. preferably <24h post symptoms onset.
- Mechanical ventilation required in 20-40% adults and continued 3-6 mo.
- Miscellaneous support: IV hydration, tube feedings, abx for ID complications
- CDC hotline: 404-639-3670; antitoxin & toxin assay - call State Health Dept or CDC
- Concern bioterrorism?: 404-639-2206 (day)/ 404-639-2880
- Antitoxin, equine: hypersensitivity reactions in 9%, anaphylaxis in 2%

Prevention

- Destroy spores w/heat 120 degrees C x 30min (pressure cooker)
- Prevent germination - lower pH, refrigerate, freeze, dry, add salt, sugar or Na nitrate
- Inactivate toxin - heat 80 degrees C x 20min or 90 degrees C x 10min
- Water-chlorine + hypochlorite = sporicidal

IMPORTANT POINTS

- Recommendations from CDC, [see www.cdc.gov/ncidod/dbmd/diseaseinfo/botulism.pdf]
- Common forms: foodborne and infant; others [rare]: wound, bioterrorism (inhalation), unclassified
- Sequence w/all forms: toxin absorbed then blood then nerve endings then cranial nerves then descending flaccid paralysis
- Major risk: respiratory failure; may require ventilatory support x 3-6 mos.
- Rx antitoxin ASAP if suspected. Get from State HD or CDC; 1 vial IV

SELECTED READINGS

Ferreira JL et al. Comparison of the mouse bioassay and enzyme-linked immunosorbant assay procedures for the detection of type A botulinal toxin in food. J. Food Prod 2004;67:203

Arnon SS, Schechter R, Inglesby T, et al. Botulinum toxin as a biological weapon. JAMA 2001;285:1059

CDC. Botulism outbreak associated with eating fermented food - Alaska, 2001. MMWR 2001;50:680

Maselli R, Bakshi N. American Assoc of Electrodiagnostic Medicine case report 16: Botulism. Muscle Nerve 2000;23:1137

Werner SB, Passaro D, McGee J, et al. Wound botulism in California, 1951-1998; recent epidemic in heroin injectors. CID 2000;31:1018

CLOSTRIDIUM DIFFICILE John G. Bartlett, M.D.

CLINICAL RELEVANCE & DIAGNOSIS

- Anaerobic gram-positive spore-forming bacillus
- Colonizes colon on 3% healthy adults and 20-30% hosp pts.
- Major known cause of antibiotic-associated colitis/diarrhea
- Risk: abx use, increased age, hospitalization comorbidities, immune suppression
- Lab dx: EIA for tox A or tox A+B (sens 70-80%, spec >98%)
- Clues: hx of abx use (especially clindamycin, cephalosporins, ampicillin, piperacillin), colitis (fever, cramps) + elevated WBC, low albumin, fecal WBCs.
- False negative EIA for toxin in 20-30%; if available cytotoxin assay superior

SITES OF INFECTION

- Colon: colitis/pseudomembranous colitis, toxic megacolon
- Extra colonic infection: rare and usually not important
- Reactive arthritis (post diarrheal): rare & not HLA-B27 linked
- Enteritis: only 7 cases reported with small bowel involvement only

TREATMENT REGIMENS

Treatment: Abx

- Principles: + toxin assay, D/C implicated abx, avoid narcotics, infection control (contact isolation) +/- metronidazole.
- Abx guidelines: IDSA, CDC, SHEA - all say metronidazole is preferred rx.
- Preferred: metronidazole 250mg PO qid or 500mg PO tid x 10d ($12/10d)
- Alt: vancomycin 125mg PO qid x 10d ($280/10d)
- Toxin assay negative and high probability: repeat test +/- treat empirically

Treatment: special considerations

- If need systemic abx for ongoing infection (other than C.difficile): use oral metronidazole + agent unlikely to cause C. difficile: IV vancomycin, macrolide, sulfa, doxycycline or aminoglycoside
- Supportive care: IV hydration or oral fluids

- Avoid antiperistaltics (Lomotil, loperamide, opiates)
- Infection control: single room, wash hands, vinyl gloves, no rectal thermometer
- Epidemics (hosp & nursing home): control abx, especially clindamycin use
- Ileus or vomiting: IV metronidazole 500mg tid +/- vanco PO (500mg qid) by NG tube or rectal tube or both.
- Surgery: total colectomy if severely ill & unresponsive to PO vanco +/- IV metro, especially toxic megacolon

Treatment: multiple relapses

- Metronidazole 250mg PO qid or vancomycin 125mg PO qid x 10d, then one of the following:
- Vancomycin 125mg QOD (pulse dose) x 6wks
- Lactobacillus GG 1 tab "culturelle" bid (CVS pharmacies) + cholestyramine 4g tid x 4-6wks
- Saccharomyces boulardi 500mg qid from day 6 of vanco x 4-6 wks
- Alt: IVIG 400mg/kg q 3 wks (experimental) or vaccine trial
- Alt: Stool from healthy donor via enema or NG tube

IMPORTANT POINTS

- Guidelines: metronidazole PO preferred - IDSA (CID 2001;32:331); SHEA (Inf Con Hosp Ep 1995;16:459) CDC (MMWR 1995;44:RR-12)
- C. difficile causes 20% of antibiotic-associated diarrheas & >95% of pseudomembranous colitis.
- Clinical clues: hx of abx + diarrhea, colitis (cramps, fever), elevated WBC, hypoalbuminemia
- Reponse to Rx is rapid: if diarrhea persists >5-7d, question dx or consider concurrent IBD, lactose deficiency, medication effect, etc. Relapses at 3-21d post metronidazole or vancomycin in up to 25%.
- Most cases not due to C. difficile caused by fecal floral change with resultant osmotic diarrhea.

SELECTED READINGS

Pepin J, Valiquette L, Alary ME, Villemure P, Pelletier A, et al. Clostridium difficile-associated diarrhea in a region of Quebec from 1991 to 2003: a changing pattern of disease severity. CMAJ 2004; Aug 31;171 (5):466-472

Pepin J, Alary ME, Valiquette L, Raiche E, Ruel J, Fulop K et al. Increasing risk of relapse after treatment of Clostridium difficile colitis in Quebec, Canada. Clin Infect Dis 2005; Jun 1:40(11):1591-1597

Mylonakis M, Ryan ET, Calderwood SB. Clostridium difficile - associated diarrhea. Arch Intern Med 2000;161:525

Gerdny DN, Johnson S, Peterson LR, et al. Clostridium difficile associated diarrhea and colitis. Inf Cont Hosp Epid 1995;16:459

Kyne L, Warny M, Oawar A, Kelly CP. Asymptomatic carriage of Clostridium difficile and serum levels of IgG antibody against toxin A. NEJM 2000;342:390

CLOSTRIDIUM SPECIES   John G. Bartlett, M.D.

CLINICAL RELEVANCE & DIAGNOSIS

- Most disease is toxin mediated: gas gangrene -alpha toxin w/ myonecrosis & sepsis. Tetanus -tetanus toxin: w/ neurotoxin. Botulism - botulinum toxin w/paralysis. Colitis - C. difficile toxin A.
- Food poisoning: enterotoxin w/ diarrhea; neutropenic enterocolitis. Alpha toxin: sepsis

- Soft tissue disease, gas formation: crepitant cellulitis; gas forming cellulitis; emphysematous cholecystitis
- Bacteremia: significant with gas gangrene or neutropenic typhilitis

SITES OF INFECTION

- GI tract: food poisoning, botulism, enteritis necroticans, typhilitis, antibiotic-associated diarrhea & colitis.
- Bacteremia: usually a contaminant except with gas gangrene or typhilitis
- Soft tissue: gas gangrene; crepitant cellulitis or necrotizing fasciitis. Tetanus: C. tetani
- Intra-abdominal sepsis: peritonitis and intra-abdominal abscess (polymicrobial); emphysematous cholecystitis

TREATMENT REGIMENS

Soft tissue

- Gas gangrene: aggressive surgery & penicillin 20mU/d IV & clindamycin 600mg IV q8h or metronidazole 500mg q6h
- Gas gangrene: hyperbaric oxygen IV; controversial & less important than immediate surgery
- Crepitant cellulitis/necrotizing fasciitis: debridement & penicillin 20Mu/d, clindamycin 1.8g IV/d, metro 2g IV or PO/d or imipenem

Toxin mediated

- Botulism: trivalent antitoxin (A/B & E) CDC: 404-639-3670
- Tetanus: tetanus toxoid & human TIG 500 IU IM & metronidazole 500mg IV q6h & benzodiazepine
- C. difficile: d/c implicated abx & metronidazole 250 mg PO q6h x 7-10 d
- Neutropenic enterocolitis: clindamycin or metronidazole or imipenem
- Neutropenic enterocolitis: surgery; most C. sordellii require surgery; most C. tertium do not.
- Clostridium perfringens type A food poisoning: supportive care, diarrhea resolves <24 hr.

Miscellaneous

- Emphysematous cholecystitis: urgent cholecystectomy; ampicillin-sulbactam, ticarcillin-clavulanate, piperacillin-tazobactam, imipenem
- Bacteremia: usually contaminant unless gas gangrene or necrotizing enterocolitis
- Mixed infection: cover mixed anaerobic infection with imipenem, beta-lactam/beta-lactamase inhibitor or combination metro/clind & cephalosporin.
- Surgery critical with gas gangrene; often important - cholecystitis, crepitant cellulitis, typhilitis

IMPORTANT POINTS

- Clostridia - normal colonic flora including C. perfringens in 50% and C. difficile in 3%
- Most blood culture isolates are not clinically important unless evidence of neutropenic enterocolitis or gas gangrene
- Most pathology is toxin mediated with toxins that have great clout - gas gangrene, botulism, tetanus, C. difficile, typhilitis
- Clostridial disease is usually a clinical dx sometimes supported by gram stain (distinctive GPB), culture of blood/soft tissue or toxin assay (C. difficile)
- ABX active vs most clostridia: PCN, amp, chloramphenicol, cefotaxime, piperacillin. Less active: cefoxitin, clindamycin, metro, ceftaz. If mixed infection suspected - need to broaden coverage.

SELECTED READINGS

Kimura AC, et al. Outbreak of necrotizing fasciitis due to Clostridium sordelli among black tar heroin users. Clin Infect Dis 2004;38:87-91

Kaiver MA, Linden JV, Whaley DN, et al. Clostridum infections associated with musculoskeletal tissue allographs. N. Engl. J. Med 2004;350:2564

Young V B, Schmidt TM. Antibiotic associated diarrhea accompanied by large scale alterations in microbiota. J. Clin Micro 2004;42:1203

CLOSTRIDIUM TETANI (TETANUS)

David Zaas, M.D. and Paul Auwaerter, M.D.

CLINICAL RELEVANCE & DIAGNOSIS

- Classic triad of rigidity, muscle spasm, and autonomic dysfunction.
- Trismus or lock jaw is the presenting complaint in 75% of cases due to masseter spasm, if extends to facial muscles causes classic "risus sardonicus"(painfully grinning face)
- Generalized tetanus: most commonly, muscles of head and neck affected first with caudal spread to entire body.
- Localized tetanus: spasm, restricted to a limited part of body due to lower toxin loads. Associated with a lower mortality.
- Incubation period from the injury to first sx averages 7-10 days (range 1-60 days).
- Waves of opisthotonos, highly characteristic and due to spasms of back musculature.
- Autonomic nervous system involvement can include labile blood pressure, arrhythmias, diaphoresis, urinary retention, and temperature dysregulation.
- Cephalic tetanus: usually localized cranial nerve dysfunction and follows head trauma or a middle ear infection. Associated with a high mortality.

SITES OF INFECTION

- Usually follows recognized injury contaminated with soil, manure, or rusted metal.
- Also can complicate burns, ulcers, gangrene, necrotic snakebites, middle ear infections, septic abortions, intramuscular injections, and surgery.
- Increasing incidence in some areas associated with high prevalence of injection drug use.
- The diagnosis is usually made clinically based on history and physical findings. C. tetani is very infrequently recovered from wounds.

TREATMENT REGIMENS

Neutralization of unbound toxin

- Human tetanus immune globulin 3000-6000 units IM for active tetanus
- Tetanus toxoid should be administered at a separate site if vaccination status is unknown or if greater than 5 years since last booster.
- For treatment of contaminated wounds please see tetanus diptheria prophylaxis module.
- Tetanus prophylaxis (500 U IM) should be given for contaminated wounds if <3 Td doses or unknown vaccination status

Removal of infection source

- Debridement of wounds should be considered when appropriate.
- Metronidazole has replaced penicillin as the antibiotic of choice due to a better safety profile and improved outcomes.
- Recommended treatment: metronidazole 7.5mg/kg q 6 hrs given IV or PO (not to exceed 4g/day)

- Alternatively, penicillin can be given in doses of 1 to 10 mU/day IV
- Other alternative antibiotics include erythromycin, tetracycline, chloramphenicol, and clindamycin.

Control of rigidity and spasms
- Sedation with benzodiazapines mainstay of treatment.
- When sedation alone is inadequate, neuromuscular blocking agents may be used in conjunction with mechanical ventilation.

Control of autonomic dysfunction
- Most importantly, aggressive fluid resuscitation of up to 8 L per day in some pts may be required.
- Alpha and beta adrenergic blockers have been used with variable results and should be used only with caution.

Supportive measures
- Intubation and mechanical ventilation are often necessary.
- Since mechanical ventilation is usually required for several weeks, early tracheotomy often performed.
- Early enteral nutritional support important.
- Use of life support measures in intensive care units has decreased mortality from nearly 50% to approximately 10%.

IMPORTANT POINTS
- Decreased prevalence in developed countries is due to successful implementation of vaccination programs.
- Vaccination schedules: Started at 2 months of age with 3 vaccinations at monthly intervals, a booster is given before age 5 and then every 10 years. (See Vaccination schedules in Appendix II.)

SELECTED READINGS

Ahmadsyah I, Salim A. Treatment of tetanus: an open study to compare the efficacy of procaine penicillin and metronidazole. Br Med J 1985;291(6496):648-50.

Galazka A, Gasse F. The present status of tetanus and tetanus vaccination. Curr Top Microbiol Immunol 1995;195:31-53

Cook TM, Protheroe RT, Handel JM. Tetanus: a review of the literature. British Journal of Anaesthesia 2001; 87(3):477-87

CDC. Tetanus surveillance-United States, 1995-1997. MMWR 1998; 47: 1-13

Anon. Tetanus among injecting-drug users--California 1997. MMWR Morb Mortal Wkly Rep 1998;47(8): 149-51.

CORYNEBACTERIUM DIPHTHERIAE

Paul Auwaerter, M.D.

CLINICAL RELEVANCE & DIAGNOSIS
- Pleiomorphic gram-positive bacillus capable causing tonsillitis/pharyngitis, cervical LN/swelling, palatal paralysis & T<103F.
- Classic gray-white membrane covering post. pharynx. Toxigenic strains capable of causing carditis and neuritis.
- Now rare, diphtheria often confused with severe strep throat, Vincent's angina or glandular fevers.
- Dx: Throat or nasopharyngeal swab. Transport rapidly & alert micro lab for special media. Rapid dx possible if lab has IFA staining of 4h cx.

- Emerging NON-TOXIGENIC strains cause endocarditis, arthritis and recurrent sore throat.

SITES OF INFECTION

- Pharyngeal: malaise, fever, sore throat with gray-white membrane covering tonsils, palate, uvula and posterior pharynx.
- Laryngeal/Bronchial: Spread of membrane can cause dyspnea and cyanosis on basis of obstruction.
- Cardiac: toxin-related ~1-2wks after illness w/ 1st deg. block, AV dissociation, arrhythmias, myocarditis. Some cardiac effects seen 10-25% pts. Myocarditis/advanced blocks = 60-90% mortality.
- Neurologic: toxin-related paralysis of pharyngeal mm., with possible CN palsies, and subsequent motor neuropathy of limbs.
- Cutaneous: Chronic, nonhealing wound w/grayish membrane. Seen in tropics. In US, homeless, alcoholics, native Americans. Most strains non-toxigenic, role in pathogenesis of ulcer often unclear.

TREATMENT REGIMENS

Diphtheria treatment

- Equine hyperimmune antiserum reduces mortality by neutralizing toxin prior to cellular entry. Critical to administer ASAP w/ presumptive Dx.
- Hypersensitivity to horse proteins determined by 1:100 dilution antitoxin scratched or pricked into skin. If neg. proceed w/ 0.02mL of 1:1000 dilution. Have epinephrine available if necessary.
- Reaction requires desensitization protocol.
- Antitoxin: 20,000-40,000U pharyngeal disease <48h; 40-60,000U nasopharyngeal; 80-120,000U for extensive disease, brawny neck or sx>72h. Give IV (severe dis.) or IM.
- ABX: Eythro 20-25mg/kg q12h IV x 7-14d OR PCN G 50,000U/kg/d div. q6h IV x 5d (or Procaine) followed PCN VK 50mg/kg/d x 5d
- Clindamycin (600mg IV q8h) probably an acceptable alternative.
- Antibiotics may decrease toxin production.
- Serum sickness occurence 10%.
- Antitoxin available from CDC (440-639-8200).
- Culture Nasopharynx 2wks after illness to ensure eradication.

C. diphtheriae carrier

- Erythromycin preferred (250-500mg qid po)

Prevention

- Primary series age>7yrs (Td, toxoids): two doses IM 4wks apart, 3rd dose 6-12 mos. later.
- Booster (Td): every 10 yrs
- Pts with clinical diphtheria should still receive toxoid immunization during convalescent phase, since infection may not be immunogenic.

IMPORTANT POINTS

- Administer antitoxin ASAP with presumptive dx. DON'T wait for confirmation.
- Most deaths in first 3-4d from asphyxiation or myocarditis.
- Public health threat. Must identify contacts and carriers to limit spread. Humans only known reservoir.
- Immunized patients may acquire disease.
- Recommendations from Chap. 193 R.R. MacGregor, Princ. and Prac. Inf. Diseases 5th ed., 2000.

SELECTED READINGS

Kneen R, Pham NG, Solomon T et al. Penicillin vs. erythromycin in the treatment of diphtheria. Clin Infect Dis. 1998 Oct;27(4):845-50

Efstratiou A, Engler KH, Mazurova IK et al. Current approaches to the laboratory diagnosis of diphtheria. J Infect Dis. 2000 Feb;181 Suppl 1:S138-45

Reacher M, Ramsay M, White J et al. Nontoxigenic corynebacterium diphtheriae: an emerging pathogen in England and Wales?. Emerg Infect Dis. 2000 Nov-Dec;6(6):640-5

Harnisch JP, Tronca E, Nolan CM, Turck M, Holmes KK. Diphtheria among alcoholic urban adults. A decade of experience in Seattle. Ann Intern Med. 1989 Jul 1;111(1):71-82

Centers for Disease Control and Prevention (CDC). Fatal respiratory diphtheria in a U.S. traveler to Haiti--Pennsylvania, 2003. MMWR Morb Mortal Wkly Rep. 2004 Jan 9; 52(53): 1285-6

COXIELLA BURNETII
John G. Bartlett, M.D.

CLINICAL RELEVANCE & DIAGNOSIS

- Obligate intracellular pleomorphic, gram-negative rod
- Zoonosis, worldwide but rare in US
- Primary reservoirs: cattle, goats, cats, sheep. C. burnetti shed in animal urine, stool, milk, birth products; highest placenta.
- Other sources: cats, dogs, ticks
- Q fever an occupational risk w/ farm animal contact; also vets, farmers, abattoir workers
- Dx: serology with IFA; acute (pneumonia) 4x rise; chronic (endocarditis) high titer phase 1

SITES OF INFECTION

- Most: asymptomatic or flu-like illness w/no dx
- Pneumonia: "atypical" - most common clinical dx
- Hepatitis: acute or chronic
- Endocarditis: especially prosthetic valves; most Q fever-related chronic fevers represent endocarditis
- Rare - pericarditis, myocarditis, encephalitis, aseptic meningitis, osteomyelitis, chronic fatigue
- Cutaneous: nonspecific rash (usually with chronic infection)

TREATMENT REGIMENS

Treatment: Abx

- Guidelines from Marrie, T (Pneumonia - PPID 2000; pg 2045) and Raoult, D et al (Endocarditis - CID 2001; 33:312)
- Pneumonia (preferred): doxycycline 100mg PO or IV bid x 14-21d
- Alt: erythromycin 1g IV q6h + rifampin 300mg PO bid
- Alt: levofloxacin 500mg PO/IV qd or gatifloxacin 400mg IV/PO qd x 14-21d or moxifloxacin 400mg/d IV/PO each 14-21 d
- Endocarditis: doxycycline 100mg IV/PO bid + chloroquine 200mg tid x 12-18mos, indefinitely or until phase I IgG Ab is < 1:200.
- Hepatitis (preferred): doxycycline 100mg PO/IV bid x 2wks (duration arbitrary)

IMPORTANT POINTS

- Guidelines for abx: T Marrie - pneumonia PPID 2000 p 2043; D. Raoult et al - endocarditis CID 2001;33:312
- Dx is serology w/seroconversion (pneumonia) or high titer (endocarditis)

- Main forms - "atypical pneumonia" (multilobar consolidation), nonspecific fever & endocarditis
- Chronic endocarditis is usually prosthetic valve endocarditis. Chronic infection often w/ "autoimmune" phenomenon, e.g., rash, (+) rheumatoid factor, positive Coombs'.
- Occupational disease from cattle, goat, sheep; also parturient cats

SELECTED READINGS

Fenallar F, Fournier P-E, Garrier, MP, et al. Risk factors and prevention of Q fever endocarditis. CID 2001;33:312

Marrie T. Coxiella burnetii. Chapter 177 IN: Principles & Practice of Infectious Disease, 5th Ed, Mandell G, Bennett J, Dolin R, Churchill Livingstone, 2000, pg 2043

Brouqui P, Dupont HT, Drancourt M, et al. Chronic Q fever: Ninety-two cases in France including 27 cases without endocarditis. Arch Intern Med 1993;153:642

Weir WRC, Bannister B, Chambers S, et al. Chronic Q fever associated with granulomatous hepatitis. J Infect 1980;8:56

Maurin M and Raoult D. Q Fever. Clin Microbiol Rev 1999;12:518

EHRLICHIA SPECIES
Paul Auwaerter, M.D.

CLINICAL RELEVANCE & DIAGNOSIS

- Tickborne illnesses: Human Monocytic Ehrlichiosis (HME) Ehrlichia chaffeensis, Amblyomma americanum (Lone Star tick) vector. Seen mostly in areas from NJ to Ill to Tx.
- Human Granulocytic Ehrlichiosis (HGE) Anaplasma phagocytophilium, Ixodes scapularis (deer tick) vector. Seen in same areas as Lyme: NE, Mid-Atlantic, Upper Midwest. Also Europe.
- HME: Suspected exposure endemic area spring-fall. Abrupt febrile, flu-like illness, HA, N/V, abd pain. Abnl LFT's, leukopenia, decr. plts. common. ~30% maculopap. rash +/- petechiae.
- Dx: Confirmed case as a) 4x rise IFA titer or >1:256 or b) PCR detection or c) visible morulae and IFA >64. Probable case if single titer 1:64-128.
- HGE: Sx similar to HME but less rash (10%). Can see leukopenia & thrombocytopenia, but neutropenia distinguishes from HME. Generally milder illness than HME. Coinfection w/Lyme or Babesia possible.

SITES OF INFECTION

- Systemic: Fever, headache, nausea, rigor, myalgia, nausea, vomiting, abdominal pain w/ average ~7d post tick-bite.
- Monocytes or lymphocytes: HME--Few pts (~7%) w/ morulae (mulberry-like clusters) in monos or lymphs.
- Granulocytes: HGE--Morulae much more common in HGE (20-80%) than in HME.
- Elderly/Immunosuppressed/asplenics at risk for severe disease--multiorgan failure incl. ARDS, renal failure, CNS abnl, coagulopathies.
- Children: HME presentation differs with rash in 67%, more frequent cytopenias, more neuro sxs.

TREATMENT REGIMENS

HME or HGE

- Do not wait for confirmatory dx, Rx w/clinical suspicion. Delayed tx may increase mortality, normally ~3% esp. in immunosuppressed.

- Doxycyline 100mg PO/IV bid standard as ddx often includes RMSF & tx empirical. Duration uncertain, but at least >3d after last fever [min. 5-7d]. Often quick clinical response <48hr except ICU pts
- Pregnancy or doxy intolerance: rifampin 600mg PO/IV qd x 7-10d for HGE. Choices for HME unclear but may respond to rif or chloramphenicol 500mg qid.
- In vitro resistance to chloramphenicol, macrolides, PCNs and AGs, and clinical data scanty, so routine use cannot be strongly recommended. Quinolones have activity, but limited clinical data.

IMPORTANT POINTS

- Recommendations based on Med Clin North Am 2002 Mar;86(2):375-92 and author's opinion.
- No randomized clinical trials exist to define optimal antibiotic choice or treatment.
- Spectrum of illness may range from subclinical to moderate to severe. About 40% HME pts require hospitalization. Abnl LFTs with leukopenia or thrombocytopenia clinical tip-off in pt w/ tick exposure
- Immune compromised pts at risk of severe illness, and common lab abnl in ICU may not trigger consideration of infection.
- Doxycycline mainstay of empirical treatment of tickborne disease since ddx often includes Lyme and RMSF.

SELECTED READINGS

Steere AC, McHugh G, Suarez C et al. Prospective study of coinfection in patients with erythema migrans. Clin Infec Dis 2003; 36: 1078-1081.

Talbot TR, Comer JA, Bloch KC. Ehrlichia chaffeensis infections among HIV-infected patients in a human monocytic ehrlichiosis-endemic area. Emerg Infect Dis. 2003 Sep;9(9):1123-7

Dumler JS, Sutker WL, Walker DH. Persistent infection with Ehrlichia chaffeensis. Clin Infect Dis 1993 17: 903

MMWR. Statewide Surveillance for Ehrlichiosis -- Connecticut and New York, 1994-1997 . MMWR June 19, 1998 / 47(23);476-480

Buller RS, Arens M, Hmiel SP, et al. Ehrlichia ewingii, a newly recognized agent of human ehrlichiosis. N Engl J Med 1999 Jul 15;341(3):148-55

EIKENELLA CORRODENS Joseph Vinetz, M.D.

CLINICAL RELEVANCE & DIAGNOSIS

- Facultatively anaerobic, fastidious, gram-negative rod, pits agar on culture plates
- Component of normal human periodontal flora
- Common component of infected human bites, esp. clenched fist injuries; rare from cat/dog bites
- Member of HACEK group of endocarditis-associated bacteria (Haemophilus spp., Actinobacillus, Cardiobacterium, Eikenella, Kingella)
- Course of infection typically indolent (>1 wk from injury to clinical manifestations of infection)
- Also cause of head and neck infections; respiratory tract infections such as aspiration pneumonia/lung abscess

SITES OF INFECTION

- Human bites: clenched fist injury most common; also affects nail biters (rare)
- Head and neck: periodontitis, floor of mouth; internal jugular septic thrombophlebitis

- Lung: lung abscess; aspiration pneumonia; septic emboli from head and neck infective thrombophlebitis
- Heart: endocarditis, particularly after IV drug abuse
- Gyn: occasionally associated with IUD

TREATMENT REGIMENS

Human bite

- Often present within polymicrobial infection
- Surgical drainage any abscess, critical for optimal management
- Severe infection: parenteral therapy: Amp/sulbactam 1.5-3g IV q6h; other beta lactam/beta lactamase inhibitors also effective
- Oral regimen: Amoxicillin/clavulanate 250-500mg po tid; 875/125mg PO bid
- Third gen. cephalosporin in standard doses as effective as beta lactam/BL inhibitor but ceftriaxone better for continued once daily outpt management
- No role for clindamycin, metronidazole
- Aminoglycosides: no role, no synergy even in endocarditis

Head and neck infections

- Same as for human bite

Endocarditis

- Drugs of choice: Third generation cephalosporins (ceftriaxone 1g IV bid, cefotaxime 1-2g IV q8h, cefepime 1-2g IV q8h)
- Insufficient clinical data for definitive recommendations
- PCN, ampicillin useful, but recent emergence of beta lactamase-producing isolates; few laboratories do sensitivity testing; prudent to avoid these agents unless in vitro susceptibility data obtained

Other sites of infection

- See human bite above
- In case of pulmonary empyema, drainage necessary

IMPORTANT POINTS

- Surgical drainage of collections essential
- Consider polymicrobial infection so that antibiotic selection also covers Strep species, S. aureus, anaerobes

SELECTED READINGS

Sheng WS et al. Eikenella corrodens infections and microbiological characteristics of the causative isolates. Eur J Clin Microbiol Infect Dis 2001;20:231-6

Berbari EF, Cockerill FR 3rd, Steckelberg JM. Infective endocarditis due to unusual or fastidious microorganisms. Mayo Clin Proc 1997; 72:532-42

Goldstein EJ. Current concepts on animal bites: bacteriology and therapy. Curr Clin Top Infect Dis 1999;19:99-111

Talan DA, Citron DM, Abrahamian FM, et al. Bacteriologic analysis of infected dog and cat bites. N Engl J Med. 1999;340:138-40

Talan DA et al. Clinical presentation and bacteriologic analysis of infected human bites in patients presenting to emergency departments. Clin Infect Dis. 2003;37:1481-9

ENTEROBACTER SPECIES
Joseph Vinetz, M.D.

CLINICAL RELEVANCE & DIAGNOSIS
- Gram-negative, aerobic bacilli of the family Enterobacteriaceae; major pathogenic spp. E. cloacae (most common), E. aerogenes, E. agglomerans
- Opportunistic, nosocomial cause of pneumonia, line sepsis, UTI, burn and surgical wound infections, neurosurgery-related meningitis
- Typically resistant to multiple antibiotics, has inducible beta-lactamase (ESBL) which can result in emergence of antibiotic resistance while on therapy
- Enterobacter sakazaki, an emerging pathogen, in premature babies and neonates, contaminates milk-based, powdered infant formulas as well as household environments
- E. sakazaki may be confused with Enterobacter cloacae; distinguished by yellow pigment production, biochemical reactions; important to recognize because of epidemiologic associations

SITES OF INFECTION
- Urinary tract: nosocomial cystitis, pyelonephritis in context of indwelling bladder catheter
- Lung: nosocomial pneumonia
- Skin/wound: colonization and infection of burns, surgical sites, may lead to sepsis; may be part of polymicrobial infection in dirty sites such as decubitus ulcer
- Bloodstream: spread from infected IV catheter or primary site of infection; endocarditis rare
- CNS: nosocomial meningitis related to neurosurgery

TREATMENT REGIMENS
Serious infections
- Double coverage with "synergistic" antibiotics recommended: e.g., beta-lactam/ betalactamase inhibitor + aminoglycoside
- Ceftazidime 2g IV q8h
- Cefepime 2g IV q8-12h
- Piperacillin 3-4g IV q4h
- Piperacillin/tazobactam 3g IV q4-6h
- Ticarcillin/clavulanic acid 3-6g (ticarcillin) IV q4-6h, up to 24 g/d
- Imipenem 500mg IV q6h
- Ciprofloxacin 400mg IV q8-12h
- Any of the above plus gentamicin or tobramycin 1.7mg IV q8h or 5-7mg IV qd or amikacin 7.5mg/kg IV q12h

UTI without systemic signs
- Remove bladder catheter; straight catheterize patient until pyuria cleared
- Single agent such as fluoroquinolone appropriate, duration typically 2 weeks

IMPORTANT POINTS
- Remove infected hardware if possible (bladder catheter, endotracheal tube, peripheral IV or central line, peritoneal dialysis catheter, etc.)
- Consider Enterobacter spp. similar to Pseudomonas aeruginosa: they both can develop resistance to antibiotics during the course of therapy, necessitating double antibiotic coverage for serious infxns

SELECTED READINGS

Lynch JP. Hospital-acquired pneumonia: risk factors, microbiology, and treatment. Chest 119(2 Suppl): 373S-384S, 2001

Chow JW, Yu VL. Combination antibiotic therapy versus monotherapy for gram-negative bacteraemia: a commentary. Int J Antimicrob Agents 11:7-12, 1999

Rochon-Edouard S et al. Comparative in vitro and in vivo study of nine alcohol-based handrubs. Am J Infect Control. 2004;32:200-4

Cordero L et al. Enteric gram-negative bacilli bloodstream infections: 17 years' experience in a neonatal intensive care unit. Am J Infect Control. 2004 Jun;32(4):189-95

Lai KK. Enterobacter sakazakii infections among neonates, infants, children, and adults. Case reports and a review of the literature. Medicine (Baltimore). 2001;80:113-22

ENTEROCOCCUS Jeremy Gradon, M.D. and Joseph Vinetz, M.D.

CLINICAL RELEVANCE & DIAGNOSIS

- Enterococci aerobic gram-positive cocci grow in short chains, part of normal colonic flora.
- Vancomycin resistant enterococci (VRE): E. faecium >> E. faecalis.
- Risk factors: prolonged hospitalization, hemodialysis, ICU stays and broad spectrum antibiotic therapy +/- vancomycin use. No reliable means to terminate VRE colonization.
- Use contact isolation to prevent nosocomial spread on hands of caregivers. VRE colonization impedes transfer of patients to long-term care facilities.
- Association of VRE with morbidity and mortality most significant in debilitated hosts.

SITES OF INFECTION

- E. faecalis: community-acquired UTI, meningitis, endocarditis or part of mixed flora in abdominal abscess around perforated viscus.
- E. faecalis and E. faecium: nosocomial urinary or central venous catheter infections, mixed flora infections in wounds, burns, and after surgery on bowel, pelvis or biliary tract.

TREATMENT REGIMENS

General considerations

- Cephalosporins and TMP-SMX ineffective against enterococci
- Combine ampicillin/penicillin with aminoglycoside (AG) for SBE and serious bacteremia. Lower dose gent (3mg/kg-day) enough for synergy but once daily AG probably inadequate if normal renal function.
- AG synergy with pen/amp lost with high level AG resistance (MIC >500-1000mcg/mL) If gent resistant, test streptomycin. Optimal Rx of SBE with high level AG resistance not defined. High dose pen?
- betalactamase production rare (use nitrocefin disc)
- VRE strains also resistant to amp (83%)
- Prolonged linezolid Rx (>2 wks) ADRS: thrombocytopenia, leukopenia, secondary drug resistance, peripheral neuropathy.
- Prolonged quinupristin/dalfopristin: muscle, joint aching
- Teicoplanin not available in US
- Removal of infected devices usually required for cure.

- Removal of infected IV catheter may result in cure regardless of the use of antibiotics.

Not VRE
- Uncomplicated urinary tract infections with susceptible strains: amoxicillin 1g PO qid.
- Pen allergy: nitrofurantoin 50-100mg qid

Serious infections/SBE without high aminoglycoside resistance
- Ampicillin 3g IV q6h plus gentamicin 1mg/kg q8h
- Penicillin G 5mU IV q6h plus gent 1mg/kg q8h
- Streptomycin 7.5mg/kg (max 500mg) q12h (if gent resistant and streptomycin sensitive).
- Pen allergy: vancomycin 1g IV q12 h plus gent 1mg/kg q8h
- Consider penicillin desensitization for serious infections
- Duration: Endocarditis 4-6 weeks; bacteremia 2 weeks

VRE
- Linezolid 600mg IV q12h (watch plt, wbc!) Switch to PO when stable.
- Daptomycin 4-6mg/kg IV qd
- Quinupristin/dalfopristin (E. faecium only) 7.5mg/kg IV q8h
- VRE UTI only: Fosfomycin 3g PO

Infections w/ high level aminoglycoside resistance
- Optimal Rx of SBE with high level AG resistance not defined. High dose PCN 24mU/d IV?
- Endocarditis Rx > 6wks and/or consider surgery if no response.

IMPORTANT POINTS
- Mortality due to enterococcal infection is as much the result of the patient's underlying status as of the infection itself.
- Contact isolation for VRE. Leave stethoscope, BP cuff in room.
- Change catheters in veins, bladder, peritoneum important, particularly w/VRE. Replacement of prosthetic valves with VRE may be necessary.
- Check for high level AG resistance
- If high dose aminoglycoside resistant consider high dose Pen or daptomycin.

SELECTED READINGS

Maki D, Agger WA. Enterococcal bacteremia: Clinical features, the risk of endocarditis and management. Medicine 1988; 67: 248: 269

Vergis EN, Hayden MK, Chow JW, et al. Determinants of vancomycin resistance and mortality rates in enterococcal bacteremia. A prospective multicenter study. Ann Intern Med 135:484-92, 2001

Zeana C, Kubin CJ, Della-Latta P, Hammer SM. Vancomycin-resistant Enterococcus faecium meningitis successfully managed with linezolid: case report and review of the literature . Clin Infect Dis. 33:477-82, 2001

Raad I, Hachem R, Hanna H et al. Prospective, randomized study comparing quinupristin-dalfopristin with linezolid in the treatment of vancomycin-resistant Enterococcus faecium infections. J Antimicrob Chemother 2004;53:646-9

Padiglione AA, Wolfe R, Grabsch EA et al. Risk factors for new detection of vancomycin-resistant enterococci in acute-care hospitals that employ strict infection control procedures. Antimicrob Agents Chemother. 2003;47:2492-8

ERYSIPELOTHRIX RHUSIOPATHIAE

Joseph Vinetz, M.D.

CLINICAL RELEVANCE & DIAGNOSIS
- Thin, pleomorphic gram-positive rod. Cause of erysipeloid

- Zoonoosis, major reservoir domestic swine, but also from wide variety of animals
- Major animal reservoirs: pigs, sheep, fish, shellfish, domestic fowl
- Major syndromes: mild skin form-erysipeloid (most common); diffuse cutaneous form (rare); sepsis/endocarditis (rare)
- Intrinsically resistant to vancomycin, which may be used empirically unless the organism is properly identified and distinguished from diphtheroids, Corynebacterium spp.

SITES OF INFECTION

- General: sepsis (rare); metastatic skin lesions (rare)
- Skin: erysipeloid (cellulitis; "Rosenbach's Rouget"): purplish-red, spreading patch, raised border, central clearing, starts at site of inoculation; can have bullous forms w/ dissemination
- Cardiovascular: endocarditis; 1/2 on normal valves, usually aortic; Large, shaggy, ulcerated vegs., often occurs in context of sepsis
- Lymph: ~10% of cellulitis cases have associated lymphangitis or regional lymphadenopathy

TREATMENT REGIMENS

Localized infection

- Penicillin; single dose of benzathine PCN 1.2mU; or PCN VK 250mg PO qid x 5-7 d; daily procaine PCN 600,000 to 1.2 mU IM per day for 5-7 d
- Erythromycin 250mg PO qid x 5-7 d
- Doxycycline 100mg bid PO x 5-7 d

Disseminated skin infection

- As for localized infection; assess for endocarditis

Sepsis/endocarditis

- Penicillin 2.4mU IV/day in 4 divided doses +/- streptomycin 1g IV/d or gentamicin 1 mg/kg IV q 8hr for first week
- Evidence for aminoglycoside limited
- Valve replacement possibly needed

IMPORTANT POINTS

- Diagnosis: Erysipeloid: culture of skin bx--lab can confuse with diphtheroids, coryneforms, but E. rhusiopathiae distinguished by H2S production; blood culture
- Prevention: education of occupational risk groups; gloves; vaccination of susceptible herds (not possible for aquatic sources)
- Organism always resistant to vancomycin

SELECTED READINGS

Fidalgo SG et al. Susceptibility of Erysipelothrix rhusiopathiae to antimicrobial agents and home disinfectants. Pathology 2002; 34: 462-465

Brooke CJ and Riley TV. Erysipelothrix rhusiopathiae: bacteriology, epidemiology and clinical manifestations of an occupational pathogen. J Med Microbiol 1999; 48:789-799

Umana, E. Erysipelothrix rhusiopathiae: an unusual pathogen of infective endocarditis. Int J Cardiol 2003; 88:297-299

Freland, C. Erysipeloid. in Infectious Diseases and Medical Microbiology; 2nd Edition, eds Braude AI, Davis CE, Fierer J. Philadelphia: Saunders, 1986

Fidalgo SG, Riley TV. Detection of Erysipelothrix rhusiopathiae in clinical and environmental samples. Methods Mol Biol. 2004;268:199-205

ESCHERICHIA COLI

Paul Auwaerter, M.D.

CLINICAL RELEVANCE & DIAGNOSIS

- Gram-negative rod, Enterobacteriaceae w/ human strains as (1) commensal bowel flora, (2) intestinal pathogenic (enteric/diarrheagenic), (3) extraintestinal pathogenic
- Predominant facultative anaerobe of normal human colonic flora
- Most common cause of UTI, neonatal meningitis, traveler's diarrhea. Seen often w/ intra-abdominal infections. Uncommon cause of nosocomial pneumonia, line-infections.
- E. coli O157:H7 spectrum - 10% nonbloody diarrhea; 90% hemorrhagic colitis, 10% (pts <10 yrs) hemolytic-uremic syndrome [HUS]; <5% w/intestinal and extraintestinal complications
- E. coli easy to grow from sterile specimens. Stool cx: only if chronic diarrhea (need reference lab to ID) or suspect O157:H7 (cx all bloody diarrhea) use sorbitol-MacConkey agar or perform Shiga EIA.
- Appx. 90% strains lactose fermenter; some diarrheagenic E. coli strains, including many of the EIEC strains, typically lactose negative. Indole test 99% (+).

SITES OF INFECTION

- GU: cystitis, pyelonephritis, renal abscess, prostatitis, PID
- GI: traveler's diarrhea (enterotoxigenic > enteroinvasive > enteroadherent strains); intra-abdominal abscess, peritonitis (secondary and SBP)
- Lung: nosocomial pneumonia
- Bloodstream : bacteremia/sepsis secondary to UTI, GI/biliary tract, venous catheter
- Skin/soft tissues: cellulitis--often in diabetics, debilitated w/ decubiti or ulcers; myositis/fasciitis, post-operative wound infections
- CNS: neonatal meningitis, occasional adult nosocomial or geriatric meningitis; brain abscess

TREATMENT REGIMENS

Uncomplicated UTI

- See "Cystitis, Bacterial," "Prostatitis, Bacterial and "Pyelonephritis" in the Diagnoses section
- Preferred agents (IDSA/AUA Guidelines): TMP-SMX DS or fluoroquinolones
- Preferred: TMP-SMX DS PO bid x 3d (Short course) if local resistance is known to be <10 - 20%
- Alt: cipro 250mg PO bid (or 500mg XR qd) x 3d; levofloxacin 250mg PO qday x 3d

Bacteremia/pneumonia/pyelonephritis/other

- Sensitivity data once known should guide abx selection.
- E. coli extended-spectrum beta-lactamase (ESBL) strains uncommon, but consider in nosocomial situations, severe infections requiring MICU care - consider initial carbapenem or aminoglycoside use.
- Ceftriaxone 1-2g IV qd or other third generation cephalosporin
- Ciprofloxacin 400mg IV q12h or 500mg PO q12h, levofloxacin 500mg PO/IV qd, moxifloxacin 400mg IV/PO qd, gatifloxacin 400mg PO/IV qd
- Ampicillin-sulbactam 3g IV q6h +/- gentamicin 1.5mg/kg/q8h or 5-7mg/kg/day IV
- Ampicillin (if sensitive) 2g IV q6h
- TMP-SMX (if sensitive) 5-10mg/kg/d divided q6-8h IV

- Alt: imipenem, meropenem, ertapenem; cefepime; cefazolin or cefuroxime (if sensitive); aztreonam; ticarcillin, piperacillin; piperacillin-tazobactam; aminoglycosides
- 7-14 d therapy common course suggested

Hemolytic-uremic Syndrome E. coli O157:H7

- HUS defined by triad of hemolytic anemia, thrombocytopenia, and renal failure. Sz may be common.
- NO antibiotics; studies suggest increase HUS in children if abx used
- No anti-motility agents
- Notify public health authorities promptly

Gastroenteritis (non-O157:H7)

- See "Traveler's Diarrhea" in the Diagnoses section
- If treatment required (severe sx): cipro 500mg PO bid; ofloxacin 300mg PO bid; norfloxacin 400mg PO bid; TMP-SMX DS PO bid; rifamixin 200mg tid - all drugs given for 3d, except bloody diarrhea x 5d.
- Do not use rifamixin 200mg tid in invasive disease.
- Laboratory confirmation of E. coli induced diarrhea usually unavailable. Most treatment is empiric.
- Dx of ETEC or EAEC requires EIA, DNA probe testing. Many strains resistant to TMP-SMX and doxycycline.
- Alt: bismuth subsalicylate 1048mg PO qid x 5d; Enteroinvasive (EIEC) amp 500mg PO or 1g IV qid x 5d; Enteropathogenic (EPEC) neomycin 50mg/kg/divided q8h or furazolidone 100mg PO qid either x 3-5 d.
- Note: rifamixin not absorbed from GI tract, so do not use if concerned of systemic disease/sepsis.

IMPORTANT POINTS

- Increasingly, E. coli resistant to ampicillin (30-45%) & ciprofloxacin (15%)
- Urine culture is not needed for management of an uncomplicated UTI
- Diagnosis of UTI should be accompanied by an abnormal urine analysis (leukocyte esterase +, nitrites +)
- If hemolytic-uremic syndrome suspected, abx should not be given; stool should be cultured on sorbitol-McConkey agar (notify microbiology) or perform EIA for shiga toxins.

SELECTED READINGS

Warren JW, et al. Guidelines for antimicrobial treatment of uncomplicated acute bacterial cystitis and acute pyelonephritis in women. Clin Infect Dis 1999; 29: 745-758

Guerrant RL, et al. Practice guidelines for the management of infectious diarrhea. Clin Infect Dis 2001; 32: 331-350

Centers for Disease Control & Prevention. Outbreaks of E. coli O157-H7 infections among children associated with farm visits - Pennsylvania and Washington 2000. Morbid Mortal Wkly Rprt 2001; 50: 293-297

Ochoa TJ, Cleary TG. Epidemiology and spectrum of disease of Escherichia coli O157. Curr Opin Infect Dis. 2003 Jun;16(3):259-63

Nataro JP, Kaper JB. Diarrheagenic Escherichia coli. Clin Microbiol Rev. 1998 Jan;11(1):142-201

FRANCISELLA TULARENSIS   John G. Bartlett, M.D.

CLINICAL RELEVANCE & DIAGNOSIS

- Small, pleomorphic, aerobic GNB
- Culture: Poor or no growth on standard media. Requires cysteine in media - thioglycolate, Legionella media. Lab hazard.
- Epidemiology: Tick exposure or contact with rabbits; aerosol - cutting hay, lawn, etc. or BIOTERRORISM
- Bioterrorism: Pneumonia+ pleuritis + hilar adenopathy; Differential - anthrax, plague
- Six clinical forms (see below) - all have incubation period 3-5d (range 1-21), abrupt onset fever
- DIAGNOSIS: DFA stain, PCR, serology +/- cult, BUT hard to grow & lab hazard

SITES OF INFECTION

- Ulceroglandular
- Glandular
- Oculoglandular
- Oropharyngeal
- Pneumonia
- Septicemia

TREATMENT REGIMENS

Post-exposure prophylaxis

- Preferred: Doxycycline 100mg PO bid or ciprofloxacin 500mg PO bid X 14d

Tularemia

- Indications: Tularemia or fever or flu-like illness within 14 days of presumed exposure
- Preferred: Streptomycin 1g IM bid or Gentamicin 5mg/kg/d x 10d
- Alternative (efficacy unproven): Doxycycline 100mg IV bid or chloro 1g IV q6h or cipro 400mg IV bid; Rx until stable then PO for 14-21d (total)
- Pregnancy: Gentamicin 5mg/kg/d IV x 10d, alt - doxy or cipro

Disease control

- Notify Infection Control or other facility contact and health dept if bioterrorism suspected
- No person-to-person transmission. No isolation
- Alert micro lab - need biological safety level 2.
- Surface decontamination - 10% bleach and soapy water
- Clothing - soapy water

IMPORTANT POINTS

- Guidelines from Johns Hopkins Center for Bioterrorism Defense Studies, JAMA 2001;285:2763
- Tularemia endemic SE, Western US & New England islands; most cases ulceroglandular, < 200/yr
- Pneumonic form - must consider bioterrorism; recent outbreak in Nantucket due to lawn mowing
- Dx: Cult & ID requires >1wk. Suspect this dx - blood & sputum, warn lab
- Epidemic pneumonia + ?bioterrorism. Differential: Tularemia, Anthrax, Q fever, Plague

SELECTED READINGS

Dennis TD, Inglesby TV, Henderson DA et al. Tularemia as a biologic weapon. JAMA 2001; 285: 2763

Cross JT, Penn RL. Francisella tularensis (Tularemia). Chapter 216 IN: Principles & Practice Infectious Diseases, 5th Ed. Mandell G, Bennett J, Dolin R, Eds. Churchill Livingston 2000; pg 2393

Dahlstrand S, Ringertz O, Zetterberg. Airborne tularemia in Sweden. Scand J Infect Dis 1971;3:7

Enderlin G, Morales L, Jacobs RP, et al. Streptomycin and alternative agents for the treatment of tularemia. CID 1994;19:42

Evans ME, Gregory DW, Schaffner W, et al. Tularemia: A 30 year experience with 88 cases. Medicine 1985;64:251

HAEMOPHILUS DUCREYI (CHANCROID)

Noreen A. Hynes, M.D., M.P.H.

CLINICAL RELEVANCE & DIAGNOSIS

- A painful genital ulcer disease with adenopathy; uncommon in United state. When occurs in U.S., usually in discrete outbreaks but endemic in some areas.
- Communicable until the ulcer heals; heals with or without Rx but Rx speeds healing. Increases risk of HIV acquisition and transmission.
- Painful inguinal adenitis (buboes) in up to 40%; may suppurate; autoinoculation of eyes and fingers occasionally seen
- Up to 10% co-infected with syphilis therefore MUST Rx for BOTH.
- Autoinoculation of nongenital sites occurs. Trauma/abrasion needed for infection. Painful ulcer + regional painful adenopathy in 1/3 of patients. Painful ulcer + suppuration = high prob. chancroid.
- Chancroid ulcer classically ragged w/ undermined edges, sharply demarcated, no induration; purulent, dirty grey base. Ulcer w/ friable base; bleeds if scraped. Men > 1 ulcer in ~50%. Many women asx.

SITES OF INFECTION

- Genitalia: Genital ulcer
- Inguinal lymph nodes: Following small, missed genital ulcer or with genital ulcer
- Conjunctivae: Autoinoculation from genitalia
- Fingers: Can follow autoinoculation or foreplay

TREATMENT REGIMENS

Regimens in pregnancy

- Ceftriaxone 250mg IM x 1
- Erythromycin base 500mg PO qid x 7d
- Azithromycin: safety and efficacy in pregnancy and lactation not established

Treatment in HIV infection

- Some experts recommend the 7-day erythromycin Rx due to slow healing in this group of patients
- Efficacy of azithromycin and ceftriaxone unknown in this group. Use only if follow up is ensured.

Management of fluctuant buboes

- Incision and drainage is probably preferred Rx in those not adequately responding to antibiotics alone.
- Bubo aspiration is simpler and safer than I&D but reaspiration often needed; sinus tracts may form.

Recommended regimens

- Azithromycin 1g PO x 1
- Ceftriaxone 250mg IM x 1

- Ciprofloxacin 500mg PO bid x 3d
- Erythromycin base 500mg PO qid x 7d

Other management considerations
- Follow-up:Re-examine all pts 3-7d after initiation of Rx. If no clinical improvement: 1) reassess dx, 2) consider coinfxn w/another STD or HIV, 3) consider non-adherence w/ Rx, 4) antibiotic-resistance
- Sex partners: All sex partners during the 10d preceding onset of sx to the present should be examined and treated regardless of symptoms
- Candidates for longer Rx and close follow-up: HIV-infected persons; uncircumcised men

IMPORTANT POINTS
- This module based on the CDC's 2002 STD Rx Guidelines (MMWR 2002; 51 (RR-6).
- Uncircumcised men may be at higher risk; take longer to cure
- No immunity develops after single infection
- More commonly diagnosed in men, esp. if partners include commercial sex workers
- Incubation is 3-5 days; may be as long as 14 days.

SELECTED READINGS

Cole LE et al. A humoral immune response confers protection against Haemophilus ducreyi infection. Infect Immun 2003; 71:6971-6977.

Schmid GP. Treatment of chancroid, 1997. Clin Infect Dis 28(Suppl 1):S14-S20. 1999.

Lewis DA. Diagnostic tests for chancroid. Sex Transm Infect 2000; 76:137-141.

Centers for Disease Control and Prevention. Sexually Transmitted Disease Surveillance, 2000. Atlanta, GA: U.S. Dept of Health and Human Services, CDC, Sept 2001

Ernst AA et al. Incision and drainage versus aspiration of fluctuant buboes in the emergency department during an epidemic of chancroid. Sex Transm Dis 1995;22:217-20

HAEMOPHILUS INFLUENZAE   Paul Auwaerter, M.D.

CLINICAL RELEVANCE & DIAGNOSIS
- Small aerobic gram-negative coccobacilli found mainly in the respiratory tract.
- Encapsulated, type B strains account for most invasive and bacteremic pneumonia.
- Non-typeable strains cause otitis media, acute exacerbations of chronic bronchitis (AECB), sinusitis and nonbacteremic pneumonia.
- Sensitivity of gram-stain and cx probably ~50% for pneumonia. Confusion may arise due to colonization which is higher especially in smokers.
- Infant vaccination has made childhood meningitis, epiglottitis, bacteremia and septic arthritis very uncommon in the US.
- 25-35% of strains worldwide produce beta-lactamase, meaning ampicillin or amoxicillin should only be used for significant infections if susceptibility is known.

SITES OF INFECTION
- Lung: AECB, community acquired pneumonia
- HEENT: epiglottis, sinus, otitis media, peri-orbital cellulitis
- Blood stream: bacteremia, rarely endocarditis
- CNS: meningitis (incidence markedly reduced with use of Hib vaccine. Rare in adults)
- Joints: septic arthritis (often weight-bearing joints)
- Eye: conjunctivitis (subtype aegyptius: Brazilian purpuric fever)

TREATMENT REGIMENS

Non-threatening infections
- Otitis media, acute exacerbation of chronic bronchitis (AECB), sinusitis
- Amoxicillin-clavulanate 500mg tid or 875mg q12h PO (with food)
- Amoxicillin 500mg tid PO. Expect resistance (25-35%), but use if sensitive or empirically treating (eg sinusitis).
- TMP-SMX DS tabs 1 tab PO q12h (some resistance ~7-10%)
- Cefuroxime 250-500mg PO q12h
- Azithromycin 500mg PO x1 then 250mg qd x 4d; clarithromycin 500mg bid or XL 2 tabs 500mg qd x 5-10d telithromycin 400mg bid x 5d
- Moxifloxacin 400mg qd, gatifloxacin 400mg qd, levofloxacin 500mg qd PO.

Meningitis
- Dexamethasone (0.15 mg/kg) 15-20 min before first dose of abx, then q6h x 4d.
- Ceftriaxone 1-2g IV qd-q12h (4g max)
- Cefotaxime 2g IV q4-6h (12g max)
- Use ampicillin [2g IV q4h] if sensitive
- Beta-lactam alternative: ciprofloxacin 400mg IV q12h or other FQ
- Peds: cefotaxime <7 days, <2 kg: 50 mg/kg IV q8h; >2 kg: 50 mg/kg IV q12h; >7 days: >2 kg: 50 mg/kg IV q6-8h; Children: 200 mg/kg/d IV divided q6h.
- Peds ceftriaxone: <7 days old, >2 kg: 50 mg/kg IV q24h; >7 days old, >2 kg: 75 mg/kg IV q24h; Children: 100 mg/kg IV divided q12-24h.
- In pediatric studies, at 24h, clinical condition & mean prognostic score significantly better in dex-treated patients. F/u exams demonstrated significant decrease in audiologic and neuro sequelae.
- Antibiotic Rx duration: 10-14d

Severe Infection
- e.g., pneumonia, epiglottis, severe cellulitis, septic arthritis
- Ceftriaxone 1-2g IV qd q12h
- Cefotaxime 2g IV q6h
- PCN alternative: ciprofloxacin 400mg IV q12h or other FQ. TMP-SMX another possibility, although some resistance described.
- Use ampicillin [2g IV q6h] if sensitive
- See specific diagnosis module for details of nonantimicrobial management.

Prevention
- Haemophilus influenzae type b (Hib) vaccine--series of four immunizations: 2, 4, 6 and 12-15mos.
- Catch-up schedule (if > 1mo. behind schedule): 0, 4 and 8 weeks final [total of 3 if > 12mos at start].
- 3 conjugate vaccines licensed, if PRP-OMP used (Pedvax HIV or ComVax) dose at 6mos not required. DTaP/Hib should not be used at 2, 4 or 6 mos, but can be used as booster thereafter.
- Some groups respond poorly to immunization, e.g., Native Alaskans.
- Absent spleen places host at increased risk for invasive H. influenzae. Hib immunization recommended prior to elective splenectomy.
- Otherwise Hib generally not recommended for those >5yrs. age.
- Post-meningitis exposure prophylaxis: Rifampin 600mg PO q12h x 4 doses
- Contact defined as spending at least 4h/d for 5/7d preceding hospitalization of index case. Rifampin only effective if taken within 7d of index hospitalization.

- Chemoprophylaxis not recommended if all household contacts under 48mos have completed Hib immunizations, unless child is immunocompromised.

IMPORTANT POINTS

- The childhood vaccination campaign using protein-conjugated H. influenzae antigens has virtually eliminated invasive H. influenzae type B infections in children in the US
- Adults usually infected with non-typeable H. influenzae, hence reason Hib immunization not recommended after age 5.
- Most H. influenzae rx'd empirically, since cx not obtained for sinusitis, AECB, OM etc. Significance of beta-lactamase production or empiric use of amp/amoxicillin unclear in these settings.
- A patient with suspected epiglottitis should never be left unattended (e.g., for x-rays etc.) - it is better to forgo the test than to leave the patient alone.

SELECTED READINGS

Shann F. Haemophilus influenzae pneumonia: Type b or non-type b?. Lancet 1999; 354: 1488-1490

Centers for Disease Control & Prevention. Progress toward eliminating Haemophilus influenzae type B disease among infants and children - United States, 1987-1997. Morbid Mortal Wkly Rprt 1998; 47: 993-998

Roson B, et al. Prospective study of the usefulness of sputum gram stain in the initial approach to community-acquired pneumonia requiring hospitalization. Clin Infect Dis 2000; 31: 869-874

Ghaffar F, et al. Effects of amoxicillin-clavulanate or azithromycin on nasopharyngeal carriage of Streptococcus pneumoniae and Haemophilus influenzae in children with acute otitis media. Clin Infect Dis 2000; 31: 875-880

Doern GV, Brown SD. Antimicrobial susceptibility among community-acquired respiratory tract pathogens in the USA: data from PROTEKT US 2000-01. J Infect. 2004 Jan;48(1):56-65

KLEBSIELLA SPECIES   Joseph Vinetz, M.D.

CLINICAL RELEVANCE & DIAGNOSIS

- Gram-negative, aerobic bacilli of the family Enterobacteriaceae. Major pathogens: K. pneumoniae, K. oxytoca
- Cause of lobar pneumonia (major syndrome), urinary tract infections, biliary and surgical wound infections (often in association with other organisms), rhinoscleroma (rare)
- Often, but not always, nosocomial pathogen
- Lobar pneumonia due to K. pneumoniae typically in debilitated, elderly, alcoholic or diabetic patients
- Lobar pneumonia often necrotic, associated with "currant jelly" sputum and abscess/cavity on chest Xray, classic "bowed fissure sign" caused by swollen upper lung lobe impinging on lower lobe
- Klebsiella spp. often resistant to many abxs, including cephalosporins (eg extended spectrum beta-lactamase/ESBL) and aminoglycosides; empiric coverage should be tailored to local resistance patterns

SITES OF INFECTION

- Lung: both nosocomial and community acquired in elderly, debilitated, alcoholic, diabetic patients
- Urinary tract: bladder and kidney, usually nosocomial, often catheter-related, may lead to sepsis

- Bloodstream: usually associated with primary organ system infection; can be peripheral IV or central venous catheter associated; neutropenic fever due to intestinal source
- Eye: endophthalmitis (rare), in association with liver abscess, diabetes
- Bone and joints: in association with decubitis ulcers leading to polymicrobial infection
- Nasal passages: Rhinoscleroma (Mikulwicz cells--foamy macrophages with ingested bacilli) due to K. rhinoscleromatis

TREATMENT REGIMENS

Urinary tract infection

- Uncomplicated UTI: Empiric oral fluoroquinolone, change according to in vitro sensitivities
- Complicated UTI: cephalosporins, advanced penicillins, fluoroquinolones as for pneumonia
- Complicated UTI: gentamicin or tobramycin 1.5mg IV q8h or 5-7mg IV qd or amikacin 7.5mg/kg IV q12h or 15 mg/kg IV qd

Pneumonia

- Ceftazidime 2g IV q8h
- Cefepime 2g IV q12h
- Piperacillin 4g IV q4h
- Ticarcillin 3-4g IV q6h
- Imipenem 500mg IV q6h
- Ciprofloxacin 400mg IV q8-12h; other fluoroquinolones in standard maximum doses
- Aztreonam 1g IV q8h

IMPORTANT POINTS

- Consider aspiration mechanism in pneumonia, with concomitant need to treat anaerobic bacteria that may be present
- Single agent appropriate for both UTI and pneumonia because emergence of resistance on monotherapy not expected
- Aminoglycosides not used in cavitary pulmonary disease

SELECTED READINGS

Paterson DL, Ko WC, Von Gottberg A, et al. Outcome of cephalosporin treatment for serious infections due to apparently susceptible organisms producing extended-spectrum beta-lactamases: implications for the clinical microbiology laboratory. J Clin Microbiol 39(6):2206-12, 2001

Meyer KS, Urban C, Eagan JA, et al. Nosocomial outbreak of Klebsiella infection resistant to late-generation cephalosporins. Ann Intern Med 119(5):353-8, 1993

Waters V et al. Molecular epidemiology of gram-negative bacilli from infected neonates and health care workers' hands in neonatal intensive care units. Clin Infect Dis. 2004;38:1682-7

Andraca R, Edson RS, Kern EB. Rhinoscleroma: a growing concern in the United States? Mayo Clinic experience . Mayo Clin Proc 68:1151-7, 1993

LEGIONELLA SPECIES

John G. Bartlett, M.D.

CLINICAL RELEVANCE & DIAGNOSIS

- Detection of Legionella from any human specimen means disease - it doesn't colonize
- Pneumonia (Legionnaires' disease) has 10-25% mortality rate
- Pontiac fever is flu-like syndrome without pneumonia, doesn't kill and doesn't require antibiotics
- Legionella is rare cause of endocarditis, wound infection, pancreatitis, sinusitis and encephalitis

- Preferred tests: Culture respiratory tract specimen (selective media) and urinary antigen for L. pneumophila serogroup 1
- Dx: Urinary antigen (detects only L. pneumophila serogroup 1, but causes ~70 - 80% of cases); alternatives: respir. secretion PCR, cx (often falsely negative & takes >3-5d), & paried serology.
- New test: PCR on respiratory secretions to detect L. pneumophila serogroups (Becton Dickenson)

SITES OF INFECTION

- Lung: pneumonia (may be lobar, patchy, interstitial)
- Systemic (Pontiac fever)
- Miscellaneous sites: endocarditis, wound infection, sinusitis

TREATMENT REGIMENS

Pneumonia

- Preferred (fluoroquinolone + rifampin): Levofloxacin 750mg/d PO or IV X 7-10d; Gatifloxacin 400mg/d PO or IV 10-14d; Azithromycin 500mg/d PO or IV 7-10d
- Rifampin 300mg PO or IV bid + any other agent listed (optional)
- Alternative: erythromycin 1g IV q6h, then 500mg PO qid 7-10d total
- Alternative: ciprofloxacin 400mg IV q12h, then 750mg PO bid 7-10d total
- Alternative: doxycycline 100mg IV q12h, then 100mg PO bid 7-10d

Other sites

- Endocarditis: fluoroquinolone (see "Pneumonia" above) + rifampin 300mg PO bid x 4-6wks. Valve replacement usually required
- Pontiac Fever: No abx (self-limited)

Outbreaks

- Most outbreaks are in hospitals and hotels; most cases are sporadic
- Identify water source by culture (50-70% of all water sources yield Legionella)
- Match water source and clinical strains by species/serogroup and location
- Intervention: 1) copper-silver ionization; 2) superheat to 60C-77C & flushing; 3) ultraviolet light for localized areas

IMPORTANT POINTS

- Information is from Stout JE (NEJM 1997;337:682) and Edelstein P (Ann Intern Med 1998;129:128)
- Legionella causes one common and important disease--Legionnaires' disease; also causes Pontiac fever and endocarditis.
- Legionnaires' disease may be epidemic or sporadic, nosocomial or community acquired. Typical host: >40, smoker, compromised CMI (cancer Rx, organ tx, steroids) See Table 11 in Appendix I
- Natural habitat is water - all water
- Intracellular pathogen - effective drugs in animal models - fluoroquinolones, macrolides, TMP-SMX, rifampin, doxycycline.

SELECTED READINGS

Bartlett JG, Dowell SF, Mandell LA, et al. Practice guidelines for community-acquired pneumonia. CID 2000;31:347

Stout JE, Yu VL. Legionellosis. NEJM 1997;337:682

Edelstein PH. Antimicrobial therapy for Legionnaires' disease: time for a change. Ann Intern Med 1998;129:128

Fenstersheib MD, Miller M, Diggins C, et al. Outbreak of Pontiac fever due to Legionella anisa. Lancet 1990;1:336

Thomas DL, Mundy LM, Tucker PC. Hot tub legionellosis. Legionnaires' disease and Pontiac fever a point-source exposure to Legionella pneumophila. Arch Intern Med 1993;153:2597

LEPTOSPIRA INTERROGANS   Joseph Vinetz, M.D.

CLINICAL RELEVANCE & DIAGNOSIS

- One of 4 spirochetes pathogenic for humans
- Zoonotic disease, transmitted by domestic animals (dogs, cattle, pigs, and more) and rodents (rats, mice)
- Transmitted in inner cities, suburban and rural areas.
- Risk factors include farming, slaughterhouse work, walking in alleys, swimming in fresh water (viz. triathletes, kayaking), being a flood victim
- May be biphasic illness: septicemic phase then immune phase (fever, meningitis)
- Consider dx with fever, elevated bilirubin, elevated creatinine, transaminases ~5-7-fold above normal
- Complications: renal failure, hemorrhage, myocarditis; mortality can be as high as 25% if untreated
- Hx: abrupt onset fever, severe leg muscle aches, in appropriate epidemiological context
- In U.S., Hawaii endemic for leptospirosis
- Diagnosis uncommon, depends on serology or culture in specialized laboratory

SITES OF INFECTION

- Systemic illness with protean manifestations; multi-organ involvement possible
- Liver: jaundice, transaminases can be normal or elevated typically no more than 5-fold to 7-fold above normal
- Renal: acute renal failure usually resolves, but may require dialysis; ATN, interstitial nephritis; RBCs, WBCs, protein seen in urine; IV fluids may obviate need for dialysis
- Pulmonary: hemorrhage; atypical pneumonia, scattered patchy infiltrates, or ARDS
- Cardiac: EKG abnormalities common; myocarditis; heart failure
- CNS: aseptic meningitis (CSF WBCs 10-1000); hyporeflexia and axonal motor weakness
- GI: intestinal hemorrhage (rare); elevated lipase, amylase mimicking pancreatitis; mimics cholecystitis leading to surgery
- Eye: conjunctival suffusion (dilated small vessels); hypopyon; uveitis
- Derm: non-specific rash can occur, not typical

TREATMENT REGIMENS

Penicillin
- 1.5 mU IV q6 hr for hospitalized patients x 5-7 d

Doxycycline
- 100mg bid IV or PO x 5-7 d

Ceftriaxone
- 1g IV q day x 5-7 d

IMPORTANT POINTS

- Definitive recent source: Levett PN; Leptospirosis; Clin Microbiol Rev. 14:296-326, 2001.
- Diagnosis: Two FDA-approved commercially available kits are available, an Indirect Hemagglutination (MRL) and a dipstick test (PanBio). The dipstick test is much better in my opinion.

- In U.S., definitive testing (culture and microagglutination test (MAT) only available at CDC through state health labs, and at Vinetz lab at the U. of Cal San Diego (joseph_vinetz@hotmail.com)
- Cultures should be obtained prior to abx; some commercial blood culture systems do not kill leptospires, and such specimens should be sent expeditiously to CDC or UCSD for specific lepto cultures.
- Epidemiology: Lepto can be transmitted to humans from vaccinated animals (e.g., cattle or dogs)--the vaccine may prevent animal illness but not the chronic carrier/transmission state

SELECTED READINGS

Vinetz JM. 10 Common Questions about Leptospirosis. Infect. Dis. in Clin. Practice 9:19-25, 2000

Vinetz JM et al. Sporadic Urban Leptospirosis. Annals of Internal Medicine 125:794-98, 1996.

Levett PN. Leptospirosis. Clin Microbiol Rev. 14:296-326, 2001

Bharti AR et al. Leptospirosis: a zoonotic disease of global importance. Lancet Infect Dis. 2003 Dec;3 (12):757-71

Panaphut T. Ceftriaxone compared with sodium penicilling for treatment of severe leptospirosis. Clin Infect Dis. 2003;36:1507-13

LISTERIA MONOCYTOGENES   John G. Bartlett, M.D.

CLINICAL RELEVANCE & DIAGNOSIS

- Small gram-positive rod; grows on routine media
- Colonizes colon in 5% of adults
- Important cause of foodborne disease in vulnerable: pregnancy, compromised CMI, elderly
- Important cause meningitis in compromised host and persons >50yrs
- Dx: cult from normally sterile site (CSF, blood, etc); serology (listeriolysin O antibody) in foodborne outbreaks

SITES OF INFECTION

- Septicemia
- CNS: Meningitis/brain abscess/rhomboencephalitis (rare)
- Pregnancy: Bacteremia with stillbirth and/or premature delivery
- Gastroenteritis
- Endocarditis
- Focal infections: Lymphadenitis, cellulitis, pneumonia, osteomyelitis, septic arthritis, conjunctivitis

TREATMENT REGIMENS

Infections

- Principles: Most common serious forms - meningitis, esp w/ defective CMI & age >50; Rx - amp +/- gent; also 3rd trimester pregnancy - same Rx
- Meningitis: Preferred (consensus choice): Ampicillin 2g IV q4-6h +/- gentamicin 1.7mg/kg IV q8h x >/- 3wks
- Meningitis: Alternative (pen allergy): TMP-SMX 3-5mg/kg (trimeth) q6h IV x >/- 3wks
- Bacteremia: Meningitis options x 2wks
- Brain abscess or rhombencephalitis: Meningitis options x 4-6wks
- Gastroenteritis: No antibiotic treatment

Prophylaxis

- Recommendations from CDC (ASM News 1993;59:444) and Medical Letter 2004;2:22

- Thoroughly cook animal source food
- Thoroughly wash raw vegetables
- Avoid unpasteurized milk and food from unpasteurized milk
- Wash hands, utensils & cutting boards used with uncooked food
- Keep ready-to-eat food cold

Prevention in high-risk persons

- High risk - pregnant women, CMI compromise (organ transplants, chronic steroids, infliximab, cancer chemo Rx, AIDS), elderly
- Avoid soft cheeses - Mexican style, feta, brie, camembert, blue cheese
- Leftover foods and ready-to-eat foods should be steaming hot
- May wish to avoid food from delicatessen counters

IMPORTANT POINTS

- Recommendations: Authors opinion & consensus from B. Lorber (see references)
- Major risks: 1) compromised CMI (steroids, transplants, cancer chemo Rx, AIDS); 2) 3rd trimester pregnancy; 3) occasional cases: age >50yrs, diabetes, ulcerative colitis, antacids, cirrhosis
- Mortality: meningitis 20%; endocarditis 50%; pregnant women 20% stillbirths
- Major source: ingestion unpasteurized milk; fresh cheeses (esp imported, soft, ripened), ice cream, raw veg, fermented raw sausages, raw/cooked poultry, raw meats, smoked fish; deli meats & hot dogs
- Think Listeria when: "diphtheroids" in CSF, meningitis in comp host or >50 yrs, fever 3rd trimester, foodborne outbreak w/ neg cult.

SELECTED READINGS

Marco F, Almela M, Nolla-Salas J, et al. In vitro activities of 22 antimicrobial agents against Listeria monocytogenes strains isolated from Barcelona, Spain. Diag Microbiol Inf Dis 2000;38:259

CDC. Diagnosis and management of foodborne illnesses. MMWR 2001;50RR-2:pg13

Lorber B. Listeria monocytogenes. Chapter 195 IN: Principles & Practice of Infect Dis, Mandell G, Bennett J & Dolin R. 5th Ed, Churchill Livingston, 2000; p 2208

Dalton CB, Austin CC, Sobel J, et al. An outbreak of gastroenteritis and fever due to Listeria monocytogenes in milk. NEJM 1997;336:100

Durand ML, Calderwood SB, Weber DJ, et al. Acute bacterial meningitis in adults. A review of 493 episodes. NEJM 1993;328:21

MORAXELLA CATARRHALIS   John G. Bartlett, M.D.

CLINICAL RELEVANCE & DIAGNOSIS

- Gram-negative diplococcus - appears identical to N. gonorrhoeae
- Grows easily on blood chocolate agar
- Colonizes upper airways in 1-5%; found only in humans
- Causes disease by contiguous spread - otitis, sinusitis, acute exacerbations of chronic bronchitis

SITES OF INFECTION

- Sinusitis
- Otitis
- Exacerbations - chronic bronchitis
- Pneumonia
- Bacteremia (<100 reported cases)
- Endocarditis

TREATMENT REGIMENS

Treatment
- Abx guideline - Med Letter 2004;2:22
- Preferred: TMP-SMX 1DS bid PO
- ALT: macrolide - erythro 500mg qid, clarithro XL 1gm/d or 500mg bid, azithro 500mg, then 250mg/d
- ALT: tetracycline - doxycycline 100mg PO/IV bid
- CEPH: cefuroxime, cefotaxime, ceftriaxone
- ALT: oral cephs - cefuroxime, cefpodoxime
- ALT FQ: moxifloxacin (Avelox) 400mg PO qd, levofloxacin (Levaquin) 500mg IV/PO, gatifloxacin (Tequin) 400mg IV/PO qd
- ALT: amox-clavulanate (Augmentin) 875mg bid PO

IMPORTANT POINTS
- Abx guidelines - Med Letter 2004;2:22
- Respiratory tract pathogen in sinusitis, otitis, AECB - rare cause pneumonia
- Produces betalactamase - 95% of strains resistant to amoxicillin
- Nearly every abx except pen and amoxicillin work (TMP-SMX, ceph, macrolide, doxy)
- Looks like meningococcus & gonococcus on GS; causes contiguous disease, not invasive disease

SELECTED READINGS

Collazos J, deMiguel J, Ayarza R. Moraxella catarrhalis bacteremia pneumonia in adults: two case reports and review of the literature. Eur J Clin Microbiol Infect Dis 1992;11:237

Lieberman D, Lieberman D, Ben-Yaakov M, et al. Infectious etiologies in acute exacerbations of COPD. Diag Microbiol Infect Dis 2001;40:95

Kilpi T, Herva E, Kaijalainen T, et al. Bacteriology of acute otitis media in a cohort of Finnish children followed for the first two years of life. Pediatr Infect Dis 2001;20:654

Biedenbach DJ, Jones RN, Pfaller MA, et al. Activity of BMS 284756 against 2,681 recent clinical isolates of Haemophilus influenzae and Moraxella catarrhalis: Report from SENTRY Antimicrobial Surveillance Program(2000) in Europe, Canada & US. Diag Microbiol Infect Dis 2001;39:245

Stefanou J, Agelopoulou AV, Sipsas NV, et al. Moraxella catarrhalis endocarditis: case report and review of the literature. Scand J Infect Dis 2000;32:217

MYCOBACTERIUM AVIUM-INTRACELLULARE (MAI, NON-HIV)

Susan Dorman, M.D.

CLINICAL RELEVANCE & DIAGNOSIS
- M. avium complex (M. avium and M. intracellulare) strains are frequent causes of mycobacterial lung disease in the USA.
- Environmental sources, especially water, are the reservoir for most human infections.
- No convincing evidence for person-to-person spread of MAI
- Commercially available nucleic acid probe test can identify cultured mycobacteria as MAI. No PCR or other rapid test FDA-approved for direct use on sputum or blood.
- M. avium and M. intracellulare are slow growing mycobacteria (10-21 days on solid media).
- Antimicrobial susceptibility testing: clinically relevant for clarithromycin; indicated for isolates from patients on prior macrolide therapy/prevention.

SITES OF INFECTION

- Pulmonary - fibrocavitary, "TB"-like: typically apical location, male predominance (50 + years old), pre-existing lung disease (smoking-related, silicosis, bronchiectasis, cystic fibrosis).
- Pulmonary - nodular (often bilateral), or isolated RML or lingula infiltrate/cavity: female predominance (40+ years old), associated with pectus excavatum/mitral valve prolapse/thoracic scoliosis
- Extrapulmonary localized (skin, soft tissue, joints, tendons, bones): less common than pulmonary disease, but may occur after trauma or environmental exposure.
- Cervical lymphadenitis: typically in children ages 1-5 years; may occur in immunocompetent children.
- Disseminated: rare except in AIDS patients; typically occurs in immunocompromised hosts (exogenous immunosuppression, SCID, IFN gamma or IL-12 pathway disorders).
- Pulmonary - "hot tub lung": diffuse lung disease with cough/fever/hypoxia. Non-necrotizing granulomatous inflammation +/- interstitial pneumonia. Pathogenesis unclear--"infection" vs. hypersensitivity.

TREATMENT REGIMENS

Pulmonary MAI Disease

- Clarithromycin + rifabutin + ethambutol (+/- aminoglycoside for first 8-12 weeks). Alternative azithromycin+ (rifampin or rifabutin) + ethambutol (+/- aminoglycoside for 8-12 wks). (AJRCCM 1997;156:S1)
- Doses: clarithromycin 500mg PO bid (250mg bid for weight < 50 kg); azithromycin 250mg/d; rifampin 600mg PO qd; rifabutin 300mg PO qd; ethambutol 25mg/kg/d for 2 months then 15mg/kg/d
- Monitor for uveitis if clarithromycin and rifabutin used together.
- Duration of treatment not definitively established. Typical duration is 18-24 months total, including 12 months after sputum culture becomes negative for MAI. Monitor sputum smear and culture monthly.
- Aminoglycoside choice: amikacin (15-20 mg/kg, 2 or 3 times per week) most active against MAI. Severity of MAI disease, immunosuppression, toxicities important in considering use of aminoglycoside.
- Thrice weekly macrolide-containing regimens for pulmonary MAI may be comparable to daily therapy and better tolerated but have not been directly compared (see references).
- Adjunctive treatment when clinically indicated: bronchial hygiene (inhaled beta agonists, mucus-clearing devices), treatment as needed for nonmycobacterial pulmonary superinfection.
- Role of surgery: no randomized studies; typically reserved for patients with poor response to medical tx and who are good surgical candidates. Should be performed in centers with extensive experience.
- Clinical expectations of treatment: symptomatic and radiographic improvement within 2-6 months, and conversion of sputum culture from positive to negative within approximately 6 months.

- Monitoring for drug adverse reactions: hepatotoxicity (rifampin, rifabutin); uveitis (rifabutin); ocular toxicity (ethambutol); nephrotoxicity and/or ototoxicity (aminoglycosides).

Hot tub lung

- Discontinuation of exposure necessary. No consensus opinion about role of corticosteroids and/or antibiotics. Anecdotal reports of rapid improvement after stopping exposure (no steroids or antibiotic)

Cervical lymphadenitis in children

- Excisional surgery without chemotherapy (success rate of > 95%).
- If surgical risk high (e.g., facial nerve involvement), clarithromycin-containing multidrug regimen is reasonable, but limited experience, optimal duration unknown
- Incisional biopsy, or use of non-macrolide-containing regimens often associated with persistent clinical disease including sinus tract formation.

Extrapulmonary localized disease

- Surgery (excisional or debridement) plus clarithromycin-containing multidrug regimen (same doses as for pulmonary disease). Optimal duration unknown.

Disseminated disease

- Clarithromycin-containing multidrug regimen (same doses as for pulmonary disease); optimal duration unknown and dependent on clinical response and predisposing factors.

IMPORTANT POINTS

- Interpretation of a single positive respiratory culture for MAI should take into account the possibility of environmental contamination.
- MAI lung disease is typically associated with persistently positive respiratory cultures, with heavy MAI growth. Most experts recommend a thoracic CT as part of diagnostic workup for pulmonary MAI.
- For pulmonary MAI disease, ATS diagnostic criteria are guidelines and applicability in specific patients should be carefully considered by an experienced clinician.
- For patients with positive MAI respiratory cultures in whom decision is made not to treat MAI, long-term close followup is essential (symptoms, repeat sputum exams, thoracic CT scans).
- For macrolide resistant dz: (moxifloxacin 400mg qd or levofloxacin 500 to 750mg qd) + ethambutol 15mg/kg/d + rifabutin 300mg qd +/- IV amikacin 10-15mg/kg/d

SELECTED READINGS

American Thoracic Society. Diagnosis and treatment of disease caused by nontuberculous mycobacteria. Am J Respir Crit Care Med 1997;156(Suppl):S1-S25.

M.D. Iseman. Medical management of pulmonary disease caused by Mycobacterium avium complex. Clinics in Chest Medicine 2002;23:633-41.

A Khoor et al. Diffuse pulmonary disease caused by nontuberculous mycobacteria in immunocompetent people (hot tub lung). Am J Clin Pathol 2001;115:755-62.

TR Aksamit. Mycobacterium avium complex pulmonary disease in patients with pre-existing lung disease. Clinics in Chest Medicine 2002;23:643-53.

RJ Wallace, Jr et al. Repeat positive cultures in Mycobacterium intracellulare lung disease after macrolide therapy represent new infections in patients with nodular bronchiectasis. J Infect Dis 2002;186:266-73.

MYCOPLASMA PNEUMONIAE   Paul Auwaerter, M.D.

CLINICAL RELEVANCE & DIAGNOSIS

- Aerobic, fastidious organism. Frequent cause of atypical pneumonia. Peaks late summer/fall, most frequent in children/young adults but also elderly; may cause epidemics (schools, barracks).
- Extrapulmonary abnormalities frequently associated with infection (see sites of infection).
- Cold agglutinin ABs occur in 50-70%, but nonspecific. These anti-I IgM ABs are directed against rbc antigen; may be associated w/ hemolysis, renal failure, Raynaud's. Peak 2-3 wks, last 2-3 mos.
- Dx: If sputum produced see PMN's without bacteria (org. lacks cell wall so does not pick up gram stain). Cold agglutinin titer 1:32 or greater supportive. Bedside cold agg. if + = equiv. titer 1:64.
- Dx: Mycoplasma IgM more specific, but commonly neg. first 7-10d. DNA detection by GenProbe or PCR on sputum ~89-95% sens./specificity compared to culture/serology; throat swabs results worse.
- Dx: Most labs do not perform mycoplasma cx routinely. Need special transport media and cx methods, then 1-2wks to show characteristic mulberry colonies on culture.

SITES OF INFECTION

- Respiratory: Appears like URI with 5-10% developing tracheobronchitis or pneumonia. Often with headache. Distinguish from virus by gradual progression of sx over 1-2d (vs. abrupt onset w/influenza).
- Resp. (2): dry cough, nontoxic ("walking pneumonia"). Often minimal exam findings compared to CXR. Pleural effusion 5-20%.
- HEENT: bullous myringitis VERY RARE w/ native infection. Frequent association only with experimental inoculation.
- Derm: Erythema multiforme in 7% esp. children. Also Stevens-Johnson, macular or morbilliform or papulovesicular rashes.
- Cardiac: arrhythmias, CHF in up to 10%. EKG changes common, esp. conduction abnl.
- Neuro: Meningoencephalitis, aseptic meningitis, Guilliain-Barre, ataxia,transverse myelitis, peripheral neuropathy. Association based on serology making true causation uncertain.
- Heme: hemolytic anemia (rarely clinically significant)
- Rheum: occasional arthritis, transient Raynaud's phenomenon.

TREATMENT REGIMENS

Pneumonia

- Often not severe, rather mild and self-limited. Antibiotics may shorten duration, though cough may linger for weeks. Beta-lactams ineffective since organism lacks cell wall.
- Usual dose duration is 2-3 weeks, but this is not based on prospective study.
- Erythromycin 250mg PO qid or doxycycline 100mg PO bid are traditional and inexpensive choices.
- Newer, more expensive drugs with excellent in vitro MIC's include: azithromycin 250mg qd, clarithromycin 250mg q12h, levofloxacin 250mg PO qd, moxifloxacin 400mg PO qd, gatifloxacin 400mg qd.
- New drugs not superior over older; however, definitive dx of mycoplasma rare at time of treatment decision.

- Dosing of FQ & adv. macrolides ~1/2 of usual empiric pneumonia doses, as M. pneumoniae very sensitive to these drugs.
- Treatment recommendations from S. Baum, Chapter 172 "Principles & Practice of Inf. Diseases," 5th ed; 2000.

Upper respiratory tract infections
- Most go undiagnosed.
- Supportive care, antimicrobials not required as infection self-limited.

Extrapulmonary disease
- Effect of antibiotics unknown, but using 10-14d of a drug listed in the pneumonia section likely prudent.

Prevention
- Outbreaks described in the military, families and long-term care facilities.
- Prophylaxis: azithromycin 500mg day 1 then 250mg days 2-5 (ZPAK) may reduce secondary attack rate.

IMPORTANT POINTS
- Problematic diagnosis since culture difficult, serology insensitive at time of patient presentation. Sputum GeneProbe or PCR probably best for rapid, accurate diagnosis but availability limited.
- Normal WBC # and clear chest exam despite pneumonia on CXR should prompt consideration of atypical pneumonias, esp. Mycoplasma.
- Bedside cold agg. test: draw blood into anticoagulant test tube, cool to 4C and formerly smooth adherence of rbcs to glass display macroscopic agglutination that reverses with warming.
- M. pneumoniae often severe in sickle cell pts w/ overwhelming infection--severe cold agglutinin disease causing digital necrosis.
- Cold agg. AB are insensitive and nonspecific for M. pneumoniae dx. Comp. fix. and anti-IgM AB more specific, but arise later in infection therefore less helpful since frequently neg. at presentation.

SELECTED READINGS

Ritkind D, Chanock R, Kravetz H et al. Ear involvement (myringitis) and primary atypical pneumonia following inoculation of volunteers with Eaton agent. Ann Otol Rhinol Laryngol 1976; 85:140

Klausner JD, Passaro D, Rosenberg J et al. Enhanced control of an outbreak of Mycoplasma pneumoniae pneumonia with azithromycin prophylaxis. J Infect Dis. 1998 Jan;177(1):161-6

Smith R, Eviatar L. Neurologic manifestations of Mycoplasma pneumoniae infections: diverse spectrum of diseases. A report of six cases and review of the literature. Clin Pediatr (Phila). 2000 Apr;39(4):195-201

Chan ED, Welsh CH. Fulminant Mycoplasma pneumoniae pneumonia. West J Med. 1995 Feb;162 (2):133-42

Fekety FR Jr, Caldwell J, Gump D, et al. Bacteria, viruses, and mycoplasmas in acute pneumonia in adults. Am Rev Respir Dis. 1971 Oct;104(4):499-507

NEISSERIA GONORRHOEAE

Noreen A. Hynes, M.D., M.P.H.

CLINICAL RELEVANCE & DIAGNOSIS
- Gram-negative appearing as diplococci, transmitted sexually or perinatally. Infects mucous membranes GU and GI tracts.

- Still remains a major bacterial STD in parts of US, particularly large cities; US rate in 2000 was 132/100,000; about 600,000 cases/yr
- Fluoroquinolone (FQ) resistance is increasing. Do not use to Rx GC in men who have sex with men or infxn acquired in Asia, the Pacific Basin, HI, CA, MA, or New York City.
- Incubation period is 3-7 days in men; unclear duration in women but maybe 10 days
- In men, usually causes symptomatic urethritis; BUT up to 25% of infections asymptomatic. Epididymitis is most frequent complication of GC in men.
- Less common complications in men include "Bull headed clap," urethral stricture, prostatitis
- Up to 50% of infections in women are asymptomatic. In women accessory gland infections, perihepatitis, perinatal morbidity, PID can occur.
- In both sexes anorectal infection, pharyngitis, conjunctivitis and disseminated infxn are seen
- Disseminated gonococcal infection (DGI) including gonococcal tenosynovitis is increasingly rare; severe DGI (meningitis or endocarditis) should be managed w/ help from an ID consultant
- Gram stains: urethral & accessory gland secretions (~95% sensitive); female cervical secretions (~50%). Don't gram stain pharyngeal secretions due to N. meningitidis. Test all sites to increase yield.

SITES OF INFECTION
- Urethra: urethritis
- Cervix: cervicitis
- Epididymis: epididymitis
- Accessory glands (Skene's, Bartholin's), Fallopian tubes: PID
- Endometrium: endometritis
- Glisson's capsule of the liver: (Fitz-Hugh-Curtis syndrome)
- Throat: pharyngitis
- Conjunctiva: conjunctivitis
- Anorectum: proctitis
- Dissemination: skin lesions, arthralgia, tenosynovitis, arthritis, hepatitis, myocarditis, endocarditis, meningitis

TREATMENT REGIMENS

Uncomplicated infxn of cervix, urethra, rectum
- Standard of Care = 2 drug regimen to Rx gonorrhea and chlamydia if chlamydia infection not ruled out.
- Cefixime 400mg PO (as 20mL of 100mg/5mL suspension - only form available) x 1 plus antichlamydial if chlamydia not ruled out (azithromycin 1g PO x 1 or doxycycline 100mg bid x 7d)
- Ceftriaxone 125mg IM x 1 plus antichlamydial if chlamydia not ruled out (azithromycin 1g PO x 1 or doxycycline 100mg bid x 7d)
- Ciprofloxacin 500mg PO x 1 plus antichlamydial if chlamydia not ruled out (azithromycin 1g PO x 1 or doxycycline 100mg bid x 7d)
- Ofloxacin 400mg PO x 1 plus antichlamydial if chlamydia not ruled out (azithromycin 1g PO x 1 or doxycycline 100mg bid x 7d)
- Levofloxacin 250mg PO x 1 plus antichlamydial if chlamydia not ruled out (azithromycin 1g PO x 1 or doxycycline 100mg bid x 7d)

- Fluoroquinolone resistance GC is increasing

Cervix, Urethra, Rectum (alternative)

- Standard of Care = 2 drug regimen to Rx gonorrhea and chlamydia if chlamydia infection not ruled out
- Spectinomycin 2g IM x 1 plus antichlamydial if chlamydia not ruled out (azithromycin 1g PO x 1 or doxycycline 100mg bid x 7d)
- Ceftizoxime 500mg IM x 1 plus antichlamydial if chlamydia not ruled out (azithromycin 1g PO x 1 or doxycycline 100mg bid x 7d)
- Cefoxitin 2g IM x 1 w/probenecid 1g PO x 1 plus antichlamydial if chlamydia not ruled out (azithromycin 1g PO x 1 or doxycycline 100mg bid x 7d)
- Cefotaxime 500mg IM x 1 plus antichlamydial if chlamydia not ruled out (azithromycin 1g PO x 1 or doxycycline 100mg bid x 7d)
- azithromycin 2g PO x 1 (Increasing resistance seen)
- Other single dose fluoroquinolones: Gatifloxacin 400mg PO, norfloxacin 800mg PO, lomefloxacin 400mg PO all x 1 appear to be safe and effective but offer no advantage over other FQ.

Uncomplicated pharyngeal infections

- Standard of Care = 2 drug regimen to Rx gonorrhea and chlamydia if chlamydia infection not ruled out
- Ceftriaxone 125mg IM x 1 plus antichlamydial if chlamydia not ruled out (azithromycin 1g PO x 1 or doxycycline 100mg bid x 7d)
- Ciprofloxacin 500mg PO x 1 plus antichlamydial if chlamydia not ruled out (azithromycin 1g PO x 1 or doxycycline 100mg bid x 7d)

Gonococcal conjunctivitis

- Ceftriaxone 1g IM once (plus saline lavage)

Special patient situations

- Men who have sex with men: Do not use FQs in confirmed or suspect cases of GC due to antibiotic resistance levels in this group.
- Areas w/high rates of fluoroquinolone resistant GC: Includes CA, HI, MA, NYC, and Pacific Basin. Use alternative treatments described above
- Pregnancy: Any regimen above except quinolones, tetracyclines, 2g azithromycin. Use erythromycin and amoxicillin in presumptive or definitive Rx of chlamydia.
- HIV infection: should receive the same treatment as HIV-uninfected persons
- Allergy, intolerance, adverse reactions: If can't tolerate cephalosporins or fluoroquinolones, use spectinomycin regimen. If used for possible pharyngeal infection, test of cure needed at 3-5d post Rx.
- Disseminated gonococcal infection (preferred): Ceftriaxone 1g IM or IV q24h until 24-48h after improvement, then change to oral Rx to complete 7d.
- Quinolone use in adolescents: Can be used in those who weigh >45kg.
- Gonococcal meningitis and endocarditis: (ID Consultation!) Ceftriaxone 1-2g IV q12h (1)in meningitis for 10-14 d; (2) in endocarditis for at least 4 wks.

Disseminated Gonnococcal Infection (DGI)

- A. Alternative initial regimens (continue initial regimen for 24-48h after clinical improvement. Then change to PO to complete 7d)
- Ciprofloxacin 500mg IV q12h X 24-48 hrs after clinical improvement; ofloxacin 400mg IV q12h X 24-48 hrs after clinical improvement; spectinomycin 2g IM q12h X 24-48 hrs after clinical improvement
- Completion of 1 week Rx regimen with cefixime 400mg PO bid or ciprofloxacin 500mg PO per day or ofloxacin 400mg PO bid

- B. Severe DGI: meningitis and endocarditis
- a) Meningitis: ceftriaxone 1-2g IV q12h X 10-14 d; b) Endocarditis: ceftriaxone 1-2g IV q12h X at least 4 weeks; c) Allergy/intolerance to cephalosporins or quinolones: spectinomycin 2g IM once.

IMPORTANT POINTS

- This module is based on the CDC's 2002 STD Rx Guidelines (MMWR 2002; 51 (RR-6) and CDC Revised Recommendations for Gonorrhea Treatment, 2004 (MMWR 2004; 53:335-8)
- Fluoroquinolones (FQ) should not be used to treat MSM with gonorrhea or anyone with infxn acquired in Asia, the Pacific Basin, HI, CA, MA, or New York City due to high rates of FQ resistant GC.
- Dual therapy for gonorrhea and chlamydia is the STANDARD OF CARE if chlamydia infection has not been ruled out at the time of Rx
- Pharyngeal and anorectal infection appear to be associated with DGI
- Anyone treated with spectinomycin must be reevaluated 3-5 days after treatment if had pharyngeal exposure (only 52% effective at this site)

SELECTED READINGS

Thiery G et al. Gonococcemia associated with fatal septic shock. Clin Infect Dis 2001;32:e92-3

Centers for Disease Control and Prevention. Increased in fluoroquinolone-resistant Neisseria gonorrhoeae among men who have sex with men---United States, 2003 and revised recommendations for gonorrhea treatment, 2004. MMWR 2004, 53(16):335-338.

Centers for Disease Control and Prevention. Oral alternatives to cefixime for the treatment of uncomplicated Neisseria gonorrhoeae urogenital infections. http://www.cdc.gov/STD/treatment/Cefixime.htm. April 30, 2004.

Fox KK et al. Gonorrhea in the HIV era: a reversal in trends among men who have sex with men. Am J Public Health 2001;91:959-64

Centers for Disease Control and Prevention. 1998. Sexually transmitted diseases treatment guidelines 2002. MMWR 2002; 51 (RR-6):1-78

NEISSERIA MENINGITIDIS   John G. Bartlett, M.D.

CLINICAL RELEVANCE & DIAGNOSIS

- Gram negative, diplococcus - grows in blood or chocolate agar or selective media - Thayer Martin
- Capsule dictates 13 serogroups - most important are A, B, C, W135 and Y
- Epidemics usually due to A, B or C serogroups; vaccines mix serogroups A, C, Y & W135 (no licensed vaccine for B)
- Usual pathogenesis: oropharynx (carriage/infection) then bacteremia, then meningitis and/or fulminant meningococcemia
- Clinical: fever + leukocytosis, (HA, altered mental status if meningitis) then petechial rash, then purpura fulminans + shock
- Culture: blood, CSF and skin (rash)

SITES OF INFECTION

- Meningitis
- Bacteremia
- Respiratory tract infection: otitis, epiglottitis, pneumonia
- Focal infection: pericarditis, urethritis, arthritis, conjunctivitis
- Chronic meningococcemia (complement deficiency in many)

Treatment Regimens

Prevention

- Prophylaxis: household, or intimate contact, med personnel with contact w/oral secretions
- Agent: rifampin 600mg qd x 2d or ciproflox 500mg x 1, or ceftriaxone 250mg IM
- Vaccine: A, C, Y, W135 for outbreaks & international travel to endemic areas (meningitis belt of Africa); offer to college freshman residing in dormitories
- New quadravalent conjugate (Menacta) for children under 11 years.

Meningococcal meningitis or bacteremia

- Guidelines from: N Rosenstein et al, NEJM 2001;344:1378
- Preferred: penicillin 18-24 mU/d IV, ceftriaxone 2g qd or cefotaxime 12g/d x 7-10d
- Alternatives: chloramphenicol 1g IV q6h x 7-10d
- Steroids: controversial - if given - dexamethasone 0.15mg/kg IV q6h x 4d starting 30min before abx

Important Points

- Guidelines are from Rosenstein NE, NEJM 2001;344:1378
- Typical presentation: abrupt fever - then petechiael rash - hemorrhagic rash - purple rash - shock
- Penicillin resistance is increasing but is not yet relevant in US - pen is preferred drug
- Virulence is determined by serogroup and serotype

Selected Readings

Yazdankhah SP, Caugnant DA. Neisseria meningitidis: an overview of the carriage state. J Med Microbiol 2004;53:821-32

Stollenwerk N, et al. Diversity in pathogenicity can cause outbreaks of meningococcal disease. Proc Natl Acad Sci USA 2004;101:102.29-34

Zimmer SM and Stephens DS. Meningococcal conjugate vaccines. Expert Opin Pharmacother 2004;5:855-63

Raghunathan PL, et al. Opportunities for control of meningococcal disease in the U.S. Ann Rev Med 2004;55:333-53

van den Beek, et al. Steroids in adults with acute bacterial meningitis: a systematic review. Lancet Infect Dis 2004;4:139-43

NOCARDIA

John G. Bartlett, M.D.

Clinical Relevance & Diagnosis

- Gram-positive branching, beaded, filamentous rod, weakly acid fast, grows on special media (Thayer-Martin) in 3-5d
- Smears & cx positive in only 1/3rd of cases; send multiple specimens & warn lab of suspected dx
- Looks like Actinomycetes sp, but - acid fast, aerobic & seen mostly in compromised hosts
- Suspect with CMI defect (AIDS, steroids, CGD, organ transplant) + indolent lung +/- CNS disease
- Dx: Gram stain + AFB stain + sputum cx; rarely seen as colonization (take [+] sputum culture seriously)
- 12 species: N. asteroides 90%, lung +/- CNS disease, N. brasiliensis = mycetoma (tropics); N. farcinica - bad prognosis

Sites Of Infection

- Lung: indolent pneumonia, abscess, fibronodular infiltrates

- Brain: abscess or granulomas
- Disseminated: bones, heart, renal, joints, retina, skin, CNS, peritonitis, endocarditis
- Primary cutaneous: sporotrichoid (non-tropics) or mycetoma (madura foot, tropics)
- Ocular; keratitis, endophthalmitis

TREATMENT REGIMENS

Sulfonamides

- Principles: Rx based on host, site of disease & in vitro activity; sulfas usually preferred, must treat for 6-12mo
- Two categories: seriously ill usually treated w/ IV imipenem or sulfa or cefotaxime all potentially combined w/ amikacin; less seriously ill treated with oral agents - esp TMP-SMX or minocycline
- Pulmonary: TMP-SMX 5-10mg/kg/d (TMP) in 2-4 doses IV x 3-6wks, then PO (1-2DS bid) x >5mo
- Pulmonary alternative: sulfisoxazole, sulfadiazine, trisulfapyrimidine 3-6g/d PO 2-4 doses or TMP-SMX 1-2 DS bid up to 2 DS tid
- CNS: AIDS, severe or disseminated disease - TMP/SMX 15mg/kg/d (TMP) IV x 3-6wks, then PO (3 DS bid) x 6-12 mo
- CNS alternative: ceftriaxone 1g bid IV or cefotaxime 2-3g q 6h IV + amikacin
- Severe disease, compromised host, multiple sites: TMP-SMX IV (above doses) + amikacin 7.5mg/kg q 12h or oral sulfas 6-12g/d
- Sporotrichoid (cutaneous): TMP-SMX 1 DS bid x 4-6mo
- Sensitivity N. asteroides: sulfa - 95%, minocycline - 90%, imipenem - 85%, amikacin - 90%, cefotax - 80%, amox/clav - 50%, cipro - 40%, ampicillin - 30%

Sulfa alternatives

- Oral: minocycline 100mg bid x > 6mo (initial Rx local disease or maintenance)
- Oral alternative if in vitro activity shown: amoxicillin-clavulanate 875/125mg bid or doxy, erythro, clari, linezolid or fluoroquinolone or combinations x >6mo
- Severe disease, AIDS: imipenem 500mg IV q 8h or meropenem (CNS) 0.5-1g q 8h, each + amikacin 7.5mg/kg q 12h IV
- Severe disease: cefotaxime 2-3g q 6-8h or ceftriaxone 1-2g/d IV +/- amikacin

Miscellaneous

- Chronic granulomatous disease - should get interferon + sulfa prophylaxis
- Surgical debridement or drainage, consider for extrapulmonary lesions
- In vitro sensitivity tests important - esp with non-sulfa therapy
- Sulfa intolerance (esp AIDS) - consider desensitization
- Sulfa Rx - some get sulfa levels 2hrs post dose - expect 100-150mg/L and Rx >6mo
- Monitor for relapse x 1yr post Rx
- Decrease/reduce immunosuppression if possible
- No person-person transmission
- Rx duration: immunocompetent - 6mo; immunosuppressed - 12mo. Immunosuppressed & continued immunosuppression - low dose abx indefinitely

IMPORTANT POINTS

- Guidelines are authors opinion and P Lerner (CID 1996;22:891)
- Rx is normally long (6-12mo) & hard (high dose sulfa, imipenem/amikacin etc); less serious - oral sulfa or minocycline from start
- Cure rates: soft tissue - 100%, pul - 90%, disseminated - 60%, CNS - 50%
- 60% compromised - diabetes, steroids, organ tx, cancer chemo Rx, AIDS; TMP-SMX/ dapsone prophy prevents

- Dx: Pulmonary +/- CNS, indolent course, Low CMI, filamentous branching, beaded, gram pos rod. CNS in 40%; if pul disease - get brain MRI.

SELECTED READINGS

Husain S, McCurry K, Dauber J, et al. Nocardia infection in lung transplant receipts. J Heart Lung Transplant 2002;21:354

Matulionyte R, et al. Secular trends of Nocardia infection over 14 years in a tertiary care hospital. J Clin Pathol 2004;57:807-12

Queipo-Zaragoza JA, et al. Nocardia infection in immunosuppressed kidney transplant recipients. Scand J Urol Nephrol 2004;38:168-73

Pintado V, et al. Nocardial infection in patients with HIV infection. Clin Microbiol Infect 2003;9:716-20

Gomez-Flores A, et al. In vitro and in vivo activities of antimicrobials against Nocardia brasiliensis. Antimicrob Ag Chemother 2004;48:832-7

PASTEURELLA MULTOCIDA   Jeremy Gradon, MD

CLINICAL RELEVANCE & DIAGNOSIS

- Aerobic to facultatively anaerobic, nonmotile small gram-negative rods commonly inhibiting oroflora of dogs/cats. Animal bites or scratches may result in cellulitis +/- bacteremia
- Commonly associated with cat bite infections
- Occasionally associated with dog bite infections
- Occasional cause of pneumonia
- Rare cause of bacteremia or endocarditis

SITES OF INFECTION

- Skin and soft tissue, cellulitis - following cat bite
- Bone/joint infections - following penetrating cat bites; septic arthritis - knee most common, esp with RA, OA or prosthetic joint
- Lung - may cause lobar pneumonia
- Bloodstream - may be primary or secondary to a bite
- Endocarditis - rare
- Other - metastatic seeding of internal organs from bacteremia

TREATMENT REGIMENS

Antibiotics

- Amoxicillin-clavulanate 500mg PO q8h or 875mg PO bid with food (preferred empirical coverage of bite wounds)
- Ampicillin-sulbactam - 3g IV q6h
- Penicillin - 500mg PO q6h or 4mU IV q4h
- Levofloxacin 500mg PO or IV qd
- Occasional strains produce beta-lactamases
- First-generation cephalosporins (e.g., cephalexin/Keflex) and clindamycin ineffective

IMPORTANT POINTS

- Pasteurella multocida does not cause "cat scratch disease," (rather that entity is caused by Bartonella henselae)
- Bite infections are frequently polymicrobial and thus amoxicillin-clavulanate will provide broad "all-comers" empirical coverage
- Pasteurella multocida is a cause of rapidly progressive infections (i.e., pt may present within a few hours of a cat bite with established severe infection)
- Keep involved extremity elevated. Involve a hand surgeon early w/ hand bite infections

- Patients with endocarditis often have no history of animal contact (11/17 cases, see Saleh reference)

SELECTED READINGS

Balestra B. Mycotic aneurysms of the aorta caused by infection with Pasteurella multocida. Clin Infect Dis 2000; 31: e1-e2

Saleh MAF, Al_madan MS, Erwa HH et al. First case of human infection caused by Pasteurella gallinarum causing infective endocarditis in an adolescent 10 years after surgical correction for truncus arteriosus. Pediatrics 1995; 95: 944-948

Hassoun PM. Dog kissing, recurrent Pasteurella pneumonia and degenerative lung disease. Inf Dis Clin Pract. 1996; 5: 79-80

Talan DA, et al. Bacteriologic analysis of infected cat and dog bites. N Engl J Med 1999; 340: 85-92

Majeed, et al. The cat and the catheter. N Engl J Med 1995; 332; 338

PEPTOSTREPTOCOCCUS/PEPTOCOCCUS

John G. Bartlett, M.D.

CLINICAL RELEVANCE & DIAGNOSIS

- Anaerobic gram-positive cocci, normal flora mouth, GI tract, genital tract, skin
- Requires uncontaminated specimen (blood, body fluid, etc) & anaerobic cx
- Gram stain: GPC seen are identical w/aerobic strep (chains) or Staph (clusters)
- Account for nearly all anaerobic GPC except Finegoldia magna (formerly P. megna)
- Common in mixed anaerobic infections at all anatomical sites
- Clinical clues: putrid discharge, gram stain- GPC + GNB, abscess, mixed infection
- Most common & important: Finegoldia magna & P. asaccharolyticus; less - P. micros & P. anaerobius
- Pathogenesis: endogenous infection - no pt-pt transmission, not infecting compromised hosts

SITES OF INFECTION

- Intraabdominal sepsis: part of mixed infection
- Lung: aspiration pneumonia, lung abscess, empyema
- Female genital tract: part of mixed infection
- Dental: part of mixed infection
- Soft tissue: ulcers, cellulitis, fasciitis
- Abscesses: brain, dental, lung, tubo-ovarian, soft tissue +/- osteomyelitis
- Endocarditis: <1% endocarditis cases
- Bacteremia: <1% bacteremias

TREATMENT REGIMENS

Treatment

- Principles: nearly all are mixed infections. Peptostreptococcus rarely cultured; sensitive to many abx, treatment usually empiric for mixed flora.
- Best abx: PCN, clindamycin, ampicillin, imipenem, BL-BLI (Augmentin, Zosyn, Unasyn)
- Also active: vancomycin, quinolones (moxi/gati/ levofloxacin), metronidazole (?), linezolid, daptomycin
- Variable activity: doxycycline, macrolides (erythro/azithro/clarithromycin), ceftazidime
- No activity: TMP-SMX, norfloxacin, aztreonam, aminoglycosides

- Caution: metronidazole not active vs. microaerophilic strep which are important in mixed infections.

Treatment: other
- Abscesses - require drainage except lung & tubo-ovarian + some brain or hepatic abscesses
- No patient-patient transmission risk: normal flora of everyone
- Host defenses - less important; not disease of compromised host
- In vitro sensitivities: rarely done except endocarditis, persistent bacteremia or osteomyelitis

IMPORTANT POINTS
- Treatment recommendations are author's opinion
- MOST INFECTIONS: Peptostreptococci found with other anaerobes + strep +/- coliforms
- Suspect organism with GS showing mixed flora; putrid states; endogenous infections; any abscess
- Cx: requires uncontaminated specimen + anaerobic cx (rarely achieved)
- ABX: nearly always empiric. Metronidazole: active vs. Peptostreptococci; not active vs. aerobic streptococci, including S. anginosus complex etc. BE CAREFUL not to narrow treatment.

SELECTED READINGS
Finegold SM, George WL, Mulligan ME. Anaerobic infections. Disease-a-Month 1985;31:8

Bartlett JG. Systemic infection involving anaerobes. CID 1993;16:S248

Sweet R, Schachter J, Landers DV, et al. Treatment of hospitalized patients with acute pelvic inflammatory disease. Am J Obstet Gynec 1988;158:736

Stone HH, Strom PR, Fabian TC, et al. Third generation cephalosporins for polymicrobial surgical sepsis. Arch Surg 1983;118:193

Bantar C, Canigia LF, Relloso S, et al. Species belonging to the Streptococcus milleri group: Antimicrobial susceptibility and comparative prevalence in significant clinical specimens. J Clin Microbiol 1996;34:2020

PLESIOMONAS
David Zaas, M.D. and Paul Auwaerter, M.D.

CLINICAL RELEVANCE & DIAGNOSIS
- Gram-negative rod; uncommon cause of gastroenteritis; children > adults, especially in tropical and sub-tropical climates
- Associated w/ drinking untreated water, eating uncooked shellfish, or travel to underdeveloped countries.
- Infection typically characterized by self-limited watery diarrhea w/ blood or mucus, abdominal pain, emesis, and fever.
- Sx usually occur within 48 hours of exposure. Dx: stool culture.
- P. shigelloides may cause both sporadic cases as well as outbreaks. Increasing incidence in summer months.
- Although normally self-limited, up to 30% may develop chronic diarrhea and abdominal pain persisting >3 weeks.
- Prevalence of P. shigelloides among patients w/ infectious diarrhea estimated from 0 to 8%.
- Highest incidence reported in traveler's returning to Japan where appx. 75% of microbiologically confirmed cases of traveler's diarrhea in 1999 due to P. shigelloides.

SITES OF INFECTION

- CNS: meningitis (rare)
- Dissemination: bacteremia/sepsis, infection more common in immunocompromised hosts--associated w/ high mortality.
- Gastrointestinal: usually Plesiomonas limited to GI tract causing diarrheal illness
- Musculoskeletal: osteomyelitis, septic arthritis--all rare
- Ocular: endophthalmitis (rare)

TREATMENT REGIMENS

Immunocompetent hosts: mild infection

- Illness usually self-limited, lasting < 2-4 d; antibiotic Rx not indicated.

Immunocompromised hosts

- Greater likelihood of dissemination and severe infections, empiric antibiotics recommended for pts w/ AIDS or other immunocompromised pts.
- Preferred: ciprofloxacin 500mg PO bid
- Ceftriaxone (1-2g IV qd) used successfully in severe cases

Immunocompetent hosts: severe infection

- Severe/protracted diarrhea or extra-intestinal disease: Rx empiric antibiotics until culture and sensitivity available.
- Abx shown to shorten the duration of sxs
- Plesiomonas chronic diarrhea (sx >3 wks), abx resolve sx.
- Preferred: ciprofloxacin 500mg PO bid (or other oral fluoroquinolone)
- Ceftriaxone (1-2g IV qd) used successfully in severe cases
- Isolates frequently express beta-lactamases, therefore PCN-resistant

IMPORTANT POINTS

- Shigelloides is the most common species of Plesiomonas reported to cause human disease. Previously known as Aeromonas shigelloides.
- Approximately 15% of cases cultured w/ a co-pathogen in addition to Plesiomonas.
- Plesiomonas shigelloides is not normal bowel flora and isolated < 0.1% of asymptomatic individuals.

SELECTED READINGS

Shigematsu M, Kaufmann ME, Charlett A, et al. An epidemiological study of Plesiomonas shigelloides diarrhea among Japanese travelers. Epidemiol Infect 2000; 125(3): 523-30.

No authors listed. Plesiomonas shigelloides and Salmonella serotype Hartford infections associated with a contaminated water supply--Livingston County, New York, 1996. MMWR Morb Mortal Wkly Rep. 1998 May 22;47(19):394-6.

Wong TY, Tsui HY, So MK, et al. Plesiomonas shigelloides infection in Hong Kong: Retrospective study of 167 laboratory confirmed cases. Hong Kong Med J. 2000;6(4):375-80.

Stock I, Wiedemann B. Natural antimicrobial susceptibilities of Plesiomonas shigelloides strains. Journal of Antimicrobial Chemotherapy 2001; 48: 803-811.

Holmberg SD, Wachsmuth K, Hickman-Brenner FW, et al. Plesiomonas enteric infections in the United States. Annals of Internal Medicine 1986; 105: 690-694.

PROPIONIBACTERIUM SPECIES Paul Auwaerter, M.D.

CLINICAL RELEVANCE & DIAGNOSIS

- Gram-positive pleomorphic rod that grows best anaerobically. Usually inhabits human skin, sebaceous glands, nasopharynx, GI/GU tracts.

- Most common, non-spore forming anaerobic rod found in clinical specimens. Frequent blood culture contaminant. P. acnes is the species most often isolated.
- Generally sensitive to penicillins, resistant to aminoglycosides.
- Commonly associated w/ acne vulgaris (see "Acne Vulgaris" in the Diagnoses section); most frequent serious infection: CNS shunt infections.
- Low virulence, and slow growth--often requiring 5-6d for significant growth in cxs.

SITES OF INFECTION

- Skin: associated with acne conditions, soft tissue infection (occasional)
- CNS: shunt infections, meningitis (post-operative), brain abscess, subdural empyema
- Renal: infectious shunt-related glomerulonephritis described, CAPD catheter infection and peritonitis
- Cardiac: endocarditis (rare)
- Ocular: endophthalmitis (usually post-cataract surgery)
- Bone: prosthetic joint infection, osteomyelitis (rare)
- Dental: caries, abscesses

TREATMENT REGIMENS

Systemic infection

- Routine anaerobic bacterial abx sensitivity testing often unavailable and problematic due to lack of standardization. Choice often empiric.
- P. acnes often susceptible to PCN, tetracyclines, chloramphenicol, erythromycin, & vancomycin (including teicoplanin)--but resistance increasing likely due to widespread abx use for acne vulgaris.
- Preferred: penicillin G 2mU IV q4h
- Alt: clindamycin 600mg IV q8h, vancomycin 1g IV q12h
- Consider removal of foreign bodies. Some success w/ retention of shunts, prostheses but no clear data to guide.
- Duration: 2-4 wks, may be able to switch to oral meds in some circumstances (soft tissue infxns).
- Note: metronidazole or tinidazole w/o activity against Propionibacterium species.

Acne vulgaris

- See "Diagnoses" section

IMPORTANT POINTS

- P. acnes mostly a contaminant, especially from blood cxs. Clinician must carefully weigh clinical situation to judge culture results.
- Do not routinely dismiss as contaminant if isolated (especially repeatedly) from CSF shunts.
- Slow growing organism, so blood and other specimen cxs often only positive after 3-5d incubation.
- Most eubacteria such as P. acnes are resistant to nitroimidazoles such as metronidazole--preferred choices: penicillins, clindamycin.

SELECTED READINGS

James WD. Clinical practice. Acne. N Engl J Med. 2005 Apr 7;352(14):1463-72

Fincher ME, Forsyth M, Rahimi SY. Successful management of central nervous system infection due to Propionibacterium acnes with vancomycin and doxycycline. South Med J. 2005 Jan;98(1):118-21

Deramo VA, Ting TD. Treatment of Propionibacterium acnes endophthalmitis. Curr Opin Ophthalmol. 2001 Jun;12(3):225-9

Cooper AJ. Systematic review of Propionibacterium acnes resistance to systemic antibiotics. Med J Aust. 1998 Sep 7;169(5):259-61

Skinner PR, Taylor AJ, Coakham H. Propionibacteria as a cause of shunt and postneurosurgical infections. J Clin Pathol. 1978 Nov;31(11):1085-9

PROTEUS SPECIES

Jeremy Gradon, MD

CLINICAL RELEVANCE & DIAGNOSIS

- Gram-negative, urease-splitting rod
- "Swarms" on moist agar (many flagella/organism)
- Second most commonly isolated Enterobacteriaceae after E. coli
- Commonest species: P. mirabilis (indole negative), other Proteus spp. are indole positive
- Causes ~ 10% of uncomplicated UTIs
- Splits urea, raising urinary pH (e.g., > 8.0) and can cause struvite stone formation
- Struvite stones can be nidus of chronic renal infection or obstruction

SITES OF INFECTION

- GU: UTI
- Abdomen: intra-abdominal infection
- Skin: burn wound infections, surgical site infections
- Other: meningitis, bacteremia, line sepsis
- Prosthetic device, bronchoscope infections

TREATMENT REGIMENS

Proteus mirabilis

- Ampicillin: 500mg PO q6h or 2g IV q6h
- Cefuroxime: 250mg PO q12h or 750mg IV q8h
- Levofloxacin 500mg PO q24h or 500mg IV q24h

Indole positive Proteus species

- Ceftriaxone 1g IV q24h
- Imipenem 500mg IV q6h
- Levofloxacin 500mg IV or PO q24h

IMPORTANT POINTS

- Reservoir often patient's own GI tract
- Need urology for management of struvite stones
- P. mirabilis intrinsically resistant to tetracycline and nitrofurantoin
- Most nosocomial Proteus infections due to indole + strains (not P. mirabilis)

SELECTED READINGS

Story P. Proteus infections in hospital. J Pathol Bacteriol 1954; 68: 55-62.

Mobley HLT, Warren JW. Urease-positive bacteriuria and obstruction of long-term urinary catheters. J Clin Microbiol 1987; 2: 2216-2217

Weinstein HJ, Bone RC, Ruth WE. Contamination of a fiberoptic bronchoscope with a Proteus species. Am Rev Respir Dis 1977; 116: 541-543

Liassine N, Madec S, Ninet B et al. Postneurosurgical meningitis due to Proteus pinneri with selection of a ceftriaxone-resistant isolate: Analysis of chromosomal class A beta lactamase HugA and its LysR-type regulatory protein Hug R. Antimicrob Agents Chemother 2002; 46: 216-219

Thakar CV, Lara A, Goel M, et al. Staghorn calculus in renal allograft presenting as acute renal failure. Urological Research 2003; 31: 414-416

PROVIDENCIA

Brian Jefferson, M.D.

CLINICAL RELEVANCE & DIAGNOSIS

- Member of Enterobacteriaceae: motile gram (-) facultative aerobic rod, same tribe as proteus and morganella spp.
- 5 species: P. alcalifaciens, P. heimbachae, P. rettgeri, P. rustigianii, P. stuartii. Proteus stuartii most common isolate causing infections in humans.
- Common constituents of nl GI flora in both humans and animals.
- P. stuartii and P. rettgeri are common causes of gram-negative bacteremia in nursing home patients. Elderly pts. w/chronic indwelling catheters at especially high risk.
- Mortality to bacteremia not excessively high w/appropriate treatment.
- Although usually a commensal organism, P. alcalifaciens implicated as an agent of enteroinvasive gastroenteritis. Most studies in children. Overseas travel may increase risk.
- Over 50% of P. stuartii infections in an academic hospital setting found to be ESBL-multidrug resistant strains.
- Increasing age, underlying neoplasm, and previous hospitalization and antibiotic therapy a risk for ESBL multidrug resistance for P. stuartii infections.
- Providencia spp. have predilection for chronically catheterized urine. P. stuartii comprises >50% of all pathogens from patients with long standing indwelling catheters.

SITES OF INFECTION

- GU: UTI, most commonly catheter associated
- Isolates recovered from urine, throat, perineum, axillae, stool, blood and wound specimens
- Bacteremia (rare): associated with older age and chronic indwelling catheters
- Nosocomial: reports of highly resistant P. rettgeri UTI outbreaks associated with chronic indwelling catheter and exposure to multiple abx
- Pulmonary: endotracheal intubation or suctioning may confer a higher risk for pneumonia

TREATMENT REGIMENS

Preferred agents

- Amikacin 7.5mg/kg IV q 12h
- Ciprofloxacin 500-750mg IV/PO q12h
- Levofloxacin 500mg IV/PO qd
- Ceftriaxone 1-2g IV q 24h. (Do not use if ESBL suspected or critically ill)
- Duration (UTI): 7d, removal of foreign material (e.g., catheter) desirable.
- Duration (bacteremia): 14 d

Alternative regimens

- TMP-SMX (Bactrim) DS 1 q12 h for 10-14 d or 20 TMP/kg/day IV q6 h.
- As a rule, multiple resistance profiles have been reported for Providencia spp. and antimicrobial testing is extremely important.

IMPORTANT POINTS

- Treatment failures: may carry chromosomal gene encoding extended-spectrum beta-lactamase (ESBL), usually induced in the presence of some but not all beta-lactam antibiotics.
- P. rettgeri can hydrolyze urea, unlike the other Providencia spp. Look for elevated urinary pH.

- P. alcalifaciens and P. rustigianii tend to be the most susceptible of the Providencia spp. P. stuartii generally is the least susceptible species to antibiotic therapy.

SELECTED READINGS

Tumbarello et al. ESBL-producing multidrug resistant Providencia stuartii infections in a university hospital. Journal of Antimicrobial Chemotherapy(2004) 53,277-282

Stock I et al. Natural antibiotic susceptibility of Providencia stuartii, P. rettgeri, P. alcalifaciens and P. rustigianii strains. J Med Microbiol 1998 Jul; 47(7):629-42

O'Hara et al. Classification, identification, and clinical significance of Proteus, Providencia, and Morganella. Clin Microbiol Rev 2000 Oct;13(4):534-46

Murata T et al. A large outbreak of foodborne infection attributed to Providencia alcalifaciens. J Infect Dis 2001 Oct 15;184(8):1050-5

Woods et al. Bacteremia due to P stuartii: Review of 49 episodes. South Med J, 89(2) Feb 1996. 221-224

PSEUDOMONAS AERUGINOSA Khalil G. Ghanem, M.D.

CLINICAL RELEVANCE & DIAGNOSIS

- Gram-negative, motile, aerobic, lactose nonfermenter responsible for pneumonia, UTI, bacteremia, post-neurosurgical meningitis & skin infections.
- Risk factors include neutropenia, diabetes, skin burns, cystic fibrosis, & AIDS.
- Primarily a nosocomial pathogen. Inhabits moist environments including soil, water (hot tubs, sinks, water faucets, respirators, disinfectants), plants, & animals.
- Dx: culture of sputum, urine, blood, abscess fluid, joint fluid, or CSF.

SITES OF INFECTION

- Respiratory: pneumonia (nosocomial, CF, AIDS) & lung abscesses.
- CV: endocarditis (IVDU); bacteremia (primary & secondary due to indwelling catheters).
- Skin: ecthyma gangrenosum (neutropenia); cellulitis (DM, IVDU, post-operative); folliculitis; abscesses; noma neonatorum (infants).
- GU: UTI/pyelonephritis (DM and hospitalized pts w/ indwelling catheters).
- ENT: otitis externa & malignant otitis externa (DM); chronic otitis media; sinusitis (AIDS).
- CNS: brain abscesses; meningitis post neurosurgical manipulation.
- Bone/joint: vertebral, sternoclavicular or pelvic bone infections (IVDU); osteochondritis of foot (following penetrating injuries through tennis shoes).
- Eye: keratitis; endophthalmitis.
- GI: diarrhea; necrotizing enterocolitis "typhlitis" (young children & neutropenia).

TREATMENT REGIMENS

Chemotherapy

- Ceftazidime 2g IV q8h
- Cefepime 2g IV q 8-12h
- Piperacillin 4g IV q4h
- Ticarcillin 3-4g IV q4-6h
- Imipenem 500mg - 1g IV q6h; meropenem 1g IV q8h
- Ciprofloxacin 400mg IV q8-12h or 750mg PO q12h (for less serious infxns); may not be wise empiric choice due to rising resistance.
- Aztreonam 2g IV q 6-8h
- Colistin 1.7mg/kg IV q8h
- Polymyxin B 0.75-1.25 mg/kg IV q12h

- Gentamicin or tobramycin 1.7-2.0 mg/KG IV q8h or 5-7 mg/kg IV qd or amikacin 7.5mg/kg IV q12h. Usually used in combination w/other antimicrobials (preferably beta-lactams).

General principles

- Isolation of infected pts, hand-washing by staff & visitors, & vigilant infection control measures may help prevent nosocomial transmission.
- In patients w/ chronic lung disease (e.g., CF), good pulmonary toilet (mucolytic agents, chest PT, postural drainage) are important adjunctive treatment measures.
- Double coverage using high doses of synergistic antibiotic combinations (e.g., B-lactam + aminoglycoside) possibly recommended, espeically for empiric concerns if Pseudomonas is suspected, especially for serious infections (see references for controversy).
- Rx of AIDS-related pseudomonas infections may require a more prolonged course of therapy to prevent chronic infections/relapses.
- Multiple resistance mechanisms occur; increasing resistance especially in CF wards and ICUs; chemotherapy based on susceptibility testing.
- Multi-drug resistant strains may be susceptible to colistin or polymixin B.
- Pseudomonas endocarditis may require surgical intervention in addition to chemotherapy.
- Pts with CF, pregnancy, burns, and critical illnesses may require higher doses of aminoglycosides. Serum drug levels should be monitored carefully.

Important Points

- Ecthyma gangrenosum (skin lesion w/hemorrhage, necrosis, & surrounding erythema) is a clue to Pseudomonas bacteremia in the neutropenic host
- Suspect malignant otitis externa in patients with DM, otalgia and facial nerve palsy (may have bilateral infections)
- Pseudomonas keratitis can complicate prolonged corneal exposure in ICU patients
- Left-sided pseudomonas endocarditis may require surgical intervention
- Advanced AIDS predisposes to P. aeruginosa pneumonia, bacteremia, endocarditis, sinusitis, skin infections, & malignant otitis externa.

Selected Readings

Safdar N, Handelsman J, Maki DG. Does combination antimicrobial therapy reduce mortality in Gram-negative bacteraemia? A meta-analysis. Lancet Infect Dis. 2004 Aug;4(8):519-27.

Lipman J, Allworth A, Wallis SC. Cerebrospinal fluid penetration of high doses of intravenous ciprofloxacin. Clin Infect Dis 2000; 31: 1131-1133

Kielhofner M, Atmar RL, Hamill RJ, et al. Life-threatening pseudomonas aeruginosa infections in patients with Human Immunodeficiency Virus infection. Clin Infect Dis 1992; 14: 403-411

Johansen PH. Pseudomonas infections of the foot following puncture wounds. J Am Med Assoc 1968; 204: 170-172

Hall JH, Callaway JL, Tindall JP, et al. Pseudomonas aeruginosa in dermatology. Arch Derm 1968; 97: 312-324

RHODOCOCCUS EQUI

Aimee Zaas, M.D. & Paul Auwaerter, M.D.

Clinical Relevance & Diagnosis

- Pleomorphic nonmotile gram + coccobacillus; variable acid-fast staining; salmon-pink colonies at 4-7 days

- Ubiquitous in environment; inhalation, local inoculation or ingestion are modes of acquisition
- Can be confused with diptheroids, Micrococcus, Bacillus (all common contaminants) or Mycobacteria
- Typically infects persons with impaired cell-mediated immunity (AIDS, corticosteroids, organ transplant)
- 10-15% of infections in immunocompetent patients
- Pulmonary infection (cavity, nodules, bronchopneumonia) most common manifestation
- HIV: patients often co-infected with other pathogens at presentation
- Social Hx: exposure to animals, particularly horses
- Dx: sputum/blood cx; may need CT guided biopsy culture or bronchoscopy
- Lab may dismiss as "diphtheroids" (contaminant); make lab aware of clinical history

Sites Of Infection

- Pulmonary infection most common: necrotizing pneumonia/abscess/cavitation
- Local spread may occur to chest wall, mediastinal lymph nodes
- Hematogenous dissemination: brain, bone, subcutaneous tissue
- Relapse after treatment often at sites of hematogenous dissemination
- Cavities tend to be thick-walled; air-fluid levels distinguish from tuberculosis/nocardia
- Other infections: wound, ocular, bacteremia, peritonitis, osteomyelitis, brain abscess, abdominal organ abscess
- HIV + patients often bacteremic at time of bronchopneumonia

Treatment Regimens

Antibiotics

- Treatment (induction) lengthy: at least 4 weeks or until infiltrate disappears;
- Some authors recommmend at least 8 weeks in immunocompromised patients
- Combination therapy with intracellular activity recommended (see below)
- Suppressive therapy 3-6 months in non HIV, often lifelong in HIV; no data on stopping if immune reconstitution on HAART
- First line: Vancomycin 1g IV q12h (15mg/kg q 12 for larger patients) OR imipenem 500mg IV q 6h PLUS
- Rifampin 600mg PO qd OR ciprofloxacin 750mg PO bid OR erythromycin 500mg PO qid
- Maintenance therapy (after infiltrate clears): ciprofloxacin 750mg PO bid OR erythromycin 500mg po qid
- Avoid penicillins/cephalosporins due to development of resistance
- Linezolid effective in vitro; no clinical reports of success
- Other agents reported with activity: azithromycin, TMP-SMX, chloramphenicol, clindamycin

Surgical

- Resection of large abscesses/necrotizing pneumonias adds to success in combination with abx

Important Points

- If relapse occurs on maintenance therapy: beware of resistant organisms
- Notify lab if suspicious of Rhodococcus - can be dismissed as a contaminant
- Mortality 20%; up to 50% in patients with AIDS
- Histopath: often shows malakoplakia -- plump epithelioid histiocytes with eosinophilic, homogenous, or granular cytoplasm
- Many drug interactions with rifampin (esp. with HAART)

BACTERIA

SELECTED READINGS

Stiles BM, Isaacs RB, Daniels TM, Jones DR. Role of surgery in Rhodococcus equi pulmonary infection. J Infection 2002; 45(1): 59-61

Bowersock TL, Salmon SA, Portis ES, et al. MICs of oxazolidinones for rhodococcus equi strains isolated from humans and animals. Antimicrobial Agents Chemotherapy 2000;44:1367-69

Perez MGV, Vassilev T, Rammerty A. Rhodococcus equi infection in transplant recipients: a case of mistaken identity and review of the literature. Transplant Infectious Diseases 2002;4:52-56

Nordmann P, Ronco E. In vitro antimicrobial susceptibilities of Rhodococcus equi. J Antimicrobial Chemotherapy 1992; 29:383-5

Kedlaya I, Ing MB, Wong SS. Rhodococcus equi infections in immunocompetent patients: case report and review. Clinical Infectious Diseases 2001;32(3):E39-46

RICKETTSIA RICKETTSII
Joseph Vinetz, M.D.

CLINICAL RELEVANCE & DIAGNOSIS

- Obligately intracellular, gram-negative agent of Rocky Mountain Spotted Fever
- Potential for rapidly lethal illness, can be difficult to diagnose. Must start presumptive Rx (doxycycline) in the right setting.
- Most (90%) but not all cases present with rash, usually after 3-5 d prodrome
- Severity ranges from undifferentiated febrile syndrome to multiorgan failure
- Classic triad: fever, headache, rash. Occurs mostly May to September in endemic areas
- Endemic areas: East of Rocky Mountains; most common in Oklahoma, Carolinas, Virginia, Maryland; also Montana, Wyoming
- Tick-transmitted: dog tick (Dermacentor); wood tick (Amblyomma)
- General lab findings: nl to low WBC; thrombocytopenia characteristic; occ. mild anemia; coagulopathy (DIC); hyponatremia in 50%; high CK, LDH with tissue injury in severe cases
- Dx: skin bx w/direct fluorescent antibody (DFA rapid, but not avail in many places); or serum indirect fluorescence assay (IFA) to detect antibodies to spotted fever group Rickettsia
- Dx: IFA often negative early in course of illness

SITES OF INFECTION

- General: fever, myalgia, sepsis syndrome
- Skin: petechial rash, begins on extremities, moves towards trunk (centripetal); endothelial cell dysfunction leads to edema of hands and feet. 50% of rashes begin after 3d of fever.
- Neuro: vasculitis; headache, focal neuro deficits, deafness, meningismus (sometimes with CSF mononuc/poly pleocytosis), delirium, abnl EEG (diffuse slowing)
- Renal: acute renal failure--ATN and/or intravasc volume depletion; may require hemodialysis
- Pulmonary: pneumonia (alveolar infiltrates); non-cardiogenic pulm edema; hyaline membrane dz (ARDS)
- Cardiac: myocardial dysfxn unusual

TREATMENT REGIMENS

Doxycycline
- Adult: 100mg PO or IV bid, x 7d or 3d after defervescence
- Drug of choice in children as well as adults given potential fatal outcome

- Rx with doxycycline or tetracycline recommended for children for 2 reasons: 1) RMSF can be life threatening; 2) a brief course of Rx is unlikely to lead to tooth problems or staining
- Adjunctive steroids not recommended

Tetracycline
- Child: 25 to 50 mg/kg/day PO in 4 divided doses

Chloramphenicol
- Adult: 500mg PO qid, 7d or 3 d after defervescence
- Child: 50-75 mg/kg/day PO in 4 divided doses

IMPORTANT POINTS
- It is better to treat empirically even if diagnosis not confirmed (but only suspected), rather that wait to prove diagnosis and then treat.
- RMSF can occur in fall or winter, primarily in Southern states
- In appropriate setting (endemic area, spring to summer season), best to treat suspected cases early before confirmation of disease
- Fewer than 20% of RMSF cases have history of known tick bite (since often pediatric)
- Dx: PCR on skin bx (not blood) useful in qualified labs; culture not routinely done-hazardous (BSL3 agent)

SELECTED READINGS

Masters EJ et al. Rocky Mountain spotted fever: a clinician's dilemma. Arch Intern Med. 2003;163:769-74

O'Reilly M et al. Physician knowledge of the diagnosis and management of Rocky Mountain Spotted Fever. Mississippi, 2002. Ann NY Acad Sci 2003; 990:295-301

Paddock CD et al. Hidden mortality attributable to Rocky Mountain spotted fever: immunohistochemical detection of fatal, serologically unconfirmed disease. J Infect Dis. 1999 Jun;179 (6):1469-76

Centers for Disease Control and Prevention. Consequences of Delayed Diagnosis of Rocky Mountain Spotted Fever in Children--West Virginia, Michigan, Tennessee, and Oklahoma, May--July 2000 . MMWR

Dalton MJ et al. National surveillance for Rocky Mountain spotted fever, 1981-1992: epidemiologic summary and evaluation of risk factors for fatal outcome. Am J Trop Med Hyg. 1995 May;52:405-13

RICKETTSIA SPECIES
Joseph Vinetz, M.D.

CLINICAL RELEVANCE & DIAGNOSIS
- Two major groups of obligately intracellular, gram neg bacteria: 1) Spotted fever group; 2) Typhus group. For Rocky Mountain Spotted Fever, see previous monograph.
- Generic syndrome: fever, headache, rash, in appropriate epidemiological context (i.e., tick bite); because lab diagnosis difficult, may need to start empiric Rx before Dx established
- Suspect in febrile travelers returning from Africa, South America and Asia, with rural, especially brush, exposure; look for skin lesions
- Spotted fever group [SPF]: R. conorii (Mediterranean spotted or Boutonneuse fever) - tick-borne, tache noire; R. africae (tick-borne), R. akari (mite-borne; rickettsialpox; found in US)
- SPF: African Tick Bite Fever - emerging dz caused by R. africae; acute febrile illness with headache, tache noire w/ regional adenitis, vesicular rash, aphthous ulcers; cattle tick vector.
- SPF infections usually non-fatal; serious illness can occur with RMSF-like syndrome (esp. R. conorii infection)

BACTERIA

- Tache noir (ulcerated, necrotic lesion at site of infectious tick bite/ black eschar) characteristic of R. conorii (usually), R. africae (may be many), R. akari (but not RMSF).
- Typhus group: R. prowazeki (epidemic typhus; louse borne; assoc'd w/ poor sanitation, eg. Burundi, Peru); R. typhi (endemic/murine typhus, fleas; in US, especially border w/ Mexico, Hawaii)
- Scrub typhus, caused by Orientia tsutsugamushi, formerly R. tsutsugamushi, transmitted by chiggers in southeast Asia; associated with inoculation eschar; can be tetracycline resistant
- Lab Diagnosis: serologic (indirect immunofluorescence assay); direct immunofluorescence on skin biopsy; polymerase chain reaction (all done in reference labs)

SITES OF INFECTION

- General: fever, headache, myalgia reflective of disseminating infection
- Liver: elevated transaminases 5-10X normal; normal or moderately elevated alkaline phosphatase; jaundice rare unless there is shock
- Skin: Inoculation eschar, "tache noire"; may be multiple esp. with R. africae; maculopapular or vesicular rash
- HEENT: occasional oral aphthous ulcers

TREATMENT REGIMENS

Doxycycline
- 100mg PO bid for 5-10d or >= 3d after cessation of fever; this applies to non-severe cases
- 100mg IV q12hr for severe cases, up to 24 hr after defervescence, followed by 2-3 d more of oral doxycycline

Tetracycline
- 500mg PO q6hr on empty stomach for 5-10d or >=3d after cessation of fever

Chloramphenicol
- 500mg PO q6hr for 5-10 d or >=3d after cessation of fever
- 50-100 mg/kg IV in 4 divided doses for severe cases in which other antimicrobials are contraindicated

Ciprofloxacin
- 500mg PO bid for 5-10d or >= 3d after cessation of fever
- Second-line choice with limited data, but some prefer for R. conorii infections.

IMPORTANT POINTS

- Laboratory diagnosis: CDC Division of Viral and Rickettsial Diseases, (404) 639-1075; also contact state health departments
- In the U.S., suspect murine/endemic typhus in south Texas, California; rickettsialpox in New York City in patients with fever, eschar, papulovesicular rash; transmitted by mites from house mice
- Suspect African tick-bite fever, Boutennouse fever, scrub typhus in patients with fever, tache noire, returning from travel to Africa, Middle East, Thailand
- Look for skin lesions, especially on legs, suggestive of inoculation eschar, which may be papules or ulcerated (tache noire)
- Maculopapular rash may appear late in the course of illness, after fever develops

SELECTED READINGS

Rolain JM, Jensenius M, Raoult D. Rickettsial infections--a threat to travellers?. Curr Opin Infect Dis. 2004;17:433-7

Gikas A, et al. Comparison of the effectiveness of five different antibiotic regimens on infection with Rickettsia typhi: therapeutic data from 87 cases. Am J Trop Med Hyg. 2004;70:576-9

Centers for Disease Control and Prevention. Murine typhus--Hawaii, 2002. MMWR 52(50):1224-26

Moreira-Galvao M.A., et al. Fatal spotted fever rickettsiosis, Minas Gerais, Brazil. Emerg Infect Dis. 2003;9:1402-5

Jensenius M, Fournier P-E, Raoult D. Tick-borne rickettsioses in international travellers. Int J Infect Dis 2004; 8:139-146

SALMONELLA SPECIES
John G. Bartlett, M.D.

CLINICAL RELEVANCE & DIAGNOSIS

- Gram-neg rod, 2-4 x 0.4-0.6um; grows on standard media for stool-need fresh specimen.
- S. typhi (typhoid fever) colonizes humans only; developing countries; 15% mortality; 400 cases/yr in US
- Salmonella (non-typhoid) one of top 2 bacterial enteric pathogens (C. jejuni is other)
- The major bacterial cause foodborne infection esp. eggs
- Clinical spectrum: colon colonization, gastroenteritis, enteric fever and focal infection
- Nontyphoid salmonella: 1-3 mil/year U.S.; most common cause foodborne diarrhea; usual sources are: meat, poultry, eggs, dairy products.
- Dx: culture blood, urine, stool; serology not useful

SITES OF INFECTION

- Typhoid fever
- Gastroenteritis
- Enteric fever
- Vascular infection
- Osteomyelitis
- Septic arthritis
- Carrier state
- Reactive arthritis

TREATMENT REGIMENS

Gastroenteritis

- Guidelines from IDSA (CID 2001;32:331). Usually no treatment
- Indications to treat: severe disease, >50yrs, prosthesis, presence of valvular heart disease or severe atherosclerosis, cancer, uremia, immunosuppressed
- Preferred - immunocompetent (if tx is indicated): TMP-SMX DS bid, cipro 500mg bid or ceftriaxone 2g IV/d all x 5-7d
- Preferred - immunosuppressed: Above x>14d

Other infections

- Abx guidelines from Med Letter (2001; 43:69)
- Typhoid fever: ceftriaxone 1-2g IV qd then cefixime (Suprax) 400mg qd - total 10-14d or ciprofloxacin 500mg bid x 10-14d. Add steroids in typhoid fever if in shock.
- Non-typhoid: serious infection: 3d gen cephalosporin or fluoroquinolone
- Bacteremia: ceftriaxone 2g IV/d or cefotaxime 2g IV q6-8h x 7-14d or ciprofloxacin 400mg IV q12h x 7-14d
- Vascular prosthesis infection: ceftriaxone, cefotaxime or fluoroquinolone (above doses) x 6wks + early removal of prosthesis or give suppressive therapy life-long
- HIV + salmonellosis: IV cephalosporin or IV fluoroquinolone, then FQ (ciprofloxacin 500-750mg bid etc) x 4wks; relapse within 6 wks: life-long abx or until immune recovery

- Osteomyelitis: ceftriaxone 2g/d, cefotaxime 2g q 6-8h or cipro 750mg bid x >4wks + remove sequestra
- Arthritis: ceftriaxone 2g/d, or cefotaxime 2g q 6-8h x 6wks
- Endocarditis: ceftriaxone 2g/d or cefotaxime 2g q 6-8h x 6wks
- UTI: ceftriaxone, cefotaxime or ciprofloxacin IV x 1-2wks, then oral cipro or TMP-SMX x 6wks + remove any obstructions

Prevention

- Avoid use of raw or undercooked eggs
- Time-temperature standards for food preparation
- Health care workers or food handlers who are long term carriers are at low risk to transmit
- Stool surveillance for food handlers is not recommended
- Food handlers - personal hygiene prevents transmission
- Carrier state (use sensitivity tests): ciprofloxacin 500mg PO bid x4-6wks or TMP-SMX 1 DS bid x6wks or amoxicillin 500mg PO tid x6wks + cholecystectomy if stones present
- Typhoid fever vaccine: Recommended for travel to developing countries, esp with rural travel & prolonged exposure
- Available typhoid vaccines in US: 1) oral, live, attenuated vaccine (Vivotif Berna vaccine/Ty21a strain) given 1 dose qod x 4d 2) Vi capsular polysaccharide given IM x 1. Either give 50-80% efficacy.

IMPORTANT POINTS

- Guidelines for enteric disease IDSA (CID 2001;33:331). Guidelines for systemic disease (Med letter 2001; 43:69)
- Abx for most gastroenteritis: prolongs carrier state & represents abx abuse
- Abx resistance is big problem - chloro, TMP-SMX & amp; more recently cephalosporin & fluoroquinolones. Need sensitivity tests to treat
- Main source: undercooked food from animals - meat, poultry, eggs
- Sickle cell pts more prone to salmonella osteomyelitis than others

SELECTED READINGS

Hennessy TW, et al. A national outbreak of Salmonella enteritidis infections from ice cream. NEJM 1996;334:1281

Spika JS, Waterman SH, Hoo GW, et al. Chloramphenicol - resistant Salmonella newport traced through hamburger to dairy farms. A major persisting source of human salmonellosis in California. NEJM 1987;316:565

Donabedian H. Long-term suppression of Salmonella aortitis with an oral antibiotic. Arch Intern Med 1989;149:1452

Freerksen E, Rosenfield M, Freerksen R, et al. Treatment of chronic Salmonella carriers. Chemotherapy 1977;23:192

Ferreccio C, et al. Efficacy of ciprofloxacin in the treatment of chronic typhoid carriers. J Infect Dis 1988;157:1235

SERRATIA SPECIES

Paul Auwaerter, M.D.

CLINICAL RELEVANCE & DIAGNOSIS

- Aerobic, gram-negative rod of Enterobacteriaceae family, Klebsiella tribe. Only S. marcescens routine cause of human disease, others (S. liquifaciens, rubidaea, dorifera) rare.

- Common cause of nosocomial infection, as often colonizes respiratory or GU tracts with GI less common except in neonates. Hand-to-hand spread implicated mostly in transmission.
- Infections described in heroin-using addicts
- May cause nosocomial outbreaks especially in neonatal units or related to contaminated equipment.

SITES OF INFECTION

- Bacteremia: usually catheter associated
- UTI: often w/ catheter or instrumentation association
- Wound Infection: post-operative complications
- Endocarditis: rare, mostly IVDU populations
- Osteomyelitis: rare, mostly IVDU populations
- Pneumonia: usually nosocomial with history of intubation, or invasive procedures. May occur as "community-acquired" pathogen in the elderly or nursing home resident.
- Septic arthritis: described after intra-articular injections
- Conjunctivitis, keratitis

TREATMENT REGIMENS

Bacteremia, pneumonia or serious infections

- Organisms frequently drug resistant. Amikacin susceptibility usually maintained often capable of synergy w/ antipseudomonal penicillins.
- Often plasmid-mediated resistance to third-gen cephs, but also described with fourth-gen cephs (cefepime) and carbapenems. ESBL strains reported. Fluoroquinolone resistance described.
- Cefepime 1-2g IV q8h, or imipenem 0.5-1.0g IV q6h or ciprofloxacin 400mg IV q 12h. Sensitivities should guide choices.
- Aztreonam, gentamicin or amikacin, piperacillin/tazobactam also often effective.
- Duration depends on clinical response, usually 7-14 days.

Endocarditis

- Choice dictated by sensitivities. Four to six week duration of parenteral therapy.

Osteomyelitis

- Choice dictated by sensitivity profile. Treat for 6-12 weeks depending upon response. Use IV treatment until stable/clinically improved (10-14d min) then may convert to PO therapy if appropriate.

IMPORTANT POINTS

- Important nosocomial pathogen implicated as both cause of actual outbreaks due to contaminated equipment as well as pseudo-outbreaks due to inability to sterilize contaminated instruments.
- Mostly likely a cause of hospital-acquired UTI, pneumonia or bacteremia. IVDUs prone to endocarditis or osteomyelitis.
- Source of recommendations: author's opinion.

SELECTED READINGS

Yu WL, Wu LT, Pfaller MA et al. Confirmation of extended-spectrum beta-lactamase-producing Serratia marcescens: preliminary report from Taiwan. Diagn Microbiol Infect Dis. 2003 Apr;45(4):221-4

Guide SV, Stock F, Gill VJ et al. Reinfection, rather than persistent infection, in patients with chronic granulomatous disease. J Infect Dis. 2003 Mar 1;187(5):845-53. Epub 2003 Feb 24

Kirschke DL, Jones TF, Craig AS et ak. Pseudomonas aeruginosa and Serratia marcescens contamination associated with a manufacturing defect in bronchoscopes. N Engl J Med. 2003 Jan 16;348 (3):214-20

Choi SH, Kim YS, Chung JW, Kim TH, Choo EJ, Kim MN, Kim BN, Kim NJ, Woo JH, Ryu J. Serratia bacteremia in a large university hospital: trends in antibiotic resistance during 10 years and implications for antibiotic use. Infect Control Hosp Epidemiol. 2002 Dec;23(12):740-7

Yu VL. Serratia marcescens: historical perspective and clinical review. N Engl J Med. 1979 Apr 19;300 (16):887-93

SHIGELLA SPECIES
Khalil G. Ghanem, M.D.

CLINICAL RELEVANCE & DIAGNOSIS

- Gram neg; family Enterobacteriaceae; 4 groups: A (S. dysenteriae) B (S. flexneri) C (S. boydii) D (S. sonnei). Causes spectrum of illness bacillary; watery diarrhea to dysentery.
- Classic Sx: fever (30%)+ abd cramps then voluminous stool [small intestinal phase]; 48h later, stools more frequent, less fever, tenesmus + blood (40%)& mucus (50%) [colonic phase].
- Sx2: duration of illness without Abx Rx lasts from 1-30d (mean of 7d). Complications rare except w/ S. dysenteriae.
- Dx: stool cx in first 48h high yield. Use MacConkey or EMB agar in addition to Shigella-Salmonella agar. Gram stain stool= in 40%, sheets of PMN; serology used for epi studies NOT dx.
- Affects children 6mo-10yrs; adults infected from kids; person-to-person mostly, but water (wells contaminated w/feces) and food (20% of cases in US) more common vectors in developing countries.
- As few as 10 organisms can cause disease hence person to person transmission is common especially w/crowding; invades mucosa but generally not beyond that, hence blood cx are usually neg.
- If no Abx used, fecal excretion lasts 1-4wks; longer term carriage documented. Amount excreted usually low hence person-to-person spread in carriers less likely.
- 60-80% of cases in the U.S. are caused by S. sonnei.

SITES OF INFECTION

- GI: small intestine (abdominal pain, watery diarrhea and fever), colon (diarrhea, tenesmus, mucus and blood)
- Eye: keratoconjunctivitis
- Joints (arthritis & post-Shigella Reiter's syndrome in pts w/HLA-B27)
- Lungs: pneumonia, usually in immunocompromised host.

TREATMENT REGIMENS

Prevention

- Safe water supply (chlorination & effective sewage rx); garbage collection; hand washing; appropriate refrigeration & cooking of food; isolating & treating cases of diarrhea.
- Contact precautions are very effective in decreasing spread.

Therapy

- Appropriate rehydration in cases of severe fluid losses.
- All infections should be treated. Use of antimicrobials shortens duration of illness and shedding; decreases risk of transmission since person-to-person is common route.
- If known sulfa sensitive: TMP (160mg)/SMX (800mg) PO q12h X3-5d

- If TMP/SMX resistant or in area of high resistance (SE Asia, Africa, S. America) or unknown susceptibility: cipro 500mg/norflox 400mg/oflox 200mg all PO bid x 3-5d.
- Alternatives include: ceftriaxone, azithromycin nalidixic acid, ampicillin depending on susceptibility patterns.

IMPORTANT POINTS

- With bloody diarrhea DO NOT USE MOTILITY AGENTS; increased risk of toxic dilatation of colon & increased carriage time.
- Specific diagnosis by stool culture is recommended.
- Empiric treatment for Shigella is recommended in an outbreak situation or w/ increased index of suspicion.
- It is recommended (see references.) to treat patients with suspected shigella infection with antibiotic therapy in view of MULTIPLE randomized trials clearly showing benefit.
- Antibiotic resistance patterns vary: resistance to TMP/SMX is increasing; quinolones are favored when susceptibility is unknown.

SELECTED READINGS

Ashkenazi S, Levy I, Kazaronovski V, et al. Growing antimicrobial resistance of Shigella isolates. J Antimicrob Chemother 2003 Feb;51(2):427-9

Replogle ML, Fleming DW, Cieslak PR. Emergence of antimicrobial-resistant shigellosis in Oregon. Clin Infect Dis 2000 Mar;30(3):515-9

Garcia-Fulgueiras A, Sanchez S, Guillen JJ, et al. A large outbreak of Shigella sonnei gastroenteritis associated with consumption of fresh pasteurised milk cheese. Eur J Epidemiol 2001;17(6):533-8

MMWR . Shigella sonnei outbreak among men who have sex with men--San Francisco, California, 2000-2001. MMWR Morb Mortal Wkly Rep 2001 Oct 26;50(42):922-6

DuPont HL, Levine MM, Hornick RB, et al. Inoculum size in shigellosis and implications for expected mode of transmission. J Infect Dis 1989 Jun;159(6):1126-8

STAPHYLOCOCCUS AUREUS   Sara Cosgrove, M.D.

CLINICAL RELEVANCE & DIAGNOSIS

- Gram-positive cocci in clusters; easily grown on blood agar or other conventional media; coagulase positive; thermonuclease positive
- Carried in anterior nares by 20-30% of population. Higher carriage rates seen in diabetes, injection drug users (IDU), HIV or dialysis pts. Carriers have > risk of subsequent infection.
- Dx: positive cx from sterile site (blood, joint, CSF), abscess or wound. Positive cx from nares = colonization, not infection
- Methicillin resistance increasing. MRSA traditionally associated w/ healthcare system interaction; community-acquired MRSA emerging as significant pathogen, esp. children, prisoners, IDUs.
- Risk factors: skin disease, venous catheters, other foreign bodies (e.g., prosthetic joints, pacemakers), IDU, hemodialysis
- Staph toxic shock syndrome (see Dx module > sepsis syndromes for details) by TSST-1 producing strains = fever, low BP, red rash & multiorgan dz. Risks: tampon use, nasal packing, surgical wounds.
- Ingestion of preformed enterotoxin causes acute, self-limited gastroenteritis. Incubation 2-6h.

BACTERIA

SITES OF INFECTION

- Bloodstream: primary risk is presence of intravascular catheter, which should be removed
- Cardiac: endocarditis occurs in 6-25% of S. aureus bacteremia; native and prosthetic valves
- Abscesses: liver, spleen, kidney; results from hematogenous seeding from bacteremia
- Skin & soft tissues: cellulitis, furucle, carbuncle, abscess, impetigo (often in combination with Strep pyogenes)
- Bone: osteomyelitis (S. aureus leading cause)
- Prosthetic devices: pacemaker leads and pocket, prosthetic joints
- Lung: nosocomial pneumonia or following influenza; septic pulmonary emboli (associated with right-sided endocarditis)
- Mucosal surfaces - related to release of TSST-1 and subsequent toxic shock syndrome
- GI: gastroenteritis
- Breast: mastitis

TREATMENT REGIMENS

Bacteremia

- Remove focus of infection whenever possible
- MSSA (preferred): oxacillin or nafcillin 2g IV q4h. Alternative for non-life threatening PCN allergy: cefazolin 1-2g IV q8h
- MRSA or life-threatening PCN allergy (preferred): vancomycin 15mg/kg q 12h [usually 1g IV q12h]
- Vancomycin alternatives (allergy or failure-none are FDA approved for S. aureus bacteremia): linezolid 600mg IV/PO q12h, quinupristin-dalfopristin 7.5mg/kg IV q12h, daptomycin 6mg/kg IV qd

Soft tissue infx

- Surgical drainage. Antibiotics indicated for cellulitis, and deep infections after debridement.
- IV abx generally not needed unless severe infection, concomitant bacteremia or systemic toxicity.
- IV antibiotic choices same as for bacteremia (except daptomycin dose is 4mg/kg IV qd)
- MSSA (oral): cephalexin 500mg PO qid, dicloxacillin 500mg PO qid, clindamycin 300-450mg PO tid, amoxicillin/clavulanate 875mg PO bid
- MRSA (oral--check susceptibilities): clindamycin 300-450mg PO tid, TMP-SMX 1-2 DS tabs PO bid, minocycline 100mg PO bid, linezolid 600mg PO bid
- Consider decolonization for recurrent soft tissue infections: 2% mupirocin ointment to nares bid for 5 days +/- Hibiclens washes.

Endocarditis

- Consult w/ cardiac surgery if patient persistently positive blood cultures, evidence of heart failure or embolic disease.
- Obtain brain & CNS vessel imaging if neurologic symptoms or persistent headache present.
- MSSA, native valve, right-sided involvement ONLY w/o embolic dz other than septic pulmonary emboli or vascular prosthesis: oxacillin or nafcillin 2g IV q4h PLUS gentamicin 1mg/kg IV q8h for 14d
- Alt: ciprofloxacin 750mg PO bid PLUS rifampin 300mg PO bid for 28 days, if isolate proven susceptible.

- MSSA, native valve, left-sided: oxacillin or nafcillin 2g IV q4h for 4-6 weeks with or w/o gentamicin 1mg/kg IV q8h for 1st 3-5 days.
- Alt: if life-threatening penicillin allergy desensitize or vancomycin 15mg/kg IV q12h with or without gentamicin 1mg/kg IV q8h for 1st 3-5 days
- MRSA, native valve, right or left sided involvement: vancomycin 15mg/kg IV q12h for 4-6 weeks
- MSSA, prosthetic valve: oxacillin or nafcillin 2g IV q4h for 6 weeks PLUS gentamicin 1mg/kg IV q8h for 1st 2 weeks PLUS rifampin 300mg PO q8h
- MRSA, prosthetic valve: vancomycin 15mg/kg IV q12h for 6 weeks PLUS gentamicin 1mg/kg IV q8h for 1st 2 weeks PLUS rifampin 300mg PO q8h for 6 weeks after blood cultures have cleared.

Toxic shock syndrome
- See "Toxic Shock Syndrome, Staphylococcus"
- Remove the focus of staphylococcal colonization or infection
- Stabilize blood pressure w/ aggressive hydration +/- pressors.
- MSSA: oxacillin or nafcillin 2g IV q4h PLUS clindamycin 600mg IV q8h.
- MRSA: vancomycin 15mg/kg IV q12h PLUS clindamycin 600mg IV q8h (if susceptible).
- Consider intravenous immunoglobulin infusions

Pneumonia
- Antibiotic choices same as for bacteremia except daptomycin cannot be used for pulmonary infections because it has poor lung penetration.

Important Points
- Community-acquired MRSA growing issue. Risk factors not predictive, isolates often sensitive to tetracylines or TMP-SMX.
- Mortality associated with S. aureus bacteremia is 20-40%.
- S. aureus bacteremia is associated with heart valve involvement in 25% when studied with transesophageal echo (TEE).
- All patients with S. aureus bacteremia should undergo at least an "adequate" transthoracic echo (TTE). TEE is preferred for patients with prosthetic valves or with inadequate TTE.
- Be alert for the development of metastatic abscess formation w/ any S. aureus bacteremia. S. aureus in urine cx should alert to the possibility of associated bacteremia.
- Patients with MRSA colonization or infection should be placed on contact precautions.

Selected Readings
Fowler VG Jr, Miro JM, Hoen B, Cabell CH, Abrutyn F, et al. Staphylococcus aureus endocarditis: a consequence of medical progress. JAMA 2005; Jun 22;293(24):3012-3021

Fridkin SK, Hageman JC, Morrison M, Sanza LT, Como-Sabetti K, Jernigan JA et al. Methicillin-resistant Staphylococcus aureus disease in three communities. N Engl J Med 2005; Apr 7;352(14):1436-1444

Von Eiff C et al. Nasal carriage as a source of Staphylococcus aureus bacteremia. N Engl J Med 2001;344:11-16

Lowy FD. Staphylococcus aureus infection. N Engl J Med 1998; 339: 520-532

DiNubile MJ. Short-course antibiotic therapy for right-sided endocarditis caused by Staphylococcus aureus in injection drug users. Ann Intern Med 1994; 121:873-876

STAPHYLOCOCCUS EPIDERMIDIS

John G. Bartlett, M.D.

CLINICAL RELEVANCE & DIAGNOSIS

- Staphylococcus epidermis--the major pathogen of coagulase-negative staph category
- Nearly always nosocomial, source is skin flora, cause is foreign body & biofilm
- # 1 cause of nosocomial bacteremia; but also #1 contaminant
- #1 infection plastic/metal-lines, valves, joints, etc.
- Cultures: need 2 positive blood cultures, or heavy growth in presence of e.g., foreign body.

SITES OF INFECTION

- IV lines, vascular grafts, valves - bacteremia
- CSF shunt: meningitis
- Dialysis catheter: peritonitis
- Prosthetic joint: septic arthritis
- Prosthetic valve: endocarditis
- Post sternotomy osteomyelitis
- Implants (breast, penile, pacemaker) local infection
- Endophthalmitis post ocular surgery

TREATMENT REGIMENS

Foreign body: general

- >80% beta-lactamase positive & methicillin-resistant. Most active - vancomycin, linezolid, daptomycin; gentamicin +/or rifampin often added.
- Standard for deep infection: vancomycin 1g IV q 12 h +/- rif 300mg bid IV/PO +/- gentamicin 3-5 mg/kg/d IV.
- Alt (if methicillin resistant): linezolid 600mg IV/PO bid; daptomycin IV 4-6 mg/kg/d; each + rifampin +/or gentamicin.
- Alt (methicillin-sensitive): oxacillin/nafcillin 1.5-3 g IV q6h, cefazolin 1-2g IV q8h, ciprofloxacin 400 mg IV q12h, clindamycin 600mg IV q8h, TMP-SMX

Site specific

- Prosthetic valve: consider valve replacement & abx 6 wks
- Peripheral line: remove line & abx 2 wks
- Central line: often keep line & abx x 2-4 wks
- Prosthetic joint: remove joint & abx 6 wks
- Dialysis cath: keep catheter (at least for first effort) & IV vanco (usually 2g IV/week (redose when level <15mcg/mL)
- Vascular graft: remove graft & abx 6 weeks
- CSF shunt: shunt removal usually recommended but variable; IV vancomycin & po/IV rifampin plus possible intravententricular vancomycin 5-20 mg/d & gentamicin 4-8 mg/d (must also give IV gentamicin).

IMPORTANT POINTS

- Guidelines from G Archer (PPID 2000; pg 2092) & Med Letter (2004;2:22)
- Most common cause bacteremia; most common contaminant in all specimens
- CDC: "Never treat a single pos blood cult for Staphylococcus epidermidis"
- Usually need foreign body plus 2 positive cultures or heavy growth to implicate as causative pathogen.
- Major cause of all hardware infections - lines, joints, implants, shunts, valves, etc.

SELECTED READINGS

Vuong C, et al. Quorum-sensing control of biofilm factors in S. epidermidis. J. Infect Dis. 2003;188:706-718

Archer G. Staphylococcus epidermidis and other coagulase-negative staphylococci; . Chapter 184 in Principles & Practice of Infectious Disease, Mandell JL, Bennett JE & Dolin R (Editors) Churchill Livingston Phil 5th Ed, 2000, pp2092-2100

Metallidis S, et al. Comp. in vitro activity of linezolid & 5 other antimicrobials against nosocomial isolates of methicillin-resist S aureus, meth resist S aureus, meth resist S epi & vanco-resis enterococcus E. faecium. J. Chemother 2003;15:442-8

Dickema DJ, Pfaller MA, Schmitz FJ, et al. Survey of infections due to Staphylococcus species: frequency and occurrence and antimicrobial susceptibility of isolate collected from the US, Canada, Latin America & Europe. Clin Infect Dis 2001;32:S114

Richards MJ, Edwards JR, Culver DH, et al. Nosocomial infections in combined medical-surgical care units in the US. Infect Control Hosp Epid 2000;21:510

STENOTROPHOMONAS MALTOPHILIA

John G. Bartlett, M.D.

CLINICAL RELEVANCE & DIAGNOSIS

- Non-fermenting gram-negative rod, easily grown on standard media. Formerly Xanthomonas maltophilia.
- Ubiquitous - found in water, soil, plants
- Nosocomial sources - distilled water, nebulizers, dialysates, contaminated disinfectants, etc.
- Risks: foreign bodies (catheters), neutropenia, broad spectrum abx, cystic fibrosis

SITES OF INFECTION

- Nosocomial pneumonia
- Bacteremia +/- septic shock & DIC
- Plastic - IV lines, CSF shunts, caths
- Skin & soft tissue - wound, burns, metastatic nodules
- Urinary tract infection
- Ecthyma gangrenosum (rare)
- Sinopulmonary infection, esp cystic fibrosis pts.
- Ocular - corneal tx, contact lens, HSV keratitis

TREATMENT REGIMENS

Treatment

- Preferred: TMP-SMX 15-20 (TMP)mg/kg/d
- Alternative: ceftazidime 2g IV q8h or ticar/clav 3.1gm IV q 4h
- Alternative: FQ - cipro 500mg PO/ 400mg IV q 12h, gatifloxacin 400 PO/IV qd, levofloxacin 500mg PO/IV qd (limited experience)
- Some experts recommend coverage with TMP/SMX plus ticar/clav.

Prevention

- Judicious abx use
- Hand washing
- Barrier precautions
- Surveillance
- Identify common source - water, equipment

IMPORTANT POINTS

- Guidelines for abx: Med Letter Treatment Guidelines (2004;2:22)
- Risks - hospitalization, plastic, multiple abx, trauma, neutropenia, cancer
- Resistant to most abx including imipenem, quinolones, aminoglycosides, cefepime
- Outbreaks: waterborne, equipment, solutions

SELECTED READINGS

Spencer RC. The emergence of epidemic multiple-antibiotic=resistant Stenotrophomonas maltophilia and Burkholderia cepacia. J Hosp Inf 1995;30(Suppl):453

Vartivaran S, Papadakis KA, Palacios JA, et al. Mucocutaneous and soft tissue infections caused by Xanthomonas maltophilia: A new spectrum. Ann Intern Med 1994;121:969

Tsiodras S, Pittet D, Carmel Y, et al. Clinical Implications of Stenotrophomonas maltophilia resistant to TMP-SMX: a study of 69 patients at 2 university hospitals. Scan J Infect Dis 2000;32:651

Micozz A, Venditti M, Monaco M, et al. Bacteremia due to Stenotrophomonas maltophilia in patients with hematologic malignancies. Clin Infect Dis 2000;31:705

Cohn ML, Waites KS. Antimicrobial activities of gatifloxacin against nosocomial isolates of S. maltophilia measured by MIC and time kill studies. AAC 2001;45:2126

STREPTOCOCCUS PNEUMONIAE

John G. Bartlett, M.D.

CLINICAL RELEVANCE & DIAGNOSIS

- Gram-positive diplococcus with capsule; grown on blood agar; capsular swelling w/ Quellung sera
- Ecologic niche: nasopharynx 5-10% adults, 20-40% of children
- Dx: proven by positive cx body fluid (blood, CSF, joint etc); supportive dx if positive gram stain or cx from respiratory specimen and/or urine antigen in adult.
- Most common bacterial pathogen of otitis, sinusitis and pneumonia, but usually not cultured in any of these.

SITES OF INFECTION

- Lung (pneumonia)
- Sinuses (sinusitis)
- Middle ear (otitis media)
- Bronchi (exacerbation of chronic bronchitis)
- CNS (meningitis)
- Peritoneum (spontaneous bacterial peritonitis)
- Pericardium (purulent pericarditis)
- Skin (cellulitis)
- Eye (conjunctivitis)

TREATMENT REGIMENS

Respiratory tract

- Pneumonia (community-acquired; IDSA guidelines CID 2003;37:1405): preferred - PCN sensitive (MIC <4): ceftriaxone 1g IV q24/q12 or cefotaxime 1-2g IV q 6-8h
- Oral agents: amoxicillin, 2-3gm/d, cefpodoxime 200mg bid, cefprozil 500mg bid, clarithro 1g qd, or 500mg bid, azithro (1500mg total dose) 500mg, then 500mg or 250mg qd, or doxy 100mg PO bid
- PCN-resistant (MIC >4): levofloxacin (Levaquin) 500-750mg IV/po qd; gatifloxacin (Tequin) 400mg IV/po qd, moxifloxacin (Avelox) 400mg IV/po; telithromycin (Ketek) 800mg PO qd

- Sinusitis (empiric - ACP Ann Intern Med 2001;134:479): amoxicillin 2-3g/d PO or doxycycline 100mg PO bid
- Otitis media (Redbook-Pediatrics 2000, pg 647): amoxicillin; Amox failures - amox/clavulanate (Augmentin)
- Acute exacerbations of chronic bronchitis (ACP Ann Intern Med 2001;134:595): amoxicillin 2-3g/d PO or doxycycline 100mg PO bid

Meningitis
- Preferred (Med Letter 2004;2:22) empiric: vancomycin 1g IV q12h (up to 4g/d) plus ceftriaxone 2g IV q12h or cefotaxime 2g IV q4h or 3g q8h
- PCN sensitive (MIC <0.2): ceftriaxone 1-2g IV q12h, or cefotaxime 2g IV q4h or 3g IV q8h
- PCN resistant (MIC >0.2) or beta-lactam hypersensitivity: vancomycin 15mg/kg q12h (usually 1g IV q12h)

Prevention (adult)
- Pneumovax (23-valent) prevents bacteremia.
- See "Pneumococcal Prophylaxis" in the Vaccines section

IMPORTANT POINTS
- Sources: Pneumonia - IDSA guidelines (CID 2003;37:1405). Sinusitis, Exac bronchitis - (CDC & ACP Ann Intern Med 2001;134:495,498,595); Meningitis - (Med Letter 2004;2:22)
- Best abx without meningitis: ceftriaxone, cefotaxime, amoxicillin (95% sensitive); high level PCN-resistance: fluoroquinolones, telithromycin
- Penicillin resistance in US: 14%; PCN-resistant strains often resist to macrolides (>60%), cephalosporins, doxycycline, TMP-SMX.
- Abx active vs 99-100% S. pneumoniae strains: vancomycin, fluoroquinolones (except ciprofloxacin), linezolid, telithromycin, daptomycin.

SELECTED READINGS

CDC. Effect of susceptibility breakpoints on reporting of resistance in Streptococci pneumoniae. United States 2003; MMWR 2004;53:152

Mandell L, Bartlett JR, Dowell SF, et al. Update of practice guidelines for the management of pneumonia in immunocompetent adults. Clin Infect Dis 2003;37:1405-33

Houck P, Bratzler DW, Nsa W, et al. Timing of antibiotic administration and outcomes for Medicare patients with community acquired pneumonia. Arch Intern Med 2004;154:637-44

Karlowsky JA, Thornsberry C, Critchley I, et al. Susceptibilities to levofloxacin in streptococcus pneumoniae, Haemophilus influenzae and Moraxella catarrhalis clinical isolates from children: results from 2000-01, 2001-02 TRUST studies in the US. US Antimicrobial Ag Chemother 2003;47:1790-7

Neurmberger E, Bishai WR. The clinical significance of macrolide-resistant Streptococcus pneumoniae. Clin Infect Dis 2004;38:99-103

STREPTOCOCCUS PYOGENES (GROUP A)

John G. Bartlett, M.D.

CLINICAL RELEVANCE & DIAGNOSIS
- Gram-positive cocci in chains, grows on blood agar - best in anaerobic conditions. Group A Strep (GAS), beta-hemolytic.
- Ecologic niche is pharynx; 2-3% of adults colonized; 15-20 % school children
- Dx: recovery from normally sterile site; ASO antibody response (rheumatic fever) anti-DNAase B (pyoderma); supportive - (+) throat cx or rapid antigen test
- Common: pharyngitis and cellulitis

BACTERIA

- Rare but devastating: toxic shock, necrotizing fasciitis (See Table 8 in Appendix I)

SITES OF INFECTION

- Pharynx (pharyngitis)
- Skin (erysipelas lymphangitis, cellulitis)
- Fascia (fasciitis)
- Muscle (myositis)
- Endometrium (puerperal sepsis)
- Lung (pneumonia) +/- early bloody effusion
- Heart valves (endocarditis)
- Toxin mediated (Scarlet fever, Toxic shock syndrome)
- Bacteremia
- Non-supparative complications (see "Acute rheumatic fever" in the Diagnoses Section), glomerulonephritis

TREATMENT REGIMENS

Pharyngitis

- Principles: GAS only causes 10-20% of adult pharyngitis - most cases are viral (including EBV & HIV); Rx criteria are clinical (Centor criteria) or antigen detection; drug - Penicillin
- Preferred (Amer Heart Assoc, Am Acad Peds, IDSA Med Letter): PCN - Benzathine penicillin 1.2mU IM x 1 or Penicillin V 500mg PO bid or tid x 10d
- Alternative: amoxicillin 750 PO bid or tid x 10d
- Pen allergy: erythromycin 500mg PO bid or tid x 10d. Alt: azithromycin 500mg, then 250mg x 5d, clarithromycin (Biaxin) 1g XR/d or 500mg bid x 5d
- Cefpodoxime proxetil (Vantin) 200mg bid x 5d
- Cefdinir 300mg bid x 5d
- Cefadroxil 500mg bid x 5d
- Loracarbef 200mg bid x 5d

Soft tissue, sepsis

- Preferred: clindamycin 600mg IV q8h + penicillin G 4mU IV q4h
- Penicillin G 2-4mU IV q4h
- Clindamycin 600mg IV q8h
- Cefazolin 1-2g IV q6-8h
- Cefotaxime 2-3g IV q6-8h or ceftriaxone 2gm/d
- Vancomycin 1g IV q12h

Special considerations

- Necrotizing fasciitis: emergent fasciotomy and debridement; repeat debridement usually necessary
- Myositis: debridement
- Toxic shock syndrome: IVIG 2 or more doses [See Toxic Shock Syndrome, Streptococcal in Diagnoses section and Table 7 in Appendix I], massive IV fluids (10-20L/d), albumin if <2g/dL, debridement of necrotic tissue
- Prophylaxis: rheumatic fever - benzathine pen 1.2mu IM q mo; pen V 250mg PO bid, erythro 250mg bid until >5yrs post-ARF & age in 20's.
- Prophylaxis: cellulitis, chronic lymphedema - clindamycin 150mg qd or TMP-SMX 1 DS/d or immediate Rx with pen V or amox 500-750mg PO bid onset of sx

IMPORTANT POINTS

- Recommendations for pharyngitis - Amer Heart Assoc (Pediatrics 1995;96:758) & IDSA (CID 2002;35:113). Deep infections - D Stevens (Cur Opin ID 1998;11:285).

- Diverse & devastating: pharyngitis; non-suppurative (ARF, Scarlet fever, nephritis); soft tissue (erysipelas, myonecrosis, lymphangitis, fasciitis); toxic shock; misc (endocard, pneum, puerperal sepsis)
- All S. pyogenes sensitive to penicillin; 5+% resistant to erythromycin; rare strains resistant to clindamycin
- Clindamycin is superior to pen in animal models of fasciitis/myonecrosis
- Predisposing factors: soft tissue (IDU, diabetes, surgery, trauma, varicella, vein donor, lymphedema); pneumonia (influenza), contacts w/GAS (pharyngitis & fasciitis)

SELECTED READINGS

Stevens D, et al. In vitro antimicrobial effects of various combinations of penicillin & clindamycin against 4 strains of Streptococcus pyogenes. Antimicro Ag Chemother 1998;42:1266

Stevens DL, Bryant AE, Hackett SP. Antibiotic effects on bacterial viability, toxin production and host response. Clin Infect Dis 1995;20:S154

Basiliere JL, et al. Streptococcal pneumonia. Recent outbreaks in a military recruit population. Am J Med 1968;44:580

Baddour LM, Bisno AL. Recurrent cellulitis after coronary by-pass surgery. JAMA 1984;251:1049

Barg NL et al. Group A streptococcal bacteremia in intravenous drug abusers. Am J Med 1985;78:529

STREPTOCOCCUS SPECIES   Paul Auwaerter, M.D.

CLINICAL RELEVANCE & DIAGNOSIS

- Clinical labs classify streptococci on the basis of hemolytic characteristics on 5% sheep blood agar (e.g., beta-hemolysis), Lancefield Group antigens and other biochemical tests
- Viridans streptococci produce alpha (green-hence viridans) hemolysis on blood agar. Oropharynx/GI tract usual niche. Common cause of dental infections, subacute bacterial endocarditis, bacteremia.
- Viridans isolated from CSF or respiratory sections are usually contaminants, but occasionally are responsible for disease.
- Group B strep (S. agalactiae): neonatal sepsis/meningitis, puerperal sepsis, chorioamnionitis; also bacteremia, septic arthritis. Found in GI/GU tracts. More common in adults w/ comorbidities.
- S. intermedius/S. anginosus/S. constellatus group ("S. milleri" no longer appropriate) have propensity for invasion, abscess production, head & Neck infections, bacteremia, meningitis/brain abscess.
- S. intermedius/anginosus/constellatus group (microaerophilic strep): rarely "contaminants" when present in blood cultures.
- Groups C, F, G Strep: bacteremia, endocarditis, septic arthritis, osteomyelitis
- Group D Strep (non-enterococcal), e.g., S. bovis. Associated with colonic malignancy. Cause of endocarditis
- Abiotrophia and Granulicatella spp (formerly known as nutritionally variant streptococci): endocarditis
- Streptococcus pneumoniae: see separate pathogen module
- Nomenclature and taxonomy of streptococci confusing because of many historical efforts at describing the class: Blood agar beta-hemolysis (1902); Lancefield carbohydrate group antigens (1933); Organization into 4 groups by hemolysis, Lancefield and phenotype testing (1937): 1. Pyogenic (beta-hemolytic incl. Group A, B, C, E, F & G); 2. Viridans 3. Lactococci (generally not human pathogens) and 4. Enterococci; rRNA gene sequencing (1990s) yielding true phylogenetic relationships.

SITES OF INFECTION

- Blood: primary bacteremia, esp. w/ neutropenia or malignancy
- Cardiovascular: endocarditis
- Head and neck: dental infections, deep neck space infections (including submandibular, retropharyngeal and lateral neck)
- Lung - pneumonia (rare) associated with oropharyngeal aspiration, abscess and empyema
- Abdomen - abscesses, cholangitis, visceral infections, GU tract
- Shock syndrome (low bp, rash, ARDS) due to viridans strep (e.g., S. mitis) described in cancer patients
- CNS: brain abscess, meningitis
- Musculoskeletal: septic arthritis, cellulitis

TREATMENT REGIMENS

Streptococcus pyogenes (Group A strep)

- See modules Streptococcus pyogenes (Group A), cellulitis, pharyngitis, acute rheumatic fever etc.

Group B streptococcus (S. agalactiae)

- Bacteremia, soft tissue infections: PCN G 10-12 mU/d x 10d [eg, give 2MU q4h or six divided doses/d]
- Meningitis (Adult): PCN G 20-30 mU/d x 14-21d
- Osteomyelitis: PCN G 10-20 mU/d x 21-28d
- Endocarditis: PCN G 20-30 mU/d x 4-6 wks AND gentamicin 1mg/kg q8h for first 2 wks
- PCN allergic: may substitute vancomycin 1g IV q 12h for PCN
- Some use gentamicin (1 mg/kg q8h IV) additionally for any serious GBS infection

Streptococcus pneumoniae (Pneumococcus)

- See modules Streptococcus pneumoniae, pneumonia-community acquired, chronic bronchitis-acute exacerbations, otitis media, sinusitis-acute, etc.

Viridans streptococci

- Cause of primary bacteremia, but up to 80% of cultures may represent contaminants or transient bacteremia. Don't dismiss in cancer pts. on chemotherapy. Continuous bacteremia = suspect endocarditis.
- Viridians group responsible for declining amt of endocarditis compared to "enteric" strep such as S. bovis and enterococci--probably due to aging population and less rheumatic heart disease
- See "Endocarditis" in the Diagnoses section for specifics
- Tetracyclines, macrolides, clindamycin with 25-50% isolates resistant; TMP-SMX >75%. Increasing resistance to beta-lactams, esp. S. mitis (>40%).
- Penicillin G 2-4 mU IV q4h +/- gentamicin for synergy 1.0 mg/kg/q8h IV
- Ceftriaxone 2g IV qd
- Vancomycin 1g IV q12h (if PCN allergic)
- Duration 10-14 days (not endocarditis)

Streptococcus anginosus group

- Group comprises 3-15% of streptococcal isolates of endocarditis. See "Endocarditis" in the Diagnosis section. For management, follow viridans Streptococci recommendations.
- Dental abscesses, sinusitis, fasciitis of head and neck: can be life threatening & require aggressive surgical management. See appropriate HEENT module for specific management.

- Bacteremia often associated with deep-seated abscess. Investigate for abscess--most often intraabdominal. Drainage is usually recommended.
- Brain abscesses often polymicrobial, but S. intermedius in 50-80%. See Brain abscess module for management.
- Implicated in aspiration pneumonia, lung abscess & empyema
- Penicillin G 2-4 million U IV q4h preferred.
- Alt: ceftriaxone 2g IV qd, clindamycin 600-900mg IV q8h or 300-450mg PO qid, vancomycin 1g IV q12h (PCN-allergic)

Group C, E, F Streptococci:
- Bacteremia, cellulitis, septic arthritis or other serious infection: PCN 12-18 milU/d IV x 10-14d
- Endocarditis: See "Endocarditis" in the Diagnoses section re: viridans streptococci recommendations for specifics.

Group D Streptococci:
- Penicillin high-level resistance not described, some strains resistant to clindamycin.
- Bacteremia: PCN 12-18 mU/d IV x 10-14d
- Endocarditis: PCN 14-18 mU/d IV x 4 weeks, may consider gentamicin 1mg/kg/d to shorten duration to 2wks, OR use if PCN MIC >0.1, and definitely if MIC >0.5 and < 2 (rare).

Abiotrophia and Granulicatella spp
- Mainly a cause of endocarditis. Many isolates with some PCN resistance. See "Endocarditis" in the Diagnoses section re: viridans Streptococci recommendations, though would not use 2wk "short-course" therapy.

General note: Criteria favoring 2-wk short course beta-lactam + aminoglycoside combination for endocarditis:
- 1. PCN sensitive oral viridans Streptococci or S. bovis, MIC <0.125mg/L)
- 2. Native valve endocarditis
- 3. No heart failure, aortic insuff., conduction abnl
- 4. No metasatic infectious foci
- 5. Quick clinical response and afebrile within 7d

IMPORTANT POINTS
- A high proportion of blood cultures growing viridans streptococci may be due to cutaneous contamination, or transient oral bacteremia.
- Penicillin-resistance w/ viridans streptococci not due to beta-lactamase production (hence no benefit from using agents such as ampicillin-sulbactam)
- S. anginosus group especially confusing as can be either beta-hemolytic or nonhemolytic. Penicillin resistance is not an issue for the S. intermedius group
- Recurrent invasive Group B Streptococcal infection described in 4% of nonpregnant adults within one year of first episode.
- Nutritionally-variant strains (Abiotrophia/Granulicatella) consider in "culture negative" endocarditis; special media historically required, though many modern broth micro systems should recover.

SELECTED READINGS

Clarridge JE, et al. Streptococcus intermedius, Streptococcus constellatus and Streptococcus angiosus ("Streptococcus milleri" group) are of different clinical importance and are not equally associated with abscess. Clin Infect Dis 2001; 32: 1511-1515

Swenson FJ, et al. Clinical significance of viridans streptococci isolated from blood cultures. J Clin Microbiol 1982; 15: 725-727

Shinzato T , Saito A. The Streptococcus milleri group as a cause of pulmonary infections. Clin Infect Dis 1995; 21: S 238-243

Pfaller MA, Jones RN, Doern GV et al. Survey of blood stream infections attributable to gram-positive cocci: frequency of occurrence and antimicrobial susceptibility of isolates collected in 1997 in the US, Canada, and Latin America... Diagn Microbiol Infect Dis. 1999 Apr;33(4):283-97

Gold JS, Bayar S, Salem RR. Association of Streptococcus bovis bacteremia with colonic neoplasia and extracolonic malignancy. Arch Surg. 2004 Jul;139(7):760-5

TREPONEMA PALLIDUM (SYPHILIS)

Noreen A. Hynes, M.D., M.P.H.

CLINICAL RELEVANCE & DIAGNOSIS

- Chancre occurs at point of introduction/contact
- Protean manifestations seen
- Preventing congenital infection is KEY! Up to 70% of untreated woman can transmit to fetus for up to 4 years
- 4 adult stages: primary, secondary, latent, tertiary. Latency period has no physical manifestations. Early latent 1 yr or less since exposure; 25% relapse to secondary stage signs; dx by serology.
- Course through stages may be more rapid in HIV-infected persons
- Lesions of syphilis resolve without treatment although person remains infected
- Consider syphilis in ANY sexually active person with a generalized rash or painless genital ulcer
- Late latent=1 yr or more after exposure without clinical findings; dx by serological tests. Tertiary syphilis=late stage; includes gumma, heart and aortic findings; neurologic disease (1-30yrs later)

SITES OF INFECTION

- Mucocutaneous areas: Chancre (primary) lesion appears 10-90 days after contact,usually 1 lesion, may be more; untreated lasts several weeks. Secondary (rash) occurs within 6 mo of primary.
- Central nervous system: Asx, meningitis (1-2yrs after infection), meningovascular (5-7yrs), general paresis & tabes dorsalis (10-20), gummatous neurosyphilis
- Cardiovascular system: aortitis (ascending)
- Bone: arthritis, osteitis, periostitis
- Liver: hepatitis
- Secondary (e.g., rash) within 6 mo of exposure; palmar-plantar copper coin rash classic; many other rash forms, condyloma latum. Other secondary sx include alopecia areata (patchy baldspots), fever.
- Ocular: uveitis, iridocyclitis, Argyll-Robertson pupil

TREATMENT REGIMENS

Primary and secondary syphilis in adults

- Recommended: benzathine penicillin (PCN) G 2.4mU IM x 1
- PCN allergy (nonpregnant, preferred): doxycycline 100 mg PO bid X 14d OR tetracycline 500mg PO qid x 14d requires well-documented close f/u.

Latent syphilis in adults

- Early latent [<1 yr infxn duration] (w/ normal CSF exam, if done): Benzathine penicillin G (BPG) 2.4 mU IM x 1

- Late latent or latent of unknown duration (w/ normal CSF exam, if done) benzathine penicillin G 2.4 mU q wk x 3wk. If any dose >2 days late, must recommence Rx from 1st dose.
- PCN allergy recommended: (1) doxycycline 100mg PO bid x 4w or (2) tetracycline 500mg PO qid x 4w

Neurosyphilis in adults

- Only penicillin is currently recommended; allergic persons should be desensitized and treated with penicillin
- Recommended: aqueous crystalline penicillin G 18-24mU/d IV, admin as 3-4mU IV q4h for 10-14d
- Alternative: procaine penicillin 2.4mU IM qd, PLUS probenecid 500mg PO qid x 10-14 d

Syphilis in HIV-infected persons

- Penicillin is the highly preferred regimen for all stages of syphilis in HIV-infected persons
- Primary, Secondary and Early Latent Syphilis: Treat with benzathine penicillin G as for HIV-uninfected persons; some experts recommend 3 weekly doses (i.e., as for late latent syphilis)
- PCN-allergic HIV + w/primary, secondary or early latent syphilis can be treated as allergic HIV-neg person (although NOT the ideal).
- Late latent syphilis or syphilis of unknown duration requires a LP to rule out neurosyphilis. All require PCN-based treatment. Desensitization required.

Syphilis in pregnancy

- Only penicillin is currently recommended. Treatment during pregnancy should be the penicillin regimen appropriate to the stage of syphilis diagnosed; desensitization required for PCN-allergic preg pt
- Some experts recommend a second dose of benzathine PCN G2.4 mU IM 1 wk after the initial dose for primary, secondary, early latent syphilis

Miscellaneous

- Parenteral penicillin G is the preferred drug for Rx of all stages of syphilis. It's the ONLY documented efficacious therapy for neurosyphilis and in pregnancy.
- Jarish-Herxheimer reaction: an acute febrile reaction, often accompanied by headache, myalgia, and rash may occur within 24 hrs of Rx; most often in early syphilis. May induce premature labor or cause fetal distress but is NOT a contraindication to treatment and should NOT delay Rx.
- Pharmacologic data suggest that ceftriaxone should be effective in treating primary and secondary syphilis. But data are limited. Optimal dose and duration has NOT been established. Single dose NOT effective. May try 1g qd for 8 to 10 days.
- For nonpregnant patients with primary or secondary syphilis, erythromycin could be used as alternative: 500mg PO qid for 2 wks. This regimen is less effective than doxycycline and tetracycline.
- There are increasing reports of documented treatment failures when azithromycin is used to treat primary or secondary syphilis or their contacts. Azithromycin should be avoided in most patients with incubating or infectious syphilis. It should not be used treatment of ANY pregnant or HIV-infected patients. Closed follow-up is required for penicillin-allergic non-HIV infected, non-pregnant patients treated with this antibiotic.
- Follow-up using quantitative non-treponemal tests should be done based upon stage of syphilis (see "Important Points")

IMPORTANT POINTS

- This module is based on CDC's 2002 STD Treatment Guidelines (MMWR 2002; 51 (RR-6).
- Primary syphilis: may be darkfield positive but serologically negative; TP-specific test (eg FTA) may be positive before RPR.
- Secondary syphilis: RPR positive in 99%
- Consider in differential dx of all genital ulcers esp in IDU or those who exchange sex for drugs or money
- Treat before lab results reported in high risk persons who may not return for results
- HIV-infected persons may have unusual serologic response, often very high titers; may be neg; but interpret results in usual manner

SELECTED READINGS

Villanueva AV, et al. Posterior uveitis in patients with positive serology for syphilis. Clin Infect Dis 2000 30:479-85

Bolan G. Management of syphilis in HIV-infected persons. The Medical Management of AIDS, Sande MA and Volberding PA (eds), 6th ed, 1999, W.B. Saunders Company, Phil PA, pp 453-465.

Gilstrap LC, Faro S. Syphilis in pregnancy. Infections in Pregnancy, 2nd ed. 1997. Wiley-Liss, New York, pp 135-149

Musher DM. Early syphilis. Sexually Transmitted Diseases, 3rd ed. Holmes KK et al (eds), 1999, McGraw-Hill, New York, pp479-485.

Swartz MN, et al. Late syphilis. Sexually Transmitted Diseases, 3rd ed. Holmes KK et al (eds), 1999, McGraw-Hill, New York, pp 487-509.

TROPHERYMA WHIPPLEI   Paul Auwaerter, M.D.

CLINICAL RELEVANCE & DIAGNOSIS

- Agent of Whipple's disease, distant relationship to actinomyces by 16s rDNA sequence. Fastidious, 0.25um rods that may appear gram +
- Rare infection, worldwide incidence est. 12 cases annually--but rate may increase with improved diagnostics (PCR/serology).
- Epidemiology not well-known, male: female 8:1, typical patient said to be Caucasian male, >40yrs living in rural environment
- Dx (1):Traditional dx by duodenal bxp demonstrating PAS-staining lg. foamy macrophages in lamina propria.
- Dx (2):PAS staining macrophages in LN, brain or other tissue; electron microscopy demonstrating rod-shaped bacteria with unique trilaminar membrane;
- Dx (3): PCR of fluid or tissue (sensitivity/specificity unknown); culture (difficult).
- Dx (4): Serology and immunostains recent discoveries & not widely available.

SITES OF INFECTION

- GI: "classical presentation" -wt. loss, fever, diarrhea, abd. pain, lymphadenopathy, arthralgia (may precede GI sx for yrs)
- CNS: dementia without other cause, personality change, hemiparesis, sz, ophthalmoplegia
- Ocular: uveitis; oculomasticatory or oculofascial-skeletal myorhthymia rare but considered pathognomonic of WD if present
- Cardiac: culture-negative endocarditis, myocarditis, pericarditis
- Less common: skeletal muscle, pulmonary, renal involvement
- Ddx: Crohn's, lymphoma, celiac disease, Still's disease, amyloidoisis, atypical mycobacteria

TREATMENT REGIMENS

Initial therapy

- Initial therapy usually parenteral to eradicate 1° disease (10-14d)
- PCN G 6-24mU IV qd in divided dose (q4h) and Streptomycin 1mg/kg IM qd (max 1gm/d)
- Alt: ceftriaxone 2g IV qd
- Steroids occasionally added for severe constitutional Sx or granulomatous process. In 1950's steroids alone without abx in Whipple's Disease helped some, but many worsened.
- Lack of good clinical trials to guide treatment, given rarity. Current recommendations garnered from case series and retrospective analysis.
- Sources:Maiwald & Relman, CID 2001; 32: 457-463; Marth & Raoult, Lancet 2003; 361:239

Long-term therapy

- One-year (or longer) total duration often suggested to prevent relapses seen with shorter term therapy
- Co-trimoxazole DS PO bid x 1 year
- Alt: Doxycycline 100mg PO bid or PCN Vk 500mg PO qid
- Other abx used: chloramphenicol, clarithromycin, fluoroquinolones
- Some physicians follow duodenal biopsies and treat only until PAS negative.
- Recent in vitro studies suggest cephalosporins, aztreonam, and fluoroquinolones were not active. Doxycycline and hydroxychloroquine judged to be bactericidal combination.

IMPORTANT POINTS

- Clinical pearls: Pts. w/ hyperpigmentation & relative hypotension may be confused with Addison's; granulomatous adenopathy may be confused with sarcoid.
- Macrophages containing MAI in pts with HIV may be confused w/ Whipple's on PAS stain.
- Arthralgia very common (>90%) and may precede GI sx in one-third. Joint complaints tend to be intermittent, migratory and transient generally of peripheral joints.
- Anemia common (90%) and may be due to B12 def. secondary to malabsorption.
- PCR of CSF, blood is decreasing need to obtain brain or other organ tissue for PAS staining.

SELECTED READINGS

Dutly F and Altwegg M. Whipple's Disease and "Tropheryma whippelii.". Clin Microbiol Rev 2001; 14 (3): 561-583

Fenollar F, Lepidi H, Raoult D. Whipple's endocarditis: Review of the Literature and comparisons with Q fever, Bartonella infection, and blood culture-positive endocarditis. Clin Infect Dis 2001; 33: 1309-16

Gerard A, Sarrot-Reynauld F, Liozon E et al. Neurologic presentation of Whipple Disease. Medicine 2002; 81: 443-457

Ghigo E, Capo C, Aurouze M et al. Survival of Tropheryma whipplei, the agent of Whipple's Disease, requires phagosome acidification. Infect and Imm 2002; 70 (3): 1501-1506

Keinath RD, Merrell DE, Vlietstra R, Dobbins WO 3rd. Antibiotic treatment and relapse in Whipple's disease. Long-term follow-up of 88 patients. Gastroenterology 1985 Jun;88(6):1867-73

VIBRIO VULNIFICUS John G. Bartlett, M.D.

CLINICAL RELEVANCE & DIAGNOSIS

- Gram-negative comma-shaped rod; 1-3 x 0.5-0.8um; easily grown on routine media

BACTERIA

- Normal marine flora in temperate climates; Gulf of Mexico (50% of oyster beds), East/West Coast
- Disease from ingestion (esp. raw oysters) or water contact with skin lesion
- Predisposed: liver disease, alcoholism, hemochromatosis (iron overload conditions)
- Dx: recovery from blood or necrotic lesion = medical emergency
- Microbiology: cx - blood (sepsis), wound (wound infection), stool (gastroenteritis)

SITES OF INFECTION

- Wound infection (cellulitis may spread rapidly with bullae, features of myonecrosis or fasciitis)
- Blood (primary septicemia)
- GI tract (gastroenteritis)

TREATMENT REGIMENS

Antibiotics

- Sepsis: doxycycline 100mg IV bid + ceftazidime 2g IV q8h or fluoroquinolone. Do not delay.
- Alternative: cefotaxime 2g IV q6h IV or ciprofloxacin 400mg IV q12h. Moxi, levo & gatifloxacin are also highly active
- Cefotaxime & minocycline are synergistic in vitro
- Gastroenteritis: role of therapy is unclear

Surgery

- Necrotic tissue: surgical debridement, fasciotomy or amputation

IMPORTANT POINTS

- Guidelines: Med Letter (2004;2:22) and G. Morris (CID 2003;37:272)
- Causes 90% of seafood-related deaths in US; esp due to raw oysters; coastal areas afflicted April-Oct; host with liver disease most at risk.
- Predisposing factor for sepsis: liver disease (80%); less common: diabetes, immunodeficiency, iron overload.
- Pathogenesis for sepsis: eat raw oysters, fever/chills in 3-7 days, then - shock + necrotic/ecchymotic bullae in 50-75%; mortality = ~55%.
- Pathogenesis for wound infection: prior/new wound + estuarine water contact, then - fever, chills & painful extremity - then bacteremia in 30%; mortality = 24%.

SELECTED READINGS

CDC. Vibrio vulnificus infections associated with eating raw oysters - Los Angeles, 1996. MMWR 1996;45:621

CDC. Vibrio vulnificus infections associated with raw oyster consumption - Florida, 1981-1992. MMWR 1993;42:405

Blake PA, Merson MH, Weaver RE, et al. Disease caused by a marine Vibrio: clinical characteristics and epidemiology. NEJM 1979;300:4

Levine WC, Griffin PM. Vibrio infections on the Gulf Coast: the result of a first year of regional surveillance. J Infect Dis 1993;167:479

Johnston JM, Becker SF, McFarland LM. Vibrio vulnificus: man and the sea. JAMA 1985;253:2850

YERSINIA PESTIS   John G. Bartlett, M.D.

CLINICAL RELEVANCE & DIAGNOSIS

- Always significant when recovered

- US: bubonic plague, ~10 cases/yr usually in NM, AR, CO, CA; pneumonic plague, 1 case per 10 yrs. in US
- Bioterrorism: epidemic of pneumonia with critically ill previously healthy adults; r/o tularemia & anthrax.
- Dx: gram stain and cx of sputum, bubo aspirate, blood
- Gram-negative bipolar rod ("safety pin"); grows on standard media, but up to 6 days to ID

SITES OF INFECTION

- Pneumonic plague
- Bacteremia
- Bubonic plague (adenopathy)
- Cutaneous
- Meningitis

TREATMENT REGIMENS

Treatment

- Indication to Rx in outbreak: persons with temp >38.5° C or new cough
- Preferred: streptomycin 1g IM bid or gentamicin IV 5mg/kg/d x 10d
- Alt: doxycycline 100mg PO or IV bid or ciprofloxacin 400mg IV bid or chloramphenicol 1g qid x10d.
- Pregnancy: gentamicin 5mg/kg/d x10d. Alt: doxycycline or ciprofloxacin x10d
- Meningitis: chloramphenicol 1g IV q6h

Treatment: prevention (bioterrorism)

- Indications: household, hospital or other close contact (definition: <2 meters of case who has been treated <48hr)
- Preferred: doxycycline 100mg PO bid x7d or ciprofloxacin 500mg bid x7d
- Alt: chloramphenicol 1g PO qid x 7d
- Pregnancy: doxycycline 100mg PO bid x 7d or ciprofloxacin 500mg PO bid x 7d
- Infection control: surgical mask, gowns, gloves & eye protection until case treated >48hrs
- Other: isolate or cohort pts; warn lab - biosafety level 2

Treatment: bioterrorism suspected

- Notify infection control and state/local health department
- Definitive dx of Y. pestis: Ft. Collins 970-221-6400

IMPORTANT POINTS

- Guidelines from Johns Hopkins Center for Biodefense Studies (JAMA 2000;283:2281)
- Bioterrorism (pneumonic): aerosol - incubation 2-4d, fever, cough +/- hemoptysis, dyspnea to DICto death day 2-6.
- Bulbonic plague: flea bites, incubation 2-8d, fever, tender bubo, bacteremia +/- DIC.
- Clinical clues bioterrorism: many healthy persons w/ pneumonia +/- hemoptysis & rapid death, r/o anthrax.
- Mortality pneumonic plague, 50-60%; bulbonic, 5-15%.

SELECTED READINGS

Inglesby TV, Dennis DT, Henderson DA, et al. Plague as a biological weapon. JAMA 2000;283:2281

Smith MD, Vinh DX, Hoa NT, et al. In vitro antimicrobial susceptibilities of strains of Yersinia pestis. Antimicrob Ag Chemother 1995;39:2153

Centers for Disease Control. Fatal human plague. MMWR 1997;278:380

Butler T. Yersinia species, Including Plague. Chapter 218 IN: Principles & Practice of Infectious Diseases, Mandell G, Bennett J, Dolin R (Eds), 5th Ed, Churchill Livingston, 2000;pg:2406

Galimand M, Guiyoule A, Gerbaud G, et al. Multidrug resistance in Yersinia pestis mediated by a transferable plasmid. NEJM 1997;337:677

YERSINIA SPECIES (NON-PLAGUE)

Khalil G. Ghanem, M.D.

CLINICAL RELEVANCE & DIAGNOSIS

- Gram-negative coccobacilli of family Enterobacteriaceae; 3 species cause human disease: pestis, enterocolitica & pseudotuberculosis.
- Other Yersiniae: fredrikensii, intermedia, kristensenii, bercovieri, mollaretti, rhodei, ruckeri, aldovae MAY cause gastroenteritis & soft tissue infections in humans.
- Transmission: contaminated food/water/blood; virulence factors: plasmid & chromosomal; reservoir: farm (pigs, cattle, sheep, chicken), mammals, pets (dog/cat), birds, environmental.
- Dx: blood cxs (virulence confirmed); stool (biotype or serotype to ascertain virulence, e.g., 1A biogroup avirulent); mesenteric LN bx & cx; pharyngeal exudate cx; serological (limited use); PCR.
- Prevention: focus on animal reservoirs; avoid undercooked meats, screen blood bank donors for acute symptoms (fevers, diarrhea).

SITES OF INFECTION

- Enterocolitica (1): GI (colitis; "pseudoappendicitis"; mesenteric adenitis; rectal bleeding; ileal perforation); SKIN: erythema nodosum (30%).
- Enterocolitica (2): JOINTS - Reiter's-reactive arthritis in 30%, 2-30d after diarrhea; HLA-B27 risk; sx last >1month in 66%; knees, ankles, toes, fingers; synovial fld: 25,000 WBC with 60-90%PMNs
- Other Yersiniae: possible cause GI (enteritis) and SKIN (soft tissue infxn). Pathogenicity still debated.

TREATMENT REGIMENS

Y. enterocolitica

- Enterocolitis & adenitis usually self-limited; no Rx unless clinically indicated. Septicemia: gentamicin 5mg/kg IV qd or divided doses. Other Abx: fluoroquinolones, chloramphenicol, doxy, TMP/SMX.
- Some isolates resistant to cephalosporins. AVOID in sick pts unless Abx susceptibility known.

Y. pseudotuberculosis

- Clinically ill patients & septicemia: ampicillin 100-200mg/kg/day; others: gentamicin; tetracycline.

IMPORTANT POINTS

- Iron overload syndromes (esp. use of deferoxamine), raw oyster ingestion & chitterlings classically associated w/ increased risk of infection with Yersiniae.
- Contaminated blood products described in cases of enterocolitica and pseudotuberculosis septicemia.
- Mortality in sepsis despite proper Rx: enterocolitica=50%; pseudotuberculosis= 75%.
- Enterocolitica resistant to PCNs whereas pseudotuberculosis sensitive. Resistance to 3rd gen cephalosporins w/ enterocolitica emerging.
- Reiter's syndrome (conjunctivitis, urethritis and arthritis) associated with Y. enterocolitica infection.

SELECTED READINGS

Merilahti-Palo R, Lahesmaa R, Granfors K, et al. Risk of Yersinia infection among butchers. Scand J Infect Dis 1991;23(1):55-61

Weber J, Finlayson NB, Mark JB, et al. Mesenteric lymphadenitis and terminal ileitis due to Yersinia pseudotuberculosis. N Engl J Med 1970 Jul 23;283(4):172-4

Sulakvelidze A. Yersiniae other than Y. enterocolitica, Y. pseudotuberculosis, and Y. pestis: the ignored species. Microbes Infect 2000 Apr;2(5):497-513

Nuorti JP, Niskanen T, Hallanvuo S, et al. A widespread outbreak of Yersinia pseudotuberculosis O:3 infection from iceberg lettuce. J Infect Dis. 2004 Mar 1;189(5):766-74.

Nesbakken T, Eckner K, Hoidal HK, et al. Occurrence of Yersinia enterocolitica and Campylobacter spp. in slaughter pigs and consequences for meat inspection, slaughtering, and dressing procedures. Int J Food Microbiol 2003 Feb 15;80(3):231-40

FUNGI

ASPERGILLUS
John G. Bartlett, M.D.

CLINICAL RELEVANCE & DIAGNOSIS

- Hyphae 2-4um wide, usually septate, 40 degree angle branching
- Ubiquitous mold, worldwide-soil, plants, cellars, marijuana
- May cause nosocomial epidemics in compromised hosts
- Dx: Lungs - CT scan; sinusitis - nasal endoscopy; cx & fungal stains - often false neg; blood cx - always neg; common contaminant.
- New test is serum galatomannan level which is standard in Europe for high risk patients; availability in US and specificity variable.
- Dx: Histopath or body fluids w/ evidence of mold or fungal invasion (usually cx neg); Lung-CT (w/ halo/crescent sign esp if neutropenic)

SITES OF INFECTION

- Pulmonary: allergic bronchopulmonary (ABPA), invasive, fungus ball (aspergilloma); Airways: laryngeal, tracheal, bronchial
- Sinusitis: allergic, fungus ball, invasive
- Endocarditis
- Otitis
- CNS: abscesses, meningitis
- Bone: osteomyelitis (often vertebral)
- Cutaneous
- Urinary tract
- Foreign body: catheter, shunt, prosthesis
- Ocular: invasive, endophthalmitis

TREATMENT REGIMENS

Pulmonary

- Invasive pulmonary: Ampho B 1.0-1.5mg/kg/d and then itraconazole 200mg bid until lung disease and underlying disease gone
- Possibly preferred: Voriconazole 6mg/kg bid IV day 1, then 4mg/kg bid IV >7d, then 200mg bid or 300mg bid for severe infection.
- Invasive pulmonary (Alt.): Itraconazole 200mg IV q 12h x 4d, then 200mg IV qd or 600mg/d PO, then 200mg PO bid (monitor Itraconazole level), or caspofungin 70mg IV, then 50mg IV qd.

FUNGI

- Salvage for ampho failures: consider voriconazole & caspofungin
- Aspergilloma: No consensus - main concern is hemoptysis
- Aspergilloma Resection - consider if adequate pulm. function, plus: sarcoidosis, compromised host, increasing IgG or hemoptysis
- Aspergilloma - other: Observe (most) bronchial artery embolism (temporizing), intracavitary amphoB (1 pos report), oral itraconazole (anecdotal successes, 5), IV ampho B (no)
- Allergic bronchopulmonary aspergillosis (ABPA): Prednisone 0.5mg/kg/d x 1wk then 0.5mg/kg qod x 5wks or itraconazole 200mg bid +/- prednisone or voriconazole 200mg PO bid +/- prednisone

ENT infections

- Sinonasal, acute invasive, comp host: Surgery + ampho B lavage + correction host defect (increased WBC, decrease steroids)
- Sinonasal chronic invasive, healthy host: Surgical debridement +/- voriconazole, itraconazole or amphoB
- Sinus fungus ball: Surgical removal
- Sinus-allergic fungal: Surgical drainage + antibacterials
- Otic infection - immunocompetent - topical cresylate, alcohol, boric acid, 5FC ointment, clotrimazole etc.; comp host - voriconazole 200mg PO bid or itraconazole 200mg PO bid

Nonpulmonary infections

- Brain abscess: Surgical drainage plus ampho B 1-1.5mg/kg/d & 5FC 100-150mg/kg/d; role unclear for voriconazole, itraconazole & lipid AmB.
- Meningitis: AmphoB 1-1.5mg/kg/d + intrathecal via Ommaya reservoir
- Bone: Surgical debridement + voriconazole or itraconazole or amphoB + rifampin or ampho B + 5FC
- Cutaneous: Itraconazole 200mg PO bid or amphotericin B; catheter-associated: remove line; burn-associated: surgical debridement
- Endocarditis: Valve replacement + ampho B
- Hepatosplenic: Lipid ampho B 5mg/kg/d and/or itraconazole 200mg PO bid

IMPORTANT POINTS

- Recommendations are from IDSA (CID 2000;30:696 and NEJM 2002;347:485)
- Voriconazole and caspofungin are replacing Ampho B as preferred treatment - less toxicity. Voriconazole is more effective.
- Forms: Allergic (lung, sinuses), saprophyte (fungal ball), superficial, foreign body (catheter etc), invasive (decreased ANC & decreased CMI- marrow/organ tx, AIDS, CGD)
- Three unique pulm syndromes: 1) fungus ball-usually observe or remove; 2) bronchoallergic-steroids +/- itraconazole or voriconazole; 3) invasive-voriconazole or highest dose ampho B (1-1.5mg/kg/d)
- Dx: Histopath or body fluids w/ evidence of mold or fungal invasion (usually cx neg); Lung-CT (w/ halo/crescent sign esp if neutropenic)

SELECTED READINGS

Soubani AO. Clinical significance of lower respiratory tract Aspergillus culture in elderly hospitalized patients. Eur J. Clin Microbiol Infect Dis 2004;23:491

Schwartz S, Thiel F. Update on the treatment of cerebral aspergillosis. Ann Hematol 2004;83 Suppl 1:S42

Kawazu M. Pros & cons of diagnostic potential of real time PCR double sandwich EIA for galactomaanan & a (1>3)-beta-D-glucan test in weekly screening for invasive aspergillosis in pts w/hematologic disorders. J. Clin Micro 2004;42:2733

Denning DW. Aspergillus species. Chapter 248 IN: Principles & Practice of Infectious Diseases. Mandell G, Bennett J, Dolin R (Eds), Churchill Livingston, 5th Ed 2000;pg2674

Denny DW. Invasive aspergillosis. CID 1998;26:781

BLASTOMYCES DERMATITIDIS   John G. Bartlett, M.D.

CLINICAL RELEVANCE & DIAGNOSIS

- Dimorphic fungus - mycelia form in nature (room temp) & yeast in tissue (37 degrees C). Yeast - 8x30um broad-based buds
- Epidemiology: found in N & S America, Europe, Africa, Asia; in US - southeast (except FL) midwest, west PA & north NYS; natural habitat - riverbanks, soil.
- Most cases: manual laborers, hunters, farmers; usually sporadic
- Pathogenesis: inhalation to pneumonia (acute, chronic, asymptomatic) +/- dissemination, especially to skin, bone/joints, GU tract.
- Dx: large yeast w/broad based bud upon wet mount w/KOH (skin, CSF, urine, BAL); tissue use PAS or silver stains; cx - Sabouraud media 30 degrees C.

SITES OF INFECTION

- Pulmonary (70-75%)
- Disseminated (10-20%)
- CNS: meningitis or brain abscess
- Bone/Joint
- GU: primarily prostate
- Cutaneous

TREATMENT REGIMENS

Pulmonary

- Life threatening: ampho B 0.7-1.0 mg/kg/d IV, total dose 1.5-2.5g or Ampho B until stable then itraconazole 200-400mg/d PO.
- Alt: Ampho B >500 mg, then itraconazole 200-400mg/d PO
- Mild-moderate: itraconazole 200-400mg/d PO x >6mos. Alt: fluconazole 400-800mg/d PO or ketoconazole 400-800mg/d PO x >6mos.

Extrapulmonary

- CNS: Amphotericin 0.7-1.0m mg/kg/d IV; total dose > or = 2g
- CNS Alt: fluconazole 800mg/d IV/PO or lipid Amphotericin
- Non-CNS, life-threatening: Amphotericin B 0.7-1.0 mg/kg/d IV; total dose 1.5-2.5g or until stable, then itraconazole 200-400mg/d.
- Non-CNS, mild/moderate: itraconazole 200-400mg/d PO
- Non-CNS alt: ketoconazole 400-800mg/d PO or fluconazole 400-800mg/d IV/PO
- Azoles alt: Ampho B 0.5-0.7 mg/kg/d IV

Treatment: immunosuppressed

- Ampho B 0.7-1.0 mg/kg/d IV; total dose 1.5-2.5g. Consider itraconazole 200-400 mg/d PO suppressive Rx until immunosuppression clears.
- Non-CNS alt: Ampho B IV, >1g then itraconazole

IMPORTANT POINTS

- Recommendations are based on IDSA guidelines (CID 2000;30:679)
- Most cases should be treated
- Endemic in SE & S Central states - MS, AK, WI
- Ampho B preferred Rx with immunosuppressed, CNS, life-threatening disease, and azole failures; itraconazole - preferred azole (monitor itraconazole levels)

• Most common presentation: indolent onset, chronic pneumonia

SELECTED READINGS

Chapman SW, Lin AC, Hendricks KA, et al. Endemic blastomycosis in Mississippi: Epidemiological and clinical studies. Semin Resp Infect 1997;12:219

Chapman S. Blastomyces dermatitidis . Chapter 255 IN: Principles & Practice of Infectious Diseases, Mandell G, Bennett J, Dolin R (Eds). 5th edition, 2000, pg 2733.

Sarosi GA, Davies SF. Blastomycosis. Am Rev Resp Dis 1979;120:911

Chapman WS, Bradsher RW, Campbell GD, Jr, et al. Practice guidelines for management of patients with blastomycosis. CID 2000;30:679

Pappas PG, Pottage JC, Powderly WG, et al. Blastomycosis in patients with AIDS. Ann Intern Med 1992;116:847

CANDIDA ALBICANS
Paul Auwaerter, M.D.

CLINICAL RELEVANCE & DIAGNOSIS

• Budding yeast, capable of >10 diseases. Causes ~100% oropharyngeal (OPC), 90% vulvovaginitis candidiasis.
• Normal commensals of skin, GI & GU tracts. Difficulty is often separating invasive disease from asymptomatic colonization.
• Common risk factors: prior abx use, immune suppression, malignancy, diabetes, malnutrition, post-surgical, catheters, TPN
• Dx: Culture normally sterile site; mucosal - typical lesion & positive KOH/gram stain
• Albicans generally susceptible to major drugs. Azole resistance seen mostly in HIV with OPC. Candida speciation is reasonably predictive guide to therapy (see also "Candida Species")
• Candida susceptibility testing not a routine test. Most helpful for guiding therapy with non-albicans Candida or if resistance suspected especially with hx of prior azole use.

SITES OF INFECTION

• Cutaneous: diaper dermatitis, monilia, intertriginous infections, balanitis, vulvitis, paronychia
• Chronic mucocutaneous candidiasis: persistent infections of the skin, nails, and mucous membranes; most pts have T-cell dysfunction/disorder
• Oropharyngeal/esophageal: thrush, esophagitis; very common w/ HIV
• Vulvovaginal: vaginitis; most common in women of childbearing age
• Blood/cardiovascular: candidemia, often catheter-related; endocarditis-prosthetic & native valves
• Genitourinary: candiduria common in catheterized patients (often not significant)
• Disseminated Candidiasis: often w/ neutropenia, malignancy or GI disease involving liver or spleen (hepatosplenic candidasis)
• Musculoskeletal: arthritis, osteomyelitis, myositis
• Ocular: endophthalmitis; screening recommended for patients with candidemia
• Neurological: meningitis

TREATMENT REGIMENS

Mucocutaneous candidiasis

• See "Candidiasis," and "Vaginal Discharge: in the Diagnoses section for specifics.
• Cutaneous candidiasis: maintain dry skin surface (frequent diaper changes), control hyperglycemia; topicals: clotrimazole, miconazole, nystatin, ketoconazole 2% all bid for 3-5 days

- Oropharyngeal Candidiasis (OPC): clotrimazole oral troches 10mg 5x/d; Nystatin [suspension 400,000-600,000U qid OR 200,000U pastilles 1-2 used 4 or 5x/d]; fluconazole 100mg qd PO. Duration 7-14d.
- OPC Alt: Itraconazole 200mg/d PO (use solution, ~66% response rate for Flu-resistant OPC), AmB 0.3mg/kd/d IV, caspofungin 70mg IV load then 50mg qd, vori 200mg PO bid
- OPC Alt: AmB 1mL oral suspension qid PO (no longer commercially available in US)
- Esophageal: Flu 200mg PO/IV qd to improvement, then 100 mg/d PO (14-21d total) or maintenance if recurrent. Alt: Vori 200mg PO/IV bid, AmB 0.3-0.7mg/kg/d IV, Caspo 50mg qd IV.
- Vulvovaginal: suppositories/topical [OTC: clotrimazole, butoconazole, miconazole, tioconazole] use short course (1-3d) for mild sx; >7-14d if severe, recurrent or abnl host.
- Vulvovaginal: Flu 150mg PO single dose (wait 3d for response); topical nystatin 100,000U/d x 7-14d. Boric acid 600mg gel capsule intravaginal qd x 14d effective esp. non-albicans.
- Chronic Mucocutaneous Candidiasis: systemic azoles or amphotericin B effective
- Relapses not uncommon, esp AIDS. Long-term suppression w/ fluconazole 200mg qd PO for OPC, avoid due to the development of resistance.

Endophthalmitis
- Uncomplicated small lesions in pts otherwise at low risk may be initially managed with flu 6-12mg/kg/d IV/PO; poor response (e.g., progression or lack of a response) should prompt change to AmB 0.7-1.0mg/kg/d IV and consideration of pars plana vitrectomy (usual when vitreitis present). Duration: 6-12 wks post-surgery.

Central Nervous System Candidiasis
- Am B (0.7-1.0mg/kg/d +/- 5-FC (25mg/kg qid); consider fluconazole in low risk patients. Treat minimum 4 weeks. Shunt removal may be required.

Gastrointestinal Candidiasis
- AmB or fluconazole (see candidemia recs) and surgical exploration/drainage in patients suspected of perforation and/or secondary peritonitis or abscess. Patients on CAPD should have dialysis catheter removed, treat 2-3 wks. Wait 2 wk minimum before replacing catheter.

Bone and Soft Tissue Infections
- Surgical debridement + AmB 0.5-1.0mg/kg/d (better studied) x 6-10wks or fluconazole 6mg/kg/d x 6-12 mos. Can add AmB to bone cement. Many start with AmB 2-3wks then change to fluconazole.

Candiduria
- Presence not necessarily equating renal tract infection as colonization common even w/pyuria. Two exceptions: always treat in renal transplant, pregnant and neutropenic patients.
- Catheter-related infection often resolves without therapy (40%). Urine cx post catheter removal can help determine need for treatment. Catheter change alone rarely effective.
- Upper tract disease (fever/ leukocytosis) requires systemic therapy. Any hardware such as stents may need to be removed for eradication.
- Persistence/recurrence or suspect source of sepsis should prompt GU tract studies. Fungal balls likely require surgical removal.
- If treatment required, preferred: fluconazole 200mg mg/d PO/IV x 7-14d
- Alt: Ampho B 0.5mg/kg/d IV x 7-14d
- Alt: 5-FC 25mg/kg PO qid x 7d ; effective but be wary of initial or emerging resistance w/ therapy. Myelosuppressive, monitor drug levels if used >7d.

FUNGI

- Alt: Amphotericin B bladder washings-50 mg/ 1L sterile water @ 40mL/hr x 5 days. Never a favorite with patients or nurses, now mostly reserved for localization purposes.
- Limited experience with caspofungin, but likely effective

Candidemia/invasive candidiasis

- Remove all percutaneous lines if suspected, although controversial in neutropenic host.
- Nonneutropenic hosts: Fluconazole 400-800mg/d IV/PO, AmB 0.6-1.0mg/kg/d IV, Caspo 70mg IV load then 50mg qd. Duration 14d after last (+) cx and sx resolution.
- Neutropenic hosts: AmB 0.7-1.0mg/kg/d or LFAmB 3-5mg/kg/d IV, Caspo 70mg IV load then 50mg/d-- all x 14d after last (+) cx and sx resolution. Alt: Flu 6-12mg/kg/d IV/PO.
- Chronic disseminated candidiasis: follow neutropenic recommendations, but conversion to Flu usual after 1-2 wks. Duration of Rx totals 3-6 mos. or calcification of radiologic lesions.
- All patients w/ candidemia to undergo ophthalmological exam to r/o endophthalmitis. Onset of disease rare after otherwise successful course of therapy.

Endocarditis

- Replacement of infected valve almost always required.
- AmB 0.6-1.0mg/kg or LFAmB 3.0-6.0mg/kg/d IV plus 5-FC 25-37.5mg/kg PO qid
- Alt: Flu 6-12mg/kg/d IV/PO or Caspo 70mg IV load then 50mg qd
- Duration: at least 6 weeks after valve replacement.
- Success w/ long-term Flu suppression reported in pts unable to undergo valve surgery.
- Histopathologic examination and culture of the valve can confirm the diagnosis and allow resistance testing.

Prevention

- Neutropenia: Flu 400mg/d or itraconazole solution (2.5mg/kg/q12h) in pts at high-risk of invasive candidiasis. Duration Rx unclear, but minimum should be for period of neutropenia.
- Solid-organ transplants: best evidence for high-risk liver transplant pts, use Flu 400mg/ d.
- ICU: Controversial, some evidence that units w/ high rates of candida infection may benefit if oral Flu 400mg/d employed.

Important Points

- See "Candida Species" for non-albicans specifics
- Rarely a laboratory contaminate. Clinical correlation of in vitro susceptibility patterns is not firmly established for most species, especially for systemic Candida infections.
- Isolation from respiratory tract rarely represents actual infection. Candida pneumonia should only be diagnosed with biopsy-proven evidence.
- "Chronic candidiasis" (The Yeast Connection) unproven as cause of chronic fatigue, non-specific sx. No benefit to stool cx or GI eradication in these pts.

Selected Readings

Dismukes WE, Wade JS, Lee JY. A randomized, double-blind trial of nystatin therapy for the candidiasis hypersensitivity syndrome. N Engl J Med. 1990 Dec 20;323(25):1717-23

Mora-Duarte J, Betts R, Rotstein C et al. Comparison of caspofungin and amphotericin B for invasive candidiasis. N Engl J Med. 2002 Dec 19;347(25):2020-9

Pelz RK, Lipsett PA, Swoboda SM et al. Enteral fluconazole is well absorbed in critically ill surgical patients. Surgery. 2002 May;131(5):534-40

Rex JH, Pfaller MA. Has antifungal susceptibility testing come of age?. Clin Infect Dis 2002; 35:982-9

Walsh TJ, Teppler H, Donowitz G et al. Caspofungin versus liposomal amphotericin B for empirical antifungal therapy in patients with persistent fever and neutropenia. N Engl J Med. 2004 Sep 30;351 (14):1391-402

CANDIDA SPECIES
John G. Bartlett, M.D.

CLINICAL RELEVANCE & DIAGNOSIS
- Yeast 4-6um, pseudomycelia, one of few fungi that grow on blood agar and in blood culture
- Most infections: endogenous from colonization - GI, GU tract, skin; also environment
- Dx: cx normally sterile site; mucosal - typical lesion & pos KOH/gram stain
- Need care w/interpreting cultures: 1/3 sputum & 1/5 BAL at Mayo yield Candida; however Candida pneumonia is very rare
- Common non-albicans spp: C. glabrata, C. guilliermondii, , C. krusei, C. kefyr, C. lusitaniae, C. parapsilosis, C. tropicalis. See separate module for Candida albicans.

SITES OF INFECTION
- Disseminated/candidemia
- Hepatosplenic
- Urinary
- Pneumonia (rare)
- Osteomyelitis
- Peritoneal, gall bladder
- Endocarditis
- Endophthalmitis
- Mucocutaneous - thrush, esophagitis, vaginitis and paronychia
- Esophagitis
- Vaginitis
- Meningitis

TREATMENT REGIMENS

Deep infections
- Principles: dx: establish Candida as pathogen; Rx: remove any foreign bodies, use Ampho B or azole
- Regimens: Ampho B 0.6-1.0mg/kg/d IV, Lipid Ampho 3-5 mg/kg/d IV, fluconazole 400-800 IV/PO/d
- Alt: voriconozole 200mg PO bid 6mg/kg IV q 12 hx2, then 4 mg/kg q 12 h Candidemia: remove line, Ampho B or fluconazole until cx neg x 14d
- Candidemia & neutropenia: remove lines; Ampho B, lipid Ampho or caspofungin
- Urinary: often (+) cx not pathologic; remove catheter; fluconazole 200 mg/d PO/IV x 7-14d or Ampho B or flucytosine
- Osteomyelitis: debride; Ampho B x 6-10 weeks
- Intra-abd: remove catheters; Ampho B or fluconazole x 2-3 wks
- Endocarditis: remove valve & Ampho B or lipid Ampho, + 5FC 25 mg/kg q6h PO
- Meningitis: remove shunt/device & Ampho B & 5FC 25 mg/kg PO q6h until signs resolved >4 wks
- Endophthalmalitis: Ampho B, fluconazole

Mucosal candidiasis
- Thrush: clotrimazole 10mg 4x/d; nystatin 2-400,000 U 5x/d or fluconazole 100-200 mg/d x 7-14 d
- Alt: itraconazole 200mg/d, caspofungin or Ampho B 0.3-0.7 mg/kg/d

- Esophagitis: fluconazole 100-200mg/d IV/PO x 14-21 d post improvement
- Esophagitis: voriconazole 4mg/kg bid IV/PO or Ampho B 0.3-0.7 mg/kg or caspofungin
- Vaginitis: topical (butoconazole, miconazole, troconazole, terconazole) x 1-7 d or fluconazole 150mg PO x 1
- Vaginitis-recurrent: fluconazole 150mg q wk, itraconazole 100mg qod or topical agent; all 6 mos.

Treatment options/issues for Rx Candida species

- Most resistant: C. glabrata (some centers 30-40% azole-resistant) and C. krusei (azole-resistant, intrinsic); C. lusitaniae (ampho-resistant, instrinsic). Some azole-resistance: C. tropicalis (~5%).
- Fluconazole: up to 800 mg/d IV/PO
- Itraconazole-capsule w/food, liquid w/empty stomach; 200-400 mg/d IV/PO
- Voriconazole: 200 to 300mg PO bid or 4mg/kg IV q12h; active vs. all Candida spp., cross-azole resistance possible.
- Caspofungin: 70mg IV, then 50mg IV/d
- Ampho B: up to 1mg/kg/d IV
- Topical Ampho: rarely indicated
- Lipid ampho: 3 to 5mg/kg/d IV

IMPORTANT POINTS

- Recommendations: IDSA (CID 2004;38:161)
- Candida is common contaminant: consider culture source, gram stain and host
- Candidiasis & foreign body: must remove foreign body
- Antifungals: Ampho always active, azoles usually preferred
- Fungal sensitivity testing recommended for deep infection, refractory and recurrent infections

SELECTED READINGS

Pappas PG, et al . Guidelines for Treatment of Candidiasis. Clin Infect Dis 2004:38:161.

Hospenthal DR, Murray CK, Rinaldi MG. The role of antifungal susceptibility testing in the therapy of candidiasis. Diag Mircobiol Infect Dis 2004;48:153-60

Mora-Duarte J. Comparison of caspofungin and amphotericin for invasive candidiasis. N Engl J Med 2002;347-2020

Rex JH, Bennett JE, Sugar AM et al. A randomized trial comparing fluconazole with amphotericin B for the treatment of candidemia in patients without neutropenia. NEJM 1994;331:1325

Rex JH, Walsh TJ, Sobel JD, et al . Practice guidelines for the treatment of candidiasis. CID 2000;30:662

COCCIDIOIDES IMMITIS
John G. Bartlett, M.D.

CLINICAL RELEVANCE & DIAGNOSIS

- Dimorphic fungus: large spherule 15-75um diameter at 37 degrees C
- Diagnostic Stains: H&E, PAS, KOH, calcofluor, (not gram); grows on standard fungal media
- Endemic in CA, AZ, TX, NM, Mexico, S. America
- Dx: 1) Identify spherule or cx, 2) (+) serology w/blood or body fluid, or 3) pos. skin test (epidemiologic purposes only)
- Serology: complement fixation titer (>1:16=disseminated); serial tests immunodiffusion, EIA (need confirmation). Neg tests don't exclude.
- Seroconversion (skin test) 3%/yr in high endemic areas
- Always pathogenic when seen on histopathalogy or cultured

SITES OF INFECTION

- Pulmonary
- Skin
- Bone & joints
- Meninges

TREATMENT REGIMENS

Acute pulmonary

- Acute pulm: Rx if high risk (AIDS, steroids, organ tx, 3rd trimester preg) or severe (wt loss 10%, sx >8wks, infiltrates >1/2 lung, CF titer >1:16)
- Rx: itraconazole 200mg bid or fluconazole 400mg/d x 3-6mo; except pregnancy - AmphoB 0.5-0.7mg/kg/d
- Bilat reticulo-nod/unilat infiltrates: AmphoB 0.7-1mg/kg/d until stable, then itra 200mg bid or fluconazole 400mg/d x >1yr
- ARDS: steroids - prednisone 60-80mg/d

Chronic pulmonary

- Pulmonary nodule: No antifungal & no surgery - observe
- Cavitary & asympt: usually observe; consider surgery if persists >2yrs, progresses >1yr or near pleura
- Cavitary symptomatic: resection or azole Rx - itraconazole 200mg bid or fluconazole 400mg/d x 8-12mo
- Ruptured cavity: lobectomy + decortication + antifungal agents
- Chronic fibrocavitary: itraconazole 200mg bid or fluconazole 400mg/d x >1yr.
- Consider surgery for response failures with significant hemoptysis and lesions that are well localized

Extrapulmonary

- Non-meningeal, preferred: itraconazole 200mg bid, fluconazole 400mg/d, ketoconazole 400mg qd
- Non-meningeal, alternative: amphotericin B 0.5-0.7mg/kg/d
- Ampho B preferred for pregnancy, lesions that worsen rapidly or are in critical loci, e.g., spinal column disease
- Meningeal: fluconazole 400-800mg/d; may give intrathecal ampho B at initial Rx; alternative: itraconazole 400-600mg. After clinical improvement, continue fluconazole 400mg/d forever
- Meningeal failure to respond to azoles or IV AmB: intrathecal amphotericin, 0.01-1.5mg

IMPORTANT POINTS

- Recommendations are from IDSA (CID 2000;30:658) and NIH (Ann Int Med 2000;133:676). Non-meningeal rx: itraconazole may be best azole for coccidioides (Ann Int Med 2000;13:676).
- Hx: incub period 7-21d - Sx: (25-50%) cough, fever, infiltrate (50%) - chronic pulm dz in 4% (nodule or cavity) or dissemination (0.5%)
- Dx: 1) identify spherule or culture C. immitis; 2) + serology in blood/body fluid; or 3) + skin test
- Risk for severe disease: low CMI (AIDS, organ tx, steroids), 3rd trimester pregnancy, large inoculum, race: Black or Filipino
- Monitor itraconazole serum levels (goal: >1mcg/mL)

SELECTED READINGS

Shibli M, Ghassibi J, Hajal R, O'Sullivan M. Adjunctive corticosteroids therapy in acute respiratory distress syndrome owing to disseminated coccidioidomycosis. Crit Care Med 2002;30:1896

Gonzalez GM, Tijerina R, Najvar LK, et al. In vitro and in vivo activities of posaconazole against Coccidioides immitis. Antimicrob Ag Chemother 2002;46;1352

Ampel NM. Coccidioidomycosis among persons with HIV in the era of HAART. Semin Resp Infect 2001;16:257

Proi LA, Tenoria AR. Successful use of voriconazole for treatment of Coccidioides meningitis. J. Antimicrob Chemother 2004;48:2341

Arnold MG, et al. Head and neck manifestations of disseminated coccidioidomycosis. Laryngoscope 2004;114:747-52

CRYPTOCOCCUS NEOFORMANS

John G. Bartlett, M.D.

CLINICAL RELEVANCE & DIAGNOSIS

- Yeastlike round fungus 5-10um w/polysaccharide capsule; reproduces by narrow-based budding.
- Epidemiology: worldwide in soil, pigeon droppings
- Common cause of disease w/reduced CMI: lymphoma, chronic steroids, transplants, AIDS w/CD4 <100; 20-30% non-AIDS pts are normal hosts
- Pathogenesis: inhaled, then pneumonia, then CNS +/- skin, bone, prostate
- Clinical: frequently, meningitis may be asymptomatic w/no fever or meningismus
- Dx: antigen + in blood in 80-95% w/meningitis & 20-50% w/other forms; also culture (blood agar); sensitivity of Ag in CSF 99%, India ink 65%.

SITES OF INFECTION

- CNS: meningitis
- Lung: pneumonitis
- GU: Prostatitis, or asx infection
- Disseminated: fungemia
- Cutaneous: nodules/vesicles (reflects dissemination)

TREATMENT REGIMENS

Meningitis AIDS patients

- Amphotericin B 0.7-1.0 mg/kg + flucytosine 25 mg/kg PO qid x 2wks, then fluconazole 400mg PO qd x 10wks, then 200mg PO qd.
- Monitor 5-FC levels to avoid bone marrow suppression.
- Alternative - above without flucytosine (esp if neutropenic)
- Alternative - fluconazole 400-800mg/d IV/PO + flucytosine 25mg/kg PO qid
- Fluconazole alternative - itraconazole (not as effective); ampho B alternative - liposomal AmB 4mg/kg/d IV
- Duration: fluconazole 200mg PO qd life long or D/C maintenance fluconazole when CD4 >200 x 6 mos and completed 10wks Rx minimum & asymptomatic
- CSF pressure OP >250mm H20: remove CSF fluid until pressure drops 50%, then daily LP with same rule until OP <200.
- CSF pressure elevation: (not recommended) steroids, mannitol, acetazolamide

Non-AIDS meningitis

- Ampho B 0.7-1.0mg/kg/d IV + flucytosine 25mg/kg/qid x 2wks then fluconazole 400mg/d x >10wks.
- Alt: Ampho B 0.7-1.0mg/kg/d IV +/- flucytosine 25mg/kg qid x 6-10wks
- Duration: as above, but continue fluconazole po (200mg/d) until immunocompetent, then D/C.

- CSF Pressure management: as above

Non-CNS (AIDS or non-AIDS)

- Must do LP to r/o meningitis
- AIDS + pneumonia + neg LP: fluconazole 200-400mg/d or itraconazole 200-400mg/d both life-long or until CD4 >200 x 6mo
- AIDS + pneumonia + neg LP alternative: fluconazole 400mg/d + flucytosine 25mg/kg qid x 10wks
- Non-AIDS, pulmonary, symptomatic & neg LP: fluconazole 200-400mg/d PO x 3-6mo
- Non-AIDS + severe pulmonary: ampho B 0.4-0.7mg/kg/d IV to 1-2g total
- Non-AIDS, pulmonary, mild-mod sx + neg LP: fluconazole 200-400mg/d PO x 3-6mo
- Antigenemia or positive urine cx & neg LP: fluconazole 200-400mg/d x 3-6mo

IMPORTANT POINTS

- Recommendations from IDSA (CID 2000 30:710)
- This fungus has great tropism for CNS; LP to r/o meningitis with any lab evidence of C. neoformans
- Often very quiet (asymptomatic) including meningitis, but meninigitis is 100% fatal w/o Rx
- Dx: meningitis - blood antigen 95% sensitive, CSF >99% sensitive, near 100% specific.

SELECTED READINGS

Archibald LK, et al. Antifungal susceptibilities of cryptococcus neoformans. Emerg Infect Dis 2004;10:143-5

Larsen RA, et al. Amphotericin B and fluconazole, a potent combination therapy for cryptococcal meningitis. Antimicrob Ag Chemother 2004;48:985-91

Mussini C, et al. Discontinuation of maintenance therapy for cryptococcal meningitis in patients with AIDS treated with HAART: an International Study. Clin Infect Dis 2004;38:565-71

Kerkering TM. The evolution of pulmonary cryptococcosis: clinical implication from a study of 41 patients with and without compromising host factors. Ann Intern Med 1981;94:611-6

Yamagudii H, et al. Fluconazole immunotherapy for cryptococcosis in non-AIDS patients. Eur J Clin Micobiol Inf Dis 1995;15:787-2

FUSARIUM

Paul Auwaerter M.D. and Aimee Zaas, M.D.

CLINICAL RELEVANCE & DIAGNOSIS

- Filamentous nonpigmented (hyaline) septated fungi with acute angle branching
- Dx: skin or tissue bx with cx (+ blood cx if immunocompromised)
- Ubiquitous in environment
- Major species: F. oxysporum and F. solani
- Most common in immunocompromised hosts, with neutropenia as strongest risk factor
- Typically presents as fever refractory to broad-spectrum antibacterial agents
- Histologically indistinguishable from aspergillus, therefore CULTURE in addition to pathology is imperative for proper dx.
- Characteristic feature is skin lesions - erythematous, nodular, ulcerated; often with central eschar
- High mortality once disseminated
- Local or disseminated infection can also occur in solid-organ transplant patients

SITES OF INFECTION

- Immunocompromised pts: skin, respiratory tract, venous catheters, GI tract are portals of entry

- 50% of disseminated fusariosis occur in acute leukemia patients
- Angioinvasiveness and adventitious sporulation (fungal growth in bloodstream) lead to disseminated infections
- 88% of Fusarium infections in immunocompromised pts have skin lesions
- Skin lesions: painful, multiple, erythema +/- central necrosis
- Skin lesions: develop over days; various stages of development
- 50% of pts have positive blood cx
- Classic portal of entry: paronychia (nailbed inflammation) in immunocompromised pt
- Immunocompetent pts: area of skin or eye trauma is portal of entry
- Immunocompetent pts: localized skin lesion or eye lesion (keratitis)
- In immunocompromised patients, infection spreads rapidly. In immunocompetent patients, infection remains localized.

TREATMENT REGIMENS

Immunocompromised patients

- Recovery from neutropenia imperative. (Many authors recommend G-CSF, whereas WBC transfusions are controversial.)
- Voriconazole, amphotericin B, or amphotericin B lipid product commercially available choices
- Voriconazole: 6 mg/kg IV q12 day 1, then either 4 mg/kg IV BID or 200-300mg PO BID. Use IV until patient is stable.
- Alt: lipid formulation amphotericin B (Abelcet, Ambisome or Amphotec) 5 mg/kg IV qd
- Alt: amphotericin B 1.0-1.5 mg/kg day
- Fusarium intrinsically resistant to many antifungals (incl. itraconazole, 5-flucytosine, fluconazole, caspofungin, and in some isolates-- amphotericin)
- New antifungals (not FDA approved): ravuconazole not effective in vitro
- New antifungals (not FDA approved): posaconazole effective in vitro; recommend compassionate use if possible in refractory cases
- Treatment duration: prolonged; no strict recommendations but most would continue therapy 6 months after recovery of neutropenia.
- Surgical debridement of large single lesions and removal of infected catheters recommended

Immunocompetent patients: skin lesion

- Surgical debridement
- Topical antifungals (natamycin) can be used
- Voriconazole 200mg PO BID for 6 months after lesion is gone

Ocular involvement

- Ocular involvement can involve cornea, retina and vitreous humor
- Immunocompromised: secondary infection due to dissemination
- Immunocompromised: intra-ocular antifungals and vitrectomy usually ineffective
- Immunocompromised: voriconazole and posaconazole may be active in the eye
- Immunocompetent: keratitis occurs after trauma or corneal surgery (LASIK), contact lens wear
- Topical: natamycin drops, referral to ophthalmology for keratoplasty and close follow-up
- Alt: topical 2% voriconazole 7 times/day used in two case reports of keratomycosis treatment (see Refs)
- Systemic: reports of successful treatment with voriconazole and posaconazole
- Combination topical and systemic therapy reports excellent success. Systemic therapy duration short (14 days) in immunocompetent.

IMPORTANT POINTS

- Immunocompromised pts: consider fusarium if fever refractory to antibacterial agents, paronychia, positive blood cultures for "mold", skin lesions with necrotic centers
- Immunocompromised patients: neutrophil recovery is critical to survival
- Keratitis: think fusarium when traditional topical agents fail; prompt referral to ophthalmology essential
- Consider posaconazole in refractory cases
- Posaconazole information/compassionate use: Schering-Plough Corporation, 2000 Galloping Hill Rd, Kenilworth, NJ 07033-0530. T: (908) 298-4000

SELECTED READINGS

Nucci M & Anaissie E. Cutaneous Infection by Fusarium Species in Healthy and Immunocompromised Hosts: Implications for Diagnosis and Management. CID 2002;35;909-20

Tiribelli M, Zaja F, Fili C, et al. Endogenous endophthalmitis following disseminated fungemia due to Fusarium solani in a patient with acute myeloid leukemia. Eur J Hematology 2002;68;314-17

Groll AH & Walsh TJ. Uncommon opportunistic fungi: new nosocomial threats. Clinical Microbiology and Infection 2001:7;8-24

Ellis D. Amphotericin B: spectrum and resistance. Journal of Antimicrobial Chemotherapy 2002; 49: Suppl S1, 7-10

Jahagirdar BN & Morrison VA. Emerging fungal pathogens in patients with hematologic malignancies and marrow/stem-cell transplants. Seminars in Respiratory Infections 2002;17:113-120

HISTOPLASMA CAPSULATUM   John G. Bartlett, M.D.

CLINICAL RELEVANCE & DIAGNOSIS

- Dimorphic fungus; yeast at 37 degrees C
- Endemic - Ohio & Miss. River valleys, present in soil, associated with birds & bats
- No human-human transmission
- Dx: positive culture (diagnostic); antigen in blood + urine (near diagnostic); serology CF >1:8 or 4x rise; also tissue stains e.g., PAS, GM, Giemsa
- Antigen assay: specificity >95%, sensitivity w/disease burden; source MiraVista Lab - T: 866-647-2847 or http://www.miravistalabs.com/

SITES OF INFECTION

- Pulmonary: acute
- Pulmonary: chronic
- Disseminated: esp marrow, liver, spleen, GI
- CNS: meningitis, abscesses
- Mediastinitis: granulomatous
- Mediastinitis: fibrosing
- Pericarditis
- Ocular

TREATMENT REGIMENS

Pulmonary

- Principles: dx (cx, antigen assay, serology, tissue stain) - Rx (itraconazole &/or Ampho B) or watch
- Recommendations from IDSA guidelines (CID 2000;31:688) & CDC (AIDS OI guidelines)
- Treat: acute pulm disease if > 1 mo symptoms or hypoxic; chronic pulm disease or, granulomatous mediastinitis & obstruction

FUNGI

- No treatment: acute - pulm dz w/ mild sx, broncholithiasis, fibrosing mediastinitis
- Acute pulm w/focal infilt + immunocompetent: observation. Sx persist >1 mo: itraconazole 200mg qd x6-12wks
- Acute pul + diffuse infilt +/- AIDS + hospitalization: Ampho B 0.7-1.0mg/kg (2g total dose), then itracon 200mg bid x 12 wks. Prednisone optional 60mg PO qd x first 2wks
- Acute + diffuse infilt + immunocompet & outpt: Itracon 200mg qd or bid x 6-12wks
- Chronic pulm + immunocompet + mild-mod disease: itracon 200mg qd or bid x 12-24mo
- Chronic pulm + immunocompet + severe dis: ampho B 0.7mg/kg/d x 12wks or longer, then itracon 200mg PO bid x 12-24wks

Extrapulmonary/mediastinal

- Disseminated +/- severe sx + AIDS: ampho B 0.7-1.0mg (2g max total), then itracon 200mg bid x 12wks (AIDS - lifetime)
- Disseminated + mild/mod sx: itracon 200mg tid x 3d, then bid x 12wks
- Meningitis: ampho B 0.7-1.0mg/kg x3 mos, then flucon 800mg/d x 9-12 wks
- Granulomatous mediastinitis + obstruction: ampho B 0.7-1.0mg/kg then itracon 200mg qd or bid
- Granulomatous mediastinitis + mild Sx >1 mo: itracon 200mg qd or bid x 6-12 mos
- Fibrosing mediastinitis + obstruction: itraconazole 200mg qd or bid x 12wks (trial) +/- stents; steroids - no use; surgery - great caution
- Pericarditis: non-steroidals x 2-12wks. Hemodynamic compromise: prednisone 60mg x 1-2wks then NSAIDs. Tamponade: surgical drainage
- Arthritis (polyarticular): non-steroidals x 2-12wks

IMPORTANT POINTS

- Guidelines from IDSA (CID 2000;31:688)
- HX: exposure, then fever + pulm sx - CXR clears or chronic pulm disease or dissemination. Severity depends upon exposure inoculum & immune response.
- Histoplasma antigen in urine - good test for disseminated disease (blood Ag test less specific); titer shows response to Rx within 2-12wks.
- Itraconazole - best azole; concerns: absorption, drug interaction & toxicity (hepatitis, CHF); measure levels, expect >1-10mcg/mL.

SELECTED READINGS

Brodsky AL, Gregg MB, Kaufman L. Outbreak of histoplasmosis associated with the 1970 Earth Day activities. Am J Med 1973;54:333

Center for Disease Control. Outbreak of acute respiratory febrile illness among college students - Acapulco, Mexico, March 2001. MMWR 2001;50:261

Hecht FM, Wheat J, Korzun AH. Itraconazole maintenance treatment for histoplasmosis in AIDS: A prospective multicenter trial. J AIDS 1997;16:100

Katarika YP, Campbell PB, Burlingham BT. Acute pulmonary histoplasmosis presenting with ARDS: effect of therapy on clinical and lab features. S Med J 1981;74:534

Dismukes WE, Bradsher RW Jr, Cloud GC, et al. Itraconazole therapy for blastomycosis and histoplasmosis. NIAID Mycosis Study Group. Am J Med 1992;93:489

PSEUDOALLERSCHERIA BOYDII

Paul Auwaerter M.D. and Aimee Zaas, M.D.

CLINICAL RELEVANCE & DIAGNOSIS

- Thin-walled, septate, branching hyphae; 2.5-5 microns. Ubiquitous; typically found in soil, sewage, brackish/polluted water.

- P. boydii is the sexual form of Scedosporium apiospermum
- Emerging infection in immunocompromised hosts
- Immunocompromised patients at risk: hematologic malignancy/BMT, solid organ transplants > AIDS patients
- Immunocompromised: mortality 77% (100% if disseminated)
- Angioinvasive; best stained with Gomori methenamine silver; obtain fungal cx and histopath on all biopsies
- Important to dx since P. boydii is Ampho B resistant
- Presentation/appearance similar to Aspergillus and Fusarium.

SITES OF INFECTION

- Immunocompetent: mycetoma at site of trauma/surgery; sinusitis; fungus ball
- Classic: brain abscess or pneumonia after near-drowning
- Endocarditis, endophthalmitis, osteomyelitis, septic arthritis (case reports)
- Immunocompromised: pneumonia/fungus ball, disseminated, brain abscess, skin lesions
- Portal of entry: inhaled or via skin trauma
- Skin lesions may be pustular, nodular, or necrotic
- Sinusitis in immunocompetent is more allergic than infectious; analogous to ABPA

TREATMENT REGIMENS

Immunocompetent

- Non-pulmonary mycetoma: debridement combined with antifungals (see below)
- Pulmonary fungus ball: no standardized regimen; surgical resection alone is reasonable if symptomatic (hemoptysis)
- Brain abscess: surgical drainage plus voriconazole (see below) for 6-12 months
- Sinusitis: usually allergic not infectious; corticosteroids, decongestants are mainstay
- No data to support antifungal use for P. boydii allergic fungal sinusitis
- Voriconazole dose (IV=PO bioavailability): 6mg/kg IV q 12 on day 1 then 4 mg/kg IV BID OR 200mg PO BID
- May increase voriconazole dose to 300mg PO bid if needed for slow/insufficient clinical response.

Immunocompromised

- 85% of isolates resistant to amphotericin B
- Combined medical and surgical approach for localized lesions
- Fungus ball/abscess (pulmonary or CNS): surgical resection PLUS voriconazole
- Voriconazole: FDA-approved for refractory/ampho-intolerant patients; experts feel this is drug of choice
- Voriconazole dose (IV=PO bioavailability): 6 mg/kg IV q12 on day 1 then 4mg/kg IV BID or 200mg PO BID
- May increase voriconazole dose to 300mg PO BID if clinical response judged slow/insufficient.
- Posaconazole: in vitro activity; case reports of successful treatment; not FDA-approved
- Traditional azoles: antifungal activity - miconazole > ketoconazole > itraconazole
- Recommend prolonged therapy with any azole: 6 - 12 months, obtaining serial imaging of affected areas
- Sinusitis: Infectious not allergic; combined surgical debridement and voriconazole for 6-12 months

IMPORTANT POINTS

- Fungal culture is imperative as histopath is indistinguishable from Aspergillus

- In vitro, caspofungin showed activity against P. boydii

SELECTED READINGS

Pfaller MA, Marco F, Messer SA, et al. In vitro activity of two echinocandin derivatives, LY303366 and MK-0991 (L-743,792), against clinical isolates of Aspergillus, Fusarium, Rhizopus, and other filamentous fungi. Diagn Microbiol Infect Dis. 1998 Apr;30(4):251-5.

Torre-Cisneros J, Gonzalez-Rutz A, Hodges MR, et al. Voriconazole for treatment of S. apiospermum and S. prolificans infections. Abstract 305, p 93. 38th Annual Meeting of the Infectious Diseases Society of America, Sept 7-10 2001; New Orleans, LA.

Gonzalez GM, Tijerina R, Najvar LK, et al. Activity of posaconazole against Pseudallescheria boydii: in vitro and in vivo assays. Antimicrob Agents Chemother 2003 Apr;47(4):1436-8

Castiglioni B, Sutton DA, Rinaldi MG, et al. Pseudallescheria boydii (Anamorph Scedosporium apiospermum). Infection in solid organ transplant recipients in a tertiary medical center and review of the literature. Medicine (Baltimore) 2002 Sep;81(5):333-48

Bonduel M, Santos P, Turienzo CF, et al. Atypical skin lesions caused by Curvularia sp. and Pseudallescheria boydii in 2 patients after allogeneic bone marrow transplantation. Bone Marrow Transplant 2001 Jun;27(12):1311-3

SPOROTHRIX SCHENCKII   John G. Bartlett, M.D.

CLINICAL RELEVANCE & DIAGNOSIS

- Endemic fungus seen globally. Present in soil and on plants, most famously rose thorns
- Most cases are occupational or vocational - farming, gardening
- Dx: cx fungus, may need multiple biopsies; (+) cx = diagnosis
- Dimorphic fungus, grows at 37 degrees C; cigar shaped 1-3 x 3-10um yeast

SITES OF INFECTION

- Lymphocutaneous
- Cutaneous
- Pulmonary
- Osteoarthritis
- Meningitis
- Disseminated

TREATMENT REGIMENS

Lymphocutaneous/cutaneous

- Indications to Rx: nearly all pts
- Lymphocutaneous (preferred): itraconazole 200mg qd x 3-6mo
- Lymphocut (alternative): SSKI increasing from 5-40 qtts tid as tolerated x3-6 mos.
- Lymphocut (Alt): fluconazole 400mg qd x 6 mo.
- Adjunctive: local hyperthermia with pocket warmer, infrared or far-infrared heater; heat to 42 degrees C daily x 2-3mo
- Monitor itraconazole levels to assure absorption - expect >1mcg/mL

Extracutaneous

- Pulmonary (preferred): ampho B 0.7-1mg/kg/d IV to 1-2 gm total dose, or itraconazole 200mg PO bid (less severe) or surgical resection
- Pulmonary (alternative): ampho B, then itraconazole 200mg PO bid
- Osteoarticular (preferred): itra 200mg PO bid x12mo
- Osteoarticular (alternative): ampho B 1-2g or fluconazole 800mg qd x 12mo
- Meningitis (preferred): ampho B 1-2g; alternative: ampho B then itracon 200mg bid or ampho B then fluconazole 800mg qd

- Disseminated (preferred): ampho B 1-2g total dose or itraconazole 200mg PO bid
- AIDS: ampho B 1-2g total dose, then itra 200mg bid
- Pregnancy: ampho B for serious infection, hyperthermia for lymphocutaneous dz.
- Monitor itraconazole levels to assure absorption - expect >1mcg/mL

IMPORTANT POINTS

- Guidelines from IDSA (CID 2000;30:684)
- Most common: lymphocutaneous: skin inoculation (soil) - skin nodule (extremity) - regional nodes develop over mos-yrs; fungus likes cold
- Extracutaneous: pulm (chronic cavity), osteoarthritis (distal joint (chronic), disseminated skin or visceral (AIDS, etc)
- Prognosis: lymphocutaneous - benign & responds to Rx; extracutaneous - morbid & hard to Rx; treat everybody
- Differential (cutaneous): pyoderma, foreign body granuloma, M. marinum, blastomycosis

SELECTED READINGS

Kauffman C, Hajjeh R, Chapman S. Practice Guidelines for the Management of Patients with Sporotrichosis. CID 2000;30:684

Kauffman CA, Pappas PG, McKinsey DS, et al. Treatment of lymphocutaneous and visceral sporotrichosis with fluconazole. CID 1996;22:46

Winn RE, Anderson J, Piper J, et al. Systemic sporotrichosis treated with itraconazole. CID 1993;17:210

Rotz LD, Slater LN, Wack MF, et al. Disseminated sporotrichosis with meningitis in a patient with AIDS. Inf Dis Clin Pract 1996;5:566

Rex JH and Okhuysen PC. Sporothrix schenckii. Chapter 250 IN: Principles & Practice of Infectious Diseases, Mandell G, Bennett J, Dolin R (Eds) 5th Ed, Churchill Livingston, 2000;pg 2695

ZYGOMYCETES Aimee Zaas, M.D. & Paul Auwaerter, M.D.

CLINICAL RELEVANCE & DIAGNOSIS

- Wide (6-16 micron), aseptate, ribbon-like, nonpigmented fungi with wide angle branching
- Classically called "mucormycosis," Mucor, Rhizopus, Rhizomucor, Absidia, Cunninghamella, Saksenea all belong to the class "Zygomycetes"
- Risk factors: ketoacidosis, neutropenia, iron overload, iron chelation drug use, IDU, prednisone
- Syndromes: rhinocerebral, pulmonary, disseminated, GI, cutaneous, allergic
- Acquisition: mainly inhalation; also skin trauma and ingestion
- Defenses: macrophages (kill spores); neutrophils (kill germinating hyphae)
- Mortality: (range 11-100%); nearly 100% for disseminated disease or in those for whom immunosuppression cannot be corrected
- Send tissue for histopathology (silver stain) and culture; blood cultures are unhelpful (never positive)
- Mincing of tissue during specimen preparation can disrupt fungal structure, impairing diagnosis

SITES OF INFECTION

- Rhinocerebral: invasive sinusitis; classic palate eschar; proceeds to involve skull base + cranial nerve palsies
- Pulmonary: localized infiltrate; angioinvasion leads to infarct/cavitation with hemoptysis (may mimic PE)

Fungi

- Disseminated: multi-organ failure, tissue infarctions due to angioinvasion
- Cutaneous: at sites of trauma; can have nailbed infections; ranges from erythema to pustules to necrotizing fasciitis (see Table 8 in Appendix I)
- Gastric (rare): necrotic gastric ulcers in immunocompromised patients consuming fermented food
- Allergic: hypersensitivity pneumonitis without invasion; exposure in malt workers, farmers
- External otitis: noninvasive superficial crusting otitis
- Rhinocerebral: MRI with gadolinium of head/skull base to define extent of disease is crucial
- GI Basidiobolomycosis: emerging infection in Arizona; abd pain, leukocytosis, inflammatory mass on imaging

Treatment Regimens

Rhinocerebral
- Aggressive surgical debridement; consult otorhinolarygologist promptly
- Lipid preparation amphotericin B 5mg/kg IV q24 hours for prolonged (>6 weeks) period (Source of recommendation: author)
- Itraconazole and posaconazole may have some activity; some authors (Mandell) recommend itraconazole for therapy
- Fluconazole and voriconazole not effective
- Echinocandins (caspofungin) not effective
- Hyperbaric oxygen helpful in case reports
- Correct underlying predisposition (acidosis, neutropenia, steroids) and stop iron chelating meds

Pulmonary
- Surgical resection of unilobar disease recommended
- Surgical resection can be helpful if massive hemoptysis present
- Lipid preparation amphotericin B 5mg/kg IV q 24 hours for prolonged period
- Correct underlying predisposition (acidosis, neutropenia, steroids) and stop iron chelating meds

Cutaneous
- Surgical resection to bleeding, uninvolved margin necessary
- Lipid amphotericin B 5 mg/kg IV q 24
- If infection is superficial in immunocompetent patient, can try topical natamycin (5% opthalmic suspension) or ketoconazole

Gastrointestinal
- Basidiobolomycosis: (see reference 5) treat with resection and itraconazole liquid 200mg PO bid for >3 months
- Surgical resection of involved areas imperative
- Lipid preparation of amphotericin B5 mg/kg IV q 24 hours
- Correct underlying predisposition
- When using itraconazole, should document absorption and monitor itraconazole levels

Selected Readings

Cloughley R, Kelehan J, Corbett-Feeney G, Murray M, Callaghan J, Regan P, Cormican M. Soft tissue infection with absidia corymbifera in a patient with idiopathic aplastic anemia. J Clin Microbiol 2002 Feb;40(2):725-7

Adam RD, Hunter G, Ditomasso J, Comerci G. Zygomycosis: emerging prominence of cutaneous infections. Clin Infect Dis. 1994;19:67-69

Ribes JA, Vanover-Sams CL, Baker DJ. Zygomycetes in human disease. Clin Microbiol Rev. 2000 Apr;13 (2):236-301.

Chakrabarti A, Das A, Sharma A, Panda N, Das S, Gupta KL, Sakhuja V. Ten years' experience in zygomycosis at a tertiary care centre in India. J Infect 2001 May;42(4):261-6

Lyon GM, Smilack JD, Komatsu KK, Pasha TM, Leighton JA, Guarner J, Colby T. Gastrointestinal basidiobolomycosis in Arizona: clinical and epidemiological characteristics and review of the literature. Clin Infect Dis 2001 May 15;32(10):1448-55

PARASITES

BABESIA SPECIES
John G. Bartlett, M.D.

CLINICAL RELEVANCE & DIAGNOSIS

- Tick-borne, protozoal cause of potentially lethal, undifferentiated syndrome, especially in splenectomized patients
- Usually transmitted in focal areas of northeast US from NY to Massachusetts; also in Midwest and Washington State
- May coinfect along with Borrelia burgdorferi and the agent of human granulocytic ehrlichiosis
- Severe illness: Old age, immunosuppressed or splenectomy
- Transmitted by Ixodes (hard bodied) ticks from May to September
- In non-immunocompromised people, illness typically mild, but parasitemia can be prolonged as detected by molecular tests

SITES OF INFECTION

- Red blood cells

TREATMENT REGIMENS

General

- Preferred: Atovaquone 750mg bid x 7d, plus azithromycin 500mg x 1, then 250mg/d x 7d OR
- Preferred: Clindamycin 600mg PO tid x 7d plus quinine 650mg PO tid x 7d
- Clindamycin regimen is tolerated better if it can be administered
- Critical illness: exchange transfusion

IMPORTANT POINTS

- Diagnosis: Usually through thin and thick blood smears stained with Giemsa or Wright-Giemsa
- Diagnosis: May be confused with Plasmodium rings, but Babesia do not have brownish pigment in cells and morphology of Plasmodium gametocytes differs from Babesia; Maltese cross/tetrads are rare.
- Diagnosis: Indirect fluorescence antibody test available at CDC, PCR available at some institutions.
- Source of guidelines: NEJM 2000;343:1454
- Symptoms: Flu-like; severe complications - CHF, renal failure, ARDS

SELECTED READINGS

Homer MJ, Aguilar-Delfin I, Telford SR 3rd, Krause PJ, Persing DH. Babesiosis. Clin Microbiol Rev 13 (3):451-69, 2000

Krause PJ, Spielman A, Telford SR 3rd, et al. Persistent parasitemia after acute babesiosis. N Engl J Med 339(3):160-5, 1998

Krause PJ, Lepore T, Sikand VK et al. Atovaquone and azithromycin for the treatment of babesiosis. N Engl J Med 343(20):1454-8, 2000

Quick RE, Herwaldt BL, Thomford JW, et al. Babesiosis in Washington State: a new species of Babesia? . Ann Intern Med 119(4):284-90, 1993

Persing DH, Herwaldt BL, Glaser C, et al. Infection with a babesia-like organism in northern California . N Engl J Med 332(5):298-303, 1995

CYCLOSPORA CAYETANENSIS   Joseph Vinetz, M.D.

CLINICAL RELEVANCE & DIAGNOSIS
- Protozoal cause of diarrhea, worldwide, more common in tropical settings
- Cause of prolonged diarrhea in travelers, often remitting and relapsing for weeks to months, ultimately self-limited
- Associated with food-borne outbreaks in the U.S., particularly raspberries from Guatemala
- Associated with water-borne outbreaks in U.S., developing world (esp. Nepal)
- Incubation period ~7d, often with antecedent flu-like illness, then nausea, anorexia, abd cramps, watery diarrhea. Fatigue and malaise may be prominent.
- In AIDS, can range from asymptomatic to severe, ascending biliary tract infection (rare)
- Dx: direct exam of stool; 8-10 uM variably acid fast oocysts; iodine stain and autofluorescence under UV improves sensitivity
- Dx: may be missed on routine exam or mistaken for Cryptosporidium, MUST request specifically from lab
- In Europe, primarily associated with travel to endemic regions

SITES OF INFECTION
- GI: small intestine (acute and chronic inflammation which can persist after cure); biliary tract (rare), gall bladder (rare)
- Systemic: Reiter's syndrome (inflammation, inflammatory oligoarthritis, sterile urethritis) can develop in setting of prolonged diarrheal illness

TREATMENT REGIMENS

Sulfa-containing regimen
- TMP-SMX 160mg/800mg (1 DS tab) PO bid x 7-10 d
- In AIDS, 1 DS tab three times a week for secondary prophylaxis

Fluoroquinolone-containing regimen
- Ciprofloxacin 500mg PO bid x 7 d (less effective than TMP-SMX)

IMPORTANT POINTS
- Source of Recommendations: Verdier et al; Hoge et al
- Can be particularly important cause of diarrhea in travelers to specific locales such as Nepal
- Does not cause fever, inflammatory diarrhea or eosinophilia
- Transmission associated also with basil, salad greens esp. mesclun lettuce
- In HIV/AIDS, associated cases, but not particularly severe disease

SELECTED READINGS
Kansouzidou A et al. Cyclospora cayetanensis in a patient with travelers' diarrhea: case report and review. J Travel Med. 2004;11:61-3

Diaz E et al. Epidemiology and control of intestinal parasites with nitazoxanide in children in Mexico. Am J Trop Med Hyg. 2003;68:384-5

Ortega YR, Sterling CR, Gilman RH, et al. Cyclospora species--a new protozoan pathogen of humans. N Engl J Med. 1993 May 6;328(18):1308-12

Herwaldt B. Cyclospora cayetanensis: a review, focusing on the outbreaks of cyclosporiasis in the 1990s. Clin Infect Dis. 2000 Oct;31(4):1040-57

Verdier RI, Fitzgerald DW, Johnson WD Jr, et al. Trimethoprim-sulfamethoxazole compared with ciprofloxacin for treatment and prophylaxis of Isospora belli and Cyclospora cayetanensis infection in HIV-infected patients. Ann Intern Med. 2000 Jun 6;132(11):885-8

ENTAMOEBA HISTOLYTICA
Joseph Vinetz, M.D.

CLINICAL RELEVANCE & DIAGNOSIS

- Protozoan parasite, cause of diarrhea, dysentery, liver abscess and other syndromes
- Occurs primarily in developing countries, but immigrants, travelers, MSM diagnosed with infection in U.S.
- Must be distinguished clinically from Entamoeba dispar, a morphologically identical parasite that is noninvasive and does not cause disease
- Onset of colitis usually gradual with symptoms > 1 wk, distinguishing it from bacterial dysentery
- Diagnosis of amebic colitis: 1) observation of red cell-containing motile trophozoites on fresh stool smear (insensitive); always heme + stool
- Dx: 2) Colonoscopy: biopsy or scraping at margin of colonic mucosal ulcer: parasite may be seen; H&E shows necrosis, classic flask-shaped ulcer
- Dx: 3) stool antigen test that distinguishes Eh from E. dispar is available, more sensitive than microscopy of stool
- Dx: 4) Serology 99% sens. for amebic liver abscess; 88% sens. for colitis, but Abs may be present yrs. later so that serology may not be useful in immigrants from Eh-endemic regions
- Dx: 5) Ultrasound of liver: cannot distinguish amebic from pyogenic abscess, but can guide aspiration if necessary
- Dx: 6) Liver abscess aspiration--yields anchovy paste-like material, lack of WBCs (due to lysis by parasite) clue to diagnosis, parasites usually not seen

SITES OF INFECTION

- Colon: dysentery, ameboma (tumor-like lesion of colonic lumen; can be confused radiographically with cecal cancer), toxic megacolon
- Liver: abscess, can rupture causing peritonitis
- Lung: empyema (right sided-direct extension from liver)
- Heart: pericarditis (direct extension from liver)
- Brain: abscess (hematogenous spread, rare)
- Skin: usually perineal, genital
- GU: recto-vaginal fistula

TREATMENT REGIMENS

Intestinal colonization

- E. dispar does not require Rx
- Luminal agents alone should be used (not absorbed)
- Tinidazole: Adults: 2g qd x 3 d; children older than 3 years, 50mg/kg PO qd (max 2g/day) for 3 days.
- Iodoquinol: 650mg PO tid x 20 d

- Paromomycin: 25-35mg/kg/d in 3 divided doses x 7 d

Invasive
- Metronidazole: 500-750mg tid x 7-10 d
- Tinidazole: Adults: 2g qd x 3-5 d; children older than 3 years, 50mg/kg PO qd (max 2 g/day) for 3-5 days.
- Liver abscess aspiration not usually necessary, does not speed recovery
- Consider adding luminal agent, otherwise relapse of extraintestinal disease may occur even months later

IMPORTANT POINTS
- Amebic colitis should be ruled out prior to diagnosis of Crohn's disease; corticosteroids will worsen amebiasis

SELECTED READINGS

E Diaz et al. Epidemiology and control of intestinal parasites with nitazoxanide in children in Mexico. Am J Trop Med Hyg. 2003;68:384-5

Hughes MA, Petri WA. Amebic liver abscess. Infect Dis Clin North Am 2000 14:565-82

Petri WA Jr, Singh U. Diagnosis and management of amebiasis. Clin Infect Dis 1999 29:1117-25

Petri WA. Entamoeba histolytica: Clinical Update and Vaccine Prospects . Curr Infect Dis Rep 2002;4:124-129

GIARDIA LAMBLIA

Joseph Vinetz, M.D.

CLINICAL RELEVANCE & DIAGNOSIS
- Protozoan parasite, causes diarrhea, abdominal cramping, bloating, flatulence, occasionally leading to chronic syndrome of diarrhea, malabsorption and weight loss
- In North America, most commonly identified fecal parasite.
- At presentation, most patients have had >7 d of diarrhea.
- Weight loss of >10 lbs during illness seen >50% pts.
- More difficult to treat in immunocompromised.
- Suspects: children attending daycare centers; travel to endemic areas; ingestion of unfiltered water while camping; fecal-oral sex contact (esp. male homosexuals); well water on farm.
- Diagnosis: stool O&P exam for cysts/trophs; antigen detection specifically only detects Giardia.
- Stools profuse, watery, become greasy and foul smelling over time; blood, pus and mucus absent.
- Typical presentation: acute onset diarrhea, bloating, flatulence, cramps, accompanied by malaise, nausea, anorexia and classically with "sulfuric belching."

SITES OF INFECTION
- GI: upper small bowel, adherent to enterocytes

TREATMENT REGIMENS

Furazolidone
- 100mg PO qid x 7-10 d
- Efficacy ~80%, lower than metronidazole; main advantage in children is availability in suspension form

- Side effects: GI, turns urine brown, mild hemolysis with G6PD deficiency, not approved for use in pregnancy

Quinacrine

- 100mg PO tid x 5-7 d
- Available only from Panorama Pharmacy, 8215 Van Nuys Blvd., Panorama City, CA 91402. Tel: (818) 988-7979
- If used in combination with metronidazole, use full doses of both drugs

Metronidazole

- 250mg tid x 5-7 d (not FDA approved, but clinical standard with widespread experience)
- Efficacy 80-95%
- In pregnancy, no consistently recommended therapy because of theoretical risk of metronidazole-induced teratogenicity (never observed)
- For refractory cases, use in combination with quinacrine has been reported effective (See Nash TE et al, references)
- In pregnancy, metronidazole has been used for trichomoniasis, teratogenic potential appears minimal, use restricted to last 2 trimesters
- When taken with alcohol, can produce disulfiram-like effect

Tinidazole

- Single 2g dose, po
- Efficacy high, >90%
- Mild side effect profile; dosing regimen enhances compliance

Albendazole

- 400mg daily for 5 d
- Off label use
- Appx. 90% efficacy rate in children, equivalent to metronidazole, in 1 small study

Paromomycin:

- 25-30mg/kg/d in 3 divided doses, x 5-10d. Efficacy low, appx. 60-70%. Can be used in pregnancy, if treatment cannot be delayed beyond delivery.

IMPORTANT POINTS

- Commonly transmitted to family members of infected child, who is likely to be in daycare setting
- May result in chronic diarrhea/wt loss even in immunecompetant individuals.
- Antigen study may be superior to multiple standard stool O&Ps for giardia detection.
- Metronidazole is the time-tested standard therapy, although tinidazole w/ qd dosing may improve compliance.

SELECTED READINGS

Nash TE, Ohl CA, Thomas E, Subramanian G, Keiser P, Moore TA. Treatment of patients with refractory giardiasis. Clin Infect Dis 2001;33:22-8

Gardner TB, Hill DR. Treatment of giardiasis. Clin Microbiol Rev 2001 14:114-28

Yereli K et al. Albendazole as an alternative therapeutic agent for childhood giardiasis in Turkey . Clin Microbiol Infect. 2004;10:527-9

Hlavsa MC, Watson JC, Beach MJ. Giardiasis surveillance--United States, 1998-2002. MMWR Surveill Summ. 2005 Jan 28;54(1):9-16

LEISHMANIA SPECIES
Joseph Vinetz, M.D.

CLINICAL RELEVANCE & DIAGNOSIS

- Protozoan causes of cutaneous ulcers and hepatosplenic/bone marrow disease in tropical and developing countries
- Zoonotic disease, transmitted from various mammals (especially dogs) to humans via bite of sand flies
- Three major syndromes: cutaneous ulcer, visceral (liver, spleen, bone marrow), mucocutaneous (metastatic from skin)
- New World leishmaniasis: transmitted in Central and South America, may be cutaneous, visceral or mucocutaneous ("espundia" aka Breda's disease)
- Old World leishmaniasis: transmitted in India, middle East, southern Europe and northern Africa along Mediterranean, sub-Saharan Africa; either cutaneous or visceral (kala-azar)
- Major opportunistic pathogen in AIDS in endemic regions, or after HIV-infected patient leaves endemic region and reactivates infection
- In Old World, cutaneous disease usually self-resolves, leaving scar
- In New World, some cutaneous disease self-resolves but some infections (due to L. braziliensis) can metastasize and reactivate later (months to years) in mucosal surfaces of the mouth and nose
- Diagnosis: cutaneous--demonstration of parasite by Giemsa stain of biopsy touch prep or section; mononuclear cell infiltrate typical; culture and PCR in specialized labs
- Diagnosis: visceral--Giemsa or DFA stain of splenic aspirate, bone marrow aspirate/ biopsy; culture (gold standard), PCR (experimental) in specialized labs

SITES OF INFECTION

- Skin: cutaneous ulcer that may or may not spontaneously resolve; may be single or multiple, usually on face or extremities where sand flies bite
- Visceral: liver, spleen, bone marrow
- HEENT: progressive, destructive mucosal lesions in nose, mouth, pharynx, larynx, months to years after primary lesion resolves

TREATMENT REGIMENS

Cutaneous
- Pentavalent antimony 20mg SbV/kg IV qd x 20 d
- Ketoconazole: appears moderately effective in Old World cutaneous leishmaniasis (80-90%); less effective in New World cutaneous leishmaniasis (~70%)
- Cutaneous leishmaniasis due to L. major (Old World) appears to respond to oral fluconazole 200mg/d x 6 wks (see reference below)
- Pentamidine 3mg/kg IV on alternative d x 4 doses, or 2 mg/kg on alternate days x 7 doses
- Miltefosine (not FDA approved) shown useful for Leishmania panamensis but less so (below response rate of standard antimonials) for L. braziliensis. See references below.

Mucosal
- Pentavalent antimony 20mg SbV/kg qd x 28 d
- Amphotericin B deoxycholate 1mg/kg qd or alternate days, total dose 20-40mg/kg

Visceral
- AmBisome (liposomal amphotericin B) 2-5mg/kg qd for total of 15-21mg/kg
- Amphotericin B deoxycholate 0.5-1.0mg/kg on alternate days or daily for total dose of 15-20mg/kg

- Pentavalent antimony 20mg of SbV/kg IV for 28 days (see "Cutaneous" for different preparations)
- Miltefosine (not FDA approved), oral, appears effective: 100mg (2.5mg/kg.d x 28 d (see references)

IMPORTANT POINTS

- Call CDC Drug Service for assistance in obtaining Pentostam (pentavalent antimony; Sodium stibogluconate): (404) 639-3670 (health care providers only)
- Guidelines from Herwaldt, Lancet, 1999 (reference below); Medical Letter (2000; 42:9; available free online www.medicalletter.com/freedocs/parasitic.pdf)
- In general, for visceral disease, it seems clear that lipid formulations of amphotericin B are as effective as antimonials or conventional amphotericin B, with less toxicity but higher cost.

SELECTED READINGS

Sundar S et al. Amphotericin B treatment for Indian visceral leishmaniasis: conventional versus lipid formulations. Clin Infect Dis. 2004 Feb 1;38(3):377-83

Soto J, Toledo J, Gutierrez P, et al. Treatment of American Cutaneous Leishmaniasis with Miltefosine, an Oral Agent. Clin Infect Dis. 2001 Oct 1;33(7):E57-61. (Accessed September 6, 2004)

Sundar S, Makharia A, More DK, et al. Short-course of oral miltefosine for treatment of visceral leishmaniasis. Clin Infect Dis 31:1110-3, 2000

Herwaldt BL. Leishmaniasis . Lancet 354:1191-9, 1999

Murray HW. Clinical and experimental advances in treatment of visceral leishmaniasis . Antimicrob Agents Chemother 45:2185-97, 2001

LICE

Noreen A. Hynes, M.D., M.P.H.

CLINICAL RELEVANCE & DIAGNOSIS

- Transmission by direct contact and by fomites; pruritis is common in all infested locations; secondary bacterial infection of excoriated areas can occur; the body louse can transmit infections.
- PUBIC LICE: #1 louse infestation in US adult; maculae ceruleae(blue spots) may be seen on trunk, thighs, upper parts of arms; pubic lice can also infest head, eyelashes (nits or crusts), axillae.
- HEAD LICE: Most commonly seen in children, ages 3-12 years, in U.S.
- PREVENTION AND CONTROL CLUES: Transmission of pubic lice NOT prevented by condom use; Body lice found in seams of clothes rather than on skin.
- Pubic lice are a marker for other STDs; Body lice are seen among displaced and homeless persons and can serve a vectors of infectious diseases; Head lice are seen in children of all socioeconomic grps
- BODY LICE: Urban trench fever (Bartonella quintana) seen in alcoholic homeless persons; Relapsing fever (Borrelia recurrentis)outbreaks in Western US; Epidemic typhus (R. prowazekii) in refugee camps
- Dual infestation with scabies not uncommon

SITES OF INFECTION

- Head (Pediculosis humanis var capitus): an infestation of head hair. Nits seen more often than lice.
- Body (Pediculosis humanis var corporis): infestation of clothing seams; can transmit infectious diseases with blood meal.

- Pubis (Phthirus pubis): an infestation of pubic>axillary>head>eyelash hair. Lice visible.

TREATMENT REGIMENS

Phthiriasis (pubic lice, crabs)

- Permethrin 1% crème rinse: Apply to affected areas and washed off after 10 minutes.
- Lindane 1% shampoo: Apply to affected area and leave in place for 4 minutes. Then, wash off thoroughly. (NOT in pregnant/lactating women or children < 2 yrs)
- Pyrethrins (0.33%) with piperonyl butoxide (4%): Apply lotion to affected DRY hair and skin. Wash off out in no longer than 10 minutes.

Pediculosis corporis

- Treat clothes, not person! Body lice found in seams of clothes rather than on skin.
- Machine wash clothes on hot cycle then iron seams

Pediculosis capitis

- Permethrin 1% crème rinse applied topically once for 10 minutes, then washed off. Nit removal with 1:1 solution of H_2O and vinegar applied to hair then run vinegar-dipped fine tooth comb through hair.
- Pyrethrins (0.33%) with piperonyl butoxide (4%): Apply lotion to cover affected DRY hair and scalp. Shampoo out in no longer than 10 minutes.
- Malathion 0.5%. USE ONLY IF RESISTANT TO ALL OTHER RX! Apply to hair, let dry naturally. (DO NOT USE ANY ELECTRIC PRODUCTS WHILE HAIR DRYING--HIGHLY FLAMMABLE). Wash off after 8-12 h. Repeat 7-10 days.

Phthiriasis palpebarum (eyelash lice)

- Petroleum jelly applied to the lids qid x 10d
- Yellow oxide of mercury, 1% applied qid x 14d

IMPORTANT POINTS

- For treatment of pubic lice, this module based on the CDC's 2002 STD Rx Guidelines; 2002 AAP Guideline for Rx of Head Lice; for other lice-- Rx based on expert opinion cited in literature.
- 2003 FDA PUBLIC HEATLH ADVISORY ON LINDANE USE: Note increased risk of neurologic side effects in the elderly, persons weighing <50 kg, and children. Use other products when possible in these groups.
- Head lice in an adult, usually means child in home. Pubic lice serve as a marker for other STDs--therefore test for them. Treat ALL contacts of persons with lice.
- Hydroxyzine 25-50mg TID-QID may be needed to control itch in addition to lice-specific RX. Topical steroids may be needed, as well.
- Secondary cutaneous bacterial infection, usually due to S. aureus, seen when extensive excoriations occur in setting of uncontrolled pruritis.

SELECTED READINGS

Ko CJ and Elston DM. Pediculosis. J Amer Acad Dermatol 2004; 50:1-18

Wooltoron E. Concerns over lindane treatment for scabies and lice. Can Med Assoc J 2003; 168:1-4.

Ashkenazi I et al. Yellow mercuric oxide: a treatment of choice for phthirasis palpebrarum. Br J Ophthalmol 1991 75:356-8

Brown S et al. Treatment of ectoparasite infections: review of the English-language literature, 1982-1992. Clin Infec Dis 1995 20(Suppl 1)S104-S9.

Centers for Disease Control and Prevention. Sexually transmitted diseases treatment guidelines. MMWR 2002; 51 (RR-6):1-78.

PLASMODIUM

Joseph Vinetz, M.D.

CLINICAL RELEVANCE & DIAGNOSIS

- Malaria caused by protozoan parasite, transmitted by mosquitoes in tropics
- Infects RBCs; damage to brain, kidney, lung, placenta
- Presents as nonspecific, generalized febrile illness
- Suspect in any febrile traveler returning from tropics
- Drug resistance common; chloroquine rarely used now in U.S.
- Prompt evaluation necessary; untreated P. falciparum malaria rapidly progresses, often fatal if untreated
- Severe P. falciparum malaria: parenteral treatment, telemetry
- P. vivax and P. ovale: dormant liver stages lasting months; potential for relapse after mos/yrs
- Severe malaria: encephalopathy, seizure, hyperparasitemia (>2.5% of RBC), pulmonary edema, renal failure
- Dx: order thin blood smear from hematology lab if history of travel to endemic area plus fever; determine parasitemia/species; obtain sequential thick and thin blood smears to firmly rule out

SITES OF INFECTION

- RBCs: for P. falciparum parasitized RBCs block brain, placenta, lung, kidney, gut post-capillary venules
- Liver (dormant stages): P. vivax, P. ovale only
- Spleen

TREATMENT REGIMENS

General principles

- Consider disease severity, geographic origin of infection, parasite species (based on blood smear)
- P. falciparum infection potentially and rapidly life threatening
- Hyperparasitemia, CNS symptoms are medical emergency requiring IV Rx

Uncomplicated P. falciparum

- Consider only if certain to tolerate PO medications:
- Quinine 650mg q8h x 3-7 d plus doxycycline 100mg bid x 7 d
- Quinine 650mg q8h x3-7 d plus pyrimethamine/sulfadoxine 3 tabs on last day of quinine
- Mefloquine 750mg once then 500mg 12 h later
- Malarone (atovaquone/proguanil) 4 tabs/d (1000mg atovaquone/400mg proguanil) for 3 d, taken with milk or fatty meal
- For known chloroquine-sensitive P. falciparum, Chloroquine phosphate 1g salt (600mg base) once, then 500mg salt (300mg base) 6h later, then 500mg salt at 24h and 48 h
- Chloroquine safe in pregnancy. Mefloquine, quinine, probably safe but not FDA-approved in pregnancy

Complicated P. falciparum

- IV quinidine: admit to telemetry unit. QT prolongation, ventricular arrhythmia, hypotension and hypoglycemia may occur.
- IV quinidine gluconate: for availability call (800) 821-0538; (317) 276-2000
- Quinidine gluconate IV 20mg salt/kg loading dose in saline over 1-2h, then constant drip of 0.02mg quinidine salt/kg/min until parasitemia < 1% or oral meds tolerated
- Start doxycycline 100mg bid along with quinidine
- Parasitemia > 5-10%, consider exchange transfusion

- Mefloquine, quinine and quinidine probably safe in pregnancy but not FDA-approved. Untreated malaria in pregnant women lethal.

Plasmodium vivax, P. ovale, P. malariae

- Chloroquine phosphate 1g salt (600mg base) once, then 500mg salt (300mg base) 6 h later, then 500mg at 24 h and 48 h
- Treatment of liver forms (vivax/ovale only): primaquine 0.5mg base/kg/d x 14d (new rec). May cause hemolytic anemia due to G6PD deficiency - test first. Contraindicated in pregnancy/breastfeeding.
- Primaquine treatment is not mandatory. Some prefer to wait for the low risk of relapse rather than face potential side-effects of the drug.

Prophylaxis (see Appendix I, Table 12)

- General recommendations for U.S. adults: most malaria-endemic regions (i.e., where chloroquine resistance is known or likely to be present)
- Atovaquone/proguanil (Malarone) 1 tab daily. Take with food or milky drink. Start 1-2d before entry to malarial region, discontinue 7d after leaving.
- Mefloquine 250mg (Lariam) 1 tab weekly. Start 1 wk prior to travel and continue weekly, always on the same day each week, preferably after the main meal, until 4 wks after return.
- Doxycycline 100mg qd. Optimally taken in evening. Start 1 wk before travel, until four wks after travel. Photosensitivity risk >3%; avoid sun, use sunscreen. Drug of choice for Thailand.
- Central America N of Panama Canal (only): Chloroquine 300mg wk. Start 1 wk before, continue 4 wk after.
- Mosquitoes bite at any time of day but anopheles mainly at night with most activity at dawn and dusk. Use sprays (DEET) and avoid thin clothing.

IMPORTANT POINTS

- Guidelines from Medical Letter (August 2004; (1189) pp. 1-12 available free online www. medicalletter.com/freedocs/parasitic.pdf)
- Falciparum malaria potentially lethal, most malaria imported, major complications arise from CNS, kidney, lung
- CDC Malaria hotline: (770) 488-7788 or (404) 639-2888
- IV quinine not available in U.S. Quinidine gluconate may not be available in some hospital pharmacies.
- Even if P. vivax diagnosed, consider possibility of co-infection with P. falciparum.

SELECTED READINGS

Ohrt C et al. Malaria prophylaxis using azithromycin: a double-blind, placebo-controlled trial in Irian Jaya, Indonesia. Clin Infect Dis 1999 28(1):74-81

Centers for Disease Control. MALARIA. http://www.cdc.gov/ncidod/dpd/parasites/malaria/default.htm

Centers for Disease Control. Malarone for Malaria Treatment and Prophylaxis . http://www.cdc.gov/travel/diseases/malaria/malarone.htm

McGready R et al. Randomized comparison of mefloquine-artesunate versus quinine in the treatment of multidrug-resistant falciparum malaria in pregnancy . Trans R Soc Trop Med Hyg. 2000 94(6):689-93

Nosten F, et al. The effects of mefloquine treatment in pregnancy . Clin Infect Dis. 1999 28(4):808-15

SARCOPTES SCABIEI VAR HOMINIS (SCABIES)

Noreen A. Hynes, M.D., M.P.H.

CLINICAL RELEVANCE & DIAGNOSIS

- Occurs in 2% to 4% of patients with HIV infection; unusual presentations common in this group.
- Cyclical epidemics often in long-term care facilities; may have a somewhat cryptic presentation in the elderly, often with only intense pruritis.
- Relapse may be more common than previously thought; urticaria can be seen even w/ small number of mites.
- Crusted scabies: an aggressive form especially in immunodeficient, debilitated, or malnourished persons; if generalized, hospitalize and get ID consult; highly contagious form esp for care providers.
- Classic scabies: pruritic rash w/excoriations; papules and linear burrows (nearly pathognomonic) in characteristic distribution at belt line, under breasts, on penis.

SITES OF INFECTION

- Interdigital web spaces of hands: classic scabies
- Flexor surfaces of the wrists and elbows: classic scabies
- Axillae: classic scabies
- Male genitalia: classic scabies
- Female breasts and inframammary folds: classic scabies
- Belt line: classic scabies
- Buttocks: classic scabies
- Generalized dermatitis: crusted scabies, bullous scabies
- Face, scalp: generalized crusted scabies

TREATMENT REGIMENS

Recommended regimen

- Permethrin cream (5%): Apply to all areas of body from the neck down and washed off after 8-14 hours

Alternative regimens

- Lindane (1%): Apply 1 oz. of lotion or 30g of cream thinly to all areas of the body from the neck down. Thoroughly wash off after 8 h. IF POSSIBLE AVOID IN ELDERLY, THOSE UNDER 50 KG WEIGHT, CHILDREN
- Ivermectin in 2 doses (of 200mcg/kg) separated by 2 wks (not FDA-approved for this indication).

Crusted scabies in immunodeficient persons

- Ivermectin 200mcg/kg once combined with Permethrin cream (5%) (NOT lindane). Repeat, if needed, after 2 wks. Ivermectin is not FDA-approved for this indication.

Pregnant and lactating women

- Lindane and ivermectin are contraindicated.

IMPORTANT POINTS

- This module based on CDC's 2002 STD Rx Guidelines (MMWR 2002; 51 (RR-6).
- Definitive dx by microscopic identification of the mite, eggs, or its feces. Scrape under fingernails or the end of a burrow.
- Common: papules, burrows, excoriations, nodules, vesicles, pyoderma, eczema. In nodular scabies the mildly pigmented, pruritic nodules may be present for months before dx.

PARASITES

- Uncommon presentations: crusts, urticaria, vasculitis, attenuated or exaggerated lesions. Generalized crusted scabies requires hospitalizaton and ID consultation.
- Pruritis may persist for 1-2 weeks after curative therapy. Clothes, bed linens decontaminated by machine washing at 60 degrees C. Insecticidal spray or powder applied to items which cannot be washed.

SELECTED READINGS

Victoria J and Trujillo R. Topical ivermectin: a successful treatment for scabies. Pediatr Dermatol 2001 18:63-4

Walker GJA and Johnstone PW. Interventions in treating scabies. The Cochrane Library,Issue 3, 2004. Chichester, UK, John Wiley & Sons, Ltd.

Woolteron E. Concerns over lindane treatment for scabies and lice. Can Med Assoc J 2003: 168:1-4

Walton SF et al. Acaricidal activity of Melaleuca alternifolia (tea tree) oil: in vitro sensitivity of Sarcoptes scabei var hominis to terpinen-4-ol. Arch Dematol 2004; 140:563-566.

Tan HH and Goh CL. Parasitic skin infections in the elderly: recognition and drug treatment. Drugs Aging 2001;18:165-76

STRONGYLOIDES STERCORALIS Joseph Vinetz, M.D.

CLINICAL RELEVANCE & DIAGNOSIS

- Nematode, cause of small intestinal infection; hyperinfection syndrome in pts given steroids, HTLV-I pts, occasionally in HIV/AIDS (likely due to steroids, inanition, HTLV coinfection)
- Acquired by larval stages penetrating intact skin, then undergoing further development
- Infection can asymptomatically last decades, activated by immune suppression
- Common scenario for hyperinfection syndrome: immigrant from developing country given high dose steroids, develops gram negative sepsis, meningitis, sometimes in presence of eosinophilia (usually not)
- Widely distributed in tropics; estimated prevalence up to 4% in U.S. South
- Can cause Loeffler-like syndrome (transient pulmonary infiltrates plus eosinophilia)

SITES OF INFECTION

- GI: nausea, vomiting, cramping, diarrhea, epigastric pain/burning, weight loss; eosinophilia is typical; usually asymptomatic with chronic infection
- Lung: Loeffler-like syndrome; in presence of immunocompromised, may have overwhelming larval invasion plus gram-negative bacterial infection
- CNS: larval invasion in superinfection syndrome, accompanied by gram negative bacterial meningitis; may be associated with peripheral and/or CSF eosinophilia
- Skin: generalized or localized urticaria; Larva currens syndrome (larvae migrating to perianal area, flank, with pruritic, serpigineous or linear urticarial lesions)
- Systemic: gram-negative sepsis, with pulmonary infiltrates, in pt. given steroids, and recent or distant immigration from strongyloidiasis-endemic region

TREATMENT REGIMENS

Ivermectin

- Drug of choice
- 200mcg/kg/day x 1-2d
- May need to be repeated or prolonged in pts with hyperinfection syndrome

Thiabendazole

- 50mg/kg/d in 2 doses (max. 3g/d) x 2 d

- Toxicity at this dose common: confusion, diarrhea, hallucinations, irritability, loss of appetite, nausea and vomiting, numbness/tingling in hands/feet

IMPORTANT POINTS

- Diagnosis may be difficult because few organisms may be present
- Diagnosis of intestinal infection: observation of larvae on direct stool smear (insensitive); Baermann test (larval concentration, specialized labs only); serology (problems with cross-reactivity)
- CNS or pulmonary infection: observation of larvae on direct wet mount examination of centrifuged CSF or BAL specimen

SELECTED READINGS

Kim AC, Lupatkin HC. Strongyloides stercoralis infection as a manifestation of immune restoration syndrome. Clin Infect Dis. 2004; 39:439-40

Wehner JH, Kirsch CM. Pulmonary manifestations of strongyloidiasis. Semin Respir Infect 1997; 12:122-129

Caumes E, Datry A, Mayorga R, et al. Efficacy of ivermectin in the therapy of larva currens. Arch Dermatol 1994;130:932

von Kuster LC, Genta RM. Cutaneous manifestations of strongyloidiasis. Arch Dermatol. 1988;124:1826-1830

Terashima A, Alvarez H, Tello R, et al. Treatment failure in intestinal strongyloidiasis: an indicator of HTLV-I infection. Int J Infect Dis 2002;6:28-30

TAENIA SOLIUM

Joseph Vinetz, M.D.

CLINICAL RELEVANCE & DIAGNOSIS

- Cestode (helminth parasite) that causes cysticercosis
- Late onset seizures (focal or generalized), chronic headache, symptomatic hydrocephalus, or radiological discovery of asymptomatic brain lesions
- Can present as calcified nodules in other parts of body
- Disease endemic throughout Latin America, Balkans, East Africa, India, China, Indonesia; often imported to U.S. years after primary infection
- Transmitted by oncospheres human to human through fecal-oral route; after ingestion of undercooked meat of intermediate host such as pigs leads to intestinal infection in humans.
- Intestinal infection in humans causes few if any symptoms but leads to transmission to other humans
- Calcified CNS lesions are dead parasites that can be epileptogenic foci
- Dx: excision of cyst, serological

SITES OF INFECTION

- Brain: active: parenchymal (CT shows one or more rounded hypodense areas of variable size, no enhancement) or extraparenchymal (subarachnoid or ventricular)
- Brain: transitional: parenchymal (hypodense lesions with enhancement, edema); encephalitic (diffuse cerebral edema, multiple small enhancing lesions); meningeal (CSF changes and serologic evidence)
- Brain: inactive: parenchymal (one or more calcifications); meningeal (hydrocephalus with normal CSF and calcifications)
- Eye: live parasites can be directly visualized, surgical removal recommended

- Spinal cord: surgical removal recommended along with chemotherapy for spinal subarachnoid disease; with degenerating intramedullary parasites, steroids + chemotherapy
- Somatic: manifests as calcified lesions on plain radiographs, no intervention
- Intestinal: humans definitive host for T. solium tapeworms; oncospheres excreted infectious to humans (auto-infection or transmission to others) leading to systemic dissemination of cysticerci

TREATMENT REGIMENS

Active parenchymal neurocysticercosis

- Anti-convulsant drugs in standard doses, titrate to effect
- Albendazole: 15mg/kg/day or 800mg/day in divided doses, usually for 28 days (variable recommendations)
- Praziquantel: 50-100mg/kg/day in 3 doses for 14 days +/- cimetidine 400mg tid to increase PZQ levels
- Corticosteroids: some use dexamethasone 6-12mg/day in divided doses prior to initiation of specific chemotherapy to reduce inflammatory response to parasites dying from drug
- Cimetidine 400mg bid or tid to increase PZQ or ABZ levels

Inactive parenchymal disease

- Phenytoin or carbamazepine in standard doses, titrated to effect, may need to be long-term in presence of calcifications for control of seizures, but perhaps short-term if lesions disappear by CT
- Anti-helminthic treatment (praziquantel or albendazole) not recommended
- Surgical intervention (shunt) to relieve intracranial hypertension

Extraparenchymal disease

- Ventricular: symptoms resulting from hydrocephalus require shunt; not all cysts require surgery; surgery may be necessary for removal of 3rd/4th ventricle cysts; ependymitis may lead to clogged shunt
- With shunt of ventricular disease, ABZ or PZQ associated with better outcome; unknown whether chemotherapy alone is effective
- Subarachnoid: anticonvulsants as needed; surgery for giant cysts in Sylvian fissure; corticosteroids for involvement of basilar cisterns, meningitis; shunting
- Spinal and ocular: surgical removal of subarachnoid lesions; chemotherapy +/- corticosteroids for inflamed intramedullary lesions

IMPORTANT POINTS

- Definitive recent source: White AC; Neurocysticercosis: Updates on epidemiology, pathogenesis, diagnosis, and management; Annu Rev Med 51:187-206, 2000.
- Diagnosis and management should be in consultation with an expert in the field
- In the U.S., neurocysticercosis may be in ddx of malignant brain tumor.
- Definitive diagnosis depends on the observation of the scolex or membranes of T. solium from tissue samples.
- More commonly, diagnosis based on clinical signs and symptoms, radiologic testing, with biopsy reserved for only the most diagnostically vexing cases.
- Serological diagnosis remains experimental and not generally available in the United States. Contact Dr. Victor Tsang at the Centers for Disease Control in Atlanta for definitive Western blot testing which can test serum and spinal fluid for vct1@cdc.gov; 770-488-4056

SELECTED READINGS

Tsang VC et al. An enzyme-linked immunoelectrotransfer blot assay and glycoprotein antigens for diagnosing human cysticercosis (Taenium solium). J Infect Dis 159;50-59, 1989

White AC. Neurocysticercosis: Updates on epidemiology, pathogenesis, diagnosis, and management. Annu Rev Med 51:187-206, 2000

Coyle CM et al. Cysticercosis. In Tropical Infectious Diseases, eds. RL Guerrant, DH Walker, PF Weller (Churchill Livingstone, Philadelphia), 1999, Chapter 95, pp. 993-1000

Chang GY, Keane JR. Visual loss in cysticercosis: analysis of 23 patients. Neurology 2001 Aug 14;57(3): 545-8

Flisser A et al. Induction of protection against porcine cysticercosis by vaccination with recombinant oncosphere antigens. Infect Immun. 2004;72:5292-7

TOXOPLASMA GONDII

Joseph Vinetz, M.D.

CLINICAL RELEVANCE & DIAGNOSIS

- Protozoan parasite with major morbidity in immunocompromised, pregnant women/fetus
- Transmitted from undercooked meat (usually beef or pork in Western countries) and from infectious oocysts in cat feces
- Encephalitis, ring-enhancing lesions in AIDS; other immunocompromised pts: also causes chorioretinitis, systemic infection, myocarditis, pneumonitis
- Congenital disease: arises by transplacental infection of fetus, causes severe CNS sequelae, chorioretinitis, systemic disease
- Primary infection usually subclinical in the immune competent, but can produce mono-like syndrome w/ painless lymphadenitis (usually cervical) - most commonly single but can be multiple or generalized
- Acute disease in normal, non-pregnant host generally self-limited, not requiring treatment
- Isolated ocular disease most commonly in otherwise healthy teenagers, young adults
- Dx (acute): antibody detection-seroconversion or 4-fold rising titers necessary to confirm new infection, IgM can last >1 yr
- Dx: direct detection of parasite by microscopy of affected tissue; culture of blood or tissue - esp. immunocompromised (rarely done, expensive), PCR (experimental)

SITES OF INFECTION

- CNS: encephalitis, visualized typically as multifocal lesions on contrast brain CT or MRI, esp. affecting basal ganglia. Radiographic appearance + therapeutic response = most diagnoses.
- Eye: chorioretinitis, can be necrotizing, important to distinguish from CMV in AIDS
- Lymph node: isolated, multiple or generalized lymphadenopathy
- Heart: myocarditis, in the severely immunocompromised
- Lung: pneumonitis, in the immunocompromised, particularly bone marrow transplant patients
- Systemic: wide dissemination particularly in congenital infection

TREATMENT REGIMENS

Primary or reactivation

- Acute disease in immunocompetent, non-pregnant patients: usually no treatment, unless visceral disease or symptoms severe or persistent
- Treatment (AIDS): pyrimethamine 50-100mg/d + leucovorin 10-20mg/d + sulfadiazine 1.0-1.5g qid x 3-6 weeks after resolution of signs/symptoms;

- (cont.) followed by pyrimethamine 25mg/d + leucovorin 15mg/d + sulfadiazine 500mg qid indefinitely (or until immune reconstitution)
- Folinic acid (leucovorin) 15-20mg qd to prevent bone marrow suppressive effect of pyrimethamine.
- 2nd line regimen: pyrimethamine 50-100mg/d + leucovorin 10-20mg/d + clindamycin 600mg qid (PO or IV).
- Alternative: Atovaquone 750mg PO q6h, azithromycin 1200-1500mg PO qd, or dapsone 100mg qd instead of sulfa when pt. sulfa-intolerant
- Treatment needed in immunocompromised patients and pregnant women
- Spiramycin 3-4 g/d in divided doses for pregnant women in first trimester to prevent transmission if mother seroconverts

Prophylaxis

- HIV only if CD4 < 100, Toxo IgG seropositive
- TMP-SMX DS PO qd
- Alternatives: TMP-SMX SS PO qd; dapsone 50mg PO qd + pyrimethamine 50mg PO qwk + leucovorin 25mg PO qwk; atovaquone 1500mg PO qd + pyrimethamine 25mg PO qd + leucovorin 10mg PO qd
- Can discontinue maintenance or prophylaxis if effective HIV virologic control on HAART, CD4 > 200 for 6 mos

IMPORTANT POINTS

- Basis for recommendations: Med Letter (March 2000)
- Rx of seroconversion in pregnancy not always effective in preventing congenital dz or sequelae

SELECTED READINGS

Simpson DM, Tagliati M. Neurologic manifestations of HIV infection. Ann Intern Med. 1994;121:769-85

Montoya JG, Liesenfeld O. Toxoplasmosis. Lancet. 2004;363(9425):1965-76.

Eskild A, Magnus P. Commentary: Little evidence of effective prenatal treatment against congenital toxoplasmosis--the implications for testing in pregnancy. Int J Epidemiol 2001;30:1314-5

Zeller V et al. Discontinuation of secondary prophylaxis against disseminated Mycobacterium avium complex infection and toxoplasmic encephalitis. Clin Infect Dis 2002;34:662-7

Beazley DM, Egerman RS. Toxoplasmosis. Semin Perinatol 1998;22:332-8

TRICHINELLA SPECIES

Khalil G. Ghanem, M.D.

CLINICAL RELEVANCE & DIAGNOSIS

- Trichinosis occurs when undercooked meat contaminated with infective larvae of Trichinella sp. eaten.
- 5 sp. cause human disease: Trichinella spiralis (most common cause), nativa, nelsoni, britovi, pseudospiralis. Differ in infectivity for humans, host reservoirs, pathogenicity, & resistance to freezing
- Most cases remain asymptomatic. Development of sx depends on the size of the inoculum. 10 larvae/g muscle= mild infection; >1000/g is life-threatening. Incubation period 5-51d.
- Week 1 [GI phase]: n/v, diarrhea & abdominal discomfort.
- Week 2 [systemic phase]: fever, eosinophilia, peri-orbital edema, subconjunctival hemorrhages, chemosis, myositis, weakness (extraocular muscles, neck muscles, then limbs), rash. Sx can last 2-3 wks.

- Most Sx disappear even w/o Rx, but mortality due to myocarditis, encephalitis, or pneumonia reported (2% of cases). Long-term sequelae include muscle aches, eye problems, & weakness.
- Dx: cardinal sx w/ hx of exposure; elevated CPK, LDH & eosinophilia (often marked). Rise in serum Ab = dx; high Ab levels can last for years, therefore acute and convalescent titers needed for dx.
- Ddx: influenza, typhoid fever, dermatomyositis, glomerulonephritis, & angioedema.
- Life Cycle: undercooked meat eaten, larvae freed, invade epithelium of small intestine & mature; larvae seed skeletal muscles via blood, mature over 3 weeks, & become infective.
- Adult worms are 1.5 x 0.05mm (male) & 3.5 x 0.06mm (females). Female worms are 2x as long as the male and 1.5x as wide.

SITES OF INFECTION

- GI: n/v/d; diarrhea may last from days to weeks.
- Musculoskeletal: inflammatory response due to larvae; myositis, tenderness, periorbital edema; peaks 5-6 wks after ingestion. Respiratory muscle involvement leads to dyspnea.
- CNS: larvae migrate through CNS tissue leading to meningitis, hemorrhages, seizures, or psychiatric disturbances; larvae cannot encyst in CNS thus prolonging symptoms.
- Cardiac: myocarditis leading to severe CHF or dysrhythmias.
- Heme: marked eosinophilia, may persist for years due to low-level release of antigen by calcified parasites in tissue. Leukocytosis common.

TREATMENT REGIMENS

Prevention

- Cook all meat (especially pork) to 60 degrees C for 4 minutes; if meat <6 inches, can freeze to -15 degrees C for 20d (except T. nativa which can withstand prolonged freezing).
- Controlling swine infections: strict control of garbage-feeding regulations, rodent control, avoiding pig exposure to dead animal carcasses, & effective barriers between pigs and wild animals.
- Close inspection of meat prior to human consumption (microscopic tests performed; recently, immunodiagnostic tests available).

Chemotherapy

- GI phase: Pyrantel 10mg/kg/d X 5d, or mebendazole 200mg/d X 5d, or albendazole 400mg/d X 3d.
- Acute severe infection: prednisolone 40-60mg/d plus albendazole 400-800mg/d or mebendazole 5mg/kg/d until fever and signs improve.
- If moderate infection, just use salicylates & bed rest for symptomatic relief.
- Late phase: no therapy available or useful.
- Recommendations from Hunter's Tropical Medicine and Emerging Infectious Diseases, 8th edition, W.B. Saunders Co., chapter 111, p 786. Also see references section (web).

IMPORTANT POINTS

- Common hosts: pigs (most common source for humans; most U.S. swine fed grains & therefore uninfected), bears, foxes, birds, horses, hyenas, lions & panthers.
- In US, ingestion of wild game (bear) most common source.

SELECTED READINGS

Cabie A, Bouchaud O, Houze S, et al. Albendazole versus thiabendazole as therapy for trichinosis: a retrospective study. Clin Infect Dis. 1996 Jun;22(6):1033-5.

Roy SL, Lopez AS, Schantz PM. Trichinellosis surveillance--United States, 1997-2001. MMWR Surveill Summ. 2003 Jul 25;52(6):1-8.

Schellenberg RS, Tan BJ, Irvine JD, et al. An outbreak of trichinellosis due to consumption of bear meat infected with Trichinella nativa, in 2 northern Saskatchewan communities. J Infect Dis. 2003 Sep 15;188 (6):835-43

Costantino SN, Malmassari SL, Dalla Fontana ML, et al. Diagnosis of human trichinellosis: pitfalls in the use of a unique immunoserological technique. Parasite. 2001 Jun;8(2 Suppl):S144-6.

Pozio E, Sacchini D, Sacchi L, et al. Failure of mebendazole in the treatment of humans with Trichinella spiralis infection at the stage of encapsulating larvae. Clin Infect Dis. 2001 Feb 15;32(4):638-42

VIRUSES

ADENOVIRUS
Khalil G. Ghanem, M.D.

CLINICAL RELEVANCE & DIAGNOSIS

- Non-enveloped virus w/ double-stranded DNA; >40 serotypes. Similar viruses found in monkeys, bovine species, & birds.
- Epidemiology: ubiquitous, worldwide; crowding is a risk factor (military personnel at high risk). Mostly respiratory spread. Some serotypes associated w/ certain syndromes (see 'Sites of Infection')
- Dx: growth in tissue culture (2-7d); PCR (rapid & sensitive); demonstration of Ag by immunofluorescence; four-fold rise in serum antibodies (usually, acute & convalescent serum required).

SITES OF INFECTION

- Clinical manifestations (1): fatal disseminated infections in neonates (serotypes 3, 7, 21, & 30 frequently involved); coryza/pharyngitis in infants (1, 2, & 5);
- Pharyngoconjunctival fever occurs in children: fever, conjunctivitis, pharyngitis, rhinitis, & cervical adenitis. Associated w/ type 3 infection.
- Eyes: epidemic keratoconjunctivitis in adults (types 8, 19 & 37). Conjunctivitis may last 1 to 4 wks. Keratitis may last several mos. Secondary spread to household contacts occurs in 10% of cases.
- Genitourinary: hemorrhagic cystitis in children & immunocompromised adults. Duration of symptoms ~ 7d.
- Gastrointestinal: infantile diarrhea-watery, associated w/fever. Intussusception in children; preceding or concurrent respiratory illness common.
- CNS: acute encephalitis or meningo-encephalitis especially in children & immunocompromised adults; chronic meningoencephalitis reported in pts w/ hypogammaglobulinemia.
- Clinical manifestations URI (1, 2, 4-6), diarrhea (2, 3, 5, 40, & 41), hemorrhagic cystitis (7, 11, & 21), pharyngo-conjunctivitis (3 & 7), & meningo-encephalitis (2, 6, 7, & 12) in children.
- Clinical manifestations (3): Immunocomp. hosts can develop pneumonia w/diss. infxn (5, 31, 34, 35, & 39), UTI/hemorrhagic cystitis, intestinal infections (42-47) & meningoencephalitis (7, 12, & 32)
- Clinical manifestations (2): URI (3, 4, & 7), pneumonia & keratoconjunctivitis (8, 19, and 37) common in adults.

- Resp: 50% asymptomatic; mild pharyngitis/tracheitis in children; type 7 can cause bronchiolitis & pneumonia in infants; mild tracheobronchitis in adults is the norm, but atypical pneumonia also occur

TREATMENT REGIMENS

Prevention

- Effective prevention was an oral vaccine used successfully in the military. Production of the oral vaccine ceased in 1994, and no vaccine is currently FDA approved.
- Oral vaccine-contained live non-attenuated adenovirus types 4 and 7 which, if given through the gastrointestinal tract, do not produce illness but do produce protective antibody responses.
- Hand washing is an effective means of prevention for all adenoviral infections.
- In an epidemic, the Standard Precautions (hand washing, antiseptic solutions, respiratory isolation) plus cohorting of both patients & staff has been effective in controlling nosocomial transmission.

Chemotherapy

- Most cases of adenoviral infections are mild, and do not require specific antiviral therapy.
- Anecdotal evidence for using various compounds currently FDA licensed for other indications in treating severe adenoviral infections can be found in the literature (see references).
- There are no randomized trials showing efficacy in humans.

IMPORTANT POINTS

- Associations between serotypes of adenoviruses & clinical syndromes exhibit some geographic variation.
- Complement-fixing Abs are group-specific & disappear within a year. Neutralizing and hemagglutination-inhibiting Abs are type-specific & may persist for appx. 10 yrs or longer.

SELECTED READINGS

Fox JP, Hall CE, Cooney MK. The Seattle Virus Watch. VII. Observations of adenovirus infections. Am J Epidemiol. 1977 Apr;105(4):362-86

Keenlyside RA, Hierholzer JC, D'Angelo LJ. Keratoconjunctivitis associated with adenovirus type 37: an extended outbreak in an ophthalmologist's office. J Infect Dis. 1983 Feb;147(2):191-8

Hong JY, Lee HJ, Piedra PA, et al. Lower respiratory tract infections due to adenovirus in hospitalized Korean children: epidemiology, clinical features, and prognosis. Clin Infect Dis. 2001 May 15;32 (10):1423-9

Echavarria M, Sanchez JL, Kolavic-Gray SA, et al. Rapid detection of adenovirus in throat swab specimens by PCR during respiratory disease outbreaks among military recruits. J Clin Microbiol. 2003 Feb;41(2):810-2

Kolavic-Gray SA, Binn LN, Sanchez JL, et al. Large epidemic of adenovirus type 4 infection among military trainees: epidemiological, clinical, and laboratory studies. Clin Infect Dis. 2002 Oct 1;35 (7):808-18

CYTOMEGALOVIRUS

Khalil G. Ghanem, M.D. and Lesia Dropulic, M.D.

CLINICAL RELEVANCE & DIAGNOSIS

- A herpes virus; up to 60-100% seroprevalence; first peak in infancy (vertical + milk); second peak in young adults; can establish latent infxn in host; difference between INFECTION and DISEASE.
- Transmitted vertically or via blood (lymphocytes and PMNs), saliva, milk, urine & sexual contact (cervical secretions and semen). Primary infxn subclinical, or mono-like +/- mild hepatitis.
- Dx1: Culture in human fibroblasts (time consuming); shell vial (monoclonal Abs to early CMV Ags in cultured cells); serology (IgM/IgG-used in dx of primary infxn only in immunocompetent host)
- Dx2: antigenemia (Ag detection in neutrophils w/Ab against CMV matrix protein pp65); PCR using primers for early antigens or for CMV DNA polymerase; can be qualitative or quantitative.
- CMV antigenemia and quantitative PCR assay may be negative in the setting of significant disease involving the GI, pulmonary or CNS systems.
- Dx of CMV disease must be made by the combination of appropriate clinical syndrome + detection of CMV in blood, plasma, or tissue in the absence of other LIKELY microbial etiology.
- In transplant pts (especially between 30-100d post txp), risk depends on type of transplant (HSCT> solid organ), type (MTX, ALG & OKT3>>steroids) & duration of immune suppression.
- Without prophylaxis, symptomatic infections occur in approx. 39% of heart-lung recipients, 25% of heart, 29% of liver and pancreas, and in 8% of kidney transplants.
- Reactivation CMV occurs in approximately 70-80% of patients after allogeneic marrow or stem cell transplantation w/o prophylaxis; 35% of those get disease.

SITES OF INFECTION

- Immunocompetent: asymptomatic or heterophile-negative mononucleosis syndrome; less often - pneumonia, hepatitis, rash, Guillain-Barre; myocarditis; meningoencephalitis; hemolytic anemia.
- Transplant: pneumonitis (up to 84% mortality in BMT); hepatitis (especially liver txp); CMV syndrome (fever, neutropenia); esophagitis, gastritis, colitis, meningoencephalitis, polyradiculopathy.
- Congenital: jaundice, HSMG, petechial rash, microcephaly, chorioretinitis. Primary infection of mother during pregnancy; risk to fetus increases from first (2%) to third trimester (28%).
- Perinatal (via milk or cervical secretions): asymptomatic; subtle effects on hearing and intelligence possible long term.
- AIDS: retinitis (CD4<50), polyradiculopathy and meningoencephalitis, esophagitis, colitis. Pts w/pneumonia, 50% have concomitant CMV in BAL: NOT CLINICALLY MEANINGFUL.

TREATMENT REGIMENS

Preventing infection

- The provision of CMV negative bone marrow, stem cells, or solid organs to CMV-negative recipients is recommended if possible.

- Giving CMV-negative or leukocyte-deplete blood products to CMV-negative transplant recipients highly effective.
- Seronegative transplant recipients who are sexually active and not in long-term monogamous relationships should use latex condoms during sexual contacts.
- Handling or changing diapers or wiping oral secretions from toddlers also represents a potential risk for CMV transmission to seronegative individuals and should be avoided.

Prophylaxis vs. pre-emptive therapy

- Prophylaxis = treat all D+ or R+ patients or only high-risk patients, D+R- or R+ patients treated with antilymphocyte antibodies (ATG, Thymoglobulin, OKT3).
- Regimens vary; ganciclovir (BM toxicity), foscarnet (renal toxicity), and oral valganciclovir (BM toxicity).
- Solid organ, ganciclovir (5mg/kg/d) or valganciclovir (450-900mg/d) x 3-6 mos. Duration depends on ability to decrease immunosuppression post-transplant.
- Pre-emptive (PE): Only Rx patients w/ CMV infection (in blood or lungs) dx as part of viral surveillance monitoring (i.e., CMV antigenemia or PCR) after transplant but do not have active disease
- PE favored by many over routine prophylaxis of all high risk transplant pts: theoretical decrease incidence of resistance & limiting side effects of drugs.
- PE well established for high risk HSCT (GVHD or history of active CMV disease); also used in high risk lung, liver, heart and kidney transplant patients.
- For HSCT, PE therapy favored because of BM toxicity from ganciclovir; twice-a-day induction doses until viral load declines (1-2 weeks) followed by maintenance (2-5 weeks) until Ag/PCR negative.

Therapy

- Immunocompetent host: usually self-limited; no specific antiviral Rx necessary.
- Solid Organ Txp: ganciclovir 5mg/kg q12h induction X 14-21 days or til documented clearance of viremia and/or significant clinical improvement; 3-6 mos maintenance to decrease rate of relapse.
- CMV IVIG often used for severe interstitial pneumonitis, relapsing or resistant CMV infections. No good prospective data in these populations.
- HSCT: pneumonia [IV ganciclovir 5mg/kg q12 x 21 d then 5mg/kg q24 x 3-4wks PLUS IVIG (500mg/kg) or CMV-IG (150mg/kg) 2x/wk x 2wks then qwk for 4wks.
- HSCT w/ CMV GI & retinitis: ganciclovir 5mg/kg q12 x 14-21d then q24 x 3-4wks or until day 100. Substitute foscarnet 90mg/kg q12h for ganciclovir 5mg/kg in case of BM suppression.
- Cidofovir has documented effectiveness in cases of CMV retinitis. Cross-resistance to ganciclovir-resistant strains relatively common, esp w/ high-level ganciclovir resistance. Limited use in Txp pts
- Consider valganciclovir for induction therapy in the absence of tissue invasive disease, because of excellent bioavailability. Studied in D+R- patients for prophylaxis.

IMPORTANT POINTS

- CMV (21%) vs. EBV (79%) causing mono-like sx: LESS tonsillopharyngitis, lymphadenopathy, splenomegaly; MORE systemic symptoms ("typhoidal") & hepatitis.
- Late CMV infxns: early use of antiviral therapy at time of engraftment delays immune reconstitution against the virus, placing the patient at risk for late (>100d) disease when Rx is d/c'd.
- Valganciclovir (pro-drug of ganciclovir) has 60-70% oral bioavailability. Effective in AIDS CMV retinitis. Clinical use in txp pts increasing.

- Cross resistance between ganciclovir and valganciclovir. Clinically, no cross-resistance between ganciclovir & foscarnet (although possible).
- Because resistance testing is time consuming, dx of resistance is made clinically based on clinical evidence of Rx failure. Modify Rx while awaiting resistance test.

SELECTED READINGS

Boivin G, Goyette N, Gilbert C, et al. Absence of cytomegalovirus-resistance mutations after valganciclovir prophylaxis, in a prospective multicenter study of solid-organ transplant recipients. J Infect Dis. 2004 May 1;189(9):1615-8.

Halwachs-Baumann G, Wilders-Truschnig M, Enzinger G, et al. Cytomegalovirus diagnosis in renal and bone marrow transplant recipients: the impact of molecular assays. J Clin Virol 2001 Jan;20(1-2):49-57

Peggs KS, Preiser W, Kottaridis PD, et al. Extended routine polymerase chain reaction surveillance and pre-emptive antiviral therapy for cytomegalovirus after allogeneic transplantation. Br J Haematol 2000 Dec;111(3):782-90

Meyers JD, Flournoy N, Thomas ED. Risk factors for cytomegalovirus infection after human marrow transplantation. J Infect Dis 1986 Mar;153(3):478-88

Bowden RA, Sayers M, Flournoy N, et al. Cytomegalovirus immune globulin and seronegative blood products to prevent primary cytomegalovirus infection after marrow transplantation. N Engl J Med 1986 Apr 17;314(16):1006-10

DENGUE VIRUS

Joseph Vinetz, M.D.

CLINICAL RELEVANCE & DIAGNOSIS

- Flavivirus (4 different serotypes) transmitted by peridomestic Aedes aegypti mosquitoes
- Spreading globally in tropics, including Hawaii and Puerto Rico, potentially Texas
- Most common mosquito-borne viral disease
- Most frequently causes undifferentiated febrile syndrome which can be confused with other infxns, e.g., malaria, leptospirosis, early pulmonary anthrax, etc.
- Small proportion of cases develop dengue hemorrhagic fever (DHF) with shock and cutaneous and mucosal hemorrhage
- Prevention: mosquito control, avoid mosquito contact (DEET, long sleeves, screens, remove stagnant water, etc)
- Recent dengue outbreak on the island of Maui, Hawaii which seems to have subsided as of Feb-March 2002
- Large outbreaks in Brazil, Thailand this year

SITES OF INFECTION

- Generalized, viremia
- CNS: unusual (<5% of cases)--encephalopathy, seizure

TREATMENT REGIMENS

Supportive care

- Symptomatic care in uncomplicated cases
- DHF: ICU care, careful attention to fluid balance and electrolytes, pressors necessary in severe cases

Prevention

- Avoid mosquito bites with personal protective measures
- No vaccine available

IMPORTANT POINTS

- Dengue is used as umbrella diagnosis; other potential causes of undifferentiated febrile syndromes must be considered depending on potential exposure history
- Cases need to be reported because of potential for transmission within U.S.
- For diagnosis, consult CDC in Fort Collins, CO or WHO Arbovirus Reference Center at University of Texas Medical Branch, Galveston, Texas (Dr. Robert Tesh or Dr. Robert Shope, (409) 772-6546)

SELECTED READINGS

Chotmongkol V, Sawanyawisuth K. Case report: Dengue hemorrhagic fever with encephalopathy in an adult. Southeast Asian J Trop Med Public Health. 2004;35:160-1

Pelaez O et al. Dengue 3 epidemic, Havana, 2001 . Emerg Infect Dis. 2004;10:719-22

Mairuhu AT et al. Dengue: an arthropod-borne disease of global importance. Eur J Clin Microbiol Infect Dis. 2004;23:425-33

Halstead SB. Pathogenesis of dengue: challenges to molecular biology. Science 239:476-81, 1988

Halstead SB. In vivo enhancement of dengue virus infection in rhesus monkeys by passively transferred antibody. J Infect Dis. 1979 Oct;140(4):527-33.

EBOLA VIRUS
Joseph Vinetz, M.D.

CLINICAL RELEVANCE & DIAGNOSIS

- Filovirus, several subtypes, cause of hemorrhagic fever, primarily in sub-Saharan Africa
- Causes epidemic disease with high mortality rate (50-90%)
- Incubation period 5-10 d
- Illness starts with fever, systemic symptoms, then prostration, progressing to death from multi-organ failure and hemorrhage ~day 10
- Diagnosis: Suspect in seriously ill traveler returning from endemic area; antigen capture ELISA and RT-PCR (experimental) performed by CDC Atlanta
- Transmitted during close contact with infected individual (skin, mucous membrane)
- Fever accompanied by sx including nausea, vomiting, abdominal pain, diarrhea, chest pain, cough, pharyngitis, photophobia, adenopathy, conjunctival injection, jaundice, pancreatitis
- Ebola outbreaks continue sporadically in Gabon, Uganda, Sudan

SITES OF INFECTION

- Bloodstream: viremia, generalized endothelial cell dysfunction leading to widespread organ damage and shock
- CNS: somnolence, delirium, coma
- Skin/mucous membranes: petechiae, hemorrhages, ecchymoses around needle puncture sites; day 5 maculopapular rash develops in most patients
- Liver: jaundice, liver failure (secondary to shock or direct involvement by virus)
- Kidney: renal failure, hemorrhage
- Lung: respiratory failure due to viral infection leading to necrosis, ARDS accompanying shock
- Gonads: orchitis, can be prolonged during convalescence

TREATMENT REGIMENS

Supportive care

- No antiviral Rx available
- Fluid/electrolyte mgmt, taking into account myocardial and pulmonary dysfunction

- In 2nd week, pt. either defervescence with marked improvement or dies in shock with multiorgan failure, often accompanied by anuria, DIC, liver failure
- Heparin for DIC, but this is controversial
- Recombinant inhibitor of factor VIIa/tissue factor may be useful adjunctive treatment, as demonstrated in Rhesus monkey model of ebola virus infection.

Prevention
- Identification of cases, epidemic
- Barrier nursing, strict contact precautions
- Use of properly sterilized medical equipment
- Protection from body fluid/skin/mucous membrane contact during preparation of dead for funeral

IMPORTANT POINTS
- Ebola virus is a Biosafety Level 4 pathogen. Patients suspected to have infection should have barrier nursing in negative pressure room. Notify public health officials.
- In endemic setting, causes epidemic disease, spread by direct contact with blood and body fluids.
- Outbreaks continue to occur sporadically in subsaharan Africa, so watch for travelers (health care personnel) from there.

SELECTED READINGS
Takada A, Kawaoka Y. The pathogenesis of Ebola hemorrhagic fever. Trends Microbiol 2001 9:506-11

Weber DJ, Rutala WA. Risks and prevention of nosocomial transmission of rare zoonotic diseases. Clin Infect Dis 2001 32:446-56

Jahrling PB et al. Evaluation of immune globulin and recombinant interferon-alpha2b for treatment of experimental Ebola virus infections. J Infect Dis 1999 179 Suppl 1:S224-34

Geisbert TW et al. Treatment of Ebola virus infection with a recombinant inhibitor of factor VIIa/tissue factor: a study in rhesus monkeys. Lancet. 2003;362:1953-8

Sullivan NJ et al. Accelerated vaccination for Ebola virus haemorrhagic fever in non-human primates. Nature. 2003;424:681-4

EPSTEIN-BARR VIRUS   Paul Auwaerter, M.D.

CLINICAL RELEVANCE & DIAGNOSIS
- Human herpesvirus, establishes latent infection
- 90% eventually infected by adult yrs., 30-50% college freshman uninfected
- Subclinical infection typical (90%), esp. children from lower socioeconomic groups. Mostly spread by asymptomatic salivary shedding.
- Primary symptomatic infection = infectious mononucleosis (IM peaks in teens and early 20's) with 30-70% adolescents/adults experiencing sx
- Ddx mononucleosis syndrome: Group A Strep pharyngitis, CMV, acute HIV, Toxo, influenza, viral hepatitis, rubella, drug reactions
- Elev. WBC (10-18K), lymphocytosis (40-60%) common. Atypical lymphocytes usually 10-30% of circulating lymphocytes.
- Dx: Heterophile antibody + 90% [Monospot], neg's may turn (+) on repeat. 10% remain neg, use EBV-specific AB: EBV capsid IgM and IgG + with neg. EBNA.
- False + heterophile rare: lymphoma, hepatitis, SLE, HIV
- EBV PCR most helpful for dx CNS lymphoma in HIV + pts. Sensitivity reported as high as 97%, specificity 98% but may be less. Also useful with EBV related meningoencephalitis.

- Positive EBNA in patients suspected of IM (<4-6wks sx) strongly argues that capsid IgM/IgG titers indicate remote infection therefore NOT supportive of EBV as cause of mono-like syndrome.
- Rash following Amoxicillin occurs >98-100% with IM.
- EBV not a proven cause of chronic fatigue. Do not check EBV titers merely as evaluation of fatigue.

SITES OF INFECTION

- Classic triad: fever, pharyngitis, lymphadenopathy (esp. posterior cervical)
- Common: elev. LFTs (ALT usually < 300), splenomegaly (50%), hepatomegaly, rash (10%)
- Uncommon: hemolytic anemia, cytopenias, pneumonitis, carditis, seizures, palsies, Guilliain-Barré, encephalitis (late)
- EBV also causes oral hairy leukoplakia (HIV), Burkitt's & other lymphomas (esp. HIV), nasopharyngeal CA, lymphoproliferative disorders (HIV, transplant, X-linked)
- Pts. > 35yrs. with IM have atypical presentations with less pharyngitis, LN. These older pts instead present as hepatitis, FUO or uncommon complications
- Not an acknowledged cause of Chronic Fatigue Syndrome
- True Chronic active EBV rare: pancytopenia, chronic LN, pneumonitis, abnl LFTs > 8wks. Prove by repeated positive EBV blood cx/PCR studies.

TREATMENT REGIMENS

Treatment

- IM usually self-limited <3wks average, rest & supportive care
- Fatigue may persist in 10-20% > 1mo
- Athletes w/ IM: No training, sports x 3wks from onset; if contact sport, e.g., football, no sports x 4wks from onset and no splenomegaly (preferably by imaging).
- Corticosteroids (Prednisone 40-60mg/d) indicated for airway obstruction, severe low plts. or hemolytic anemia. Some give for severe pharyngitis or constitutional sx (controversial).
- Acyclovir/ganciclovir: No role in IM. Reduces viral shedding in mouth.

IMPORTANT POINTS

- Pharyngitis and abnl LFTs tip-off toward IM rather than GAS pharyngitis
- Roommates, household contacts no increased risk IM.
- Life-threatening IM complications: tonsillar airway obstruction (early), splenic rupture (1-2 wks), encephalitis (typically >1mo after onset of sx)
- EBV-specific ABs. helpful esp. heterophile neg IM:EBV capsid IgM & IgG + with neg. EBNA=IM-if Sx<4-6wks EBV excluded if + EBNA since EBNA only expressed >6wks acute infection as latency established
- EBV - Chronic Fatigue Syndrome, DON'T draw serologies for chronic fatigue sx--no data to support as cause

SELECTED READINGS

Schuler, J. G. and H. Filtzer. Spontaneous splenic rupture. The role of nonoperative management . Arch Surg 1995;130(6): 662-5

Steeper, T. A., C. A. Horwitz, et al. Heterophil-negative mononucleosis-like illnesses with atypical lymphocytosis in patients undergoing seroconversions to the human immunodeficiency virus. Am J Clin Pathol 1988;90(2): 169-74

Taga TH, et al. Diagnosis of Atypical Cases of Infectious Mononucleosis. Clin Infect Dis 2001;33: 83-88

Rickinson, A. B. and D. J. Moss. Human cytotoxic T lymphocyte responses to Epstein-Barr virus infection. Annu Rev Immunol 1997;15: 405-31

Torre, D. and R. Tambini. Acyclovir for treatment of infectious mononucleosis: a meta-analysis. Scand J Infect Dis 1999;31(6): 543-7

HANTAVIRUS

Joseph Vinetz, M.D.

CLINICAL RELEVANCE & DIAGNOSIS

- Two major syndromes in humans: Hantavirus pulmonary syndrome [HPS-restricted to New World); Hemorrhagic fever with renal syndrome [HFRS-Asia, Europe]
- Rodent-borne viruses in the Bunyaviridae family, associated with specific rodent reservoirs
- Transmission to humans through inhalation of aerosolized saliva, urine or feces of reservoir host
- Hantaviruses known to cause HPS carried by the New World rats and mice, family Muridae, subfamily Sigmodontinae; these rodents are not found in urban sites
- In US, most common pathogenic Hantavirus is Sin Nombre virus, cause of cardiopulmonary syndrome; mostly in southwestern US (mainly Arizona, Colorado); also elsewhere (Vermont)
- In U.S., high case fatality rate (30-50%)
- Initially manifests as undifferentiated febrile illness, with fulminant progression to ARDS-like picture typically in previously healthy young adults
- In Old World: nonspecific febrile prodrome, signs of endothelial and hem. dysfunction, hemorrhage, back pain, retroper. fluid accum, hypotension, shock, oliguric renal failure
- Diagnosis: serology, PCR, rarely viral isolation

SITES OF INFECTION

- Lung: pulmonary edema, respiratory failure
- Cardiac: the pulmonary edema in U.S. Hantavirus disease can be cardiogenic associated with myocardial depression associated with viral infection of the heart.
- Kidney: U.S.-may complicate shock but usually not primary renal disease: Old world disease, Hantaan-type virus in Asia or Puumula virus in Europe; renal failure in association with hemorrhagic fever
- Heme: hemoconcentration; thrombocytopenia; severe left shift with myelocytes, promyelocytes characteristically seen on peripheral smear, important for early clinical suspicion and diagnosis

TREATMENT REGIMENS

Supportive therapy

- Early recognition important for directing intensive care
- Management of fluid status critical to reduce risk of respiratory failure

Antiviral drugs

- None demonstrated to be clinically effective
- Ribavirin has anti-viral activity in vitro
- Ribavirin has significant toxicities and has not been shown in clinical trials to be effective

IMPORTANT POINTS

- Very important for early diagnosis is to examine peripheral smear for evidence of severe left shift; presence of thrombocytopenia, myelocytes, hemoconcentration and hypocapnia strongly suggest HPS
- CDC (9/96) case definition: temp >38.3C, bilat diffuse interstitial infiltrates resembling ARDS, oxygen requirement w/i 72hrs of hospitalization

- Lab confirmation by detection of Hantavirus-specific (HS) IgM or rising titers of HS IgG; or HS RNA by PCR; or HS antigen seen on immunohistochemistry.

SELECTED READINGS

Centers for Disease Control and Prevention. Hantavirus pulmonary syndrome--Vermont, 2000. MMWR Morb Mortal Wkly Rep 2001 Jul 20;50(28):603-5

Ramos MM, Overturf GD, Crowley MR, et al. Infection with Sin Nombre hantavirus: clinical presentation and outcome in children and adolescents. Pediatrics 2001 Aug;108(2):E27 (http://www.pediatrics.org/cgi/reprint/108/2/e27.pdf)

Centers for Disease Control and Prevention. Update: Outbreak of Hantavirus Infection -- Southwestern United States, 1993 . Vol 42, No 23;441 06/18/1993 http://www.cdc.gov/mmwr/PDF/wk/mm4223.pdf

Centers for Disease Control and Prevention. Hantavirus pulmonary syndrome--United States: updated recommendations for risk reduction. MMWR Recomm Rep. 2002 Jul 26;51(RR-9):1-12

Chapman LE et al. Discriminators between hantavirus-infected and -uninfected persons enrolled in a trial of intravenous ribavirin for presumptive hantavirus pulmonary syndrome. Clin Infect Dis 2002;34:293-304

HERPES SIMPLEX VIRUS   Noreen A. Hynes, M.D., M.P.H.

CLINICAL RELEVANCE & DIAGNOSIS

- Primary infection asymptomatic in 2/3 of both HSV-1 and 2. Genital HSV increases risk of HIV transmission/acquisition.
- Most HSV is acquired from an infected, asymptomatic source of infection. Neonatal infection risk 40% in primary genital HSV; 2%-5% if post primary shedding at delivery.
- Acute immunosuppression reactivates HSV w/in 2 wks.
- HSV-1 leading cause of sporadic encephalitis in US adults. Benign recurrent lymphocytic meningitis can follow recurrence of genital HSV by 5-7 days.
- Severe recurrent genital, perirectal sx commonly seen w/AIDS esp. low CD4s and high viral loads. HIV-infected, esp w/ AIDS need longer treatment and/or higher dose for episodic cutaneous HSV.
- 15% of E. multiforme follows recurrent HSV w/ sx. Cutaneous HSV worse in pts with abnormal skin, e.g., eczema-varicelliform eruption.
- HSV keratitis is a nonprimary infection; can be sight threatening
- HSV tracheobronchitis most common in elderly and intubated pts. HSV esophagitis in immunocompromised pts must be differentiated from other causes.
- Acylovir resistance: Uncommon; disease progression limited to compromised host; in lab-confirmed HSV, if no clinical response, change Rx. Resistance testing not routinely recommended.

SITES OF INFECTION

- Oro-facial: Primary gingivostomatitis or recurrent stomatitis or herpes labialis
- Genital: genital ulcer disease
- Finger: Herpetic whitlow
- Eye: Follicular conjunctivitis, keratitis, acute retinal necrosis syndrome, endophthalmitis
- Other skin areas: Eczema herpeticum
- Central nervous system: Sporadic encephalitis, meningoencephalits, aseptic meningitis; sacral radiculopathy, aseptic meningitis, benign recurrent lymphocytic meningitis (Mollaret's meningitis)
- Esophagus: Esophagitis
- Lung: Pneumonia

- Liver: Hepatitis
- Rectum: Proctitis

Treatment Regimens

CNS

- Encephalitis: Acyclovir 10mg/kg IV q8h x 14-28d
- Acute meningitis: Acyclovir 10mg/kg IV q8h x 7-10d
- Benign recurrent lymphocytic meningitis: Acyclovir 10 mg/kg IV q8h x 7-10d followed by daily suppressive therapy

Ocular

- Follicular conjunctivitis: trifluridine or acyclovir and/or corticosteroids (ophthalmology consultation)
- Keratitis: trifluridine or acyclovir and/or corticosteroids (ophthalmology consultation)
- Endopthalmitis: Topical acyclovir and steroids (ophthalmology consultation)

Immunosuppressed

- Prophylaxis for acute immunosuppression in organ and bone marrow seropositives: Initiation-- Acyclovir 5 mg/kg IV q8h x 7d. Follow-up--Acyclovir 200-400mg PO tid-5x/d x 1-3 mo
- Episodic Rx of recurrent infection in HIV-infected:(All for 5-10d). Acyclovir 200mg PO 5x/d OR Acyclovir 400mg PO tid OR Famciclovir 500mg PO bid OR Valacyclovir 1 g PO bid
- Daily suppressive Rx in HIV-infected: Acyclovir 400-800 mg PO bid-tid OR Valacyclovir 500mg OR Famciclovir 500 mg bid

Antiviral resistant strains

- Foscarnet 40mg/kg IV q8h until clinical resolution
- Topical cidofovir gel 1% for genital or perirectal lesions qd x 5 d may be tried (local pharmacy must compound).

Mucocutaneous

- Burn wound: Acyclovir 5mg/kg IV q8h x 7d, then 200mg PO 5x/d x 7-14d
- Esophagitis regimens: Acyclovir 400-800mg PO 5x/d x 7-10d OR Acyclovir 5mg/kg IV tid x 7-10d
- Genital HSV and proctitis--1st clinical episode: All Rx for 7-10d. Acyclovir 400mg PO tid OR Acyclovir 200mg PO 5x/d OR Famciclovir 250mg PO tid OR Valacyclovir 1g PO bid
- Genital HSV and proctitis--episodic Rx: All for 5d. Acyclovir 400mg PO tid OR Acyclovir 200mg PO 5x/d OR Acyclovir 800mg PO bid OR Famciclovir 125mg PO bid OR Valacyclovir 500mg PO bid x 3-5d
- Genital HSV or proctitis--suppressive daily therapy for recurrent disease. Acyclovir 400mg PO bid OR Famciclovir 250mg PO bid OR Valacyclovir 500mg PO qd OR Valacyclovir 1g PO qd
- Severe genital HSV or proctitis: Acyclovir 5-10mg/kg IV q8h x 5-7d or until clinical resolution. Suppressive therapy thereafter, if indicated
- Genital HSV in pregnancy: Acyclovir per above regimen w/initial HSV or highly symptomatic recurrent HSV. Give IV w/life-threatening infection.
- Herpes labialis prophylaxis: Acyclovir 400mg PO bid OR Famciclovir 250mg PO bid OR Valacyclovir 250mg PO bid OR Valacyclovir 500mg PO qd or Valacyclovir 1000mg PO qd
- Stomatitis: Acyclovir 400mg PO tid x 7-10d OR Acyclovir 200mg PO 5x/d x7-10d OR Famciclovir 250mg PO tid x 7-10d OR Valacyclovir 1g PO bid x 7-10d

Important Points

- This module is based on: 1) for STDs--the CDC's 2002 STD Rx Guidelines and 2) for non-STD HSV -- literature-based expert opinion

- 50%-80% of adults are HSV-1 seropositive; 20%-40% of adults are HSV-2 seropositive. HSV-1: Herpes labialis most common form of recurrent HSV-1 BUT 30% of genital HSV is HSV-1.
- The psychological impact of genital HSV cannot be overstated; 60% report being "devastated" when 1st told their Dx
- 33% women, 10% men have meningitis with primary genital HSV.
- Visceral involvement and dissem. HSV can be life-threatening in HIV-infected. Encephalitis rare in HIV but life-threatening complication of HSV; presentation often atypical.

Selected Readings

Cinque P et al. The role of laboratory investigation in the diagnosis and management of patients with suspected herpes simplex encephalitis: a consensus report. The EU concerted Action on Virus Meningitis and Enceph. J Neurol Neurosurg Psychiatry 1996, 61:339-345.

Steiner I and Biran I. Herpes simplex encephalitis. Curr Treat Options Infect Dis 2002, 4:491-499

Kimberlin DW and Rouse DJ. Genital herpes. N Engl J Med 2004; 350:1970-7.

Corey L et al. Once-daily valacyclovir to reduce the risk of transmission of genital herpes. N Engl J Med; 2004 350:11-20.

Filen F et al. Duplex real-time polymerase chain reaction assay for detection and quantitation of herpes simplex virus type 1 and herpes simplex virus type 2 in genital and cutaneous lesions. Sex Transmit Infect; 31:331-6.

HHV-6 / HHV-7

Khalil G. Ghanem, M.D.

Clinical Relevance & Diagnosis

- Members of the betaherpesvirus family, closely related to each other & CMV. HHV-6 has 2 subtypes: A and B.
- >90% of adults sero + for both viruses. Primary infection: HHV-6 first yr of life; HHV-7: age 2-3 years. Transmission via saliva and ? vertically.
- HHV-6 infects mature T-lymphocytes (CD4>CD8), monocytes, macrophages, megakaryocytes & glial cells; remains dormant in PBMCs. HHV-7 infects T-lymphocytes (CD4>>CD8).
- Sx: primary infx: asymptomatic; undifferentiated febrile illness; exanthem subitum (roseola infantum) [HHV-6 >>HHV-7]; febrile seizures.
- Sx: reactivation: occurs in both immunocompetent and immunocompromised, however, disease ASSOCIATIONS have been made in the compromised host mainly.
- Dx: serology [cross reaction between the 2 viruses common]; quantitative PCR [not yet available commercially] detects both latent and active viruses; more recently HHV-6 antigenemia assay introduced.

Sites Of Infection

- Primary HHV-6: asymptomatic; febrile illness (20-40% of ER visits by infants 6mo-2yrs); roseola infantum (fever, facial rash appears after fever then spreads); seizures (17% of kids w/primary infxn).
- Reactivation HHV-6 in immunocompetent: ASSOCIATION with infectious-mononucleosis-like syndrome and histiocytic necrotizing lymphadenitis.
- Associations w/reactivation HHV-6 in BMT: interstitial pneumonitis, encephalitis, marrow suppression, rash, GVHD, graft failure, fever, thrombotic microangiopathy, CMV reactivation.

VIRUSES

- Associations w/reactivation HHV-6 in solid organ transplant: interstitial pneumonitis, encephalitis, marrow suppression, rash, fever, rejection, CMV reactivation, fungal infection.
- Primary HHV-7: asymptomatic, febrile illnesses; roseola infantum (less common than HHV-6) and febrile seizures (up to 75% of infants w/primary infxn).
- Associations w/reactivation HHV-7: Reactivation of CMV disease in renal transplant recipients and possibly increased risk of graft rejection.

TREATMENT REGIMENS

In vitro data

- Both HHV-6 & 7 are susceptible to ganciclovir, foscarnet and cidofovir and much less susceptible to high doses of acyclovir.

In vivo

- Currently, there are NO formal treatment recommendations.
- No prospective studies on type or effects of treatment in setting of prophylaxis or reactivation in transplant patients.
- Disease associations rather than causation in HHV-6 and 7 infected patients make the interpretation of case reports of successful therapy problematic.
- Case reports of successful prophylaxis and therapy are provided in "References" below.

IMPORTANT POINTS

- Due to the strong association with increased CMV reactivation, it is vital to monitor patients carefully for CMV, & to treat aggressively [see "Cytomegalovirus"].
- HHV-6 has been associated with both chronic fatigue syndrome and multiple sclerosis. NO DEFINITIVE CAUSAL RELATIONSHIP HAS BEEN ESTABLISHED WITH EITHER DISEASE.
- The various types of reactivation syndromes described in both HHV-6 and HHV-7 are ASSOCIATIONS. Albeit some of the associations are strong, no CAUSAL relationship has been proven.
- If trying to determine whether to treat a presumed HHV-6 complication, one must weigh the hazards of therapy (e.g., BM toxicity w/ ganciclovir, renal toxicity w/ foscarnet) with the potential benefits.
- In the setting where no prophylaxis or treatment regimens have been advocated, routine monitoring for HHV-6 & 7 infections is not recommended.

SELECTED READINGS

Carrigan DR, Drobyski WR, Russler SK, et al. Interstitial pneumonitis associated with human herpesvirus-6 infection after marrow transplantation. Lancet 1991 Jul 20;338(8760):147-9

Knox KK, Carrigan DR. In vitro suppression of bone marrow progenitor cell differentiation by human herpesvirus 6 infection. J Infect Dis 1992 May;165(5):925-9

Tanaka-Taya K,. Reactivation of human herpesvirus 6 by infection of human herpesvirus 7. J Med Virol 2000 Mar;60(3):284-9

Boutolleau D, Fernandez C, Andre E, et al. Human herpesvirus (HHV)-6 and HHV-7: two closely related viruses with different infection profiles in stem cell transplantation recipients. J Infect Dis 2003 Jan 15;187(2):179-86

Locatelli G, Santoro F, Veglia F, et al. Real-time quantitative PCR for human herpesvirus 6 DNA. J Clin Microbiol 2000 Nov;38(11):4042-8

HHV-8

Joel Blankson, M.D., Ph.D.

CLINICAL RELEVANCE & DIAGNOSIS

- Human gamma herpes virus
- Probable cause of HIV-associated Kaposi sarcoma (KS); typically characterized by violaceous vascular lesions on skin, mucous membranes and/or viscera (e.g., GI tract, and lungs).
- HHV-8 is the probable cause of classic KS (non-HIV-associated). This variant is usually limited to skin and typically affects elderly Mediterranean and East European men.
- Probable cause of endemic African KS. Presentation varies from skin lesions only to aggressive systemic disease
- Associated with multicentric Castleman's disease, a lymphoproliferative disorder mostly seen in HIV+ patients: characterized by B-type symptoms, lymphadenopathy, hypergammaglobulinemia.
- Associated with primary effusion lymphoma; a non Hodgkin's Disease B-cell lymphoma mostly seen in HIV+ patients. Presents with body-cavity-based effusions in the absence of a solid tumor.
- Has been associated with KS as well as a febrile illness with bone marrow failure in transplant patients
- HIV-associated KS is seen mostly in homosexual men. HHV-8 found in saliva and semen. An unknown cofactor may be involved in transmission.
- Pulmonary KS typically presents with dyspnea, cough, chest pain or hemoptysis. Gastrointestinal KS can cause abdominal pain, obstruction or hemorrhage.

SITES OF INFECTION

- HHV-8 DNA detected in peripheral blood mononuclear cells, and in endothelial cells and spindle cells in KS lesions in skin, mucocutaneous membranes and viscera.
- HHV-8 DNA has been detected in transformed B cells in multicentric Castleman's Disease.
- HHV-8 DNA detected in B cells of primary effusion lymphoma (pleural, pericardial, or peritoneal)
- HHV-8 viremia reported in transplant patients
- HHV-8 DNA has been detected in saliva and semen

TREATMENT REGIMENS

Kaposi sarcoma (local disease <25 lesions)

- Cryotherapy, radiation therapy, surgery
- Topical alitretinoin has been shown to have approximately 35% partial response. 0.1% gel applied to affected site 2-4x/d
- Intralesional injections with vinblastine has 60-90% clinical response rate. 0.2-0.3mg/mL: 0.1mL/0.5 cm2 lesion.

Kaposi sarcoma (systemic disease)

- Combination chemotherapy
- A survival benefit has been demonstrated in a retrospective study in pts treated with protease inhibitor based antiretroviral therapy and chemotherapy versus chemotherapy alone.
- Protease inhibitors have antiangiogenic effects and have been effective in treating KS in animal models. Relapse of disease has been seen in patients when PIs were replaced with NNRTIs.
- Paclitaxel 100mg/m2 every 2 weeks was associated with a 59% response rate

- Pegylated liposomal doxorubicin 40mg/m2 q2w has been shown to be more effective than chemotherapy with 58% response rate.
- Alpha interferon and antiretroviral therapy: In one study, ddI 200mg BID with alpha interferon at either 1 mU or 10 mU sc qd was associated with 40% or 55% response rate respectively.
- Angiogenesis inhibitors are being used in clinical trials with some success. In one study thalidomide 200-1000mg (median dose 600mg) qd resulted in a 40 % partial response rate.

Multicentric castleman's disease

- Combination chemotherapy
- Alpha-interferon at 5MU three times a week was reported to cause prolonged remission in a case report
- Anti-IL6 antibody has been useful in alleviating symptoms due to IL-6 overproduction (one of HHV-8 genes encodes a viral variant of this cytokine)
- Ganciclovir at 1.25mg/kg qD or 5 mg/Kg IV BID or valganciclovir at 900mg PO BID caused remission of disease in a recent report of 3 HIV+ patients.
- A case series showed that the initiation of HAART did not prevent relapse of disease, but may prolong survival.

Primary febrile illness with BM failure

- A reduction in immunosuppressive therapy in conjunction with foscarnet 80 mg/kg BID x 2 weeks was successful in a transplant patient

IMPORTANT POINTS

- HHV-8 mostly causes disease in immunocompromised individuals. First line of therapy should probably be HAART in HIV infected patients or reduction of immunosuppressive therapy in transplant patients
- Treatment with PI based HAART has been associated with decreased mortality in pts receiving chemotherapy for systemic KS
- Protease inhibitors may have direct effect on KS due to antiangiogenic properties. It may therefore be beneficial to include this class of drugs in HAART regimens when treating patients with KS.
- Interferon-alpha probably is effective in KS because it has both antiviral and immunomodulatory effects.
- Pulmonary KS can be life-threatening and should be treated immediately

SELECTED READINGS

Chang Y, Cesarman E, Pessin MS, Lee F, Culpepper J, Knowles DM, Moore PS. Identification of herpesvirus-like DNA sequences in AIDS-associated Kaposi's sarcoma. Science. 1994;266:1865-9

Hengge UR, Ruzicka T, Tyring SK, Stuschke M, Roggendorf M, Schwartz RA, Seeber S. Update on Kaposi's sarcoma and other HHV8 associated diseases. Part 2: pathogenesis, Castleman's disease, and pleural effusion lymphoma. Lancet Infect Dis 2002;2:344-52

Hengge UR, Ruzicka T, Tyring SK, Stuschke M, Roggendorf M, Schwartz RA, Seeber S. Update on Kaposi's sarcoma and other HHV8 associated diseases. Part 1: epidemiology, environmental predispositions, clinical manifestations, and therapy. Lancet Infect Dis. 2002;2:281-92.

Krown SE, Li P, Von Roenn JH, Paredes J, Huang J, Testa MA. Efficacy of low-dose interferon with antiretroviral therapy in Kaposi's sarcoma: a randomized phase II AIDS clinical trials group study. J Interferon Cytokine Res 2002;22:295-303

Kumari P, Schechter GP, Saini N, Benator DA. Successful treatment of human immunodeficiency virus-related Castleman's disease with interferon-alpha. Clin Infect Dis. 2000;31:602-4.

HTLV I/II

Joel Blankson, M.D./Ph.D.

CLINICAL RELEVANCE & DIAGNOSIS

- Human Type C Retroviruses, most infections are asymptomatic
- HTLV-I endemic in Caribbean, southern Japan, parts of Africa, South America; transmitted by breast feeding, contaminated blood products, IDU, sexual contact
- HTLV-II endemic in IDUs
- HTLV-I infection has 5% lifetime risk of adult T cell leukemia (ATL). ATL presents with type B symptoms, lymphadenopathy. Skin involvement (plaques, nodules) common.
- HTLV-I infection has 0.5 -2% lifetime risk of HTLV-I associated myelopathy/tropical spastic paraparesis (HAM/TSP): Progressive disease with leg stiffness, weakness, low back pain, bladder dysfunction
- HTLV-I infection may result in immunosuppression, associated with strongyloides hyperinfection, and decreased reactivity to PPD
- HTLV-II not definitively been shown to cause human disease
- HTLV-I may accelerate the progression to AIDS in HTLV/HIV-I coinfected patients
- Transplant recipients of organs from asymptomatic HTLV-I seropositive patients have developed HAM/TSP

SITES OF INFECTION

- CD4+ T cells are the main target of HTLV-I infection
- HTLV-II infects peripheral blood mononuclear cells
- In ATL, circulation of monoclonal transformed CD4+ T cells bearing HTLV-I provirus
- HTLV-I infected CD4+ T cells found in CSF of pts with HAM/TSP

TREATMENT REGIMENS

ATL

- Conventional chemotherapy
- Small prospective phase II trial showed encouraging results with AZT (1g PO qd) and alpha interferon (9 mU SQ qd)

HAM/TSP

- Corticosteroids, cyclophosphamide, alpha-interferon, IVIG, plasmapheresis, and danazol have been used with inconsistent results
- AZT (1-2g qd) or 3TC (150mg bid) alone, or AZT (250 mg bid) and 3TC (150mg bid) used in three small studies. While decreases in proviral HTLV-I load were seen, symptoms did not improve in most pts

Asymptomatic HTLV-I/II infection

- No evidence for treatment

IMPORTANT POINTS

- >95% of patients seropositive for HTLV-I will not develop disease
- HTLV-II has not been definitively shown to cause a disease process
- CDC recommends that pts with asymptomatic infection not breast feed, donate blood, or share needles. Latex condoms should be used.
- Asymptomatic infections probably should not be treated. HTLV genome is integrated into host DNA, therefore it is probably impossible to eradicate infection
- Higher proviral loads have been associated with development of HAM/TSP.

SELECTED READINGS

Toro C, Rodes B, Poveda E, Soriano V. Rapid development of subacute myelopathy in three organ transplant recipients after transmission of human T-cell lymphotropic virus type I from a single donor. Transplantation 2003;75:102-4

Jacobson S. Immunopathogenesis of human T cell lymphotropic virus type I-associated neurologic disease. J Infect Dis. 2002;186 Suppl 2:S187-92. .

Thorstensson R, Albert J, Andersson S. Strategies for diagnosis of HTLV-I and -II. Transfusion. 2002;42:780-91.

Hermine O, Allard I, Levy V, Arnulf B, Gessain A, Bazarbachi A. A prospective phase II clinical trial with the use of zidovudine and interferon-alpha in the acute and lymphoma forms of adult T-cell leukemia/lymphoma. Hematol J. 2002;3(6):276-82.

Brites C, Alencar R, Gusmao R, Pedroso C, Netto EM, Pedral-Sampaio D, Badaro R. Co-infection with HTLV-1 is associated with a shorter survival time for HIV-1-infected patients in Bahia, Brazil. AIDS 2001;15:2053-5.

HUMAN PAPILLOMAVIRUS (HPV)

Noreen A. Hynes, M.D., M.P.H.

CLINICAL RELEVANCE & DIAGNOSIS

- Recurrent respiratory papillomatosis: a disease primarily of larynx; 2 forms -- juvenile onset (transmitted from mother during passage through birth canal) and adult-onset, believed to be an STD.
- Epidermodysplasia verruciformis: rare; probably autosomal recessive; disseminated cutaneous warts early in life with frequent malignant transformation
- Other uncommon forms: Buschke-Lowenstein tumors (giant condylomas); Bowenoid papulosis; Bowen's disease; Erythroplasia of Queyrat (on the glans penis)
- The HPVs are widespread worldwide; >80 types recognized with specific clinical manifestations. Some types have oncogenic potential.
- Common warts: Verruca vulgaris; most common type of cutaneous wart; most prevalent in young children; usually on the hands; brown, exophytic, hyperkeratotic papule
- Uterine cervical HPV: Produces squamous cell abnormalities most frequently found on Papanicolaou smear; strongly associated w/cervical cancer; > 95% of cervical CA contain HPV DNA of oncogenic types
- Anogenital warts: Condylomata acuminatum; genital HPVs are most common STD worldwide; 500,000 persons/yr in US acquire symptomatic warts; visible warts usually not associated w/ oncogenic type
- Plantar warts: Verruca plantaris; 2nd most common wart; most common in adolescents/young adults; thrombosed capillaries upon paring down distinguish from callus
- Flat warts: Verruca plana; most common in children; occur on face, neck, chest, flexor surfaces of forearms and legs
- Cutaneous Warts (common, plantar, flat): mostly seen in children/adolescents but may be occupational hazard in butchers, fish handlers, and meat packers. Usually asymptomatic except if at wt-bearing frequent friction site. Spontaneous resolution of 50-90% within 1-5 years.

SITES OF INFECTION

- Mucosa: genitalia in areas of coital friction; perianal area, mouth, cervix
- Larynx: recurrent respiratory papillomatosis
- Cutaneous surfaces: plantar warts, common warts

TREATMENT REGIMENS

Cutaneous warts
- Most will resolve spontaneously
- Hand warts. Self application of salicylic and lactic acid, collodion at 1:1:4, qd x up to 12 wks. (Cure rate about 70%)
- Hand warts: cryotherapy q wk x 3 (70% cure)
- Plantar warts: 40% salicylic acid tape kept in place x several days followed by debridement while the wart is still damp followed by cryotherapy or caustics application (30-70% trichloroacetic acid)
- Plantar warts: direct destruction using carbon dioxide laser, acids; snipping or curettage of filiform warts is alternative
- Flat warts: Tretinoin (retinoic acid cream 0.05%) qd w/ or w/out topical 5% benzoyl peroxide or topical 5% salicylic acid cream until cured
- Flat warts: Topical 5-fluorurocil cream (1% or 5%) qd until resolved

External anogenital warts: common treatments
- Approach to Rx: Response to treatment is variable and no single pt-applied or provider-applied treatment is considered better than another. For a single pt, different options may need to be tried.
- PT-applied: Polofilox 0.5% solution or gel. Apply w/ cotton swab (solution) or finger (gel) to visible warts BID x 3d, no Rx x 4d. Repeat cycle up to 4 cycles. Not to exceed 0.5 mL/d; Rx area NTE 10 sq cm.
- PT-applied: Imiquimod 5% cream. Apply w/finger qhs, 3x/wk for up to 16 wks. Wash Rx area 6-10h after Rx with mild soap and H20.
- Provider-applied: Trichloroacetic acid (TCA) or bichloroacetic acid (BCA) 80% -90%. Apply small amt to warts; air dry. Powder area with talc or sodium bicarb to remove unreacted acid. Repeat Q wk
- Provider-applied: Cryotherapy with liquid nitrogen or cryoprobe. Repeat q 1-2 wks
- Provider-applied: Podophyllin resin 10-25% in compound tincture of benzoin. Place small amt on q wart and allow to air dry. Limit to 0.5mL solution or 10 sq cm warts per session. Pt to wash off in 1-4h
- Provider-applied: TCA or BCA 80-90%. Apply a small amt to warts; let dry to white "frosting" appearance; powder w/talc, Na bicarb (baking soda) or liquid soap to remove unreacted acid. Repeat q wk.
- Provider-applied: surgical removal by tangential scissor or shave excision, curettage, or electrosurgery
- Alternative provider-applied: Intralesional interferon
- Alternative provider-applied: Laser surgery

Other HPV-associated diseases
- Epidermodysplasia verruciformis: Consultation w/an expert needed. Malignant changes managed w/surg techniques, cryotherapy, 5-FU ointment. PO retinoids or intralesional IFN improve, do not cure
- Recurrent respiratory papillomatosis: Endoscopic cryotherapy or laser surgery. Intralesional cidofovir may hold promise. Avoid tracheostomy--can spread disease to distal respiratory tract

Referral for management
- Cervical warts, rectal mucosal warts, oral warts, suspected laryngeal warts
- Suspected cancerous lesions
- Epidemeroplaysia verruciformis
- Bowen's disease and Bowenoid papulosis

- Buschke-Lowenstein tumors
- Erythromplasia of Queyrat

Anogenital-related warts: special considerations

- Pregnant women: Liquid nitrogen only recommended Rx. Avoid imiquimod, polyphyllin, and podophylox
- Cervical warts: Must be managed in consultation with an expert. High-grade squamous intraepithelial lesions (SIL) must be excluded before Rx started.
- Vaginal warts: TCA or BCA 80-90% applied only to warts; small amt to warts, let dry to white "frosting" appearance, then powder w/talc, Na bicarb to remove unreacted acid. Repeat q wk prn.
- Immunosuppressed patients: Use same Rx as for non-immunosuppressed. May need longer, more freq Rx due to lower response or non-response.
- Subclincal genital hpv infection without exophytic warts: Routine use of 3-5% acetic acid to identify these areas NOT recommended. In absence of coexistent SIL, Rx NOT RECOMMENDED
- Squamous cell carcinoma in SITU: refer to an expert for Rx
- Urethral meatal warts: Provider-applied (Cryotherapy or Podophyllin resin 10-25%) or Pt-applied (Podofilox 0.5% solution or gel or Imiquimod 5% cream) can be tried as for anogenital warts (limited data)
- Oral warts: Provider-applied cryotherapy or surgical removal only.

Important Points

- This module is based on 1) for STD HPV --CDC's 2002 STD Rx Guidelines; 2) 2004 NIH/ NCI Interim Guidance (cervical testing); 3) Other HPV-related areas--expert opinion in the peer-reviewed literature
- Ddx of anogenital warts: condylomata lata (secondary syphilis), molluscum contagiosum, seborrheic keratosis, lichen planus, "pink pearly penile papules", and neoplastic lesions
- No one Rx for anogenital HPV is better than another; recurrences common after RX. Topical therapies for anogenital warts should NOT be used if wart burden exceeds 10 sq cm
- Majority of women with "high risk" HPV types (e.g., 16 and 18) do not develop cervical cancer. External warts anogenital warts in women is NOT an indication for colposcopy
- NEW APPROACH: May add HPV DNA test (HDT) to cervical cytology (CC) in women >29 yr; rescreen in 3 yr if both tests neg; in 6-12 mo if CC neg, HDT pos for high risk types. Colpo if either pos on repeat

Selected Readings

Beutner K et al. Genital warts and their treatment. Clin Infect Dis 1999;28(Suppl1):S37-56.

Beutner K et al. Imiquimod, a patient-applied immune-response modifier for treatment of external genital warts. Antimicrob Agents Chemother 1998, 42:789-94.

Ho G, et al. Natural history of cervicovaginal papillomavirus infection in young women. N Engl J Med 1998; 338:423-428.

Marrazzo JM et al. Genital human papillomavirus infection in women who have sex with women. J Infect Dis 178:1504-9. 1998.

Palefsky J et al. Prevalence and risk factors for human papillomavirus infection of the anal canal in human immunodeficiency virus (HIV)-positive and HIV-negative homosexual men. J Infect Dis. 177:361-7. 1998.

JC/BK VIRUS

Khalil G. Ghanem, M.D.

Clinical Relevance & Diagnosis

- BK and JC DNA polyomaviruses; cause hemorrhagic cystitis, progressive multifocal leukoencephalopathy (PML), respectively; mainly immunocompromised hosts (AIDS, steroids, transplants).
- Acquired in childhood/adolescence; 60-80% adults sero+; persist in kidney; asymptomatic viruria in immunosuppression (appx. 50%) + pregnancy (3%). Transmission: saliva, placenta, ?urine, ?blood, ?sex.
- Sx: primary infxn - asymptomatic; mild URI sx (30%) with BK.
- Dx (1): PCR CSF (JC) urine (BK & JC); urine epithelial cell cytology SUGGESTIVE ("Decoy Cells"); MRI suggestive (white matter T2 intense); definitive: JC (brain bx), BK (kidney bx)[immunohistochemistry]
- Dx (2): clinical picture (immunocompromised host + symptoms) + radiographic (PML) + suggestive lab finding (PCR/urine cytology). Serology NOT helpful. Renal bx for BK recommended.

Sites Of Infection

- JC: CNS [PML: hemiparesis (42%),cognitive (36%), visual (32%),ataxia, aphasia, cranial nerves, sensory];? CNS malignancies
- BK: GU (hematuria, hemorrhagic cystitis, ureteric stenosis, interstitial nephritis); LUNG (URI); ?EYE(retinitis); ?LIVER (hepatitis); ?neoplasia; ?CNS.

Treatment Regimens

BK virus

- Asymptomatic: no Rx. Symptomatic: no effective Rx. If possible, decrease immunosuppression.

JC virus

- Asymptomatic: no Rx. PML: no good therapy; in AIDS antiretroviral medications may help; ?cidofovir (5mg/kg baseline, week 1 then q 2 weeks).

Important Points

- For both viruses, a diagnosis should not be made on the basis of PCR data alone. Combine clinical, radiographic, laboratory data.
- Controversy re: optimal therapy for PML. HAART Rx in AIDS favored. Data on cidofovir is observational & conflicting. No prospective randomized trials.

Selected Readings

Safdar A, Rubocki RJ, Horvath JA, et al. Fatal immune restoration disease in HIV type 1-infected patients w/ progressive multifocal leukoencephalopathy: impact of antiretroviral therapy-associated immune reconstitution. Clin Infect Dis 2002 Nov 15;35(10):1250-7

Marra CM, Rajicic N, Barker DE, et al. A pilot study of cidofovir for progressive multifocal leukoencephalopathy in AIDS. AIDS 2002 Sep 6;16(13):1791-7

Garcia De Viedma D, Diaz Infantes M, Miralles P, et al. JC virus load in progressive multifocal leukoencephalopathy: analysis of the correlation between the viral burden in cerebrospinal fluid, patient survival, and the volume of neurological lesions. Clin Infect Dis 2002 Jun 15;34(12):1568-75

Bogdanovic G, Priftakis P, Hammarin AL, et al. Detection of JC virus in cerebrospinal fluid (CSF) samples from patients with progressive multifocal leukoencephalopathy but not in CSF samples from patients with herpes simplex encephalitis, enterovi. J Clin Microbiol 1998 Apr;36(4):1137-8

Wyen C, Hoffmann C, Schmeier N, et al. Progressive Multifocal Leukoencephalopathy in Patients on Highly Active Antiretroviral Therapy: Survival and Risk Factors of Death. J Acquir Immune Defic Syndr. 2004 Oct 1;37(2):1263-1268

MEASLES

Paul Auwaerter, M.D.

CLINICAL RELEVANCE & DIAGNOSIS

- Until routine immunization, rubeola virus most common and highly infectious of childhood diseases. Morbillivirus, RNA virus of paramyxoviridae group, respiratory spread with subsequent viremia.
- Diagnosis usually clinical based on febrile illness, characteristic rash and/or Koplik's spots (irreg. red spots w/tiny blue-white specks on buccal/lingual mucosa).
- Measles EIA IgM helpful for acute infection; IgG to screen immune status. Tissue/secretions may be cultured for virus and/or identified by IFA. Nasopharyngeal aspirate IFA offers rapid dx.
- Related paramyxoviruses, metapneumovirus, and Hendra virus newly described agents of resp. illness; Nipah virus cause of encephalitis.
- Still a worldwide problem, up to 1 million deaths annually in developing world. Eradication difficult despite WHO efforts.

SITES OF INFECTION

- Skin/Systemic: Characteristic disease progression. Prodrome of fever, cough, coryza, conjunctivitis followed by flat macular rash fusing to form blotches first over chest/trunk then to limbs.
- Pulmonary: pneumonitis (giant-cell pneumonia). Atypical measles-now rare-pneumonitis as hallmark w/hypersensitivity-like rxn in recipients of killed-measles vaccine exposed to native measles.
- CNS: Post-infectious encephalitis occurs 1:1000 w/15% mortality. Subacute sclerosing panencephalitis (SSPE) very rare >1:300,000 occurring years after measles.
- Secondary Complications: otitis media, bronchopneumonia, croup, bronchitis. Most deaths from measles occur in malnourished children succumbing to pneumonia.
- Other: entire illness lasts up to 10d. Pts may also experience diarrhea, vomiting, lymphadenopathy, abdominal pain, pharyngitis, splenomegaly, leukopenia, and thrombocytopenia.

TREATMENT REGIMENS

Children

- Most well children may be observed without intervention.
- Consider Vitamin A 200,000IU PO x 2d
- Supplementation recommended for children ill enough to be hospitalized (6mos-2yrs) or if suffering from neurological/ophthalmological complication, malnutrition or immunodeficiency (>2yrs).
- Repeat Vitamin A dosing at 4 weeks if suffering from eye disease.

Adults

- Supportive care. Disease tends to be more severe than in pediatric populations.
- Some experience w/ribavirin used parenterally (20-35mg/kg/d x 7d) in adults w/ severe pneumonitis (CID 1994;19(3):454). Also available by aerosol, oral--but little clinical data for measles.
- Note: IV ribavirin only available from ICN pharmaceutical [only emergency use for hemorrhagic fever]: (800) 556-1937

Prevention

- Two dose schedule in US: routine vaccine w/ MMR at 12mos (once maternal antibody lost) with repeat either at ages 4-5 (ACP) or by 12 yrs (AAP).

- Birth prior to 1957, believed immune because of native acquired infection.
- Measles vaccine does NOT appear to be linked with development of autism, multiple sclerosis, inflammatory bowel disease, etc.
- Suspected exposure (e.g., contact w/ known case) in susceptible: immunize w/ vaccine (if no contraindication) within 72h of exposure = disease prevention.
- Exposure: if age <1yr, pregnant, immunocompromised or susceptible prophylax w/IM standard pooled immune globulin. 0.25 mL/kg healthy individuals or 0.5mL/kg immunocompromised, max dose 15mL.
- If receive gammaglobulin, immunize 6mos thereafter.
- Since vaccines (MMR or Attenuvax) are live attenuated viruses, they ar contraindicated in pregnancy, immunodeficiencies, lymphoma/leukemia, AIDS.
- Vaccine can be given to HIV+ if asx (CD4 >200) and immunization warranted.

IMPORTANT POINTS

- Measles not endemic in US since 1997 as most cases imported, outbreaks do occur. Koplik spots may help differentiate febrile illness (like influenza) as they can be seen in prodrome prior to rash.
- HIV, immune suppression, cancer or vitamin A deficiency/malnutrition all risks for severe measles.
- Measles cases (suspected or confirmed) should be reported promptly to local public health authorities.
- Vaccine immunity may wane, but 95% protection commonly quoted; however since 1989 two dose vaccine schedule used to decrease risk of infection with 2-5% who fail to seroconvert after one dose.

SELECTED READINGS

Anon. American Academy of Pediatrics Committee on Infectious Diseases: Vitamin A treatment of measles. Pediatrics 1993 May;91(5):1014-5

Rahmathullah L, Underwood BA, Thulasiraj RD et al. Reduced mortality among children in southern India receiving a small weekly dose of vitamin A. N Engl J Med 1990 Oct 4;323(14):929-35

MMWR. Measles outbreak among internationally adopted children arriving in the United States, February-March 2001. MMWR Morb Mortal Wkly Rep 2002 Dec 13;51(49):1115-6

van den Hof S, Conyn-van Spaendonck MA, van Steenbergen JE. Measles epidemic in the Netherlands, 1999-2000. J Infect Dis 2002 Nov 15;186(10):1483-6

Gremillion DH, Crawford GE. Measles pneumonia in young adults. Am J Med 1981;71:539-42

MOLLUSCUM CONTAGIOSUM

Ciro R. Martins, M.D. and David Kouba, M.D.

CLINICAL RELEVANCE & DIAGNOSIS

- MCV is a poxvirus of genus, Molluscipox
- Large brick- or ovoid-shaped double-stranded DNA virus
- Two subtypes, MCV I and MCV II result in indistinguishable lesions
- Three populations affected: 1) self-limited disease in children; 2) as an STD in adults; 3) patients with AIDS
- Some studies have shown increased prevalence in patients with CD4 nadir <50/mm3, during the first two month of immune reconstitution with HAART, only to resolve when CD4 counts rise above 250/mm3.
- Transmitted by skin-to-skin contact, and to a lesser degree by fomites

Viruses

- Clinical presentation: 2-3mm, firm, umbilicated, pearly papules with waxy surface. Usually asymptomatic. Infrequently: Larger, coalescent lesions (giant molluscum) in immunocompromised hosts.
- Ddx: AIDS consider cryptococcosis or histoplasmosis
- Immunocompetent hosts: ddx = verrucae, nevi, papular granuloma annulare, pyogenic granuloma.
- Symptoms may include: pruritus and associated dermatitis
- Diagnosis: largely based on clinical grounds. If diagnosis is in question, biopsy/histopathology is definitive. May appear similar to cryptococcosis in AIDS patients.
- Histopathology: Molluscum bodies (Henderson-Patterson Bodies) visible in cytoplasm of epithelium

Sites Of Infection

- Children: lesions most commonly on skin folds and genital region
- AIDS: typical lesions commonly on face/neck, or may be disseminated. Large disfiguring, fungating lesions (giant molluscum) are possible.
- Lesions may spread within plaques of atopic dermatitis, especially those treated with topical immunosuppressive agents, such as tacrolimus or pimecrolimus

Treatment Regimens

Children

- Often self-limited and does not need treatment. Most cases resolve in 6-9 months.
- If treatment is desired: curettage, manual expression, liquid nitrogen, trichloroacetic acid, keratolytics, imiquimod, retinoids, electrodessication, tape stripping, laser or cantharidin can be used.
- Only two controlled studies have demonstrated superior efficacy to placebo, multiple uncontrolled studies have demonstrated efficacy for most destructive techniques.
- Most studies are based upon small case series and open-label studies of the aforementioned modalities.
- The only double blinded studies have tested imiquimod and podophyllotoxin - both result in significantly improved cure rate versus placebo.
- Imiquimod is applied at night for 12 hours, three evenings per week for 4-6 weeks, or clinical clearance. Tretinoin 0.05% cream is applied qhs.
- Other non-specific destructive methods should be performed as infrequently as possible, such as every other month.
- Eczema molluscatum is the development of MCV infection in sites treated with topical calcineurin inhibitors. Withdrawl of either the pimecrolimus or tacrolimus is the first step in treatment.

Immunosuppressed patients

- Uncomplicated molluscum is a common nuisance but may represent a serious cosmetic/quality of life problem in the AIDS population.
- Local destructive methods and immunomodulatory agents used, but main goal is to contain spread.
- Localized, minimal disease: curettage, cryotherapy, electrocauterization, KOH solution, trichloroacetic acid, cantharidin or imiquimod cream or photodynamic therapy w/ visible light-activated ALA.
- To keep minor lesions under control, regular cryotherapy in the office, followed by patient-applied imiquimod is preferred. Larger or clustered lesions, trichloroacetic acid/PDT may be necessary.

- Giant molluscum resistant to all known therapies. Cryotherapy, CO2 laser, tretinoin and TCA have all been used, and are generally unsuccessful.
- Lesions usually resolve spontaneously and completely when CD4 counts rise above 200-250/mm3 with HAART.
- Dosing schedules for imiquimod may need to be increased to qhs, and destructive treatments should be performed more regularly in order to keep the infection under control.
- For recalcitrant infections, especially in immunosuppressed patients, combining therapeutic modalities may be a superior alternative to any one treatment.

IMPORTANT POINTS

- In children, treatment is usually unnecessary and aggressive destructive modalities may increase chance of scar.
- In AIDS patients, disseminated cryptococcosis and histoplasmosis may also present as firm umbilicated papules, similar to molluscum.
- In AIDS patients, it is important to keep lesions under control because if they evolve into giant molluscum, they are very recalcitrant to treatment.
- In-office curettage/cryotherapy is preferred initial treatments for most cases of molluscum (adults). Adjunctive use of imiquimod at home improves outcomes and may be necessary if many lesions appear.
- For children, it is critical to reassure the parents that this is a benign condition of childhood that will resolve spontaneously.

SELECTED READINGS

Cronin T.A., Resnik B.I., Elgart G., et al. Recalcitrant giant molluscum contagiosum in a patient with AIDS. J Am Acad Dermatol. 1996; 35:266-7

Syed TA, Goswami J, Ahmadpour OA, et al. Treatment of molluscum contagiosum in males with an analog of imiquimod 1% in cream: a placebo-controlled, double-blind study. J Dermatol. 1998 May;25 (5):309-13.

Syed TA, Lundin S, Ahmad M. Topical 0.3% and 0.5% podophyllotoxin cream for self-treatment of molluscum contagiosum in males. A placebo-controlled, double-blind study. Dermatology. 1994;189(1): 65-8.

Moiin A. Photodynamic therapy for molluscum contagiosum infection in HIV-coinfected patients: review of 6 patients. J Drugs Dermatol. 2003 Dec;2(6):637-9.

Silverberg N. Pediatric molluscum contagiosum: optimal treatment strategies. Paediatr Drugs. 2003;5 (8):505-12.

PARAINFLUENZA VIRUS John G. Bartlett, M.D.

CLINICAL RELEVANCE & DIAGNOSIS

- RNA enveloped virus w/5 antigenically distinct types (1, 2, 3, 4A, 4B)
- Respiratory tract; esp. URI, seasonal. Bronchitis common, pneumonia uncommon (seen in children, immunocompromised adults, elderly)
- Most common in pediatric population; most severe infections in children & compromised hosts
- Type 1: big outbreaks, autumn, odd yrs - '03, '05, '07
- Type 2: follows type 1
- Type 3: spring and summer
- Type 4A & B: rare
- Dx and cx (gold standard), DFA, PCR--all of respiratory secretions--and serology (EIA)

- Adults: healthy host - 10% of all URIs; complications - immunodeficiency, cystic fibrosis, COLD

SITES OF INFECTION

- Respiratory tract: URI w/pharyngitis (85% of parainfluenza cases), sinusitis, bronchitis, otitis, pneumonitis
- Aseptic meningitis: rare
- Severe immunodeficiency: disseminated disease

TREATMENT REGIMENS

Treatment

- Guidelines from: Hall CB (NEJM 2001;344:1917)
- Experimental: ribavirin for organ/marrow transplants w/pneumonia (experimental) and poor response in stem cell txp pts. Has been given by aerosol route and orally (30-45mg/kg/d PO).
- Experimental: aerosolized steroids +/- systemic steroids (effective in pediatric croup)
- URI Rx: see "Upper Respiratory Infections" in Diagnoses

IMPORTANT POINTS

- Guidelines from Hall CR (NEJM 2001;344:2001)
- Paraflu causes only respiratory tract infections commonly. Rare aseptic meningitis and rare disseminated infection occur in compromised hosts.
- Adults - 10% of URIs + pneumonia in peds, elderly and comp. host
- Transmission pt-pt in peds and onc/transplant units
- No specific Rx. Dx tests are insensitive in adult disease

SELECTED READINGS

Hall CB. Respiratory syncytial virus and parainfluenza virus. NEJM 2001;344:1917

Englund JA, Piedra PA, Whimbey E. Prevention and treatment of respiratory syncytial virus and parainfluenza viruses in immunocompromised patients. Am J Med 1997;102:61

Glezen WP, Greenberg SB, Atmar RL, et al. Impact of respiratory virus infections on persons with chronic underlying conditions. JAMA 2000;283:499

Nichols WG, Corey L, Gooley T, et al. Parainfluenza virus infection after hematopoietic stem cell transplantation: risk factors, response to antiviral therapy and effect on transplant outcome. Blood 2001;98:573

Elizaga J, Olavarria E, Apperley J, et al. Parainfluenza virus 3 infection after stem cell transplant: relevance to outcome of rapid diagnosis and ribavirin treatment. Clin Infect Dis 2001;32:413

PARVOVIRUS B19

Khalil G. Ghanem, M.D.

CLINICAL RELEVANCE & DIAGNOSIS

- Single-stranded DNA virus causes erythema infectiosum/"fifth disease" (children), pure red cell aplasia (sickle cell disease, immunocompromised), arthropathy, hydrops fetalis.
- Infects erythroid progenitor cells; predominant immune response humoral; (+)IgG antibodies associated w/ protection.
- Transmission: respiratory, blood, mother to fetus; high risk contacts (attack rates): students (50%), teachers (30%), day-care (9%), homemakers (9%), other women (4%). Peaks late winter-early spring.
- Dx: IgM (85%+ w/ erythema infectiosum or aplastic crisis; turns neg <3mos); IgG (2wks post infection; lifelong); PCR most sensitive (NOT diagnostic alone). Giant pronormoblasts blood/BM suggests dx.

• Dx (2): serology may be negative in immunocompromised.

SITES OF INFECTION

• JOINTS: 60% females, 30% males, 10% kids: MCP joint (75%), knees (65%), wrists (55%), ankles (40%); immune mediated; may persist >1mo esp. women.
• SKIN: Erythema infectiosum (fifth disease): facial erythema ("slapped cheek"), circumoral pallor (18 days after infection); reticular rash (trunk/limbs).
• BONE MARROW: transient aplasia (pts w/ thalassemia, hemolytic anemia); chronic pure red cell aplasia (immunosuppressed, esp HIV, transplant, sickle cell); hemophagocytic syndrome (immunocompromised).
• FETUS: Hydrops fetalis (pregnant with acute infection: risk ~1.6%; highest between 11-23 wks gestation); anemia; thrombocytopenia.
• OTHER: CNS (encephalopathy); LIVER (hepatitis); HEART (myocarditis).

TREATMENT REGIMENS

Immunosuppressed

• Chronic pure red cell aplasia: IVIG 0.4g/kg/day for 5 days or 1g/kg/day for 2-3 days; may need to repeat monthly.

Immunocompetent

• No Rx usually; NSAIDs for arthropathy; blood products for transient aplasia; weekly U/S for infected pregnant women; cordicentesis and intrauterine transfusions for hydrops fetalis.

IMPORTANT POINTS

• Once the rash appears, the patient is no longer infectious.
• If pregnant woman exposed, check IgG level; if + reassure pt she is immune. If -, risk small but if infected, follow with weekly ultrasound.
• Pregnant women who work in outbreak setting (teachers, child care) should be sent home.
• Parvo B19 may present with symmetrical arthritis identical to rhematoid arthritis. Parvo B19 arthritis NOT DESTRUCTIVE. RF MAY be positive with B19.
• Presence of B19 DNA NOT diagnostic of acute infection. DNA may persist in blood and joints for months to years. Dx based on clinical findings AND lab findings.

SELECTED READINGS

Norbeck O, Papadogiannakis N, Petersson K, et al. Revised clinical presentation of Parvovirus B19-associated intrauterine fetal death. Clin Infect Dis, 2002; 35(9):1032-1038.

Brown T, Anand A, Ritchie LD, et al. Human parvovirus in pregnancy and hydrops fetalis. N Engl J Med, 1987;316(4):183-6

Anderson LJ, Gillespie SM, Torok TJ, et al. Risk of infection following exposures to human parvovirus B19. Behring Inst Mitt, 1990; 85:60-63.

Cartter ML, Farley TA, Rosengren S, et al. Occupational risk factors for infection with parvovirus B19 among pregnant women. J Infect Dis, 1991; 163(2):282-285.

Woolf AD, Campion GV, Chishick A, et al. Clinical manifestations of human parvovirus B19 in adults. Arch Int Med, 1989; 149(5):1153-1156

RABIES

Khalil G. Ghanem, M.D.

CLINICAL RELEVANCE & DIAGNOSIS

- SS-RNA, enveloped Lyssavirus causes rabies, a uniformly fatal encephalitis of humans and other mammals. Domestic dog main reservoir worldwide. Raccoons, foxes, bats, skunks in US.
- Total US human rabies cases: appx. 5/year. Bats most common source of infxn in U.S. 39 cases from bats in last 50 yrs (51% no history of bite). 4-15% of bats in U.S. infected.
- Incubation: 1-3mths (range: dys-yrs). Sx (1) Prodome (4-10d): fever, HA, malaise, personality changes, pain /paresthesia at bite & myoedema.
- Sx (2): 2 forms: furious [80%-hydrophobia, delirium, agitation, Sz, aerophobia] paralytic [20%-ascending paralysis; meningismus, confusion]. Both: coma after 2-14d then death.
- Dx: DFA bx specimen nape of neck above hairline (50% + 1st wk, higher thereafter). RT-PCR on tissue/saliva. CSF (5-30 lymphs; oligoclonal bands). Neutralizing Ab (50% d8, 100% d15). MRI neg usually.
- Ddx: HSV encephalitis, tetanus, strychnine, or other toxin, acute inflam polyneuropathy, transverse myelitis, polio, PML.
- Ascending paralysis of rabies may be confused with polio.

SITES OF INFECTION

- CNS: hallucinations, confusion, anxiety, biting, hydrophobia, autonomic dysfxn, SIADH.
- CV: arrhythmias, myocarditis, CHF.
- GI: bleeding, N/V, ileus.

TREATMENT REGIMENS

Pre-exposure prophylaxis

- Vaccination of pets; vaccinating high risk (vets, lab workers, spelunkers, travelers to areas with high prev): 3 IM or ID (d 0, 7, 21 or 28). Booster q2-3yrs if continued risk.
- 4 licensed rabies vaccines: all equally safe & efficacious. Neutralizing Abs produced 7-10d after vaccine & last for 2-3 yrs.
- Can check serostatus to guide rebooosting schedule. No need to check serostatus after treatment in non-immunocompromised hosts.
- Specific pre-exposure prophylaxis recommendations and vaccine info: CDC/ACIP recommendations at: http://www.cdc.gov/ncidod/dvrd/rabies/Prevention&Control/ACIP/ACIP99.htm

Post-exposure prophylaxis (PEP)

- Wound care w/ 20% soap solution and irrigation with povidone iodine (risk decreased by 90%).
- Contact public health official immediately; if healthy dog/cat, observe x 10d. If pet develops sx, sacrifice to check DFA for rabies. If +, Rx patient (see below). If skunk/bat/raccoon IMMEDIATE Rx.
- Bites of squirrels, hamsters, gerbils, guinea pigs, rats, mice, chipmunks, rabbits: almost never require PEP but consult local health official.
- PEP: Rabies Immune Globulin RIG (20IU/kg) [all at wound site if possible, if not, give IM at site other than vaccine site) AND vaccine: 1mL IM deltoid d 0,3,7,14, 28.
- If pt previously vaccinated w/i last 3 yrs, then DO NOT GIVE RIG; only wound cleansing and vaccine on days 0 and 3. If immune status unsure, treat fully with all three measures.

- In rabies-endemic areas: minor exposures: (licks of broken skin/minor abrasions w/o bleeding): vaccinate while observing animal). Major exposures: (licks of mucosa/transdermal bites): Both Rig & vaccine.

Therapy

- Supportive care; no currently approved antivirals. All pts until recently succumb to dz, usually w/i 14d sx onset despite supportive measures (which may prolong lifespan by 50%, i.e., 30 days).
- Vaccine + drug-induced coma/ventilator support and ribavirin likely now the standard of care based upon reports of survival [MMWR Dec 2004 reference].

IMPORTANT POINTS

- Very often, no history of bite/scratch/exposure making early dx VERY difficult.
- Most cases in U.S. are of bat exposure; all U.S. cases in last 10 years from dogs/cats were imported. Transmission via organ transplantation documented.
- Location of bite modifies risk of rabies: facial bites assoc. w/ higher risk than extremity bites. Early suturing may be deleterious (especially facial wounds).
- Rabies virus isolated from human saliva, hence theoretical risk of human to human transmission. PEP recommended if bite/scratch/sexual contact with rabid pt.
- In U.S. intradermal vaccination currently approved for pre-exposure prophylaxis ONLY.

SELECTED READINGS

Khawplod P, Wilde H, Tepsumethanon S, et al. Prospective Immunogenicity Study of Multiple Intradermal Injections of Rabies Vaccine in an Effort to Obtain an Early Immune Response without the Use of Immunoglobulin. Clin Infect Dis 2002 Dec 15;35(12):1562-5

Smith J, McElhinney L, Parsons G, et al. Case report: Rapid ante-mortem diagnosis of a human case of rabies imported into the UK from the Philippines. J Med Virol 2003 Jan;69(1):150-5

Dutta JK. Bite by a dog under provocation: is it free from risk? . J Indian Med Assoc 2002 May;100 (5):330-1

Aguilar-Setien A, Leon YC, Tesoro EC, et al. Vaccination of vampire bats using recombinant vaccinia-rabies virus. J Wildl Dis 2002 Jul;38(3):539-44

Chang HG, Eidson M, Noonan-Toly C, et al. Public health impact of reemergence of rabies, New York. Emerg Infect Dis 2002 Sep;8(9):909-13

RESPIRATORY SYNCYTIAL VIRUS

John G. Bartlett, M.D.

CLINICAL RELEVANCE & DIAGNOSIS

- Enveloped RNA paramyxovirus; respiratory tract pathogens in humans
- Peds major causes: otitis, croup, pneumonia, asthma
- Healthy adult: URI +/- fever, sinusitis, asthma, otitis, acute exacerbation of chronic bronchitis
- Adult pneumonia: 4% of all cases; increased rate in elderly, transplant, cancer or chemo Rx
- Epidemics: annual in peds - Nov to mid-May; nosocomial - peds, nursing homes, transplant/onc wards
- Dx: viral culture (sens 60-90%, 3-7 days)
- Dx: sputum/throat DFA - low sensitivity (15%) in adults

SITES OF INFECTION

- Upper respiratory tract may occur +/- sinusitis, otitis
- Bronchi: bronchitis, bronchiolitis, asthma

- Lung: pneumonia
- CNS: meningitis, encephalitis (rare)
- Cardiac: myocarditis (rare)
- Derm: exanthem (rare)

TREATMENT REGIMENS

Treatment
- Experimental and only for immunosuppressed adult: ribavirin (30-45mg/kg/d) PO if started early (experience in stem cell & marrow tx is poor)
- Experimental: RSV immune globulin (RSVIG) 1.5g/kg IVIG with high RSV Ab titer

Prevention
- Infection control: handwashing, gown and gloves

IMPORTANT POINTS

- Guidelines: Hall CB (NEJM 2001;344:1917; PPID Mandell G, 5th Ed 2000, pg 1782)
- Pneumonia in elderly, organ tx, HIV, cancer chemo Rx
- Diagnostic tests in adults (cult, DFA, PCR) not sensitive, best is BAL viral cx
- High lethality in onc & transplant pts - consider ribavirin +/- RSV immune glob (both experimental)
- Epidemiology: staff w/child or pt w/URI can transmit to oncology pt, then oncology unit etc.

SELECTED READINGS

Neuzil KM, et al. Winter respiratory viruses and health care use: a population based study in northwest U.S. CID 2003;37:201

van Waensel JB, et al. Dexamethasone for treatment of patients mechanically ventilated for lower respiratory tract infection caused by respiratory syncytial virus. Thorax. 2003 May;58(5):383-7

Hashem M and Hall CB. Respiratory syncytial virus in healthy adults: the cost of a cold. J Clin Virol 2003;27:14

Torrence PF, Powell LD. The quest for an efficacious antiviral for RSV. Antivir Chem Chemother 2002;13:325

McCurdy LH, et al. Clinical features and outcomes of paramyxoviral infection in lung transplant recipients treated with ribavirin. J Heart Lung Transplant 2003;22:745

VARICELLA-ZOSTER VIRUS   Paul Auwaerter, M.D.

CLINICAL RELEVANCE & DIAGNOSIS

- DNA virus member of Herpesviridae family. Humans only known reservoir. Primary infection spread by respiratory route with latency established in nerves. By adulthood 90-95% infected (prevaccine era).
- Primary infection=chickenpox=fever<103F, malaise may precede rash (maculopapules, vesicles, scabs) occurring in crops. Hallmark is appearance of lesions in all stages.
- Immunosuppressed (e.g., leukemics): increased skin lesions often hemorrhagic. Greater risk visceral disease, dissemination (35-50%).
- CNS complications most feared. Cerebellar ataxia children <15 [1:4000] generally benign. Encephalitis 0.1-0.2%, in adults (5-20% mortality). Pneumonitis more common with adults/immunosuppressed.
- Herpes zoster=shingles=reactivation from latency in dorsal root ganglia. 20% lifetime risk, mainly elderly; increased rates if immune suppressed. Dermatomal unilateral eruption, thoracolumbar >freq.

VARICELLA-ZOSTER VIRUS

SITES OF INFECTION
- Cutaneous (primary or reactivation)
- CNS (primary) ataxia; encephalitis (primary or secondary), cerebral angitis (secondary), meningitis, transverse myelitis, Reye's
- Pneumonitis (primary)
- Herpes Zoster Ophthalmicus (CN V) +/- keratitis, iridocyclitis (secondary). Acute retinal necrosis, mainly HIV (secondary). Involve ophthalmology consultation.
- Ramsay Hunt Syndrome: geniculate ganglion = facial palsy, aural vesicles, taste abnl ant. 2/3 tongue (secondary)
- Disseminated (viscera +/- skin): >mortality with primary infection than dissemination as a result of secondary reactivation.

TREATMENT REGIMENS

Primary disease: varicella (chickenpox)
- Normal children/adolescents (uncomplicated) require no antiviral treatment. Avoid scratching skin which may precipitate secondary bacterial infection/cellulitis. No ASA (Reye's Syn. risk).
- Normal Adult: Rx within 24hr onset of exanthem for efficacy. Acyclovir 800mg PO qid x 5d
- Varicella pneumonia: acyclovir 10-12mg/kg q8h, or valacyclovir 1g PO tid or famciclovir 500mg PO tid all for 7-10 days.

Prevention of varicella/chickenpox
- Varicella zoster immune globulin (VZIG) only to those at high risk (newborns 5d prior or 2d after delivery, leukemics not immunized, pregnant women, persons w/ immunodeficiencies or immune suppressed).
- Risk=exposure to chickenpox or shingles + no hx of prior varicella or neg. serology. Give VZIG 5 vials (6.25mL) by 96h preferably <48h. No data suggest effectiveness of VZIG in Rx severe disease
- Postexposure prophylaxis should be within 3d exposure and could include acyclovir (40-80mg/kg) or vaccine (if not contraindicated) that offer efficacy of 70-85% vs 90% for VZIG.
- Varicella vaccine: Adults 0.5cc SQ x 2 doses, separated 4-8wks. Protection is 70-90% against infection and 95% against severe disease.
- Indications for susceptibles: healthcare workers, household contacts of immunosuppressed, young adults in dorms or military, nonpregnant women in childbearing yrs, susceptible teens & adults.
- Vaccine contraindications: pregnancy, immunosuppressive conditions, active TB, recent blood products with plasma (passive immunity problems), h/o rxns to gelatin or neomycin.
- Adults often uncertain of prior chickenpox hx. VZV Serology + in 70-90% of adults who believe they did not have varicella, so check serology prior to vaccination in suspected nonimmune.
- Susceptible staff in hospitals with exposure to VZV incl. localized zoster should avoid contact with high-risk pts. for 8-21d after exposure.

Varicella/Chickenpox Adult Immunosuppressed
- Acyclovir 10mg/kg IV q 8h x 7-10d
- Some clinicians will use more bioavailable oral therapy in stable patients to avoid hospitalization, e.g., valacyclovir 1g PO tid or famciclovir 500mg PO tid 7-10d.

- Varicella pneumonia: acyclovir 10-12mg/kg q8h, or valacyclovir 1g PO tid or famciclovir 500mg PO tid all for 7-10 days.

Zoster/shingles

- Normal host: valacyclovir 1g PO tid or famciclovir 500mg PO tid or acyclovir 10mg/kg IV q8h all x 7d.
- Disseminated zoster or immunosuppressed host: acyclovir 10mg/kg q8h x 7d although some use valacyclovir 1g PO tid or famciclovir 500mg PO tid in stable patient.
- Acyclovir-resistant VZV: Foscarnet 40mg/kg q8h IV x 10d. Most acyclovir resistant VZV strains are also resistant to ganciclovir and famciclovir.
- There is little apparent efficacy Rx zoster if beyond 72hr of presentation. Indications for treatment also include pain at presentation, age >50, immunosuppressed host or dissemination.
- Normal host: multiple studies show benefit up to > 2fold reduction in pain if antivirals used <72h of rash presentation. May add prednisone 60mg PO qd w/ taper over 10-21d.
- Recent study (see Oxman ref) showed that adult Oka/Merck vaccine (higher dose than licensed peds vaccine) reduced incidence and severity of zoster and PHN. Vaccine needs to be approved by FDA.

Postherpetic neuralgia

- Defined as pain present >120 days following rash. Pain < 30d= acute herpetic neuralgia; 30-120d=subacute herpetic neuralgia.
- PHN more likely in elderly, those with severe pain at presentation of rash. 20% pts >50yrs have pain beyond 6mos despite early antiviral Rx of shingles.
- Four first-line therapies, none clearly superior and often used in combination but multiple Rx use not well studied and increases adverse reactions.
- Gabapentin: start 100-300mg qhs or 100mg tid then titrate by 100mg tid as tolerated. Trials suggest 1800-3600mg daily target for benefit. SE: somnolence, dizziness, gait issues, cognitive impairment.
- Lidocaine patch 5% (Lidoderm): Use up to 12h daily, up to three patches. Don't use over open lesions. Min. lidocaine systemic absorption, mild rash usually only side effect. Relief usually by 2wks.
- Opioids: Published trials used either controlled-release oxycodone (up to 60mg daily) or morphine (up to 240mg). Many short- or long-acting preparations available.
- TCAs: Many types but nortriptyline best tolerated in elderly. Start 10-25mg qhs titrate to 75-150mg. Multiple SE: cardiac, anticholinergic, uses P450 2D6 pathway. Check levels if dose >100mg.
- Other options for refractory patients: capsaicin 0.025-0.075% cream qid, nerve blocks, spinal cord stimulation, intrathecal methylprednisolone (all non-FDA)

Important Points

- Mortality of primary VZV low in children but higher in adults.
- Dx for chickenpox or shingles mainly clinical. Ddx includes smallpox (distinguish because VZV has lesions in all stages), impetigo by Gr A strep; HSV; vesiculation due to enterovirus.
- If confusing can perform Tzanck smear of vesicle (multinucleated giant cells), viral cx, immunofluor. stains of fluid/histopath, PCR. Varicella IgM w/primary infection.
- Zoster Rx only if <72hr from initial rash lesion, pain w/ rash, >50yrs, immunosuppressed or disseminated disease. Rx >72hr of uncertain benefit, but help if new vesicles forming.
- No American professional societies have formulated management guidelines for zoster.
- Recommendations in this module based upon: NEJM 2002 347(5):340; MMWR Recomm Rep 1999 48(RR-6): 1; Ann Intern Med 1999 130:922 and author opinion.

SELECTED READINGS

Oxman MN, Levin MJ, Johnson GR et al. A caccine to prevent herpes zoster and postherpetic neuralgia in older adults. NEJM 2005 352: 2271

Behrman A, Schmid DS, Crivaro A, Watson B. A cluster of primary varicella cases among healthcare workers with false-positive varicella zoster virus titers. Infect Control Hosp Epidemiol 2003 Mar;24(3): 202-6

Kilgore PE, Kruszon-Moran D, Seward JF, et al. Varicella in Americans from NHANES III: Implications for control through routine immunization. J Med Virol 2003;70 Suppl 1:S111-8

Masur H, Kaplan JE, Holmes KK, et al. Guidelines for preventing opportunistic infections among HIV-infected persons--2002. Recommendations of the U.S. Public Health Service and the Infectious Diseases Society of America. Ann Intern Med 2002 Sep 3;137(5 Pt 2):435-78

Klassen TP, Belseck EM, Wiebe N, Hartling L. Acyclovir for treating varicella in otherwise healthy children and adolescents. Cochrane Database Syst Rev 2002;(4):CD002980

WEST NILE VIRUS

John G. Bartlett, M.D.

CLINICAL RELEVANCE & DIAGNOSIS

- Mosquito-borne flaviviral infection: cause of epidemic encephalitis.
- WNV infection: 80% asymptomatic; 20% sx w/fever, lymphadenopathy, GI sx, myalgia, HA, +/- rash; CNS sx in 1/150 WNV infections
- Risk: Endemic area, June-Nov, mosquito; elderly, immune suppressed - prone to neuro complications. Transmission reported by blood transfusion, organ txp.
- CNS sx (often overlapping): encephalitis (fever, altered MS, paresis, Parkinson-like, seizure) &/OR aseptic meningitis, esp w/paresis
- Asymmetric flaccid weakness described/polio-like; CSF pleocytosis helps distinguish from Guillain-Barre.
- Lab serum/CSF: EIA IgM +/- plaque reduction neutralization assay; RNA PCR - less sensitive; CSF protein 100-1000, WBC 5-1500, mostly lymphs
- Prevention: mosquito control, avoid mosquito contact (DEET, long sleeves, screens, remove stagnant water, etc.)

SITES OF INFECTION

- Viremia (1st week)
- CNS: encephalitis, meningitis, radiculomyelitis
- Other: diarrhea, rash, LN (cervical usual)

TREATMENT REGIMENS

Encephalitis

- Principles: SUSPECT w/epidemic + encephalitis or fever + paresis
- Supportive care
- Dx: serology; report positive results to Health Dept.

Experimental

- Ribavirin (up to 4g IV/d), interferon alpha 2b (3mil units/d) or hyperimmune globulin (available in Israel and NIH trial)

IMPORTANT POINTS

- Recommendations: see CDC for most up-to-date: www.cdc.gov/ncidod/dvbid/westnile
- Most have asymptomatic seroconversion or "flu" sx - fever, HA, myalgia +/- rash; CNS w/encephalitis/ myelitis in 1/150, esp elderly (but mean age 55 in 2002)
- Clues - epidemiology; sx - fever + confusion &/or paresis, hyporeflexia

Viruses

- Must r/o HSV (MRI/CT- ?temporal lobe, CSF PCR) - most should get rapid IV acyclovir awaiting dx; no specific tx for any other viral encephalitis including West Nile Virus.
- WNV experimental Rx - ribavirin, interferon, hyperimmune globulin

Selected Readings

CDC. Guidelines for surveillance, prevention and control of West Nile virus--U.S. MMWR 2000;49:25

Cunha B. West Nile encephalitis. Infect Dis Practice 1999;23:85

Lanciotti RS. Origin of the West Nile virus responsible for an outbreak of encephalitis in the northern U.S. Science 1999;286:2333

CDC. Update: West Nile Virus. MMWR 2000; 49: 1044

CDC. Serosurveys for West Nile Virus Infection - New York & Connecticut Counties 2000. MMWR 2001; 58:37

A

APPENDIX I

Table 1a. Definitions for the Diagnosis of Infective Endocarditis According to the Duke Criteria*

Definite infective endocarditis

  Pathologic criteria

    Microorganisms: demonstrated by culture or histologic examination in a vegetation, *or* in a vegetation that has embolized, *or* in an intracardiac abscess, *or*

    Pathologic lesions: vegetation or intracardiac abscess present, confirmed by histological examination showing active endocarditis

  Clinical criteria, using specific definitions listed in Table 2
      2 Major criteria, *or*
      1 Major and 3 minor criteria, *or*
      5 Minor criteria

Possible infective endocarditis
  Findings consistent with infective endocarditis that fall short of "definite" but are not "rejected"

Rejected
  Firm alternate diagnosis for manifestations of endocarditis, or

  Resolution of manifestations of endocarditis, with antibiotic therapy for 4 days or less, *or*

  No pathologic evidence of infective endocarditis at surgery or autopsy, after antibiotic therapy for 4 days or less

*See Table 1b for definitions of terminology.

Reprinted from Durack DT, Lukes AS, Bright DK. New criteria for diagnosis of infective endocarditis: utilization of specific echocardiographic findings. Duke Endocarditis Service. *Am J Med*. 1994;96(3):200-209. Copyright © 2004, with permission from Excerpta Medica, Inc.

Table 1b. Definitions of Terminology Used in the Duke Criteria

Major criteria

- Positive blood culture for infective endocarditis
  - —Typical microorganism for infective endocarditis from 2 separate blood cultures

    *Viridans streptococci,** *Streptococcus bovis,* HACEK[†] group

    OR

    Community-acquired *Staphylococcus aureus* or enterococci, in the absence of a primary focus

    OR
  - —Persistently positive blood culture, defined as recovery of a microorganism consistent with infective endocarditis from:
    - (1) Blood cultures drawn more than 12 hours apart, *OR*
    - (2) All of 3 or a majority of 4 or more separate blood cultures, with first and last drawn at least 1 hour apart
- Evidence of endocardial involvement
  - —Positive echocardiogram for infective endocarditis
    - (1) Oscillating intracardiac mass, on valve or supporting structures, *OR* in the path of regurgitant jets, *OR* on implanted material in the absence of an alternative anatomic explanation, *OR*
    - (2) Abscess, *OR*
    - (3) New partial dehiscence of prosthetic valve

      OR
  - —New valvular regurgitation (increase or change in preexisting murmur not sufficient)

Minor criteria

- Predisposition: predisposing heart condition, *OR* intravenous drug use
- Fever: temperature at least 38.0ºC (≥100.4ºF)
- Vascular phenomena: major arterial emboli, septic pulmonary infarctions, mycotic aneurysm, intracranial hemorrhage, conjunctival hemorrhages, Janeway lesions
- Immunological phenomena: glomerulonephritis, Osler nodes, Roth spots, rheumatoid factor
- Microbiological evidence: positive blood culture but not meeting major criteria as noted above,[‡] *OR* serologic evidence of active infection with organism consistent with infective endocarditis
- Echocardiogram: consistent with infective endocarditis but not meeting major criteria as noted above

---

* Including nutritional variant strains.

† HACEK indicates *Haemophilus* species, *Actinobacillus actinomycetemcomitans, Cardiobacterium hominis, Eikenella* species, and *Kingella kingae.*

‡ Excluding single positive cultures for coagulase-negative staphylococci and organisms that do not cause endocarditis.

Table 2a. Miscellaneous Causes of Fever of Unknown Origin (FUO)

Etiology	Clues to the diagnosis
Common	
Drug fever	—
Thromboembolism	Dyspnea, chest pain (blood-gas measurements may remain normal). Patient recovering from pelvic surgery or parturition at greatest risk
Alcoholic liver disease	Hepatomegaly, increased serum aspartate aminotransferase levels
Factitious fever	Absence of diurnal temperature variation, discrepancy between concomitant oral and rectal temperature measurements
Cryptic hematoma	Recent history of blunt trauma or anticoagulant therapy
Rare	
Occult dental infection	Poor dentition, history of recent dental procedure
Familial Mediterranean fever	Episodic fever with abdominal pain, serositis, skin rash, arthritis
Idiopathic pericarditis	—
Subacute granulomatous thyroiditis	—
New causes	
Kikuchi's disease	Histiocytic necrotizing adenitis, leukopenia, elevated serum transaminase levels, splenomegaly
Hypergammaglobulinemia IgD syndrome	Periodic and prolonged fevers, rash, large joint arthritis
IgD syndrome	—

Table 2b. Historical Clues in FUO

Exposure	Possible diagnosis
Birds	Salmonellosis, psittacosis, tuberculosis
Cats	Cat scratch fever, Q fever, toxoplasmosis
Dogs	Leptospirosis
Cattle	Brucellosis, Q fever, leptospirosis
Rodents	Leptospirosis, relapsing fever
Ticks	Ehrlichiosis, Lyme disease
Travel	Malaria, tularemia, tuberculosis
Sexual	HIV, hepatitis, gonorrhea, syphilis
Spelunking	Relapsing fever
Dairy products	Salmonellosis, yersinial infection, brucellosis, Q fever
Chicken, pork	Salmonellosis, yersinial infection
Shellfish	Salmonellosis

Table 2c. Physical Examination Findings in FUO

Evaluation	Finding
Vital signs	High fever with slow pulse
Head*	Nasal discharge and sinus tenderness
	Nodules or reduced pulsations in temporal artery
	Oropharyngeal ulceration
	Tender tooth
Thyroid*	Enlarged, tender
Ocular	Conjunctivitis
	Roth's spots
	Icterus
Lymphatic system	Abnormality of any nodes, including the epitrochlear and supraclavicular nodes
Heart	Murmur or changes in heart sounds
Abdomen	Splenomegaly
	Hepatic enlargement or tenderness
	Flank tenderness or swelling
Anus and rectum*	Perirectal or prostatic tenderness or fluctuance
Genitalia*	Epididymal nodule
	Testicular nodule
	Cervical discharge and uterine tenderness
Joints	Stiffness, swelling, redness
Lower extremities	Deep venous tenderness, swelling
Skin and mucous membranes	Rash
	Petechiae with vasculitis (palpable purpuric lesions)
	Purpura with petechiae
	Janeway's spots
	Osler's nodes

* Mackowiak PA, Durack DT: *Mandell, Douglas, and Bennett's Principles and Practice of Infectious Diseases*, ed 5. Edited by Mandell GL, Bennett JE, Dolin R. Philadelphia: Churchill Livingstone; 2000:623-33.

Possible diagnosis

Typhoid fever, Legionnaires' disease, brucellosis, factitious fever

Sinusitis

Temporal arteritis

Disseminated histoplasmosis

Apical abscess

Thyroiditis

Fungal infection, tuberculosis

Subacute bacterial endocarditis, leukemia

Hepatitis, cholestasis

Infectious mononucleosis, other systemic infection, lymphoma

Endocarditis

Various viral and bacterial diseases, lymphoma, lymphoreticular neoplasm

Hepatic infection or intra-abdominal abscess

Perinephric or intrarenal abscess

Abscess

Disseminated granulomatosis

Periarteritis nodosa

Pelvic inflammatory disease

Rheumatic disease

Thrombophlebitis

Drug fever, viral infection

Collagen vascular disease

Meningococcal or gonococcal bacteremia

Subacute bacterial endocarditis

Subacute bacterial endocarditis

Table 2d. Routine Laboratory Tests for FUO

Test	Finding	Significance
Complete blood count (CBC) with differential	Leukocytosis, leukopenia, anemia, thrombocytopenia	Wide range of underlying diseases
Erythrocyte sedimentation rate (ESR)	Elevation	Infection or collagen vascular disease
Liver enzyme (transaminase and alkaline phosphatase) levels	Elevation	Hepatitis, hepatic abscess or tumor, cholestasis
Syphilis serology	Positive	Syphilis
HIV screen	Positive	HIV infection (requires confirmatory test)
Urinalysis with culture	Presence of pathogens	Urinary-tract infection
Blood culture	Presence of pathogens	Bacteremia, especially bacterial endocarditis
Stool examination	Parasites or ova	Parasitic infection
Mantoux skin test	Positive	Tuberculosis
Chest film	Infiltrates	Tuberculosis or malignancy

Table 3. Cervicitis Treatment Algorithm

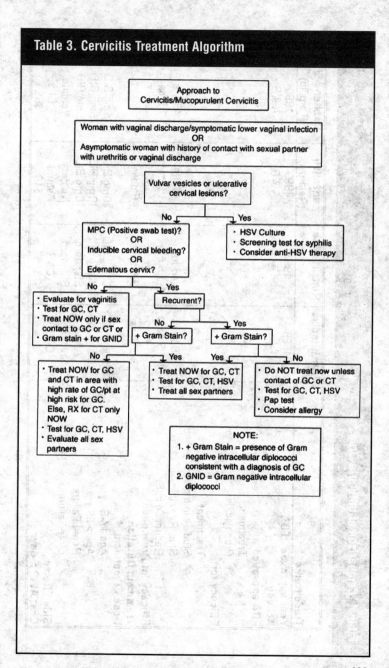

Approach to
Cervicitis/Mucopurulent Cervicitis

Woman with vaginal discharge/symptomatic lower vaginal infection
OR
Asymptomatic woman with history of contact with sexual partner
with urethritis or vaginal discharge

Vulvar vesicles or ulcerative
cervical lesions?

No → | Yes →

Yes:
· HSV Culture
· Screening test for syphilis
· Consider anti-HSV therapy

No:
MPC (Positive swab test)?
OR
Inducible cervical bleeding?
OR
Edematous cervix?

No → | Yes →

No:
· Evaluate for vaginitis
· Test for GC, CT
· Treat NOW only if sex
  contact to GC or CT or
· Gram stain + for GNID

Yes:
Recurrent?

No → | Yes →

No:
+ Gram Stain?

No → | Yes →

No:
· Treat NOW for GC
  and CT in area with
  high rate of GC/pt at
  high risk for GC.
  Else, RX for CT only
  NOW
· Test for GC, CT, HSV
· Evaluate all sex
  partners

Yes:
· Treat NOW for GC, CT
· Test for GC, CT, HSV
· Treat all sex partners

Yes:
+ Gram Stain?

Yes → | No →

No:
· Do NOT treat now unless
  contact of GC or CT
· Test for GC, CT, HSV
· Pap test
· Consider allergy

NOTE:
1. + Gram Stain = presence of Gram
   negative intracellular diplococci
   consistent with a diagnosis of GC
2. GNID = Gram negative intracellular
   diplococci

Table 4. Comparison of Influenza Drugs

	Amantadine	Rimantadine	Zanamivir (Relanza)	Oseltamivir (Tamiflu)
Trade Name				
Year approved - FDA	1966	1993	1999	1999
Activity	A	A	A & B	A & B
FDA approved				
Treatment	+	+	+	+
Prophylaxis	+	+	-	+
Efficacy for:				
Treatment	+	+	+	+
Studies in high risk patients	-	-	-	-
Start Rx within	48 hrs	48 hrs	48 hrs	48 hrs
Reduction in Sx	1-1.5 days	1-1.5 days	1-1.5 days	1-1.5 days
Efficacy for Prevention	+	+	+	+
Treatment Duration	3-5 days	3-5 days	5 days	5 days
Dose - Treatment				
Age 14-64 yrs	100mg BID	100mg BID	10mg BID	75mg BID
Age > 65 yrs	100mg BID	100mg BID	10mg BID	75mg BID
Renal Failure	Adjust	Standard	10mg BID	75mg BID
Liver Failure	Standard	Standard	No data	No data
Side Effects	CNS	CNS	Asthma	GI
Cost AWP 5 days	$1	$16	$49	$55

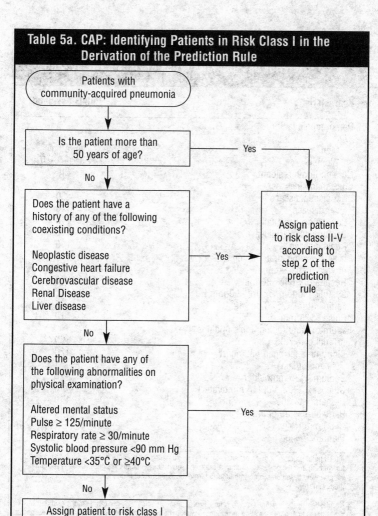

Table 5a. CAP: Identifying Patients in Risk Class I in the Derivation of the Prediction Rule

Patients with community-acquired pneumonia

↓

Is the patient more than 50 years of age? — Yes →

No ↓

Does the patient have a history of any of the following coexisting conditions?

Neoplastic disease
Congestive heart failure
Cerebrovascular disease
Renal Disease
Liver disease

— Yes → Assign patient to risk class II-V according to step 2 of the prediction rule

No ↓

Does the patient have any of the following abnormalities on physical examination?

Altered mental status
Pulse ≥ 125/minute
Respiratory rate ≥ 30/minute
Systolic blood pressure <90 mm Hg
Temperature <35°C or ≥40°C

— Yes →

No ↓

Assign patient to risk class I

In step 1 of the prediction rule, the following were independently associated with mortality: an age of more than 50 years, five coexisting illnesses (neoplastic disease, congestive heart failure, cerebrovascular disease, renal disease, and liver disease), and five physical-examination findings (altered mental status; pulse, ≥125 per minute; respiratory rate, ≥30 per minute; systolic blood pressure, <90 mm Hg; and temperature, <35°C or ≥40°C). In the derivation cohort, 1372 patients (9.7 percent) with none of these 11 risk factors were assigned to risk class I. All 12,827 remaining patients were assigned to risk class II, III, IV, or V according to the sum of the points assigned in step 2 of the prediction rule (see Tables 5b and 5c).

Table 5b. CAP: Point Scoring System for Step 2 of the Prediction Rule for Assignment to Risk Classes II, III, IV, and V

Characteristic	Points Assigned*
Demographic factor	
Age	
Men	Age (yr)
Women	Age (yr) - 10
Nursing home resident	+10
Coexisting illnesses†	
Neoplastic disease	+30
Liver disease	+20
Congestive heart failure	+10
Cerabrovascular disease	+10
Renal disease	+10
Physical-examination findings	
Altered mental status ‡	+20
Respiratory rate ≥30/min	+20
Systolic blood pressure <90 mm Hg	+20
Temperature <35° C or ≥40° C	+15
Pulse ≥125/min	+10
Laboratory and radiographic findings	
Arterial pH <7.35	+30
Blood urea nitrogen ≥30mg/dl (11 mmol/liter)	+20
Sodium <130 mmol/liter	+20
Glucose >250mg/dl (14 mmol/liter)	+10
Hematocrit <30%	+10
Partial pressure of arterial oxygen <60 mm Hg§	+10
Pleural effusion	+10

* A total point score for a given patient is obtained by summing the patient's age in years (age minus 10 for women) and the points for each applicable characteristic. The points assigned to each predictor variable were based on coefficients obtained from the logistic-regression model used in step 2 of the prediction rule.

† Neoplastic disease is defined as any cancer except basal- or squamous-cell cancer of the skin that was active at the time of presentation or diagnosed within one year of presentation. Liver disease is defined as a clinical or histologic diagnosis of cirrhosis or another form of chronic liver disease, such as chronic active hepatitis. Congestive heart failure is defined as systolic ar diastolic ventricular dysfunction documented by history, physical examination, and chest radiograph, echocardiogram, multiple gated acquisition scan, or left ventriculogram. Cerebrovascular disease is defined as a clinical diagnosis of stoke or transient ischemic attack or stroke documented by magnetic resonance imaging or computed tomography. Renal disease is defined as a history of chronic renal disease or abnormal blood urea nitrogen and creatinine concentrations documented in the medical record.

‡ Altered mental status is defined as disorientation with respect to person, place, or time that is not known to be chronic, stupor, or coma.

§ In the Pneumonia PORT cohort study, an oxygen saturation of less than 90 percent on pulse oximetry or intubation before admission was also considered abnormal.

Table 5c. Comparison of Risk-Class–Specific Mortality Rates in the Derivation and Validation Cohorts*

Risk Class (No. of Points)†	MedisGroups Derivation Cohort		MedisGroups Validation Cohort		Pneumonia PORT Validation Cohort					
					INPATIENTS		OUTPATIENTS		ALL PATIENTS	
	no. of patients	% who died	no. of patients	% who died	no. of patients	% who died	no. of patients	% who died	no. of patients	% who died
I	1,372	0.4	3,034	0.1	185	0.5	587	0.0	772	0.1
II (≤70)	2,412	0.7	5,778	0.6	233	0.9	244	0.4	477	0.6
III (71-90)	2,632	2.8	6,790	2.8	254	1.2	72	0.0	326	0.9
IV (91-130)	4,697	8.5	13,104	8.2	446	9.0	40	12.5	486	9.3
V (>130)	3,086	31.1	9,333	29.2	225	27.1	1.0	0.0	226	27.0
Total	14,199	10.2	38,039	10.6	1,343	8.0	944	0.6	2,287	5.2

*There were no statistically significant differences in overall mortality or mortality within risk class among patients in the MedisGroups derivation, MedisGroups validation, or overall Pneumonia PORT validation cohort. The P values for the comparisons of mortality across risk classes are as follows: class I, P=0.22; class II, P=0.67; class III, P=0.12; class IV, P=0.69; and class V, P=0.09.

†Inclusion in risk class I was determined by the absence of all predictors identified in step 1 of the prediction rule. Inclusion in risk classes II, III, IV, and V was determined by a patient's total risk score, which was computed according to the scoring system shown in Table 5b.

Alternative to PSI: "CURB" severity score (Confusion, Urea >19mg/dL (7 mmol/L), Respiratory rate ≥30/min, and low Blood pressure (diastolic blood pressure <60 mm Hg or systolic blood pressure ≤90 mm Hg). Give one point for each feature present. CURB score <2 qualifies as low severity, and patient may qualify for outpatient therapy.

Table 6. Diagnostic Criteria for Staphylococcal Toxic Shock Syndrome

1. Temperature greater than 38.8°C

2. Systolic blood pressure ≤90 mm Hg for adults, less than the 5th percentile for children, or >15 mm Hg orthostatic drop in diastolic blood pressure or orthostatic dizziness/syncope

3. Diffuse macular rash with subsequent desquamation

4. Three of the following organ systems involved:

   Liver: bilirubin, AST, ALT more than twice the upper normal limit

   Blood: platelets <100,000/mm^3

   Renal: BUN or creatinine more than twice the upper normal limit or pyuria without urinary tract infection

   Mucous membranes: hyperemia of the vagina, oropharynx, or conjunctivae

   Gastrointestinal: diarrhea or vomiting

   Muscular: myalgias or CPK more than twice the normal upper limit

   Central nervous system: disorientation or lowered level of consciousness in the absence of hypotension, fever, or focal neurologic deficits

5. Negative serologies for measles, leptospirosis, and Rocky Mountain spotted fever. Blood or CSF cultures negative for organisms other than *Staphylococcus aureus*

AST, aspartate transaminase; *ALT*, alanine aminotransferase;
BUN, blood urea nitrogen; *CPK*, creatine phosphokinase;
CSF, cerebrospinal fluid.
Source: *MMWR.* 1980;29:229.

Table 7. Diagnostic Criteria for Streptococcal Toxic Shock Syndrome

1. Isolation of group A streptococci:
   From a sterile site for a *definite* case
   From a nonsterile site for a *probable* case

2. Clinical criteria:
   Hypotension *and* two of the following:

Renal dysfunction	Liver involvement
Erythematous macular rash	Soft-tissue necrosis

Source: *JAMA.* 1993;269:390.

Table 8. Necrotizing Fasciitis Treatment Algorithm

Necrotizing Fasciitis:
Rapid Evaluation to Establish Diagnosis

1. Supportive care – IV fluids etc.
2. Culture blood and any drainage
3. Initiate antibiotics
4. Surgical consult
5. Define lesion with CT scan if not previously done and necessary

Debride Lesion

Strep Fasciitis

Anaerobes

Diagnosis based in Gram stain and culture

Diagnosis based in putrid discharge. Gram stain showing mixed culture

Modify antibiotic therapy – Clindamycin, Penicillin G or both

Modify antibiotic therapy – Clindamycin, Penicillin G or both

Daily reevaluation by surgeon to extend debridement

Table 9. Peri-Operative Antibiotic Prophylaxis to Prevent Surgical Site Infection

NOTE: Never "split" doses; give the full dose at one time!

DOSING: Antibiotics should **NOT be given more than 2 hours prior to incision.**

Weight (kg)	Cefazolin q2-4h (cardiac q2h)	Cefotetan q8h	Vancomycin q12h	Clindamycin q8h	Metronidazole q8h	Gentamicin	Doxycycline q12h
<70 kg	2 g	2 g	1 g	600 mg	500 mg	5 mg/kg	200 mg
71-99	2 g	2 g	1.25 g	600 mg	500 mg	5 mg/kg	200 mg
>100	2 g	2 g	1.5 g	600 mg	500 mg	5 mg/kg	200 mg
Administration	IV push	IV push	1 hour infusion	10-20 minute infusion	1 hour infusion	30 minute infusion	1 hour infusion

ALSO RE-DOSE FOR EVERY 1500 CC OF BLOOD LOSS OR HEMODILUTION.

Note: Patients receiving pre-op antibiotics to prevent an SSI generally do NOT need additional antibiotics for endocarditis prophylaxis. Patients with orthopedic hardware also do not appear to need additional prophylaxis beyond what is recommended for the case. There are no recommendations for antibiotics for these patients in cases where they are not indicated for SSI prevention.

Procedure	Prophylaxis Recommendations	PCN Allergy Alternate Prophylaxis
Gynecologic surgery		
Cesarean section	Uncomplicated procedures: No prophylaxis needed. Complicated: Cefazolin 2 g IV after cord clamping OR Metronidazole 500 mg IV after clamping	
Hysterectomy (abdominal or vaginal)	Cefotetan 2 g IV pre-op	PCN allergy: Clindamycin 600 mg IV pre-op
Repair of cystocele or rectocele	Cefotetan 2 g IV pre-op	PCN allergy: Clindamycin 600 mg IV pre-op
Dilation and curettage	Uncomplicated procedures: No prophylaxis needed. Complicated: Cefotetan 2 g IV pre-op	PCN allergy: Clindamycin 600 mg IV pre-op
Orthopedic surgery		
Joint replacement	Cefazolin 2 g IV pre-op	PCN allergy: Vancomycin 1 g IV pre-op
Open reduction of fracture	Cefazolin 2 g IV pre-op. Continue for 72 hours in closed hip fractures (open fractures should be treated as infected with cefazolin 2 g IV q8h for 10 days)	PCN allergy: Vancomycin 1 g IV pre-op and at 12 hours
Lower limb amputation	Cefotetan 2 g IV pre-op	PCN allergy: Gentamicin 5 mg/kg IV PLUS clindamycin 600 mg IV pre-op
Spinal fusion	Cefazolin 2 g IV pre-op	PCN allergy: Vancomycin 1 g IV pre-op
Arthroscopic surgery, laminectomy	No data to support prophylaxis	No data to support prophylaxis
General surgery		
Cholecystectomy (open or laparoscopic; benefit less clear in laparoscopic cases)	Cefotetan 2 g IV pre-op recommended for: pt age > 60, previous biliary surgery, acute symptoms, jaundice	PCN allergy: Clindamycin 600 mg IV with or without gentamicin
Inguinal hernia repair	Uncomplicated: Prophylaxis not recommended Complicated, recurrent or emergent: Cefotetan 2 g IV	PCN allergy: Clindamycin 600 mg IV with or without gentamicin

Table 9. Peri-Operative Antibiotic Prophylaxis to Prevent Surgical Site Infection (Cont.)

Procedure	Prophylaxis Recommendations	PCN Allergy Alternate Prophylaxis
General surgery (cont.)		
Colon surgery/ Whipple procedure	Neomycin and erythromycin 1 g each PO at 1, 2, and 11 pm the day before surgery. If no PO antibiotics, then give cefotetan 2 g IV pre-op (some use both PO and IV regimens)	PCN allergy: Clindamycin 600 mg IV PLUS gentamicin 5 mg/kg IV pre-op
Appendectomy (uncomplicated; if complicated or perforated treat as peritonitis)	Cefotetan 2 g IV pre-op	PCN allergy: Clindamycin 600 mg IV pre-op
Penetrating abdominal trauma	Cefotetan 2 g IV pre-op; continue 2 g IV q12h for 24 hours.	PCN allergy: Clindamycin 600 mg IV PLUS gentamicin 5 mg/kg IV pre-op
Mastectomy	Not recommended	Not recommended
Esophageal cases	Cefotetan 2 g IV pre-op	PCN allergy: Clindamycin 600 mg IV pre-op
Thoracic surgery		
All cases except esophageal	Cefazolin 2 g IV pre-op	PCN allergy: Clindamycin 600 mg IV
Esophageal cases	Cefotetan 2 g IV pre-op	PCN allergy: Clindamycin 600 mg IV pre-op
Urologic surgery		
Transrectal prostate biopsy, urethral instrumentation	Gatifloxacin 400 mg PO	
Radical, retropubic prostatectomy OR nephrectomy	Cefazolin 2 g IV pre-op	PCN allergy: Clindamycin 600 mg IV pre-op
Prostatectomy (TURP or peritoneal)	If sterile urine: Gatifloxacin 400 mg PO/IV pre-op only if high-risk procedure. No data to support prophylaxis if pre-procedure urine cultures are sterile and procedure is low risk	
Radical cystoprostatectomy OR anterior exeneration	Cefotetan 2 g IV pre-op	PCN allergy: Clindamycin 600 mg IV pre-op
Head and neck surgery		
Major procedure with incision of oral or pharyngeal mucosa	Clindamycin 600 mg IV +/- Gentamicin 5 mg/kg IV pre-op Alternative: Cefuroxime 1.5 g IV pre-op	
Tonsillectomy, rhinoplasty	No data to support prophylaxis	No data to support prophylaxis
Cardiothoracic surgery		
Median sternotomy	Cefazolin 2 g IV pre-op and 2 g IV q2h intra-op	PCN allergy: Vancomycin 1 g IV pre-op
Vascular surgery		
All cases	Cefazolin 2 g IV pre-op	PCN allergy: Vancomycin 1 g IV pre-op
Neurosurgery		
Craniotomy (including shunt placement)	Cefazolin 2 g IV pre-op; repeat 2 g q4h intra-op	PCN allergy: Clindamycin 600 mg IV pre-op and one dose 4 hours later
Endoscopic procedure		
PEG tube placement	Cefazolin 2 g IV pre-procedure	PCN allergy: Clindamycin 600 mg IV PLUS gentamicin 2 mg/kg IV pre-procedure

Table 10a. Recommended Adult Immunization Schedule, United States, 2003-2004 by Age Group

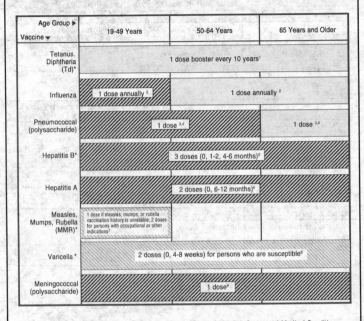

Age Group ▶ Vaccine ▼	19-49 Years	50-64 Years	65 Years and Older
Tetanus, Diphtheria (Td)*	1 dose booster every 10 years¹		
Influenza	1 dose annually ²	1 dose annually ²	
Pneumococcal (polysaccharide)	1 dose ³,⁴		1 dose ³,⁴
Hepatitis B*	3 doses (0, 1-2, 4-6 months)⁵		
Hepatitis A	2 doses (0, 6-12 months)⁶		
Measles, Mumps, Rubella (MMR)*	1 dose if measles, mumps, or rubella vaccination history is unreliable; 2 doses for persons with occupational or other indications⁷		
Varicella *	2 doses (0, 4-8 weeks) for persons who are susceptible⁸		
Meningococcal (polysaccharide)	1 dose⁹		

See Footnotes for Recommended Adult Immunization Schedule, by Age Group and Medical Conditions, United States, 2003-2004 listed after Table 10b.

	For all persons in this group		Catch-up on childhood vaccinations		For persons with medical/ exposure indications

*Covered by the Vaccine Injury Compensation Program. For information on how to file a claim call 800-338-2382. Please also visit www.hrsa.gov/osp/vicp. To file a claim for vaccine injury contact: U.S. Court of Federal Claims, 717 Madison Place, N.W., Washington, D.C., 20005, 202-219-9657.

This schedule indicates the recommended age groups for routine administration of currently licensed vaccines for persons 19 years of age and older. Licensed combination vaccines may be used whenever any components of the combination are indicated and the vaccine's other components are not contraindicated. Providers should consult the manufacturers' package inserts for detailed recommendations.

Report all clinically significant postvaccination reactions to the Vaccine Adverse Event Reporting System (VAERS). Reporting forms and instructions on filing a VAERS report are available by calling 800-822-7967 or from the VAERS website at www.vaers.org.

For additional information about the vaccines listed above and contraindications for immunization, visit the National Immunization Program website at www.cdc.gov/nip or call the National Immunization Hotline at 800-232-2522 (English) or 800-232-0233 (Spanish).

Approved by the Advisory Committee on Immunization Practices (ACIP), and accepted by the American College of Obstetricians and Gynecologists (ACOG) and the American Academy of Family Physicians (AAFP)

Table 10b. Recommended Adult Immunization Schedule, United States, 2003-2004 by Medical Conditions

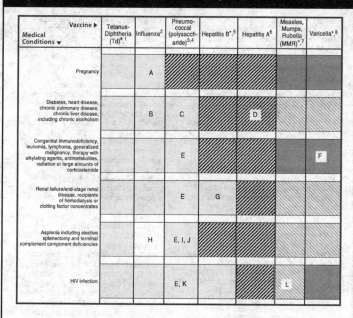

Medical Conditions ▼ / Vaccine ►	Tetanus-Diphtheria (Td)*,1	Influenza2	Pneumo-coccal (polysacch-aride)3,4	Hepatitis B*,5	Hepatitis A6	Measles, Mumps, Rubella (MMR)*,7	Varicella*,8
Pregnancy		A					
Diabetes, heart disease, chronic pulmonary disease, chronic liver disease, including chronic alcoholism		B	C		D		
Congenital immunodeficiency, leukemia, lymphoma, generalized malignancy, therapy with alkylating agents, antimetabolites, radiation or large amounts of corticosteroids			E				F
Renal failure/end-stage renal disease, recipients of hemodialysis or clotting factor concentrates			E	G			
Asplenia including elective splenectomy and terminal complement component deficiencies		H	E, I, J				
HIV infection			E, K			L	

See Special Notes for Medical Conditions below— also see Footnotes for Recommended Adult Immunization Schedule, by Age Group and Medical Conditions, United States, 2003-2004 listed on next page.

- ▨ For all persons in this group
- ▨ Catch-up on childhood vaccinations
- ▨ For persons with medical/exposure indications
- ▨ Contraindicated

Special Notes for Medical Conditions

A. For women without chronic diseases/conditions, vaccinate if pregnancy will be at 2nd or 3rd trimester during influenza season. For women with chronic diseases/conditions, vaccinate at any time during the pregnancy.

B. Although chronic liver disease and alcoholism are not indicator conditions for influenza vaccination, give 1 dose annually if the patient is age 50 years or older, has other indications for influenza vaccine, or if the patient requests vaccination.

C. Asthma is an indicator condition for influenza but not for pneumococcal vaccination.

D. For all persons with chronic liver disease.

E. For persons <65 years, revaccinate once after 5 years or more have elapsed since initial vaccination.

F. Persons with impaired humoral immunity but intact cellular immunity may be vaccinated. *MMWR.* 1999;48(RR-06):1-5.

G. Hemodialysis patients: Use special formulation of vaccine (40 ug/mL) or two 1.0 mL 20 ug doses given at one site. Vaccinate early in the course of renal disease. Assess antibody titers to hep B surface antigen (anti-HBs) levels annually. Administer additional doses if anti-HBs levels decline to <10 milliinternational units (mIU)/mL.

H. There are no data specifically on risk of severe or complicated influenza infections among persons with asplenia. However, influenza is a risk factor for secondary bacterial infections that may cause severe disease in asplenics.

I. Administer meningococcal vaccine and consider Hib vaccine.

J. Elective splenectomy: vaccinate at least 2 weeks before surgery.

K. Vaccinate as close to diagnosis as possible when CD4 cell counts are highest.

L. Withhold MMR or other measles-containing vaccines from HIV-infected persons with evidence of severe immunosuppression. *MMWR.* 1998;47(RR-8):21-22; *MMWR.* 2002;51(RR-02):22-24.

1. **Tetanus and diphtheria (Td)**—Adults, including pregnant women with uncertain histories of a complete primary vaccination series, should receive a primary series of Td. A primary series for adults is 3 doses: the first 2 doses given at least 4 weeks apart and the 3rd dose, 6-12 months after the second. Administer 1 dose if the person had received the primary series and the last vaccination was ≥10 years ago. Consult *MMWR*. 1991;40(RR-10):1-21 for administering Td as prophylaxis in wound management. The ACP Task Force on Adult Immunization supports a second option for Td use in adults: a single Td booster at age 50 years for persons who have completed the full pediatric series, including the teenage/young adult booster.
Guide for Adult Immunization, 3rd ed. ACP. 1994:20.

2. **Influenza vaccination**—Medical indications: chronic disorders of the cardiovascular or pulmonary systems including asthma; chronic metabolic diseases including diabetes mellitus, renal dysfunction, hemoglobinopathies, or immunosuppression (including immunosuppression caused by medications or by human immunodeficiency virus [HIV]) requiring regular medical follow-up or hospitalization during the preceding year; women who will be in the second or third trimester of pregnancy during the influenza season. Occupational indications: healthcare workers. Other indications: residents of nursing homes and other long-term care facilities; persons likely to transmit influenza to persons at high-risk (in-home care givers to persons with medical indications; household contacts and out-of-home caregivers of children birth to 23 months of age or children with asthma or other indicator conditions for influenza vaccination; household members and care givers of the elderly or adults with high-risk conditions); and anyone who wishes to be vaccinated. For healthy persons aged 5-49 years without high-risk conditions, either the inactivated vaccine or the intranasally administered influenza vaccine (Flumist) may be given.
MMWR. 2003;52(RR-8):1-36; *MMWR*. 2003;53 (RR-13):1-8.

3. **Pneumococcal polysaccharide vaccination**—Medical indications: chronic disorders of the pulmonary system (excluding asthma), cardiovascular diseases, diabetes mellitus, chronic liver diseases including liver disease as a result of alcohol abuse (e.g., cirrhosis), chronic renal failure or nephrotic syndrome, functional or anatomic asplenia (e.g., sickle cell disease or splenectomy), immunosuppressive conditions (e.g., congenital immunodeficiency, HIV infection, leukemia, lymphoma, multiple myeloma, Hodgkins disease, generalized malignancy, organ or bone marrow transplantation), chemotherapy with alkylating agents, antimetabolites, or long-term systemic corticosteroids. Geographic/other indications: Alaskan Natives and certain American Indian populations. Other indications: residents of nursing homes and other long-term care facilities.
MMWR. 1997;46 (RR-8):1-24.

4. **Revaccination with pneumococcal polysaccharide vaccine**—One time revaccination after 5 years for persons with chronic renal failure or nephrotic syndrome, functional or anatomic asplenia (e.g., sickle cell disease or splenectomy), immunosuppressive conditions (e.g., congenital immunodeficiency, HIV infection, leukemia, lymphoma, multiple myeloma, Hodgkins disease, generalized malignancy, organ or bone marrow transplantation), chemotherapy with alkylating agents, antimetabolites, or long-term systemic corticosteroids. For persons 65 and older, one-time revaccination if they were vaccinated ≥5 years ago and were <65 years at the time of primary vaccination. *MMWR*. 1997;46 (RR-8):1-24.

5. **Hepatitis B vaccination**—Medical indications: hemodialysis patients, patients who receive clotting-factor concentrates. Occupational indications: healthcare workers and public-safety workers who have exposure to blood in the workplace; persons in training in schools of medicine, dentistry, nursing, laboratory technology, and other allied health professions. Behavioral indications: injecting drug users, persons with more than one sex partner in the previous 6 months, persons with a recently acquired sexually transmitted disease (STD), all clients in STD clinics, men who have sex with men. Other indications: household contacts and sex partners of persons with chronic HBV infection, clients and staff of institutions for the developmentally disabled, international travelers who will be in countries with high or intermediate prevalence of chronic HBV infection for more than 6 months, inmates of correctional facilities. *MMWR*. 1991;40(RR-13):119. (www.cdc.gov/travel/diseases/hbv.htm)

6. **Hepatitis A vaccination**—For the combined HepA-HepB vaccine, use 3 doses at 0,1, and 6 months. Medical indications: persons with clotting-factor disorders or chronic liver disease. Behavioral indications: men who have sex with men, users of injecting and noninjecting illegal drugs. Occupational indications: persons working with HAV-infected primates or with HAV in a research laboratory setting. Other indications: persons traveling to or working in countries that have high or intermediate endemicity of hepatitis A. *MMWR*. 1999;48 (RR-12):1-37. (www.cdc.gov/travel/diseases/hav.htm)

7. **Measles, Mumps, Rubella vaccination (MMR)**—Measles component: Adults born before 1957 may be considered immune to measles. Adults born in or after 1957 should receive at least 1 dose of MMR unless they have a medical contraindication, documentation of at least 1 dose, or other acceptable evidence of immunity. A second dose of MMR is recommended for adults who:
   - have been recently exposed to measles or are in an outbreak setting
   - were previously vaccinated with killed measles vaccine
   - were vaccinated with an unknown vaccine between 1963 and 1967
   - are students in postsecondary educational institutions
   - work in healthcare facilities
   - plan to travel internationally

   Mumps component: 1 dose of MMR should be adequate for protection. Rubella component: Give 1 dose of MMR to women whose rubella vaccination history is unreliable and counsel women to avoid becoming pregnant for 4 weeks after vaccination. For women of childbearing age, regardless of birth year, routinely determine rubella immunity and counsel women regarding congenital rubella syndrome. Do not vaccinate pregnant women or those planning to become pregnant in the next 4 weeks. If pregnant and susceptible, vaccinate as early in postpartum period as possible.
   MMWR. 1998;47 (RR-8):1-57; *MMWR.* 2001;50:1117.

8. **Varicella vaccination**—Recommended for all persons who do not have reliable clinical history of varicella infection, or serological evidence of varicella zoster virus (VZV) infection who may be at high risk for exposure or transmission. This includes healthcare workers and family contacts of immunocompromised persons, those who live or work in environments where transmission is likely (e.g., teachers of young children, day-care employees, and residents and staff members in institutional settings), persons who live or work in environments where VZV transmission can occur (e.g., college students, inmates and staff members of correctional institutions, and military personnel), adolescents and adults living in households with children, women who are not pregnant but who may become pregnant in the future, international travelers who are not immune to infection. Note: Greater than 95% of U.S. born adults are immune to VZV. Do not vaccinate pregnant women or those planning to become pregnant in the next 4 weeks. If pregnant and susceptible, vaccinate as early in postpartum period as possible.
   MMWR. 1996;45(RR-11):1-36; *MMWR.* 1999;48(RR-6):1-5.

9. **Meningococcal vaccine (quadrivalent polysaccharide for serogroups A, C,Y, and W-135)**—Consider vaccination for persons with medical indications: adults with terminal complement component deficiencies or with anatomic or functional asplenia. Other indications: travelers to countries in which disease is hyperendemic or epidemic ("meningitis belt" of sub-Saharan Africa, Mecca, Saudi Arabia for Hajj). Revaccination at 3-5 years may be indicated for persons at high risk for infection (e.g., persons residing in areas in which disease is epidemic). Counsel college freshmen, especially those who live in dormitories, regarding meningococcal disease and the vaccine so that they can make an educated decision about receiving the vaccination. *MMWR.* 2000;49(RR-7):1-20. Note: The AAFP recommends that colleges should take the lead on providing education on meningococcal infection and vaccination and offer it to those who are interested. Physicians need not initiate discussion of the meningococcal quadrivalent polysaccharide vaccine as part of routine medical care.

Table 11. Legionella

	Legionnaire's Disease	Pontiac Fever
Site	Pneumonia	Flulike illness without pneumonia
Incubation period	2-10 days	24-48 hours
Sx	Chills, fever, dyspnea, headache	Chills, fever, headache, myalgias
Diagnosis	Culture resp. secretion, urine antigen, serology	Serology, culture common source
Epidemiology	Sporadic and epidemic	Epidemic
Risk	Predisposed – age >40, smokers, compromised CMI	Attach >90% including young & healthy
Outcome	Mortality 15-25%	Recovery in ≤1 wk

Note: *Legionella pneumophila* serogroup 1 is predominant cause of both Legionnaire's Disease and Pontiac Fever.

Table 12: Malaria Prophylaxis

Provide antimalarial drug dosages, schedules, and warnings

Advise patients that antimalarial drugs are most effective if taken exactly on schedule without skipping doses and that their drug should be continued post-travel for the most complete protection. Antimalarial drugs should be purchased before travel; drugs purchased overseas may not be manufactured according to United States standards and may not be effective. They may also be dangerous, contain the wrong drug or an incorrect amount of active drug, or be contaminated.

Halofantrine (marketed as Halfan) is widely used overseas to treat malaria. CDC does not recommend the use of Halfan because of serious cardiac complications, including deaths. Travelers should be advised to avoid Halfan unless they have been diagnosed with life-threatening malaria and no other options are immediately available.

Overdosage of antimalarial drugs can be fatal. Parents should be advised to keep drugs in childproof containers out of the reach of children.

Drugs used in the prophylaxis of malaria

Drug	Usage	Adult dose	Pediatric dose	Adverse reactions and contraindications
Atovaquone/ proguanil (Malarone®)	Primary prophylaxis* in areas with chloroquine-resistant or mefloquine-resistant *Plasmodium falciparum*	Adult tablets contain 250 mg atovaquone and 100 mg proguanil hydrochloride. 1 adult tablet orally, daily	Pediatric tablets contain 62.5 mg atovaquone and 25 mg proguanil hydrochloride. 11-20 kg: 1 tablet 21-30 kg: 2 tablets 31-40 kg: 3 tablets ≥40 kg: 1 adult tablet daily Note: Adult tablets contain 250 mg atovaquone and 100 mg proguanil hydrochloride.	Contraindicated in persons with severe renal impairment (creatinine clearance <30mL/min). Atovaquone/proguanil should be taken with food or a milky drink. Not recommended for children <11 kg, pregnant women, and women breast-feeding infants weighing <11 kg.
Chloroquine phosphate (Aralen® and generic)	Primary prophylaxis* only in areas with chloro-quine-sensitive *P. falciparum*	300 mg base (500 mg salt) orally, once/week	5 mg/kg base (8.3 mg/kg salt) orally, once/week, up to maximum adult dose of 300 mg base	May exacerbate psoriasis.
Doxycycline (many brand names and generic)	Primary prophylaxis* in areas with chloroquine-resistant or mefloquine-resistant *P. falciparum*	100 mg orally, daily	≥8 years of age: 2 mg/kg up to adult dose of 100 mg/day	Contraindicated in children ≤8 years of age and pregnant women.

Table 12: Malaria Prophylaxis (Cont.)

Drug	Usage	Adult dose	Pediatric dose	Adverse reactions and contraindications
Hydroxy-chloroquine sulfate (Plaquenil®)	An alternative to chloroquine for primary prophylaxis* only in areas with chloro-quine-sensitive *P. falciparum*	310 mg base (400 mg salt) orally, once/ week	5 mg/kg base (6.5 mg/kg salt) orally, once/week, up to maximum adult dose of 310 mg base.	See chloroquine comment.
Mefloquine (Lariam®) and generic)	Primary prophylaxis* in areas with chloroquine-resistant *P. falciparum*	228 mg base (250 mg salt) orally, once/ week	5-10 kg: ⅛ tablet orally, once/week 10-20 kg: ¼ tablet once/week 20-30 kg: ½ tablet, once/week 30-45 kg: ¾ tablet once/week >45 kg: 1 tablet, once/week Note:The recom-mended cardiac dose of mefloquine mefloquine is 5 mg/kg body weight once weekly. Approxi-mate tablet trac-tion is based on this dosage. Exact doses for children weighing less than 10 kg should be prepared by a pharmacist.	Contraindicated in persons allergic to mefloquine and in persons with active depression or a previous history of depression, generalized anxiety disorder, psychosis, schizophrenia, other major psychiatric disorders, or seizures. Not recommended for persons with conduction abnormalities
Primaquine	An option for primary prophylaxis* in special circumstances. Call Malaria Hotline (770-488-7788) for additional information.	30 mg base (52.6 mg salt) orally, daily	0.6 mg/kg base (1.0 mg/kg salt) up to adult dose, orally, daily	Contraindicated in persons with G6PD deficiency. Also contra-indicated during preg-nancy and lactation unless the infant being breastfed has a docu-mented normal G6PD level. Use in consul-tation with malaria experts.

Table 12: Malaria Prophylaxis (Cont.)

Drug	Usage	Adult dose	Pediatric dose	Adverse reactions and contraindications
Primaquine	Used for terminal prophylaxis[†] to decrease risk of relapses of *P. vivax* and *P. ovale*. Indicated for persons who have had prolonged exposure to *P. vivax* and *P. ovale* or both	30 mg base (52.6 mg salt) orally, once/day for 14 days after departure from the malarious area. Note: The recommended dose of primaquine for terminal prophylaxis[†] has been increased from 15 mg to 30 mg for adults.	0.6 mg/kg base (1.0 mg/kg salt) up to adult dose orally, once/day for 14 days after departure from the malarious area. Note: The recommended dose of primaquine for terminal prophylaxis[†] has been increased from 0.3 mg/kg to 0.6 mg/kg for children.	Contraindicated in persons with G6PD deficiency. Also contraindicated during pregnancy and lactation unless the infant being breastfed has a documented normal G6PD level.

[*] *Primary prophylaxis* refers to the use of antimalarial drugs to prevent symptoms associated with the blood stage infection; these drugs are taken before, during, and for a period of time after travel in the malaria-risk area.

[†] *Terminal prophylaxis* refers to the use of primaquine to lower the risk of relapse from liver stage infection with *Plasmodium vivax* or *P. ovale*. Primaquine is taken after departure from the malaria-risk area.

APPENDIX II

Table 13. Protocol for Trimethoprim-Sulfamethoxazole Desensitization

Day	Dose	Quantity, TMP-SMX
1	1 mL of 1:20 pediatric suspension	0.4 mg/2 mg
2	2 mL of 1:20 pediatric suspension	0.8 mg/4 mg
3	4 mL of 1:20 pediatric suspension	1.6 mg/8 mg
4	8 mL of 1:20 pediatric suspension	3.2 mg/16 mg
5	1 mL of pediatric suspension	8 mg/40 mg
6	2 mL of pediatric suspension	16 mg/80 mg
7	4 mL of pediatric suspension	32 mg/160 mg
8	8 mL of pediatric suspension	64 mg/320 mg
9	1 tablet	80 mg/400 mg
10*	1 double-strength tablet	160 mg/800 mg

* After day 10, administer 1 tablet double-strength TMP-SMX on Monday, Wednesday, and Friday for *Pneumocystis carinii* prophylaxis, or 2 tablets daily for the treatment of isosporiasis.
TMP-SMX: trimethoprim/sulfamethoxazole.

Table 14. Protocol for Beta-Lactam Oral Desensitization*

Stock penicillin G drug concentration (mg/mL)	Dose no.[†]	Amount (mL)	Drug dose (mg)	Cumulative drug (mg)
0.5	1	0.05	0.025	0.025
	2	0.10	0.05	0.075
	3	0.20	0.10	0.175
	4	0.40	0.20	0.375
	5	0.80	0.40	0.775
5.0	6	0.15	0.75	1.525
	7	0.30	1.50	3.025
	8	0.60	3.00	6.025
	9	1.20	6.00	12.025
	10	2.40	12.00	24.025
50	11	0.50	25.00	49.025
	12	1.20	60.00	109.025
	13	2.50	125.00	234.025
	14	5.00	250.00	484.025

* Perform only in setting optimized for intensive care with bedside supply of epinephrine, parenteral antihistamines, and corticosteroids and with ability to emergently intubate the airway and perform cardiac resuscitation.

† Interval between doses is 15 minutes.

Adapted from Wendel GD Jr., et al. *N Engl J Med*. 1985;312(19):1229-1232.

APACHE II Score (sum of A + B + C)

		Points
A	APS points	
B	+ Age points	
C	+ Chronic health points	
	Total APACHE II Score	

Interpretation of Score:

0 to 4 = ~4% death rate	20 to 24 = ~40% death rate
5 to 9 = ~8% death rate	25 to 29 = ~55% death rate
10 to 14 = ~15% death rate	30 to 34 = ~75% death rate
15 to 19 = ~25% death rate	Over 34 = ~85% death rate

A. Total Acute Physiology Score (APS)
Refer to Total Acute Physiology Score (Table 15b).

Glasgow Coma Scale
(circle appropriate response)

Eyes open
4 - Spontaneously
3 - To verbal
2 - To painful stimuli
1 - No response

Verbal - nonintubated
5 - Oriented and controversed
4 - Disoriented and talks
3 - Inappropriate words
2 - Incomprehensive sounds
1 - No response

Motor response
6 - To verbal command
5 - Localizes to pain
4 - Withdraws to pain
3 - Decorticate
2 - Decerebrate
1 - No response

Verbal - intubated
5 - Seems able to talk
3 - Questionable ability to talk
1 - Generally unresponsive

B. Age Points

Assign points to age as follows:	Points
≤44 years	0
45-54 years	2
55-64 years	3
65-74 years	5
≥75 years	6

C. Chronic Health Points

If the patient has a history of severe organ system insufficiency or is immunocompromised assign points as follows:

a. for nonoperative or emergency postoperative patients - 5 points

or

b. for elective postoperative patients - 2 points

DEFINITIONS

Organ insufficiency or immunocompromised state must have been evident prior to this hospital admission and conform to the following criteria:

Liver: Biopsy-proven cirrhosis and documented portal hypertension; episodes of past upper GI bleeding attributed to portal hypertension; or prior episodes of hepatic failure/encephalopathy/coma

Cardiovascular: New York Heart Association Class IV

Respiratory: Chronic restrictive, obstructive, or vascular disease resulting in severe exercise restriction, ie, unable to climb stairs or perform household duties; or documented chronic hypoxia, hypercapnia, secondary polycythemia, severe pulmonary hypertension (>40 mm Hg), or respirator dependency

Renal: Receiving chronic dialysis

Immunocompromised: The patient has received therapy that suppresses resistance to infection, eg, immunosuppression, chemotherapy, radiation, long-term or recent high-dose steroids, or has a disease that is sufficiently advanced to suppress resistance to infection, eg, leukemia, lymphoma, AIDS

Chronic Health Points =

Table 15b. Apache II APS Points

Total Acute Physiology Score (APS)
(Choose the worst value in the past 24 hours)

Physiologic Variable	High Abnormal Range				0	Low Abnormal Range			
	+4	+3	+2	+1	0	+1	+2	+3	+4
Temperature, rectal (°C)	≥41	39-40.9		38.5-38.9	36-38.4	34-35.9	32-33.9	30-31.9	≤29.9
Mean arterial pressure (mm Hg)	≥160	130-159	110-129		70-109		50-69		≤49
Heart rate (ventricular response)	≥180	140-179	110-139		70-109		55-69	40-54	≤39
Respiratory rate (nonventilated or ventilated)	≥50	35-49		25-34	12-24	10-11	6-9		≤5
Oxygenation: A-aDO₂ or PaO₂ (mm Hg)									
a) FiO_2 ≥0.5: record A-aDO_2	≥500	350-499	200-349		<200				
b) FiO_2 <0.5: record only PaO_2					PO_2 >70	PO_2 61-70		PO_2 55-60	PO_2 <55
Arterial pH* (if no ABGs record serum HCO_3 below)	≥7.7	7.6-7.69		7.5-7.59	7.33-7.49		7.25-7.32	7.15-7.24	<7.15
Serum sodium (mmol/L)	≥180	160-179	155-159	150-154	130-149		120-129	111-119	≤110
Serum potassium (mmol/L)	≥7	6-6.9		5.5-5.9	3.5-5.4	3-3.4	2.5-2.9		<2.5
Serum creatinine (mg/100 mL) (double point score for acute renal failure)	≥3.5	2-3.4	1.5-1.9		0.6-1.4		<0.6		
Hematocrit (%)	≥60		50-59.9	46-49.9	30-45.9		20-29.9		<20
White blood count (total/mm³) (in 1,000s)	≥40		20-39.9	15-19.9	3-14.9		1-2.9		<1
Glasgow Coma Score (GCS)	15 minus actual GCS [see Glasgow Coma Scale]								
Total Acute Physiology Score (APS)	Sum of the 12 individual variable points								
* Serum HCO_3 (venous-mmol/L) (Not preferred, use if no ABGs)	≥52	41-51.9		32-40.9	22-31.9		18-21.9	15-17.9	<15

Reprinted with permission from Knaus WA, Draper EA, Wagner DP, et al, "APACHE II: A Severity of Disease Classification System," *Crit Care Med.* 1985; 13(10):818-829.

654

Table 16. GFR and MDRD Calculations

IBW:	Men:	$50.0 + (2.3 \times \text{height in inches over 5 feet})$
	Women:	$45.5 + (2.3 \times \text{height in inches over 5 feet})$
CrCl:	Men:	$\dfrac{(140 - \text{age}) \times \text{IBW (kg)}}{\text{Scr (mg/dL)} \times 72}$
	Women:	estimated CrCl male $\times 0.85$
BSA:		$0.007184 \times \text{height (cm)}^{0.725} \times \text{weight (kg)}^{0.425}$
GFR:		$0.81 \times \text{CrCl} \times 1.73/(\text{BSA})$
MDRD:		$186 \times \text{Scr (mg/dL)}^{1.154} \times \text{age (years)}^{-0.203} \times 1.212 \text{ (if Black)} \times 0.742 \text{ (if Female)} \times 1.73/\text{BSA}$

IBW: Ideal Body Weight
CrCl: Creatinine Clearance
BSA: Body Surface Area
GFR: Glomerular Filtration Rate
MDRD: Modification of Diet in Renal Disease

Table 17. Aa Gradient

$$Aa = (BP - pH_2O) \times FiO_2 - (1.25 \times PaCO_2) - PaO_2$$

At sea level and room air:
$$Aa = 150 - (1.25 \times PaCO_2) - PaO_2$$

BP: barometric pressure
pH_2O: partial pressure of water at body temperature (47 mm Hg at 37°C)
FiO_2: fraction of inspired oxygen